Developmental Psychopathology and Family Process

Developmental Psychopathology and Family Process
Theory, Research, and Clinical Implications

E. Mark Cummings
Patrick T. Davies
Susan B. Campbell

FOREWORD BY DANTE CICCHETTI

THE GUILFORD PRESS
New York   London

©2000 The Guilford Press
A Division of Guilford Publications, Inc.
72 Spring Street, New York, NY 10012
www.guilford.com

Printed in the United States of America

This book is printed on acid-free paper.

Last digit is print number: 9   8   7   6   5   4   3   2   1

Library of Congress Cataloging-in-Publication Data

Cummings, E. Mark.
    Developmental psychopathology and family process:
theory, research, and clinical implications / by E. Mark Cummings,
Patrick T. Davies, Susan B. Campbell.
        p. cm.
Includes bibliographical references and index.
ISBN 1-57230-597-5
    1. Child psychopathology. 2. Child development. 3. Family—
Psychological aspects. 4. Family—Mental health. I. Davies, Patrick T.
II. Campbell, Susan B. III. Title.

RJ499.C86 2000
618.92'89—dc21   00-034831

About the Authors

E. Mark Cummings, PhD, is Professor of Psychology at the University of Notre Dame. He received his BA from Johns Hopkins University and MA and PhD from UCLA in 1977. He has published widely in journals concerned with developmental psychology, family psychology, child clinical psychology and psychiatry, and developmental psychopathology. Dr. Cummings has been a coauthor and coeditor on a half dozen books, including *Children and Marital Conflict: The Impact of Family Dispute and Resolution* (with Patrick T. Davies; Guilford Press, 1994). His work is broadly concerned with relations between adaptive and maladaptive family functioning and children's normal development and risk for the development of psychopathology. Dr. Cummings is principal investigator or coprincipal investigator of NICHD- and NIMH-funded prospective longitudinal studies on relations between family processes and child development. He has served as associate editor of *Child Development* and on the editorial boards of numerous journals, including *Child Development*, *Developmental Psychology*, the *Journal of Family Psychology*, *Parenting: Science and Practice*, the *Journal of Emotional Abuse*, and *Personal Relationships*.

Patrick T. Davies, PhD, is Assistant Professor of Psychology in the Department of Clinical and Social Sciences in Psychology at the University of Rochester. He received his PhD in developmental psychology from West Virginia University in 1995. Dr. Davies is coauthor (with E. Mark Cummings) of *Children and Marital Conflict: The Impact of Family Dispute and Resolution* (Guilford Press, 1994). His research is geared toward understanding children's close relationships, particularly within contexts of family discord, interparental conflict, parent–child relations, and family risk (e.g., parental depression, alcohol problems). Dr. Davies is principal investigator on an NIMH-funded longitudinal study concerned with relations between family process, emotional security, and child adjustment. He is an editorial board member of *Development and Psychopathology* and *Child Development*.

Susan B. Campbell, PhD, received her doctorate in psychology from McGill University in 1969. From 1970 until 1976 she was Director of the Department of Psychology at the Montreal Children's Hospital and Assistant Professor of Psychology at McGill University. Dr. Campbell joined the faculty of the Department of Psychology at the University of Pittsburgh in 1976, where she is currently Professor of Psychology. From 1985 until 1996 she served as the chair of the Clinical Psychology Program. Dr. Campbell has served on numerous editorial boards and review committees. She has held elective offices in the International Society for Research in Child and Adolescent Psychopathology and the Section on Clinical Child Psychology of the American Psychological Association (now Division 53), including president in 1997. Dr. Campbell is currently the editor of the *Journal of Abnormal Child Psychology*. She is also the principal investigator of the Pittsburgh site of the 10-site NICHD Study of Early Child Care and Youth Development, a longitudinal study of development from birth through adolescence. She is the author of *Behavior Problems in Preschool Children: Developmental and Clinical Issues* (Guilford Press, 1990), currently being updated for a second edition.

Foreword

Developmental psychopathology is an evolving interdisciplinary scientific field that seeks to elucidate the interplay among the biological, psychological, and social-contextual aspects of normal and abnormal development across the life course. During the three decades that have elapsed since its emergence, theory and research in the field of developmental psychopathology have contributed to dramatic knowledge gains in the multiple domains of child and adult development. In particular, there has been an emphasis on increasingly specific process-level models of normal and abnormal development, an acknowledgment that multiple pathways exist to the same outcome and that the effects of one component's value may vary in different systems, and an intensification of interest in biological and genetic factors related to the development of maladaptation and psychopathology. Furthermore, theory and research in the developmental psychopathology tradition have been influential in informing the formulation, implementation, and evaluation of prevention and intervention efforts.

Influenced by the theoretical expositions of a number of prominent developmentalists, theorists have highlighted the importance of viewing the development of psychopathology within a continuously unfolding, dynamic, and ever-changing context. Increased recognition of the effects of social contexts not only on psychological but also on biological structures and processes has emerged. Despite advances that have occurred, the full incorporation of a contextual focus into empirical research, even among developmental psychopathologists who are sensitive to the importance of understanding contextual influences on children and families, has proven to be a challenging endeavor. Thus, given the relative paucity of research integrating contextualism and developmental psychopathology, the present volume by Cummings, Davies, and Campbell is a significant and long-overdue contribution to the field.

When considering the role of context in children's development, the family environment is one of the most significant contextual influences and, due in part to its proximity to the child, the one that has received the most attention in the scientific literature. The conceptualization of family processes and child psychopathology within a developmental psychopathology framework as depicted in the present volume does much to advance thinking and to promote much-needed further research in this area. A developmental psychopathology perspective can be used as a guide for informing future basic and applied empirical research on family contexts, and also in consideration of how other contextual influences may interact with the child's family environment. In order to encourage the full realization of the potential inherent in a comprehensive assessment of family processes and child psychopathology, an explication of an overarching model of contextual influences and child development is valuable.

Drawing on the work of Bronfenbrenner, my colleagues and I have written extensively about an ecological–transactional analysis of children and their contexts, as well as conceptualized ecological contexts as consisting of a number of nested levels with varying degrees of proximity to the individual. The *macrosystem* includes cultural beliefs and values that permeate societal and family functioning. The *exosystem* consists of the neighborhood and community settings in which families and children live. The *microsystem* incorporates the family environment that children and adults create and experience. Finally, the level of *ontogenic development* includes the individual and his or her biological and psychological functioning. Michael Lynch and I have hypothesized that these levels of the environment interact and transact with each other over time in shaping individual adaptation and maladaptation. Accordingly, context and children's functioning are conceptualized as mutually influencing each other, and transactions between children and their contexts are viewed as allowing for continuity as well as providing opportunities for change over time.

The ecological–transactional model elucidates the challenges that will confront researchers as they strive to understand the contextual influences on children's development and their relation to the emergence of psychopathology. Specifically, a thorough understanding of children's development requires an assessment of elements from each level of the ecology over time. Clearly, some levels of children's ecologies may be more difficult to assess directly than other levels. However, some recognition of the mutually influencing nature of contextual levels must be present. Although this volume focuses on child development within the family context, the authors are very knowledgeable regarding the interplay that occurs across contexts and, drawing from the roots of developmental psychopathology, they successfully incorporate this understanding into their discussions of the risk and protective factors that influence development over time.

Developmental Psychopathology and Family Process: Theory, Research, and Clinical Implications provides a rich analysis of extant theory and research on family influences and child development, including both psychopathology and resilience. The reader is helped to navigate a theoretically rich framework, challenged to grapple with difficult issues related to methodology, and provided with the "state of the art" knowledge derived from empirical research. The incorporation of a section on the clinical implications of this body of work serves to realize the full potential inherent in a developmental psychopathology perspective.

In closing, it is gratifying to see this eminent group of developmentalists directing their attention toward further elucidating the critical role of the family context in influencing the course of development. This work represents an important step toward more fully conveying the role of the family context on emotional and behavioral development, as well as toward informing the provision of clinical interventions for children and families.

DANTE CICCHETTI, PhD
Mt. Hope Family Center
University of Rochester

Contents

PART III. CLINICAL IMPLICATIONS

Developmental Psychopathology and Family Process

Introduction

We begin by describing two hypothetical cases meant to illustrate a number of the issues addressed in this volume. They provide a perspective on the early development, family context, and course of problems in children who follow very different pathways, despite the fact that both show superficially similar problem behavior in toddlerhood. In addition to the differences in the clinical picture, these children also illustrate different constellations of risk and protective factors evident over time, and these have implications for the clinical formulation of the problem, the diagnosis, and treatment planning.

Jimmy was born after a difficult pregnancy and delivery to Mr. and Mrs. M, a family already experiencing problems that reflected ongoing marital conflict, paternal alcohol abuse, and difficulty balancing the demands of parenting their 2-year-old daughter and working full-time. Jimmy's mother had not really wanted another child at this time because she already felt overwhelmed, and she had not taken time from her hectic schedule (working as a sales clerk) to get adequate prenatal care during her pregnancy. In addition, she was a heavy smoker and often nauseated and dizzy during the early months of her pregnancy. Jimmy was born full term, but small for gestational age, possibly due to his mother's smoking and lack of good prenatal care and nutrition. As an infant, Jimmy was jittery and easily startled, and also difficult to soothe when upset. Although his health and feeding improved over the course of the first few months, his developmental milestones seemed slightly delayed. By the time he was 2, he was walking appropriately for his age, but his language development was still somewhat delayed, suggesting neurodevelopmental immaturity. Moreover, he remained a tense and difficult youngster, who often threw temper tantrums and was hard to control, especially when he was frustrated and did not get his way. His problems appeared to be exacerbated by his parents' inconsistent management style. At times, his parents, especially his father, yelled at Jimmy and spanked him; at other times, they were fairly solicitous and affectionate; Jimmy's mother also felt guilty about her inability to comfort him. At these times, Mrs. M was often more likely to let Jimmy have his way, whereas his father was more often strict and unyielding. His mother blamed herself for his language problems, further fueling her feelings of guilt and making it difficult for her to set consistent limits. Mr. M also blamed his wife for Jimmy's problems, thinking that she was not strict enough, and at times, his use of harsh physical punishment led to parental fights over child rearing.

Jimmy's parents had had a stormy marriage from the start. Mr. M had a history of hyperactivity and attention problems that had never been diagnosed. As an adult, he was still quite easily angered and had a volatile temper and poor impulse control. He, also, was a late talker and had had some learning problems in school. Mrs. M was also somewhat labile in emotional control, but she tended to become quiet and withdrawn when upset, but then to lash out at her husband, who would then go on a drinking binge and stay out all night. Parental fights were often noisy, and on a few occasions, Jimmy and his sister witnessed physical exchanges between their parents.

Because Mrs. M needed to work to make ends meet, both children were in child care, where the caregivers had a difficult time controlling Jimmy, who often got into fights with other children over toys. By the time Jimmy was 3, he had been expelled from several child care settings, and Mrs. M was at her wits' end, not sure what to do. When Jimmy was 5 and he entered kindergarten, he had a difficult time making friends with other children his age. Because he was so easily angered and aggressive, other children did not want to play with him. At times, Jimmy was quite withdrawn from his peers, but at other times, he lashed out. This made him easily victimized by stronger boys who picked on him and teased him, leading to frequent conflicts. Jimmy, often the last child picked as a playmate or partner, was becoming increasingly moody, angry, sullen, and withdrawn both at home and school. In addition, his schoolwork was very poor. Jimmy's parents were contacted by the school psychologist, who wished to assess Jimmy for special class placement. Although the parents sought help for Jimmy's problems from time to time, whenever the therapist tried to deal with their marital difficulties and Mr. M's binge drinking, they dropped out of treatment. By the time Jimmy was 14, he was failing miserably in school, had few friends, and had been arrested several times for shoplifting, vandalism, and drug use.

Jimmy illustrates a child with multiple interacting risk factors that began prenatally and continued forward, changing with development but still placing him at risk for persistent and serious problems in adjustment. Thus, biological risk (possible genetic predisposition for several disorders—reading and language delay, alcoholism, hyperactivity, antisocial personality; pregnancy and neonatal complications; possible neurodevelopmental delay) in interaction with multiple environmental risk factors (e.g., inconsistent, harsh parenting; maternal depression and distress; paternal impulsivity and alcohol abuse) set the stage for a cascade of developmental processes likely to predict a poor outcome in adolescence.

Jimmy's early irritability and difficult temperament made him more of a challenge than other infants, something that his already vulnerable and stressed parents were also less able to deal with adequately. Over the course of the first year, one would predict that Jimmy's parents would be inconsistent in their responses to his needs, sometimes becoming overly solicitous and intrusive, while ignoring at other times his crying for long periods. Theoretically, one would expect that these early experiences with unresponsive and unpredictable parenting would be reflected in insecure attachments to both parents in toddlerhood. Thus, by age 12 to 15 months, Jimmy had learned that the world was not a predictable and safe place and that his needs might or might not be met, depending upon his parents' moods and other ongoing events (e.g., Were his parents fighting? Was his dad drinking? Was his mom depressed?).

Jimmy entered child care feeling anxious and insecure, fueling his competition with other children for adult attention and becoming difficult with caregivers. Furthermore, because of the instability in both caregivers and child care settings, his expulsion from several child care centers only fed his feelings of insecurity, anger, rejection, and fearfulness. This was more difficult for Jimmy because these feelings were not balanced by a sense of comfort and security at home, and they also spilled over to influence his relationships with other children, also feeding into peer difficulties that were to become long-standing.

In addition, Jimmy's experiences with parental conflict, inconsistent parenting, severe physical punishment, and paternal drinking were associated with a number of other processes, including modeling aggressive and highly emotionally charged responses to conflict with others; expectations of rejection and hostility from peers; a limited repertoire of positive, socially competent behaviors; and feelings of low self-esteem. These feelings were reinforced by his day-to-day experiences of rejection from peers and teachers, and the lack of emotional and instrumental support at home. Moreover, at home, Jimmy and his sister often had to play quietly to avoid their father's angry outbursts, and his sister, a quiet, well-behaved child, often tried to intervene in parental disputes or to comfort her younger brother when he became upset.

From a clinical perspective, there are multiple potential diagnoses that Jimmy might receive at different stages of his development, including oppositional disorder, depression, attention deficit disorder, and learning problems, and these might or might not inform treatment decisions. In addition, he and his family are certainly candidates for a range of treatments, and there is also little question that had she been identified as a high-risk mother during her pregnancy, Mrs. M and her family would have been candidates for a variety of prevention programs. In child care and kindergarten, Jimmy would have been a candidate for several types of prevention programs geared to aggressive and noncompliant children entering school, if they were available in his community, as well as programs for children with potential academic and learning problems.

In contrast to Jimmy, Jenny was born full term without problems and was a pleasant and easy baby. Her parents, both highly educated and eager to have a child, were delighted with her. However, Mrs. G had a history of depressive episodes and being at home alone with a new infant all day triggered a bout of major depressive disorder about 3-months postpartum that did not easily remit. Indeed, despite ongoing psychotherapy, Mrs. G continued to feel trapped at home with Jenny, while Mr. G pursued his career and even received a promotion at work. Mrs. G's resentment about taking a break from her career led to frequent disagreements, and the marital distress that came and went prior to the birth of Jenny became a more chronic aspect of the marital relationship. Because Jenny had such a sunny disposition, however, even when Mrs. G felt depressed, it was difficult not to be responsive to Jenny's smiles and coos. Indeed, Jenny became the only positive aspect of the troubled marriage between Mr. and Mrs. G.

When Jenny was 1 year old, Mrs. G returned to work and placed her in child care at a high-quality center. In addition, she spent time with her maternal grandparents, with whom she had a very warm and loving relationship. Jenny continued to develop normally; by 18 months, she was quite talkative; she continued to be a happy, sociable child through age 30 months, but as she approached her third birthday, Jenny became more and more willful and determined. She often threw temper tantrums when her goals were thwarted, and this occurred much more frequently at home, where, because of their own marital problems and work stresses, her parents had limited patience to redirect her or to negotiate a compromise. Jenny's relationship with her mother became quite tense; it was made more complex by the fact that Jenny was usually quite cooperative with her grandparents, who were able skillfully to prevent her from losing control. In child care, Jenny had formed an especially close relationship with one of her caregivers and she enjoyed being around other children, looking up to some of the 4-year-olds and easily becoming engaged in play with peers and in ongoing structured group activities. In these environments, Jenny thrived. She received a good deal of emotional support and stimulation from extended family and caregivers, which went a long way to protect her from some of the stresses at home.

By the time Jenny entered school, she seemed to be a well-adjusted, well-functioning child who excelled academically and socially. At the same time, however, problems at home worsened. Her parents' marriage continued to deteriorate and her mother had another serious episode of depression requiring hospitalization. Her parents separated and reunited several times, and their preoccupation with their own problems meant that they had less and less energy to devote to Jenny. Although they sought marital therapy and never actually divorced, the tension between them was unmistakable. However, as a 6-year-old, Jenny had a hard time understanding what was happening at home and felt guilty that she had caused her parents' distress and her mother's depression. In an unconscious effort to deal with her guilt, Jenny became overly good, often trying to comfort her mother and intervene in parental disputes. At the same time, she managed to function adequately at school with peers, and with extended family, so it was not until much later, when Jenny was an adolescent dealing with her own feelings of sadness and loss over the perfect family she never had, low self-esteem, and hopelessness, that it was evident how much of a toll her early family experiences had taken on her mood and overall adjustment.

By adolescence, Jenny clearly met diagnostic criteria for depression. Moreover, given the early family situation, she might well have been a candidate for preventive intervention, regarding both the marital situation and her mother's depression. Her parents were certainly in need of marital therapy, which they sought but did not follow through. This case illustrates the complex transactions between risk and protective factors, continuity and discontinuity in developmental patterns of adaptation, and the interactions between biological vulnerability and early experiences that may predict outcome in some children, even when they seem to be well functioning at some points in and across development in some contexts but not others.

These two examples illustrate developmental patterns in childhood that are often reported but not easily explained. Clearly, adequate accounts of childhood problems require consideration of many aspects of children's lives, including their characteristics, their families, and their social settings. Furthermore, in order to help Jimmy, Jenny, and other children, it is not enough simply to document that these patterns exist. It is necessary to understand the individual, biological, social, familial, and other processes that underlie and explain their development. In addition to laying the foundation for more effective clinical practice, such understanding also has implications for conceptualizing problems and devising new clinical interventions, including both prevention and treatment; that is, an in-depth understanding of the developmental processes and pathways that precede and account for the development of clinical disorders may make it possible to intervene effectively in mental health problems well before they become serious and difficult to reverse, or even to prevent the development of serious problems in individuals at risk for disorder.

Consistent with these concerns, the field of developmental psychopathology provides exciting new directions for addressing the complex issues surrounding the development of problems in children. Unlike more traditional approaches to child psychopathology, developmental psychopathology is concerned with more than the description, diagnosis, and treatment of disordered behavior. Rather, the focus is on understanding patterns of adaptation and maladaptation during development, including factors that protect the individual against negative outcomes, as well as those factors that increase vulnerability to problems; that is, the field is concerned with "the study of the origins and course of individual patterns of behavioral maladaptation, whatever the age of onset, whatever the causes, whatever the transformation of behavioral manifestation, and however complex the course of the developmental pattern may be" (Sroufe & Rutter, 1984, p. 18). Moreover, this approach has important theoretical, research, and clinical implications regarding the conceptualization, study, and treatment of psychopathology. It also highlights new directions in intervention, especially prevention and early intervention, as well as in the treatment of diagnosed disorders.

Returning to our examples, a developmental psychopathologist would want to understand how Jimmy and Jenny adapted to the demands of their family, school, and peer group, and would try to identify the factors that both helped and hindered their healthy adaptation. The relations between their particular biological, social, emotional, and cognitive responses, and normal adaptational patterns at each successive stage of development, would be important to delineate. For example, why, in Jenny's case, did being an easy baby seem so inconsistent with her tantrum behavior and other problems in toddlerhood, as well as her later depression? Why was Jimmy's adolescent outcome so predictable from difficult behavior at such an early age? A developmental psychopathologist would want to understand the multiple and complex interacting processes that over time accounted for the maladaptive behavior shown by both Jimmy and Jenny at particular points in development, on the assumption that diagnoses and decisions about particular clinical intervention strategies would be informed by the answers to these questions.

WHAT MAKES THE DEVELOPMENTAL PSYCHOPATHOLOGY PERSPECTIVE UNIQUE?

Developmental psychopathologists are, thus, asking different questions than those currently asked in clinical psychology, psychiatry, and mental health. The developmental psychopathologist is concerned with identifying the dynamic processes that underlie the course of development. It follows that psychopathology is conceptualized as "developmental deviation," which is defined in relation to nondisordered development, and that treatment is best informed by an understanding of underlying processes and their developmental trajectory over time. Disorder is not something that one "has," that is, a pathogenic entity: rather, disordered behavior is seen as developing over time from complex transactions among genetic, biological, and psychosocial processes that influence adaptation at particular developmental transition points. Accordingly, differential diagnosis is (ideally) of secondary interest, since it is removed from the level of analysis truly needed to understand disorder and to suggest the most effective treatment; that is, a diagnosis describes a cluster of symptoms or maladaptive behaviors, but it tells us little about the underlying processes that led up to the problem itself, although it is these very processes that ultimately must be modified in treatment.

Furthermore, the model for the development of disorder encompasses a multiplicity of positive (e.g., protective) and negative (e.g., risk) influences on development and a complex interplay among these influences, as was evident from the case examples. Thus, a broader causal net is cast in order to explain disorder. Accordingly, causal models to assess and explain the dynamic processes underlying development must be much more complex conceptually than in other approaches. This also means that greater demands and requirements are placed on the methodological tools employed in developmental psychopathology research in order to assess these processes with sufficient accuracy and precision, as well as in a developmentally appropriate manner. Moreover, it is important to take into account the demands and definition of context (e.g., family, community, ethnicity, and culture) in interpreting and evaluating children's patterns of adaptation and maladaptation. Thus, the interplay among influences leading to disorder is understood from a developmental perspective, with development conceptualized in terms of pathways that emerge over time. By contrast, in the classical medical model, disorders are seen as discrete and developmentally static, with relatively little weight given to the contexts of development when arriving at a diagnostic classification. In addition, disorders are implicitly viewed as arising from singular or particular endogenous pathogens (Sroufe, 1997).

Finally, because disorders have developmental histories that almost always predate their identification and emergence as serious problems, from a developmental psychopathology perspective, it is not optimal to wait to intervene until disorders become sufficiently severe and ingrained to merit a diagnosis. Thus, developmental psychopathology provides a strong theoretical foundation for prevention and early intervention as ways to decrease both the prevalence of psychopathology in children and the severity of problems once they are identified.

THE THEMATIC FOCUS: CHILDREN AND FAMILIES

This volume focuses on the relations between family functioning and child development as they relate to psychopathology and resilience in children and adolescents. The field is defined expansively, with cogent arguments made for the integration of multiple disciplines and methodologies and the goal of understanding the development of psychopathology more completely (see, e.g., the two-volume *Handbook of Developmental Psychopathology* [Cicchetti & Cohen, 1995b]). For example, some researchers have contended that "developmental psychopathologists should investigate . . . ontogenetic, biochemical, genetic, biological, physiological, cognitive, socio-cognitive, representational, socioemotional, environmental, cultural, and societal influences on behavior" (Cicchetti & Cohen, 1995a, p. 5). Although we recognize the virtue of this point, in this volume, we cannot attempt to examine all these factors. Rather, we focus on the family as a central context for understanding the development of children's adjustment problems from a developmental psychopathology perspective. Instead, we are concerned with explicating the core principles of this field, how they may be applied to research, and their implications for clinical practice. In other words, the goal is to convey the fundamental theory and science of developmental psychopathology, including its application to research and practice, with emphasis placed on the particular context of children's development in families.

A Focus on Children's Development

There are marked differences between the disorders of childhood and adulthood (Achenbach, 1988), and it has been argued that not all adult disorders are best understood as disorders of development (Wakefield, 1997). The developmental psychopathology approach is particularly pertinent to the study of childhood disorders. Achenbach (1982) stated, for example, that "a developmental approach can shed light on all phases of the life cycle, but is crucial for understanding problems of childhood and adolescence" (pp. 1–2). Thus, although the models for the study of human development from a developmental psychopathology perspective have implications for understanding life-span development (both normal and abnormal) in all of its complexity (Cicchetti & Toth, 1991), the focus of this volume is on childhood adjustment and maladjustment. Outcomes of interest in terms of children's adjustment are also broadly defined. Some researchers study diagnosed disorders; others study more dimensional measures of adjustment and maladjustment. Consistent with the developmental psychopathology focus on adaptation and maladaptation, we are concerned with adjustment problems defined at both the dimensional and categorical level.

Family Influences

This volume has special relevance to those concerned with family relationships and children's social and emotional development. The complexity of interrelations among family subsystems, genetic inheritance, and broader social contexts and ecologies makes the study of causal relations in children's normal development and in the development of psychopathology as a function of family factors particularly challenging. This field is especially likely to benefit from the developmental psychopathology approach, which provides a sophisticated framework for unraveling causal processes in development. Although family systems approaches are prevalent, they rarely consider relations between family processes and child development in the context of developmental time. Furthermore, systematic accounts of family functioning in the developmental psychopathology literature are typically limited to relatively narrow substantive areas (e.g., divorce, child maltreatment). These considerations also reflect the need at this time for a more integrative approach to understanding children's development in families.

CONTEXTS OF DEVELOPMENT: ETHNICITY, CULTURE, AND OTHER ECOLOGICAL DETERMINANTS

The influence of family must also be understood in the context of neighborhood, ethnicity, culture, and other ecological influences (Parke & Buriel, 1998); that is, a contextual emphasis in developmental psychopathology underscores that family (e.g., parenting) and developmental processes (e.g., children's emerging coping and response patterns) may have different implications for children in different cultural and ecological contexts. Thus, with regard to the previous vignettes, if Jenny were raised in a different culture, such as a collectivist or communal culture in the Far East, would the sequelae of being too good be similar or different? Likewise, if Jimmy were raised in a dangerous, poverty-ridden, disorganized community (e.g., neighborhood, school), could his aggressive behavior be adaptive in this context, or, at the least, be considered less maladaptive? While research on these dimensions of context is at an early stage, the importance of this question merits emphasis, and we return to it throughout this volume.

POSITIVE PROCESSES AND OUTCOMES

There is renewed appreciation of the importance of healthy family functioning to child development, but what constitutes healthy family functioning? While the focus of clinical and family psychology is often on psychopathology, children's competence, fulfillment, and happiness, not just the avoidance of mental illness, are the true goals of parents for their children. How can we factor these matters, as well as concerns about adversity or psychopathology, into our thinking about children's development in families? What models or frameworks can guide our thinking, both in terms of general processes of development in families and of risk processes that underlie the development of psychopathology? Given its concern with both the positive and negative sides of human development, and the entire spectrum of outcomes and pathways, from the normal to the extremely pathological, developmental psychopathology as a discipline is particularly well suited to advance understanding of these questions and issues.

THE AUDIENCE FOR THE BOOK

A Source Book

Scholars, practitioners, or other experts working in the mental health field or related disciplines are likely to find this volume of particular interest. For professional groups, this volume can serve as a timely sourcebook that provides an accessible introduction to this emerging and influential perspective on the origins and causes of psychopathology, and how psychopathology can be better conceptualized as a developmental phenomenon, a problem for scientific study, and a focus for prevention and treatment. There are few books in developmental psychopathology and even fewer books in clinical psychology, abnormal psychology, developmental psychology, or developmental psychopathology that take a systematic family focus. Our primary goal is to illustrate the value of current themes and principles in the developmental psychopathology approach to current and future issues in the substantive area of family relationships and child development. Thus, we have made every effort to incorporate new studies and research programs, and to highlight promising directions for new empirical research. Clinical child psychologists, developmental psychologists, child psychiatrists, family psychologists, social workers, marriage and family therapists, and other interested professionals in mental health, social science, or biomedical disciplines will be likely to find this material especially timely and informative. The material may also be of interest to selected scholars more broadly concerned with models for mental health science and practice.

A Text for Advanced Courses or Advanced Training

This volume may also serve as a text for graduate-level instruction, or a primary or supplemental text for courses that aim to provide advanced training for professionals. The book is suitable for graduate education in the disciplines mentioned earlier, and as a foundation for continuing education for professionals active in mental health or biomedical disciplines. Every effort has been made to make the material as accessible as possible, including the presentation of case material and concrete examples. The book can also be used as a text in undergraduate courses, but the level of the material is probably only suitable for honors' courses or advanced undergraduate courses. The material is likely too advanced for most students without significant background in the field, such as undergraduate students in large introductory or lower-division courses, and also may be too difficult for others without significant background in the social sciences or related disciplines.

PLAN FOR THE BOOK

This volume has two interrelated goals: (1) to articulate key principles and practice implications of the emerging field of developmental psychopathology, which may thus serve as a sourcebook for understanding those developmental science concepts that are relevant to clinical work as well as to research on nonclinical issues and samples; and (2) in the particular context of the family, to advance understanding of relations between families and child development, including factors that increase risk for psychopathology and those that foster happiness, competence, and positive adjustment. The volume is presented in three parts, each reflecting major areas of activity within the field:

Part I: Theory—the assumptions, concepts, and methods of the discipline that provide a foundation for an understanding of the processes underlying child development, including the development of psychopathology in children; Part II: Research—illustrations of the applications of these principles to research through the discussion of research on children's development in families; and Part III: Clinical Implications—issues relevant to mental health practice, including directions in nosology and diagnosis, prevention, and treatment that emerge from this approach to understanding psychopathology in children.

In Part I, we examine the core theoretical and methodological proposals of the developmental psychopathology approach. While the significance of developmental psychopathology as an approach to understanding human development is widely recognized, the underlying concepts and principles are sometimes cast in a manner that is vague, abstract, and quite complex. A fundamental goal of this volume is to make these terms and their resulting implications for the broader area of family psychology and child development more explicit and accessible to a wider audience.

Chapter 1 begins with the question "What is developmental psychopathology?", and draws comparisons to other mental health disciplines. The fundamental assumptions that are inherent, but rarely explicit, about the nature of human development are next examined. Much of what follows in terms of the content of developmental psychopathology as an approach ultimately derives from these assumptions, and the implications of these assumptions are essential for students to appreciate the fundamental direction of this field.

Chapter 2 is concerned with the gaps in understanding that are vital to the clinical science and practice addressed by this approach. In particular, this field is concerned with discovering the processes of adaptation and maladaptation that account for relations between contexts of development and the developmental outcomes of individuals. The study of childhood disorders requires a second generation of research that moves beyond simply charting correlations between risk factors and diagnostic outcomes, to research that begins to uncover the causal processes that account for normal development and the development of psychopathology. As we will see, process-oriented research assumes that development does not proceed from risk factors to clinical diagnosis, but, rather, posits that continuities or changes in patterns of reactions to daily experiences act over time (i.e., adaptations, maladaptations) as causal links between risk events and the development of psychopathology. The cases of Jimmy and Jenny begin to illustrate underlying continuities, discontinuities, and processes that are the hallmark of this approach. The value of considering normal and abnormal together is examined as it contributes to process-oriented levels of understanding. Finally, the chapter illustrates what is meant by a process-oriented framework for the study of human development.

In Chapter 3, we examine the ambitious and rigorous methodological requirements that must be met if we are to advance our understanding of the processes and contexts of normal development and the development of psychopathology. Multimethod and multidimensional research directions are seen as essential to uncovering the multiple processes that underlie development. To explicate this vital point and to provide guidance for future research from this perspective, the strengths and weaknesses of the various and different approaches to methodology are considered at length.

The next chapter examines the state of current thinking about how pathways of human development across the life course can be conceptualized (Chapter 4). Clinical problems are sometimes treated as if they were a-developmental, that is, as if experiential history and developmental stages were not important to an understanding of the problems. This assumption may not be directly stated but is often implicit in therapeutic or theoretical models (e.g., studying only college students to glean general principles of human functioning). In fact, the way an individual responds to events is a function of past history or experience, as well as current experiences. It is also an error to assume that pathways between early and later development are relatively simple and straightforward (e.g., early depression predicts later depression). For example, Jimmy's early problems might forecast a range of outcomes, including depression and the antisocial behavior he actually showed. In addition, apparently benign beginnings (e.g., a "too-good" child in a home with parental psychopathology) can have ominous "sleeper effects" (e.g., predict risk for later problems, as in the example of Jenny mentioned at the outset). Moreover, during development, an individual may move back and forth between pathways of adjustment and maladjustment, as in Jenny's case, or show different constellations of problems at different ages, as in the example of Jimmy. The assumptions of a pathways model provide a launching point for considering fundamental issues of continuity and discontinuity, the interplay between nature and nurture, the importance of considering pathways of development from the perspective of the whole individual in the context of the family as opposed to group averages, and the need to consider the stage or period of development. These issues are essential to the conceptualization of pathways of development from birth through late adolescence and are amply illustrated by the two cases discussed at the outset.

Perhaps the best known, and most influential, insights from the developmental psychopathology tradition are the concepts of risk and protective factors, vulnerability and resilience (Garmezy, 1985). The last chapter in this section is concerned with these notions (Chapter 5). Notably, while the terms have an intuitive appeal and have acquired common currency in mental health circles, many individuals may not be aware of the precise definitions of these constructs, or of ongoing debates about their conceptualization. The developmental psychopathology approach posits a fundamentally different conceptualization of these influences than do traditional approaches to mental health research and practice; that is, risk and protection are conceptualized as processes, not static traits. For example, Cowan, Cowan, and Schulz (1996, p. 9) have noted, "Traditionally, risk was conceived in static terms as a marker, a stressor, or a 'factor' predicting undesirable outcomes. . . . Risks should be thought of as process. The active ingredients of a risk lie not in the variable it-self, but in the set of processes that flow from the variable, linking specific risk conditions with specific dysfunctional outcomes." Another, related topic is the need to conceptualize mediators and moderators that may account for the re-lations between risk factors and childhood disorders. These matters are con-sidered both at a definitional level of analysis and in terms of statistical con-cepts and models appropriate to testing these more complex characterizations of the factors influencing human development.

Part II illustrates the value of this approach for the study of specific peri-ods and contexts of development, in this instance, the study of an important period of human development (childhood) in terms of a specific context (the family). While the developmental psychopathology approach is theoretically applicable across the life span, and is relevant to multiple contexts (family, school, peer group, community), each period of the life span, and each context of development, raises distinct issues and questions. This part of the book il-lustrates how process-oriented study in the particular context of children's de-velopment in families is informed by the principles of developmental psycho-pathology.

Part II begins with a framework or model for considering the multiple in-fluences within the family on children's development. While these influences are interrelated, each is considered, in turn, for the purposes of exposition, in-cluding the multiple dimensions of parent–child relations that have been linked to child development (Chapters 6 and 7), and relations between marital functioning and child development (Chapter 8). To the extent possible, given the current state of knowledge, core themes of the developmental psychopath-ology perspective relevant to process-oriented study are considered, including (1) research indicating how family factors may predict the development of children's problems; (2) perspectives on the role of family factors based on re-search on normal and abnormal samples; (3) research and theory about pro-cesses underlying relations between family influences and child outcomes; (4) evidence for trajectories or pathways of adjustment, that is, a developmental framework; and (5) identification of dimensions of risk and vulnerability, and protection and resilience, associated with particular aspects of family func-tioning, that is, a risk/protective model. Returning to the framework presented at the outset, a closing chapter illustrates how this model applies to a group of high-risk children, that is, children in families with major parental depression (Chapter 9).

Part III is concerned with the clinical implications of a developmental process approach, particularly as illustrated by the study of children's devel-opment in families. Ways in which clinical practice can benefit from the devel-opmental psychopathology tradition are considered, including how diagnostic formulations might better reflect the dynamic nature of mental health prob-lems in development and in family context. The developmental psychopath-ology framework also has obvious implications for the prevention and treat-ment of children's problems. These specific directions for practice, guided by the latest research and theory about the nature, onset, and development of clinical problems in children, have promise for new conceptualizations of children's problems and their amelioration (Chapters 10 and 11). The results of several innovative and comprehensive approaches to prevention and intervention are considered, particularly with regard to children's aggression and externalizing problems. The volume closes with a brief Epilogue to acknowledge issues that could not be considered in greater depth due to space limitations, including the applicability of this approach to more serious psychopathology, the policy implications of this perspective, and future directions for research and practice.

In summary, this volume offers an extensive treatment of the many facets and implications of the developmental psychopathology approach for understanding child development and treating the clinical disorders of childhood. The goal is to provide an articulate and accessible, but nonetheless thorough, grounding in these advanced concepts about the nature of child development, the application of these notions to the study of specific research topics (e.g., children's development in families), and the extension of these concepts to the reduction of the incidence and severity of clinical disorders in children. Thus, the aim is to provide an introduction that is useful for educators, researchers, and practitioners.

PART I

Theory

What Is Developmental Psychopathology?

*T*here are many disciplines and specialties concerned with both the science and practice of adjustment and mental health within psychology. The American Psychological Association alone supports over 60 divisions devoted to various approaches, domains, and interest areas in psychology, many of them with relevance to mental health. Moreover, there are numerous disciplines outside psychology concerned with mental health issues, including psychiatry, social work, marriage and family therapy, pediatrics, and sociology. Thus, the important question arises: What is the particular concern of developmental psychopathology? Why is it necessary? What does it add in relation to other disciplines? How or in what ways can one distinguish it?

DEFINITION

Developmental psychopathology is not a narrow specialty area, but, rather, is a broadly conceptualized approach to understanding the complexities of human development. Consistent with our previous discussion, the field is best defined in terms of its primary goal, that is, achieving a science that can unravel the dynamic–process relations underlying pathways of normal development and the development of psychopathology. This fact makes the area exciting because it ambitiously tackles some of the most important research and practice questions about the human condition. On the other hand, the atypical way in which the field defines itself creates an impression that it is elusive and ill defined. Moreover, in important respects, the field of developmental psychopathology is a work in progress, still being shaped and developed. Accordingly, it remains flexible, open, and responsive to new research, methodology, and practice directions, but with "permeable" boundaries that may not fulfill the requirements that some expect of an area of study.

Nonetheless, developmental psychopathology has advanced an important redefinition of research in child psychopathology and has also changed how many developmental psychologists and experimental psychopathologists think about their subject matter. Precisely because boundaries are usually not permeable, with disciplines, regrettably, sometimes competitive rather than cooperative, lack of communication, even among areas that share many common interests, is all too common. Developmental psychopathology breaks the traditional mold because it fosters a spirit of inclusivity and collaboration rather than exclusivity.

Multidisciplinary research on common topics is the ideal, based on the assumption that the optimal study of the processes underlying child development *requires* that multiple factors, domains, and variables be examined, and that understanding will emerge from cross-fertilization and integration across multiple disciplines. In other words, it is assumed that the examination of the full range of critical processes underlying child development *necessitates* a collaborative enterprise that spans disciplinary boundaries. Thus, with the purpose of maximizing the articulation of developmental process across multiple domains, developmental psychopathology crosses the traditional boundaries of social, psychological, and biological sciences.

Given the pertinence of developmental psychopathology to clinical child research and practice in particular, comparisons of this area to more traditional approaches to clinical problems and issues merit some consideration. Notably, these comparisons apply to models of clinical psychology rooted in the traditional medical or disease models, and certainly to psychiatry. While the notions of multifactorial causation are evident in some current directions in medical research, the medical model remains very strong in psychiatry and in the study of child psychopathology, especially among those espousing biological views. While acknowledgments are sometimes made about the importance of considering a broad causal net, and for the study of process, the classical disease model is still often tacitly assumed and serves as the guide for diagnosis and treatment. Thus, disorders are viewed as discrete entities and as emerging due to singular endogenous pathogens, with any identified physiological elements of the disturbance presumed to be causes rather than simply markers or correlates (Sroufe, 1997). By contrast, as we will see, the developmental psychopathology perspective emphasizes multifactorial causation and the importance of identifying the dynamic processes that underlie disturbance.

To begin, the developmental psychopathology perspective is more integrative than traditional disciplines concerned with research and practice on child psychopathology. First, developmental psychopathology combines elements of abnormal psychology, clinical child psychology, psychiatry, child psychiatry, and developmental psychology (Cicchetti & Cohen, 1995a; Sroufe & Rutter, 1984), and fosters inclusion of a variety of other relevant disciplines, such as molecular biology and behavioral genetics (Rende & Plomin, 1990). This is because the processes underlying human development and maladaptive functioning are presumed to be influenced by a broad causal net and therefore require the inclusion of multiple scientific perspectives for full understanding to occur.

Second, the developmental psychopathology approach is concerned with multiple outcomes, including normal, at-risk, and abnormal samples. By contrast, traditional research on psychopathology has often focused on individuals with diagnosable disorders. As we will see later, a key principle of the developmental psychopathology approach is that one should not only study psychopathology, but also that the study of the normal, at-risk, and clearly abnormal groups is mutually informative and essential to a more complete understanding of developmental processes (Sroufe, 1990).

Third, developmental psychopathology is concerned with the entire range of influences on human development, including both positive and negative factors, and the entire range of outcomes, including adaptation (i.e., resiliency) as well as maladaptation (i.e., psychopathology) in the face of adversity; that is, unlike some approaches to the study of psychopathology that focus on negative influences (e.g., abuse) and negative outcomes (e.g., diagnostic classification), positive (e.g., protective) factors and positive outcomes (e.g., competence, despite risk) are also prime considerations in the developmental psychopathology approach.

Recognition of both positive and negative influences is essential because the interplay between them determines child development (Egeland, Carlson, & Sroufe, 1993; Masten, Best, & Garmezy, 1990; Masten & Coatsworth, 1998). For instance, a child facing an adverse family environment, including, for example, parental depression or abuse, may function in a positive manner, evidencing elevated social competence due to intra- or extraorganismic strengths. As another example, otherwise adverse experiences in life may include hidden positive elements that foster resiliency in individuals. Thus, a parent with depression may remain emotionally responsive to a child, fostering a secure parent–child emotional bond that helps protect the child despite the challenges of having a parent with major depression (Cummings & Davies, 1994a). In research and practice on psychopathology, the positive has often been neglected due to an understandable concern with undesirable events and outcomes.

Fourth, unlike some scientific and clinical approaches that may describe, treat, or conceptualize psychopathology as if it were a static entity (e.g., something a person "has"), developmental psychopathologists delve into the dynamic, ontogenic processes that underlie psychopathology. The assumption is that psychopathology results from a complex interplay of multiple influences that change over the course of human development. Accordingly, risk factors and patterns of adaptation to risk are constantly changing, with implications for current as well as future functioning. Problem behaviors or full-blown symptoms may be apparent at one point in development but not at another;

that is, developmental process is assumed to be subject to complex changes on multiple dimensions. Moreover, it is an error to assume that all individuals receiving a given diagnosis (e.g., depression) experienced the same history or have the same prognosis (Harrington, Rutter, & Fombonne, 1996). On the contrary, the assumption is that there are multiple pathways to the same outcome at a given point in time; that is, the intra- or extraorganismic processes underlying the same diagnosis for different individuals at a given point in time may be quite different (Cicchetti & Cohen, 1995a; Rutter, 1986), and, therefore, may require different interventions and hold different prognoses. Accordingly, developmental psychopathologists are concerned with explicating the complex interplay of influences in the ontogenesis of patterns of adaptation and maladaptation over the life course of human development, with implications for both prevention and treatment.

Fifth, and relatedly, in considering diagnosis or nosology, emphasis is placed on understanding maladaptation as an outcome of development, and not on maladaptation as a disease entity, as in the medical model (Sroufe, 1997). As we have noted, these ideas differ from traditional views of the development of children's adjustment problems. Labeling or categorizing abnormal behavior is not the same as explaining how or why maladaptation occurs; that is, maladaptation, when it occurs, evolves over time and prior adaptation interacts with current situations in predicting current functioning. Moreover, "disorder" does not necessarily lie within an individual but may in some instances be due to social contexts, at least in part (e.g., families, communities, or society as a whole may be "dysfunctional"); that is, what is viewed as "disorder" may be due to the interaction between the individual and the environment (Jensen & Hoagwood, 1997), and may in some respects actually reflect the successful adaptation of individuals to difficult circumstances (Wakefield, 1997).

Finally, greater breadth is indicated with regard to theory, methodology, and possible mechanisms of development than is typical, or even acceptable, in traditional approaches to the study of psychopathology, which may focus only on specific causal models (e.g., cognitive models; radical operant behaviorism). Multidomain and multicontextual approaches to the study of the causes, origins, and the course of development of normalcy and disorder are advocated (see Cicchetti & Cohen, 1995b), including consideration of dynamic, reciprocal interactions between social contexts and individuals over time.

In summary, important elements distinguish the developmental psychopathology perspective from more traditional approaches to science and practice in child psychopathology. The concepts are exciting, offering promise for a more complete understanding of human development. We return to each of these issues and consider in-depth their implications throughout this book. However, at this point, we turn to further considerations about the nature and definition of the developmental psychopathology approach, particularly with regard to its relation to several other, closely related disciplines.

IS IT A DISCIPLINE?

Developmental psychopathology has been variously referred to as a "science" (McCorda, 1993), a "discipline" (Cicchetti, 1990a, 1993), a "macroparadigm" (Achenbach, 1990), a "perspective" (Richters & Cicchetti, 1993), an "approach" (Richters & Cicchetti, 1993), a "domain" (Sroufe & Rutter, 1984), and a "subdiscipline" (Sroufe & Rutter, 1984). Perhaps, given its breadth and lack of unique curriculum or methodology, developmental psychopathology is more properly considered a field rather than a discipline or science, but, nonetheless, a field with a distinct contribution to make to clinical science. While the scope of developmental psychopathology overlaps with many other disciplines, it is also distinct from other approaches to mental health science and practice, including sibling disciplines such as developmental psychology and clinical psychology. By the same token, it is often considered as a perspective or field in its own right by scientists in other disciplines. Just as the principles of developmental psychology may be referred to as a "developmental" perspective within the context of a science such as psychiatry or abnormal psychology, so, too, can the assumptions of developmental psychopathology be considered as a "perspective" or "approach" in the context of other sciences. However, the incorporation of principles and themes of developmental psychopathology by other disciplines does not diminish its significance as a field or domain. Rather, this incorporation is testimony to its broad applicability and utility, and its success in fostering more advanced study of the processes underlying human development.

Its breadth and scope, however, are at the heart of the difficulty in reaching consensus on a definition (Cicchetti & Cohen, 1995a). For example, as we noted earlier, Cicchetti and Cohen (1995a) asserted that "it is generally agreed that developmental psychopathologists should investigate functioning through the assessment of ontogenetic, biochemical, genetic, biological, physiological, cognitive, social-cognitive, representational, socioemotional, environmental, cultural, and societal influences on behavior" (p. 5). For a single scientist or research group, this task is no doubt overwhelming. In making the task more manageable, each scientist underscores different levels of study, themes, and substantive domains (e.g., cultural, emotional, genetic, social) within developmental psychopathology. Thus, developmental psychopathology is not made up of a single, restrictive set of theories or perspectives or procedures. Rather, it can be considered a "macroparadigm" that acts as a framework for understanding developmental process from a number of perspectives and at different levels of analysis, ranging from theories of behaviorism, attachment, family systems, evolution, ethology, and information processing (Achenbach, 1990).

Nevertheless, developmental psychopathology embodies a core set of principles and assumptions. The "psychopathology" component, derived from clinical and abnormal psychology, reflects a concern with individual differences in maladaptive patterns of functioning. Influenced by developmental psychology, the "developmental" component reflects a concern with charting developmental trajectories in functioning, including explanations for both continuity and discontinuity in development (Rutter, 1988). The resulting notion of development over time is more complex than simply whether there is simple continuity in behavior between time 1 and time 2. Rather, the concern is with the "origins and course of individual patterns of behavioral maladaptation, whatever the age of onset, whatever the causes, whatever the transformations in behavioral manifestation, and however complex the course of the developmental patterns may be" (Sroufe & Rutter, 1984, p. 18).

However, developmental psychopathology is not an additive, overlapping combination of developmental and clinical psychology. Developmental psychology is concerned with the study of group averages, or age changes in group averages, within normal, healthy populations in the primary pursuit of understanding universal processes operating in the course of normal child development (Sroufe & Rutter, 1984). A resulting cost has been the relative neglect of the study of individual differences in developmental functioning and trajectories, especially with regard to maladaptive or abnormal behavior (Hinde, 1992). Developmental psychopathology extends the developmental framework to understand individual as well as group differences in the developmental course of disorders.

Clinical child psychology has emphasized nosology and treatment, and relations between risk factors and diagnoses. A resulting cost has been relative neglect of (1) the specific processes that account for how and why risk results in diagnoses, (2) developmental processes that may underlie the emergence of psychopathology over time, and (3) insights that might be gained from comparisons between abnormal and normal functioning (Cicchetti, 1984). Developmental psychopathology extends the study of psychopathology to the conceptualization of the processes underlying the occurrence of psychopathology. Thus, the simultaneous focus on normal and abnormal functioning over time requires the integration of elements from both developmental and clinical sciences.

Interestingly, the challenge of integrating developmental psychological and clinical psychology may also have an historical basis. Thus, Burack (1997) has noted that both disciplines were academic outsiders:

> At the most basic level, there was no common ground for the disciplines of development and psychopathology since they evolved independently, both primarily outside the domain of academic psychology. Neither is inherently compatible with mainstream academic psychology, with its roots in the methodologically rigorous frameworks of the 19th-century. (p. 143)

Thus, developmental psychopathology provides new and increasingly sophisticated frameworks and theories for understanding, studying, explaining, and assessing developmental pathways, and directing prevention and intervention programs toward ameliorating developmental processes underlying the onset of disorder. Furthermore, the emphasis is on explaining the ontogenesis of psychopathology by describing the interplay of intrapsychic, interpersonal, and ecological influences on adjustment over time. Bridging fields of study, and spanning childhood in tracing pathways of development, the aim is to articulate the processes underlying adaptation and maladaption toward developing increasingly specific process-level models. Next, we consider fundamental assumptions and theory about the nature of human development that underlies the models of the developmental processes from the perspective of the developmental psychopathology tradition.

THEORETICAL ASSUMPTIONS ABOUT THE NATURE OF HUMAN DEVELOPMENT

The Principles and Assumptions of Contextualism

Every perspective on child development is inevitably guided by a set of assumptions about and representations of how the world operates. The origins and course of adaptation and maladaptation consist of a complex array of interrelationships among events, objects, and organisms. In order to achieve understanding of complex processes, it is necessary to make assumptions about the nature of human development, which imparts a degree of simplification and global organization to thinking about the world (Biglan, 1995). In the process of organizing the world, these assumptions, in turn, affect and color all steps of scientific practice, including the nature of our theories and hypotheses, the use of research designs and statistics, and the interpretation of research findings.

Understanding the underlying assumptions is thus essential to appreciating fully the implications of the model for human development posited by a theory or approach, such as the developmental psychopathology approach. Such understanding may also shed light on the depth of the differences between the developmental psychopathology approach and various other approaches to understanding development of psychopathology in children. Thus, a treatment of the model for human development that underlies developmental psychopathology is also pertinent toward answering the question, "What is developmental psychopathology?"

Systems or ways of seeing the world in psychology have been referred to as worldviews (Reese & Overton, 1970; Overton & Horowitz, 1991). A worldview organizes the world by representing phenomena in terms of a root metaphor and adopting guidelines or rules for seeking the truth. Put more simply, adopting a worldview addresses two main questions: "What do I think the world is like?" (root metaphor) and "How do I recognize the truth?" (truth criterion).

One major worldview is contextualism (Biglan, 1995; Cicchetti & Aber, 1998). The assumptions and principles of contextualism are held by many developmental psychopathologists in thinking about the processes of development over time. For example, a 1998 special issue of *Development and Psychopathology* (*10*[2]) was devoted to highlighting the importance of this theme. In contextualism, the ongoing act in its context is used as the metaphor to understand development. Developmental processes are represented "as if" they were ongoing acts that are embedded in the contexts. Both the act and context, themselves, are also richly intertwined with the past events, future events, and contexts of varying scope or breadth.

Thus, contextualism conceptualizes development as the ongoing interplay between an active, changing organism in a dynamic, changing context. Activity and change are thus basic, essential parts of development; that is, developmental processes are not reducible to a large number of disconnected, microscopic elements and explainable by the effect of some environmental force filtered through parts of a passive organism (i.e., a machine). Nor can dynamic developmental processes be fully captured as a fixed universal sequence of qualitative changes at some irreducible, wholistic level of functioning that are guided by and culminate in a telos or final form of functioning. Rather, contextualism regards development as embedded in series of nested, interconnected wholes or networks of activity at multiple levels of analysis, including the intraindividual subsystem (e.g., interplay between specific dimensions within a domain such as affect or cognition), the intraindividual system (e.g., interplay between biology, cognition, affect), the interpersonal (e.g., family or peer relationship quality), and ecological or sociocultural system (e.g., community, subculture, culture). Thus, development regulates and is regulated by multiple factors, events, and processes at several levels that unfold over time.

Contextualism further underscores that an act-in-context has a purpose or goal that is complexly intertwined with the context. From this perspective, any act or set of acts performed by the child cannot be definitively classified as broadly adaptive or maladaptive because, according to the principle of holism, each act gains a significant part of its meaning and functional value in relation to the goals embedded in the stream of historical, proximal, and future contexts. Ascertaining the adaptive value of any act or behavior is relative; that is, it depends on evaluating its success in relation to a given goal within a given context. For example, apportioning much of the limited psychological and physical resources to a specific goal may be adaptive in increasing the probability of achieving one goal, but the remaining depleted resources may not be sufficient to meet successfully the demands of other adapatational tasks. As a more specific example, the relational strategy of dismissing or devaluing the significance of close relationships (e.g., parent–child attachment) may be adaptive, in the short term, by reducing the threat posed by a chronically rejecting caregiver and ultimately regaining some semblance of felt security, but it may hold long-term maladaptational value by forging negative internal working models of interpersonal relationships that ultimately compromise teens' abilities to successfully establish and maintain romantic relationships. Thus, maladaptation is viewed as a product of the transaction between children's intraorganismic characteristics, adaptational history, and the current context (Sroufe, 1997).

Each child's individual attributes, adaptational histories, and past and current experiences also make each individual and his or her developmental course to some degree unique (Biglan, 1995; Biglan & Hayes, 1996). Accordingly, the model for development posited by contextualism is not simply restricted to accepting the notion that one cause can have only one outcome; instead, organism–context transactions are expected to lead to multiple, diverse patterns of cause and effect. Thus, in accordance with the many-to-one conception of cause and effect, contextualists accept the notion that multiple causes can result in a single outcome or, in the terminology of developmental psychopathology, *equifinality*. Furthermore, the concept of one-to-many relations in contextualism refers to the assumption that a single cause can result in multiple endpoints or, in the terminology of developmental psychopathology, *multifinality* (Cicchetti & Rogosch, 1996). Thus, developmental psychopathologists emphasize flexibility, innovation, and diversity in achieving understanding and optimizing development. At the level of conceptualization, this is illustrated by eschewing preconceived, narrow assumptions of development and maladaptation.

On the other hand, change and diversity in organism–context transactions are expected to take an orderly form (Baltes, Staudinger, & Lindenberger, 1999); that is, the organizational perspective on developmental process that is implicit in the perspective on contextualism adopted by many developmental psychopathologists also logically leads to the acknowledgment of order, holism, and interrelations between events and facts (e.g., Pepper, 1942).

In summary, an understanding of human development requires an appreciation of change, discontinuity, and adaptation, as well as stability and continuity. Thus, some domains of development may be usefully regarded as a series of quantitative changes in sets of discrete observable behaviors or as a progression of qualitative or higher-order (i.e., patterns or organizations of functioning) changes in functioning. Likewise, depending on the specific research question or goal of analysis, maladaptation may be usefully conceptualized as lying along the same quantitative continuum, but at a different point, as adaptation (e.g., Seifer, 1995) or as a psychopathological condition that is qualitatively distinct from forms of normality. At the methodological level, the multiplicity of research questions and conceptualizations of development within contextualistic models dictate diversity and multiplicity in methodological design (Sullivan, 1998; Willet, Singer, & Martin, 1998) and multiple, diverse ways to analyze development (e.g., Cook et al., 1995; Willett, Singer, & Martin, 1998).

Related Assumptions in the Theory about the Nature of Development

Taken as a set, these contextualist guidelines are sometimes referred to as systems theories (e.g., ecological or family; Bronfenbrenner, 1986; Cox & Paley,

1997; Minuchin, 1974) or organizational approaches (e.g., Cicchetti, 1991; Sroufe, 1990). Next, four closely related assumptions about human development that derive from the contextualistic worldview, and therefore underlie the developmental psychopathology approach, are examined: an active child; multiple, diverse causes of development; holism; and orderly change and directionality.

An Active Organism

Developmental psychopathologists strongly endorse the contextualistic assumption that humans are active contributors to their own development; that is, individuals play a major role in their own development. Environment does not simply create experience; people also create their experiences and their own environment in a changing world (Zigler & Glick, 1986). The notion that individuals actively affect their own development has in recent years found relatively wide acceptance in principle. However, it is still often not fully understood at a conceptual level or adequately articulated in research. Accordingly, several examples of the implications of the assumptions are considered here.

As one example, while external events are assumed to influence development powerfully, the principle of *constructivism* posits that people's cognitive or internal representations of events are not mirror images of the actual events. In an important sense, objective reality is not the central issue because people construct what they know on the basis of (1) their perceptions of relations between their own actions and events, and not simply the events themselves; (2) their previous belief systems; and (3) the meaning that these events hold for their own well-being. For example, children with differing temperamental attributes, emotional states, psychological adjustment, or experiential histories formulate very different appraisals and interpretations of identical interpersonal situations, for example, the same marital conflict scenario (Cummings & Davies, 1995; Davies & Cummings, 1995).

Another, related notion that follows from the assumption of an active organism is that people seek out and make choices about the contexts within which they prefer to live (i.e., niche selection). For example, links between stressful life events and conduct disturbances do not just reflect stressful life events that set the stage for later antisocial behavior. In fact, individuals with antisocial tendencies have been shown to seek out actively risky contexts that increase their exposure to stressful events (e.g., delinquent peer groups, violent television; Huesmann, Eron, Lefkowitz, & Walder, 1984).

As a further example, niche selection is not the only means by which individuals actively determine their own environments, however. People with different dispositions also evoke very different reactions from people and situations. For example, by violating implicit and explicit rules of social conduct, antisocial individuals come to elicit negative reactions from others, which serves to further alienate them from society and strengthen their antisocial behavior and tendencies toward others (Crick & Dodge, 1994; Moffitt, Caspi, Dickson, Silva, & Stanton, 1996).

Multiple, Diverse Causes of Development

Development psychopathologists conceptualize that development is guided by the mutual interplay between the multifaceted, changing child and the multidimensional, dynamic context. It is the temporal and contextual richness afforded by the integration of these two pathways in understanding development that sets contextualism as embodied in the developmental psychopathology perspective apart from other philosophies about the nature of human development. For example, even unidirectional "main effect" models of socialization underscore the significance of parents and dimensions of family context for the development of children; that is, the pathway between context and children's development. Likewise, the assumption that children play a key role in shaping their own subsequent experiences has been widely accepted for years, even among developmental psychopathologists who do not espouse contextual models. Thus, it is the notion of an interplay between a changing child and a changing world that distinguishes contextualism from other approaches to articulation of issues pertaining to causality in human development.

The increased richness that concerns taking into account temporal factors in development can be seen in the conceptualization of development as regulated by the lengthy, unfolding streams of transactions between organismic and contextual characteristics. Tracing the history of these chains of processes holds one key to understanding the development of psychopathology. For example, data from the classic Isle of Wight study support the notion that the intergenerational transmission of parenting difficulties results from lengthy transactions between individuals and their familial and extrafamilial contexts over time (Quinton & Rutter, 1988; Rutter, 1989b). Parenting difficulties increased the probability that girls would be intermittently placed in group homes throughout their childhood. After the girls left these homes during adolescence, the community offered them little opportunity or support, with one of their only options being to return to the very family that was evaluated as being severely inadequate for raising children. Experiencing these lengthy histories of limited opportunities, instability, and turmoil increased girls' vulnerability to feelings of helplessness, emotional distress, and psychological difficulties. With little perceived control over their own lives, they failed to plan effectively for the future adult tasks of work, marriage, and family. Thus, as a way of escaping from the burdens and stress of the uncontrollable turmoil in their lives, these girls frequently rushed impulsively into romantic relationships with deviant men from similarly adverse environments. As a result, they were particularly at risk for becoming pregnant or married to these deviant, unsupportive men. This, in turn, further excerbated their psychosocial difficulties (e.g., depression) and, in the process, severely compromised their child-rearing practices. Thus, what started as parenting difficulties set in motion a long chain of organism-in-context transactions characterized by negative, reciprocal cycles of influence between the constraints (e.g., limited opportunities) and stress posed by various contexts and children's evolving coping and problem-solving strategies.

The increased richness with regard to taking into account the effects of contextual factors can be seen in efforts toward eludicating the interplay between risk factors and processes at several different levels of analysis (i.e., biological, psychological, interpersonal, ecological). The evolutionary theory of socialization outlined by Belsky, Steinberg, and Draper (1991) exemplifies attempts to capture the influence of context at multiple levels (i.e., ecological, interpersonal, psychological, biological). In brief, the theory hinges on the assumption that successive adaptations to environments develop, in part, to ensure the dissemination and survival of the individual's genes. Strategies for reproductive success, however, are expected to differ across contexts, and the outcomes that result in terms of the relative survival of the individual's genes may be to some extent counterintuitive (i.e., the seemingly optimal child-rearing environments may not yield the greatest reproductive success). For example, in one proposed pathway, high levels of ecological (e.g., poverty, financial strain) and familial (e.g., marital discord) stress compromise the more proximal child-rearing environment and set in motion psychological liabilities characterized by insecure attachment relationships, negative internal working models, and internalizing and exernalizing symptoms. This pattern of psychosocial vulnerability is hypothesized further to promote early maturation and puberty (see Holmbeck, 1996; Steinberg, 1988), laying the foundation for early sexual activity, early and multiple pregnancies, unstable romantic relationships, and low investment in child rearing. This lengthy transaction of factors at multiple levels of developmental context actually promotes reproductive success because it is difficult in such adverse contexts to miss the developmental window of maximal fertility and biological sustenance. By contrast, in the second hypothesized pathway, optimal child-rearing environments (i.e., sensitive parenting) that are facilitated by access to adequate resources and support in the ecological and familial contexts permit children to forge secure attachment relationships and positive internal working models of social worlds. This constellation of healthy ecological, familial, and psychological characteristics delay maturation, puberty, and, ultimately, sexual activity. Hence, the interpersonal orientation, trust, and delayed sexual activity set in motion by earlier familial and ecological factors, while promoting more enduring, supportive mating relationships characterized by greater parental investment, actually may result in reduced reproductive successes, that is, fewer children, than the pathway characterized by high ecological and familial stress.

Holism

Another fundamental principle of the developmental psychopathology approach is holism. The principle of holism posits that interdependency among parts exists in any system. Thus, development cannot be understood by dissecting the system into a series of parts because each component gains critical meaning and purpose from the other parts. *Synthesis* is the rule in holism; that is, parts must be examined in the fabric of the whole.

For example, it has been shown that the meaning and function of emotional expressions are inextricably embedded within interpersonal and development contexts (Campos, Mumme, Kermoian, & Campos, 1994; Thompson, 1994; Thompson & Calkins, 1996; Thompson, Flood, & Lundquist, 1995). Thus, according to current emotion research and theory, emotion is not reducible to a focus on mere subjective feelings. Rather, as Campos, Campos, and Barrett (1989) cogently articulate, emotions "are processes of establishing, maintaining, or disrupting relations between the person and the internal or external environment, when such relations are significant to the individual" (p. 395). Put another way, "Emotion is the way the event, the person, and the person's appreciation of the significance are interrelated" (p. 395). As such, emotion cannot be understood apart from the goals of the individual and the context within which the individual is acting.

To take a specific example, smiling in very early infancy is tied to biological functions. However, as the infant reaches the second year of life and beyond, smiling becomes complexly intertwined not only with developmental progressions but also with the nature of the social context. While smiling may specifically reflect genuine happiness in some contexts, smiling may also reflect anxiety and arousal when it is embedded within stressful social contexts (e.g., prolonged separation from parents in late infancy, exposure to parental anger) or interwoven in a larger organization of behaviors marked by high levels of emotional dysregulation (e.g., expression of anger, distress), aggression, and withdrawal (Sroufe & Waters, 1977b; Thompson, 1994; Thompson & Calkins, 1996). Furthermore, as children reach the preschool and elementary school years, they increasingly "use" smiling as a social tool for hiding their disappointment from others, repairing interpersonal interactions, or deceiving others (Cole, Zahn-Waxler, & Smith, 1994). Understanding the meaning of smiling can only be explicated through the specification of goals within the context in which it occurs.

Making matters more complex, children's smiling must sometimes be interpreted in terms of broader family functioning. For example, mother–child interaction occurs in the context of a family whole, with reciprocal interdependencies existing between the mother–child, father–child, marital, and sibling subsystems (Emery, Fincham, & Cummings, 1992). The meaning of smiling in mother–child interaction thus cannot be ascertained without knowledge of the workings of the whole family. Thus, a child may smile at the mother because the mother seems upset following a marital conflict or disciplining a sibling.

Moreover, some theorists have formulated even more elaborate ecological models that place family process firmly within the larger whole of community, culture, and society. In this regard, Bronfenbrenner's ecological theory (1979, 1986) provides an excellent illustration of holism at three larger levels of analysis: (1) the mesosystem, targeting the interplay between the family and community contexts such as day care, peer groups, and school; (2) the exosystem, focusing on external influences (e.g., parental employment, parent support networks) that indirectly affect children primarily by shaping parenting and family processes; and (3) the chronosystem, charting the effects of timing (e.g., age, stage of development), continuity (e.g., chronicity of stressor), and changes and transitions in contexts over time (e.g., divorce, school entry). However, while holism certainly raises awareness about the complexities of development, it also raises important questions. What are the boundaries of holism? How far must we go to provide a reasonable account of holism in development? No scientist or research group can feasibly untangle the underpinnings of holism at every one of these levels at the same time.

In resolving this dilemma, developmental psychopathologists often relax strong, restrictive assumptions of holism in favor of more contextualist views espousing *floating* holism. According to this notion, choosing the "whole" to study is, in part, arbitrary. Components of any whole that is studied are themselves wholes. For example, while parent–child attachment is a component of the "whole" of the family system, it is also a whole that warrants study in itself. This hierarchical, nested structure of part–whole relations can be further extended in both directions toward the more specific (e.g., components of attachment such as appraisals of parents and emotional reactivity) and more general (e.g., family system as a part nested in the larger whole of the community or neighborhood). Since an element is itself a whole, floating holism asserts that the elements and the whole may both be appropriate areas of inquiry depending on the goals of the researcher. As a result, developmental psychopathology is appropriately studied at several diverse levels of process, including cultures and subcultures, communities and schools, families and familial dyads, and individuals and their subsystems of functioning (e.g., emotion, physiology, cognition).

Orderly Change and Directionality

A focal issue in the study of human development from the perspective of the developmental psychopathologist is the search for continuity and change, including the early prediction of later outcomes. Thus, the developmental psychopathologist makes the assumption that development follows pathways of continuity and change during development; that is, development has directionality. However, notions of orderly change and directionality from a contextualistic perspective do not involve merely the search for one-to-one correspondences between cause and effect during development, or the simple addition of elements to individuals' psychological repertoires as they get older. Matters are more complex. Development is orderly and evidences directionality in the sense that "it proceeds from a state of relative globility and lack of differentiation to a state of increasing differentiation, articulation, and hierachic integration" (Werner, 1957, p. 126), which is referred to as the *orthogenetic principle* (Werner, 1948). However, orderly change and directionality are posited to be the product of complex balance or interplay among several distinct processes over the course of time in the individual's development.

Thus, the process of *differentiation* posits that development moves in an orderly fashion from a relatively simple, diffuse form toward an increasingly differentiated, complex organization consisting of multiple dimensions, levels, and hierarchies. For example, smiling becomes increasingly differentiated in form of communicative intent and sensitivity to context as children get older.

However, because parts of any system or whole mutually influence each other, differentiation occurring in one psychological system (e.g., cognitive systems) leads to changes in other psychological systems (neurophysiological, emotional, and social systems), and new organizations are formed in response to these changes. Accordingly, a second, and opposing, aspect of directionality is that differentiation coupled with reciprocal influences among multiple systems leads to *hierarchical integration*. In other words, as functioning becomes increasingly distinct and specific through differentiation, groups of specific functions are successively recombined into increasingly complex psychological systems that together form new, coherent wholes. Novelty and qualitative change in psychological functioning thus emerge through the increasing specificity (i.e., differentiation of skills and knowledge) and recombination (i.e., reintegration) of psychological systems (Lerner, 1979; Zigler & Glick, 1986).

An excellent example of the orthogenetic principle is reflected in the growth of cells in prenatal human development. Initially, after fertilization, the process of cell division results in the production of a large number of undifferentiated cells that are identical in form and function. As cell division progresses, however, cells become increasingly differentiated in form, function, and location within the body. In the first stage, cells "specialize" into three major layers of cells consisting of the ectoderm, mesoderm, and endoderm. These groups of cells become increasingly distinct and specific, with ectodermal cells, for instance, developing more specifically into skin, sense organ, and nervous system cells, which themselves become ever more specialized within systems (e.g., development of brain and spinal cord cells in the central nervous system). Through this growth process, classes of these cells are qualitatively distinct from each other. Paralleling this differentiation is the process of hierarchical integration. Groups of cells, which were initially undifferentiated at a single, unidimensional level of organization, are now nested within hierarchies of concentrically larger subsystems (e.g., intestinal tract) and systems (e.g., digestive system) (Glick, 1992).

Analogously, the developmental psychopathologist conceptualizes the development of psychological adaptation and maladaptation similarly, focusing on identifying qualitative change, differentiation, and hierarchical integration among psychological systems. Thus, development is directional in nature, impelled toward increasing complexity among its parts and systems (Cicchetti, 1991).

The development of emotion regulation in early childhood provides another example. The development of emotion regulation is reflected in an orderly series of qualitative, as well as quantitative, changes based on the differentiation and integration of neurophysiological, cognitive, linguistic, and psychosocial domains of functioning (Kopp, 1982, 1989). During early infancy, infant emotions are largely caused by neurophysiological states such as hunger, cold, and pain. In a similar vein, the methods infants have for regulating emotions are largely involuntary, preprogrammed reflex patterns (e.g., involuntary hand-to-mouth movement, finger sucking). However, around 3 months, infants begin to experience a qualitative shift in emotion regulation, so that between 3 and 9 months, infants learn to regulate their affect purposefully and actively.

Increasing differentiation and complexity in the motoric, cognitive, and visual systems allow infants to (1) engage in purposeful head turning, reaching, and grasping; (2) discriminate facial features of people; (3) decipher simple emotion displays by others; (4) develop an emergent understanding of links between their own actions, the behavior of their caregivers, and changes in their emotional states. The process by which these newly differentiated skills are integrated hierarchically into a qualitatively different mode of emotion regulation is illustrated in infant–caregiver interactions. For example, when mothers are intrusive and negative in interactions, the integration of (2), (3), and (4) allows infants to perceive the aversive nature of the interaction and use emotional signals in an attempt to elicit more desirable caregiver behavior (e.g., fretting, crying). Eventually, if the negative interactions are prolonged, infants may cope by turning away, which is a product of integrating skills (1), (2), and (3) (Cohn & Tronick, 1983).

Another qualitative change occurs around the end of the first year (10–18 months). While earlier in development infants were predominantly guided by sensorimotor processes, at this point infants make substantial progress in their responsivity and adaptiveness to social contexts. Intentionality, awareness, and goal-directedness are organizing themes of this stage. Significant motoric advances, including the emergence of walking and the refinement of motor activities (e.g., reaching, grasping), open up whole new experiences in exploring the physical and social worlds. These new realms of exploration are also met with increasingly fine-grained cognitive distinctions between the physical self, the social world, and the physical world. As infants make further advances in differentiating among familiar people and strangers in the social world, they begin to internalize the complexities of their attachment relationships with caregivers in the form of cognitive representations (Cicchetti, Ganniban, & Barnett, 1991; Kopp, 1989).

In conjunction with cognitive and motor advances, neurophysiological growth in brain (i.e., frontal lobe) development results in more successful, diverse ways of managing and expressing emotions (Thompson, Flood, & Lundquist, 1995). First, emotional experiences become increasingly differentiated as infants begin to express more specific emotions such as anger, jealousy, and fear. Second, affect is organized around a delicate balance of goals pertaining to interpersonal affiliation, attachment to caregivers, preserving a sense of security, and exploration of the environment (Belsky & Cassidy, 1994). Third, ways of managing emotion are increasingly flexible as infants intentionally solicit social interchanges as a means of maintaining positive affect, use significant others as a source of information in ambiguous social situations (e.g., social referencing), construct and execute specific plans for obtaining assistance and support from caregivers (e.g., attachment strategies), and rely on play and exploration to distract themselves from stressful events. Reorganizations in emotion regulation skills continue to occur across the life span. Thus, toddler, preschool, and early childhood periods are each characterized by lawful reorganizations of emotion regulation skills that are supported, in part, by further differentiation in social, linguistic, and cognitive systems (Cole, Michel, & Teti, 1994; Kopp, 1989).

While searching for developmental processes marked by orderly change is an important theme in developmental psychopathology, it is critical to note that contextually guided models define development more broadly than increasing differentiation and hierarchical integration *within* psychological systems. First, the orthogenetic principle has usefully extended to identify regularities of change in the relationship between the organism (i.e., children and their psychological systems) and context (Lerner & Kauffman, 1985). As children grow older, contexts also become increasingly differentiated. Thus, the development in early infancy primarily occurs in the context of dyadic caregiver–child relations designed to satisfy the biological needs (e.g., hunger, protection) of the infant. Over time, the context for development becomes increasingly differentiated and complex as the broader family system, neighborhood, peer, community, school, and subcultural domains assume greater salience in children's lives (Boyce et al., 1998). The complexity that results from increasing disaggregation of contexts also requires considerable hierarchical integration, especially in the form of negotiating a balance of involvement in and across these contexts. For example, a key task during adolescence is to negotiate a balance between participation in extrafamilial contexts that signify autonomy (e.g., peers, romantic relations) while still maintaining cooperative, supportive partnerships in the family). Second, from a contextualistic perspective, development is not simply defined as a direction toward improvements in functioning. Rather, development is more broadly regarded as *change* in psychological systems or relations between psychological systems and contexts across the life span, which may or may not reflect "progress" (Baltes, Reese, & Nesselroade, 1988). To take a clear-cut example, as individuals reach later adulthood, there are decreases, rather than increases, in certain aspects of psychological functioning (e.g., motoric, sensory). Thus, in this broader conceptualization, development is regarded as not only improvement or even the maintenance of adaptive capacities in the face of adversity (i.e., resilience), but also changes associated with how individuals regulate loss of functioning when resilience can no longer be achieved (see Baltes, Staudinger, & Lindenberger, 1999).

CONCLUSION

This chapter, in addressing the question, "What is developmental psychopathology?", describes how the developmental psychopathology approach differs from other perspectives on child psychopathology and, relatedly, articulates the assumptions about the nature of human development that are inherent in this approach. The breadth and scope of subject matter embraced may to some readers give the appearance that the discipline is ill defined and perhaps not yet well articulated. Of course, it is the case that the science of understanding childhood psychopathology is very much a work in progress and perhaps only in an early stage of development. On the other hand, it is precisely this level of breadth, scope, and vision, however unsettling, that is essential to undertake the highly challenging task of achieving an advanced understanding of childhood psychopathology. Moreover, this approach is inclusive rather than exclusive with regard to the various disciplines concerned with child development and child psychopathology, based on the assumption that multiple disciplinary perspectives are needed to achieve advanced understanding of childhood psychopathology, and that many approaches offer significant merit with regard to advancing the task as hand. Thus, developmental psychopathologists seek to foster a true integration across disciplines toward the goal of a broadened understanding of the causal net that accounts for normal development and the development of psychopathology. In the chapters that follow, we seek to articulate further this vision.

CHAPTER TWO

Identifying the Dynamic Processes in the Development of Psychopathology

Three-year-old Billy comes from a home with an alcoholic father. His parents are unhappily married and his mother suffers from depression. Thus, his background is linked with the development of a variety of behavior problems, including anxiety, depression, conduct disorders, and, later, alcoholism. However, *will Billy* develop these problems? Which ones is he likely to develop, if any? What are the early signs? What can be done to ameliorate the risk for later disorder?

Ten-year-old Joan comes from a seemingly ideal family background. Her parents are happily married, and her older sibling, Patrick, is popular and well functioning both at home and in school. Her background suggests she should be socially competent and happy. However, Joan is very aggressive and disruptive in school and has problems in interacting with both her parents and her brother. Why is she having these problems? Could they have been predicted with more information about the family? What can be done about them now?

These examples raise difficult questions for both practitioners and researchers concerned with childhood problems. Unfortunately, the research literature on the prediction of problems based upon such risk factors offers limited guidance for the individual case. This fact illustrates an important point: There is an urgent need for more complex and sophisticated models for understanding how individuals develop, models that consider the operation of multiple factors and their interaction over time, and that identify the causal process(es) that underlie relations between experiential events and child development. Models are needed not only to advance understanding of the children's disorders in the present but also to predict the development of future disorders in children *before they develop* based on possibly problematic, but nonpathological, current functioning (i.e., providing a foundation for prevention; recall the case of Jane, who seemed well-functioning but developed later problems). Prevention can be cheaper and more effective than later treatment, especially among high-risk groups (Coie, Terry, Lenox, Lochman, & Hyman, 1995). The field of developmental psychopathology, reflecting its emphasis on developmentally guided approaches to childhood disorder, is interested in detection and treatment even before syndromes crystallize into clinically significant disorders in children (Sroufe, 1989). Developmentally guided models can thus serve two purposes: insights into the nature and course of child development, especially the development of disorder, and sounder bases for prevention and treatment of childhood disturbances (Cicchetti & Cohen, 1995a).

Put another way, much is known about the associations between family experiences and child development. Some of these relations have been demonstrated over and over again. For example, insecure parent–child attachment has repeatedly been shown to predict less than optimal socioemotional behavior (Colin, 1996). It can be said that a "first generation" of research has successfully mapped many basic relations in human development, including numerous factors associated with risk for the development of disorders (Fincham, 1994). However, the strategy of documenting associations between predictors and outcomes, with no more empirical demonstration than that, has reached a point of diminishing returns. Further replications of well-known associations between risk factors and childhood disorders will not provide notable new advances in understanding.

More is needed; in fact, a "sea change" in approach to the study of relations between risk factors and child outcomes is required. This is where the conceptual advances offered by the developmental psychopathology approach become relevant. This field reflects a "second generation" of social science research that aims to advance the field beyond simply documenting correlations toward increased insights into processes and pathways that underlie normal development and the development of psychopathology. Rutter (1988) has called particular attention to the importance of mechanisms, processes, and chains of causality, rather than simple statistical associations. Thus, risk factors (e.g., parental depression, marital conflict, dysfunctional parenting, or insecure attachment) are not the variables causing childhood disorder per se, but are indicators of more complex processes that affect individual adaptation (Rutter, 1990).

As we will see, the field of developmental psychopathology provides concepts, models, and methodologies to advance this "second generation" of process-oriented understanding of child psychopathology. This second generation of research thus builds upon the foundation laid in charting associations between child and family factors provided by earlier research and moves the field forward by generating more sophisticated explanatory models about the course and prediction of normal development and the development of psycho-pathology. Among the goals of this second generation of process-oriented re-search on childhood disorders are to (1) identify and understand the causal agents underlying child disorders as dynamic organizations of social, emo-tional, physiological, genetic, cognitive, and/or other processes; (2) explicate the broader causal net (e.g., multiple processes, risk and protective factors) that accounts for child disorders and the nature of the interrelations between these factors as causal agents; and (3) identify the familial, community, ethnic, cultural, interpersonal, and other contexts that influence causal processes and the interrelations between the various dimensions and levels of social contexts (Bronfenbrenner, 1979). Notably, an understanding of context is also impor-tant to the interpretation and evaluation of whether children's functioning is best viewed as adaptive or maladaptive, that is, this evaluation depends to some extent on the social contexts in which the child is functioning (Wake-field, 1997). Finally, this second generation of research on the dynamic pro-cesses underlying childhood disorder holds promise to provide a broader and more informative foundation for prevention, intervention, and therapy, a mat-ter addressed at some length later in this volume (Chapters 10 and 11).

THE STUDY OF THE PROCESSES UNDERLYING THE DEVELOPMENT OF PSYCHOPATHOLOGY

What is meant by "process-oriented" study, and why is it relevant to practice as well as science concerns? The aim of process-oriented research is to de-scribe the specific responses and patterns in the context of specific histories or developmental periods that account over time for normal versus clinically sig-nificant outcomes. Moreover, investigators are interested in process at dy-namic level of analysis. Dynamic process refers to children's functioning in terms of the particular, often complex, organizations of social, emotional, cognitive, physiological, and other processes that reflect children's interac-tions or functioning over time (e.g., moment to moment) in particular con-texts. Thus, the goal of a process-oriented approach is not simply to identify causal factors at the level of global or marker variables, or some other broad and static characterization, but, rather, the aim is to characterize how and why the psychological, physiological, or other factors operate over time as dy-namic processes.

Notably, developmental psychopathologists are interested in explaining both diagnosed disorders and dimensions of poor adjustment (Cicchetti & Cohen, 1995a). Categorical approaches are likely to put the emphasis on more severe disorders and to be of greater immediate interest to practitioners; that is, such categories have a high degree of clinical utility. Dimensional mea-sures of adjustment, on the other hand, provide a more continuous perspective on degrees of adjustment, from normal to abnormal, and are likely to be of particular interest to theoreticians and researchers for that reason. However, those receiving a formal clinical diagnosis (e.g., depression) are also highly likely to score in the clinical range on valid and reliable dimensional measures of adjustment (e.g., depressive symptomatology); thus, the two approaches are complementary and may be particularly heuristic when used together.

Returning to a consideration of the importance of understanding the processes that underlie adjustment, having a depressed parent has been shown statistically to predict increased risk for a range of adjustment problems in children but does not directly, immediately, or even necessarily, result in adjustment problems in the offspring of depressed parents (Cummings & Davies, 1994a). It is not that simple. These relations are probabilistic, not certain. Moreover, risk depends upon the effects of varied familial environments and genetic diathesis, on children's adaptive and maladaptive functioning in daily situations; that is, risk is almost certainly not global or uniform, or unchanging, but is related to whether children develop specific patterns of responding (e.g., cognitive, emotional, physiological, neurological) in specific experiential contexts (e.g., stress, loss, challenge, relationship conflict, relationship insecurity) that over time and across the years lay a foundation for the development of the pattern of symptomatology that is classified clinically as an adjustment problem. In fact, the actual diagnosis of an adjustment problem may not be made until years after the first exposure to risk, for example, due to living with a depressed parent beginning in infancy or early childhood. The issue is to identify the early processes leading to a developmental course that later on reflects poor adjustment. An example is the relation between insecure attachment and parental depression. Some evidence indicates that children with depressed mothers are more likely to develop insecure attachment relationships in early childhood than children whose mothers are not depressed (Teti, Gelfand, & Pompa, 1990). Insecure attachment, resulting initially from the lack of responsive parenting associated with the symptomatology of depression, may set in motion a series of social and emotional processes that are linked with the later development of disorder (Cummings & Cicchetti, 1990; Radke-Yarrow, Cummings, Kuczynski, & Chapman, 1985).

It follows that a central aim of this field is to articulate the changing patterns of responding that underlie relations between risk and the development of mental health disorders. Another goal is to describe the pathways, not just outcomes, in child development that constitute the trajectories toward good and poor outcomes at particular transitions or periods. Moreover, outcomes at one point in time may or may not presage later outcomes, depending on what transpires subsequently during development; that is, one cannot predict future development based upon one risk factor, or even several risk factors, as evidenced at a single point in time. Understanding at this level of analysis can shed light on the causal processes leading to different developmental pathways. This level of understanding is needed to advance more specific theoretical models about the etiology of children's problems and to inform clinical prevention and intervention. For example, two individuals may evidence similar functioning at one point in time but, due partly to subsequent family events, may have very different outcomes later. Consider the following example:

Robin and Staci were both securely attached to their parents, and were both well functioning as toddlers. However, Staci's parents both lost their jobs, and marital problems developed between her mother and father in the face of the ensuing adversity. Over time, Staci's parents became less responsive to her needs, and less attentive to the management of discipline problems posed by Staci's increasingly disruptive behavior. On the other hand, Robin's parents faced little adversity. Her mother received a major promotion at work, and her parents' marriage was happy and rewarding for them both. Both parents remained warm and responsive toward Robin, and the management of family matters was constructive and functioned smoothly. When assessed again at age 5, Robin was still securely attached to both parents, and she was well above average in social competence. However, Staci was insecurely attached and scored in the clinical range on a measure of adjustment problems.

This scenario illustrates an important point: Developmental trajectories are not linear and may change over time. This principle is called *multifinality*. Inherent within the principle is the assumption that development is neither a static process nor predetermined by early events or characteristics. Quite the contrary, development is dynamic, involving a constant transaction between the family and other events, and children's own characteristics, so that pathways of development in a comparison of two individuals who are similar at one point in time may diverge later, resulting in quite different outcomes at a later assessment. This example thus illustrates the point that one cannot simply draw a straight line between predictors at time 1 and outcomes at time 2. As developmental processes are in constant motion in interaction with the environment, one must know what transpires between time 1 and time 2, and the individuals responses to these events, in order to account for children's adjustment over time. However, it is also important to consider the patterns of adaptational and maladaptational responding that came to characterize how Robin and Staci responded to everyday situations:

At age 4, Robin responded well to everyday situations. She felt secure about herself, so that when day-to-day things went wrong in the family, she was able to remain calm and think through solutions. She felt loved and lovable, and did not get very upset when teased by peers or when her parents (sometimes) disagreed. Staci, on the other hand, was very insecure, readily became upset when she perceived any threat, and tended to see problems even when there were none (she thought her teacher did not like her, even though that was not true). She was rarely able to think through problem situations, and adults who knew her were concerned about her.

It is critical to appreciate this piece of the puzzle concerning the causal processes that accounted for Robin's and Staci's development. It was not just that unfortunate things happened in Staci's family but not Robin's. Staci's behavior gradually changed in response to what happened around her, whereas Robin's early, positive pattern remained the same.

Similarly, a pair of individuals may function quite differently at one point in time but, due to family circumstances and other factors, end up with similar adjustment at a later point in development.

> Ann and Amy were from very different family circumstances, and at 6 years of age, their functioning was dissimilar. Ann was from an affluent family background, with parents who had an intact marriage and optimally managed both child-rearing and emotional relations with Ann. Amy, on the other hand, was from more difficult circumstances, with a single-parent father who had experienced an acrimonious divorce. During assessment at age 6, Ann was well-adjusted, whereas Amy evidenced internalizing problems in the clinical range when assessed on a rating scale of common problems. However, over the next several years, Amy was able to take advantage of her social and athletic skills to develop good social relations with classmates, and her parents (ex-spouses) learned ways to interact much more amicably in facing custody-related decisions and problems. For example, Amy's noncustodial mother gradually came to contribute faithfully to child support, even though she had remarried and had another child. An assessment conducted when both children were 10 years of age indicated that Ann, whose family circumstances had continued as stable, supportive, and positive, still scored as well-adjusted, but Amy was now also assessed as well-adjusted and above average in social competence.

In this instance the two individuals came to converge, rather than diverge, in terms of adjustment during the course of development. This principle is termed *equifinality*. However, Ann and Amy reached the same point by very different routes. Ann faced little adversity growing up, whereas Amy, despite early adversity, gradually adapted in positive ways to her improving circumstances, with ever-increasing regulatory capacities and improved representations of family, self, and others. Thus, positive or negative outcomes are not the result of single causal chains of events during development. Individuals may end up at quite similar places even with very different starting points as a result of changing patterns of adaptation or maladaptation to daily life. Thus, there is neither one set of events that leads to good adjustment, nor one set of events that leads to various negative outcomes (e.g., depression, conduct disorder), but a continual pattern of change in transaction with everyday circumstances.

Moreover, adaptation involves the quality of integrations across multiple behavioral and biological systems within the child, defined by specific patterns of responding to stresses and other events at specific points in time. Children are not simply buffeted by events during development. On the contrary, their self-initiated patterns of adaptations, or maladaptations, in response to circumstances underlie their current adjustment and serve as the starting point for future development. Thus, in the previous example, Amy may have become a well-functioning adolescent because she was able to develop her own internal resources, even if family circumstances had not improved, or because support from peers helped her overcome family adversity.

Thus, while clinical assessments may present a deceptively simple picture of relatively seamless outcomes, for example, a "straightforward" diagnosis of conduct disorder, such classifications are relatively crude shorthands for describing potentially diverse patterns of adaptation and maladaptation. It is the mechanisms and processes that guide children's functioning in everyday settings, not the shorthand label or categorical clinical diagnosis, or even a dimensional score on a reliable and valid scale of internalizing or externalizing disorders, that constitute the critical level of analysis. Ultimately, this level of analysis is necessary for both understanding the child's current functioning and predicting later adjustment.

Developmental psychopathology is groundbreaking and influential, but not unique, in calling attention to the importance of understanding the processes of functioning that underlie child development, as opposed to simple associations between relatively global descriptors of risk or adjustment. A variety of perspectives in psychology and related disciplines in recent years have aimed at advancing a process-oriented understanding of child development and functioning (Cairns, Elder, & Costello, 1996; Gottlieb, 1991a). Thus, from a developmental science perspective, Cairns (1990) has stated, "Maturational, experiential, and cultural contributions are inseparably coalesced in ontogeny. Hence developmental studies should be multi-level, concerned with ontogenic integration." (p. 5). Acknowledgment of this common enterprise is important, because fostering work that spans disciplinary boundaries is one goal of developmental psychopathology. Nonetheless, developmental psychopathology is one of the most important, influential, and well-articulated of the various complementary movements, one of the most vital in continuing to break new ground, and perhaps the most relevant perspective for clinical science and practice.

TOWARD ADVANCING CLINICAL SCIENCE FOR CHILDREN

Given the importance of developmental psychopathology to clinical science as it relates to children's problems, it is important to consider the contribution of this field to that discipline. Great strides have been made over the past several decades. Numerous genetic, familial, individual, experiential, ecological, and societal factors associated with increased risk for mental health problems have been identified. This rich knowledge base of associations among variables has provided an invaluable foundation for clinical practice as well as clinical science.

For example, it is now known that dispositions underlying proneness to depression or alcoholism are heritable, so that if one has a parent with depression or alcoholism, one is at increased risk to develop these disorders. However, it is also known that many familial and environmental variables are significant in the so-called transmission of disorder within families, so that finding disorders in offspring of parents with psychopathology is not evidence solely for genetic transmission. Moreover, a broad band of childhood disorders typically associated with such problems in the parents strongly points to the critical role of family environments. As another example, low socioeconomic status is linked with increased risk for a variety of emotional, behavioral, physiological, and other health risks, due to the multiple disadvantages associated with lower socioeconomic status.

The list of associations or correlations that have been established among familial, genetic, individual, experiential, ecological, and societal risk factors and negative psychological or other health-related outcomes has become a very long one. Accordingly, our understanding of basic relations between risk variables and mental health outcomes is much greater than in the past, even the relatively recent past.

However, there remain major gaps in our understanding of clinical disorders that limit both science and practice. Typically, as we have noted, identifying a single risk factor increases, perhaps only marginally, the statistical probability that a negative outcome will occur. Moreover, many individuals experiencing a risk factor for a disorder will not develop the disorder; furthermore, some people who do not experience the risk factor *will* develop the disorder. For example, many individuals with depressed or alcoholic parents will not develop adjustment problems, including depression and alcoholism, respectively, and some without affected parents *will* develop these syndromes. Moreover, the data suggest that parental depression, in particular, is a risk factor associated with a range of outcomes and there is much less specificity than this example suggests at first glance (i.e., it partly depends on the age and gender of the child, co-occurring risk factors, etc.). Similarly, many children from humble socioeconomic backgrounds will not experience negative psychological or health-related outcomes, and others from affluent socioeconomic backgrounds *will* experience such outcomes.

It is clear that it is not enough to know that a risk factor may sometimes lead to a negative outcome. It is important to know how and why these risk factors apply, for which particular individuals, the role of past history, current age, and the prognosis for the future. Moreover, the same set of risk factors may be associated with many different negative outcomes; specificity is the exception rather than the rule. Identifying correlations between risk factors and outcomes also does not explain *how* or *why* the disorder occurs, so that insights into the processes underlying the disorder are modest. Scientific models are limited when constrained to single or small numbers of influences, when the processes accounting for outcomes are not examined, or when such models do not consider time and periods of the life course.

Similarly, clinical practice is informed in a limited way by research findings that reveal only a glimpse of the psychological and other factors that are operating to influence adaptation, and that may, or may not, be pertinent to many individual cases in all their complexity. Focus on single variables, or small sets of variables, can even be misleading. It is also critical to have information about the causal processes that account for associations between risk factors and outcomes. For example, it is hardly a service if a child of a depressed parent believes he or she is doomed to develop adjustment problems, including, possibly, depression, based upon learning about the correlation between parental depression and child adjustment; obviously, that is far from the truth. Knowing only risks or probabilities also tells the therapist little about which aspects of the individual's functioning merit special attention in prevention or intervention efforts. Thus, a second generation of research on trajectories of normal development and the development of psychopathology is needed to advance our understanding of clinical processes and to inform clinical intervention.

The concern with processes underlying child development distinguishes current directions in developmental psychopathology from past work that used this terminology. Earlier work tended to focus on nosology and classification rather than processes that account for pathways of normal development and the development of psychopathology (Sroufe & Rutter, 1984). While such issues are highly significant to clinical science, they are not at the heart of the unique contribution of developmental psychopathology, as it is presently conceptualized, to understanding the etiology of disorder. Thus, differential diagnosis (e.g., classification of disorders) is of secondary interest to the developmental psychopathologist (Sroufe & Rutter, 1984). On the other hand, treatment techniques and systematic tests of the efficacy of treatments have a role to play in understanding process. In contrast to earlier works concerned with childhood disorders, the present work in developmental psychopathology benefits from the substantial advances over the past decade in the conceptualization of processes and pathways of development.

Admittedly, a complete study of the processes that influence development, and that underlie relations between risk and outcomes, is an inherently difficult task. There are many possible processes and pathways that may occur, and that may be important for the development of children's problems. A comprehensive assessment of the mechanisms and processes that underlie outcomes in the context of risk factors ultimately will require multidisciplinary, multi-generational, multidomain, and multicontextual measurement strategies.

Much recent research has emphasized the search for the possible underlying processes and mechanisms that account for childhood disorders. Notably, the journal *Development and Psychopathology* regularly publishes research pertaining to the multiple processes of adaptive and maladaptive functioning that may underlie the development of adjustment problems in children. For example, entire special issues have been devoted to reports concerning cutting-edge research on adaptive and maladaptive emotional (e.g., Kobak & Ferenz-Gillies, 1995; Rubin, Coplan, Fox, & Calkins, 1995) and self-regulatory (e.g., Dahl, 1996; Eisenberg et al., 1996; Porges, 1996) responses, pathways (e.g., Campbell, Pierce, Moore, Marakovitz, & Newby, 1996; Harrington, Rutter,

& Fombonne, 1996; Shaw, Owens, Vondra, Keenan, & Winslow, 1996), and contexts of development (e.g., Boyce et al., 1998; Cicchetti, Rogosch, & Toth, 1998; Lynch & Cicchetti, 1998a). Reflecting the multidisciplinary tone of the field, the journal also regularly publishes articles and has devoted special issues to physiological systems and processes possibly related to adaptive and maladaptive functioning, including the possible role of neural plasticity and activity (e.g., Courchesne, Chisum, & Townsend, 1994; Fox, Calkins, & Bell, 1994), brain development (e.g., Trevarthen & Aiken, 1994), stress adaptation (e.g., Benes, 1994; Post, Weiss, & Leverich, 1994); neuroendocrine activity (e.g., Hart, Gunnar, & Cicchetti, 1995), and temperament (e.g., Derryberry & Reed, 1994; Rothbart, Posner, & Rosnicky, 1994). These recent research directions reflect the assumption that sophisticated, multidimensional models ultimately hold the key to understanding the development of childhood disorder.

Another important source for cutting-edge research on multiple processes and mechanisms associated with the development of childhood disorder is the two-volume *Handbook of Developmental Psychopathology* (Cicchetti & Cohen, 1995b). Again, this work, which spans nearly 2,000 pages of small-print text, reflects the basic assumptions of the field, that is, that understanding at a process level of analysis based upon the assessment of multiple dimensions of functioning is essential to understanding adaptation and maladaptation in child development. This work, as well as the articles published in the journal *Development and Psychopathology* provide excellent selections for advanced courses that may be used to supplement the coverage of fundamental themes provided by the current text. Obviously, extensive coverage of the many specific processes that may underlie risk for adjustment problems in children is beyond the scope of this primer; thus, these publications are highly recommended as additional sources.

However, while fostering the examination of many subspecialities for possible gaps in understanding developmental processes and mechanisms, the field also emphasizes the importance of finding the common ground across research traditions with regard to critical underlying processes and encourages investigators to move toward the integration of findings and methods across different approaches to the study of process. This is in contrast to focusing on only one process or small set of processes as providing a "silver bullet" toward understanding children's disorders. The "silver bullet" approach makes sense only if one assumes a disease or medical model for childhood disorder. It does not make sense if one assumes that complex patterns of adaptation and maladaptation, integrated in an individual's transactions with the environment during development, ultimately account for what is classified in clinical shorthand as a clinical or psychiatric syndrome. Comprehensive, inclusive assessment of functioning across multiple domains is required if one assumes the developmental psychopathology perspective about the origins of childhood disorder. Such analyses most certainly account for more variance in explaining the processes that underlie child adjustment and may even be essential for relatively complete accounts of the development of many childhood disorders. Multidomain and multidimensional assessment of functioning is also likely to be most productive and informative from the perspective of those with practice interests; that is, answering "how" and "why" questions provides more informative directions for intervention than simply labeling a syndrome that is then associated with certain recommended interventions. Admittedly, the field, and the science of mental health research, is a long way from accomplishing this lofty goal, but its ultimate accomplishment is a central mission of the developmental psychopathology field.

CONSIDERING THE NORMAL AND ABNORMAL TOGETHER

One reason for considering the normal and abnormal together is to advance a full and complete model for phenomena and interrelations among variables; that is, examination of the generalizability of phenomena and processes requires their broad-based study in multiple contexts and in multiple groups. As Cicchetti and Cohen (1995a) have stated:

> When extrapolating from abnormal populations with the goal of informing developmental theory, however, it is important that a range of populations and conditions be considered. The study of a single psychopathological or risk process may result in spurious conclusions if generalizations are made solely based on that condition or disorder. . . . However, if we view a given behavioral pattern in the light of an entire spectrum of diseased and disordered modifications, then we may be able to attain a significant insight into the processes of development not generally achieved through sole reliance on studies of relatively more homogeneous nondisordered populations. (p. 11)

However, there are other conceptual bases for considering the normal and abnormal together, including issues pertaining to understanding the etiology and causality of disorder, and the definition of what is normal versus abnormal; that is, deviant behavior can only be defined in relation to normal behavior. Accordingly, the study of both normal and abnormal groups, and high- and low-risk groups, is assumed to be necessary in order to explain and understand children's problems and their development over time. As we have noted, the assumption is that a disorder is not a category, but rather reflects a set of maladaptive processes that emerge in transaction with the contexts of children's development. Thus, it follows that one can only understand what is abnormal by comparison to what is normal. How can one possibly hope to have a simple "gold standard" for what is normal or abnormal when faced with complex, ever-changing patterns of development? That is, it is assumed that disorder is not a well-defined entity, as in the medical model. On the contrary, it is assumed that a disturbance or disorder can only be understood relative to something else, not in an absolute sense. Highlighting the centrality of this perspective on abnormality to the study of adjustment problems, Sroufe (1990) argued for considering the normal and abnormal together as the "essence" of developmental psychopathology.

Relative to the sibling disciplines of developmental psychology, clinical child psychology, and psychiatry, developmental psychopathology takes a much broader approach to understanding the interplay between normality and abnormality. On the one hand, developmental psychology has commonly followed the narrow assumption that normal and abnormal development operate along the same continuum. On the other hand, clinical psychology and psychiatry have typically been guided by the assumption that above some threshold, abnormal behavior becomes indicative of a diagnostic entity, and at this level of dysfunction the behavior is qualitatively different from or discontinuous with normality (Rutter, 1996). Since a defining feature of developmental psychopathology is its explicit presumption that considering normal and abnormal development together is mutually informative, developmental psychopathologists make no assumptions about whether normal and abnormal functioning are continuous or discontinuous. Rather, they consider that a focus on both perspectives is more likely to lead to greater insights about both normality and abnormality. For example, Achenbach (1997) has noted:

> [One] need not assume that *all* pathological functioning is on a continuum with normal functioning. It is quite possible, for example, that some pathological functioning is qualitatively different and has categorically different determinants from normal functioning. To determine what is abnormal in the sense of being maladaptively deviant, however, we need to know what is normal in the sense of typifying people who are adapting reasonably well. (p. 93)

Developmental taxonomies that differentiate between types of alcoholics provide a nice illustration of this dual conceptualization (Sher, 1991). Antisocial alcoholics, for example, evidence drinking problems early in development, exhibit considerable antisocial behavior and impaired functioning across several domains, and have a poor prognosis for recovery. The etiological processes (e.g., robust genetic transmission, highly adverse experiential histories) and symptoms (e.g., antisocial behavior, functional impairment) thus seem to be qualitatively different from normative drinking patterns, even during the heavy drinking period of late adolescence and early adulthood. In contrast, the adaptational patterns of many nonantisocial alcoholics may best be considered as extreme variations of normality. While members of this group clearly have drinking problems, their late onset of drinking, the low rate of co-occurring psychological problems, and relatively harmonious psychosocial histories (e.g., cohesive family) closely resemble the profiles of nonalcoholic individuals. As extensions of drinking patterns in adolescence, the alcohol problems of this lower-risk group are commonly resolved in "maturing out" processes of young adulthood.

This example also makes the point that considerations of what is normal versus abnormal should take into account the children's developmental period. Clearly, the normal behaviors of infants, preschoolers, school-age children, adolescents, and young adults vary considerably. To take a simple example, it is quite normal for infants to suck their thumbs, but it is not normal for young adults to do so. Thus, one must use different comparisons for each developmental period in assessing what is normal and abnormal. Moreover, assessments based on multiple domains of responding may add to prediction and understanding. Thus, Achenbach (1997) has stated:

> Developmental changes make it imperative to obtain data on healthy and unhealthy criterion groups for each developmental period in order to take into account changes of what is pathognomic. . . . In addition to developmental changes in the prevalence and pathognomicity of particular problems and competencies, *patterns* of problems and competencies may vary over the course of development in ways that require different standards for judging what is normal versus abnormal. (pp. 98–99)

Cicchetti and Cohen (1995a) trace the origins of the notion that psychopathology is "a distortion, disturbance, or denigration of normal functioning" (p. 3) to historical work in the disciplines of embryology, psychiatry, neuroscience, and ethology (see also Cicchetti, 1990a, 1990b). Freud was particularly influential in emphasizing the connection between the normal and abnormal, and stressed the notion of a continuum of normality–abnormality (note, however, that the notion of a continuum is not an assumption made *explicitly* by developmental psychopathologists). Knowledge about the normal and abnormal also enrich each other because a truly integrative understanding of child development can be seen as requiring that one take into account the entire range of possible deviant and normal forms of children's functioning. In addition, findings from the study of abnormality can inform the study of normality, and visa versa. Thus, Glick (1997) has noted, "Just as normative developmental principles have been instrumental for elucidating many facets of psychopathology, findings from the research with disordered adults and with children and adolescents having special needs have enhanced understanding of normal processes" (p. 242).

Moreover, an assumption of the developmental psychopathology perspective is that during development, abnormality does not simply appear, but emerges gradually due to successive deviations from normative expectations over time, as a result of transactions between the child and noxious family and other circumstances. By contrast, the reification of disease entities is still very strong in psychiatry. Thus, despite change, there is an assumption of at least some element of coherence to the course of individual development; that is, development is characterized as involving a series of progressive adaptations or maladaptations to changing circumstances or situations (Sroufe & Rutter, 1984). It follows that a principle task is to define "families of developmental pathways" that may be associated with the development of children's problems with a high or low probability, or some level of intermediate probability. Disorder is seen as resulting from a series of maladaptive "choices" over time. However, it is always possible to make more adaptative choices and to move back toward normal developmental trajectories. Thus, developmental psychopathology is concerned with how normal development informs our understanding of abnormal development and the relationships between those pathways that lead to psychopathology and those that do not, but the boundary or division between normality and abnormality is blurred and not rigid or impassable.

Thus, Sroufe (1990) contended that the starting point for the study of abnormal development is always a consideration of normal development. Maladaptation is seen as inherently a function of development, and the course of developmental process, that occurs over time and in interaction with the environment (Sroufe & Rutter, 1984). Defining disorder as a "developmental deviation" is quite different from claiming that disorder is something one "has" or "gets" (Sroufe, 1990). Thus, one cannot compartmentalize disorder away from normal development in the way that is implied by treatments from a psychiatric perspective. Disorder may also emerge quite systematically from earlier functioning that is not classified as disordered at that earlier time. Therefore, another goal for an optimal science of the development of psychopathology in children must be to uncover pathways of development that appear normal at a given point in time but have the significant probability of predicting deviation from normality (i.e., adjustment problems) at a later point in time. A goal, therefore, is to anticipate adjustment problems even years before they seemingly "appear" full-blown (which, of course, is assumed to be a case of misunderstanding the directions of earlier pathways that were mistakenly seen as benign).

Thus, returning to the first example we presented at the start of the book, Jane, in response to her struggling parents' marriage and the disorganized family environment associated with that marriage, was doing everything she could to help. However, her apparently "superadjusted" behavior masked very high levels of underlying emotional insecurity and distress. Moreover, the very pattern of behavior she adopted to help her parents and family certainly must have increased the already great burdens on her emotional functioning caused by her parents' problems, and therefore prevented, or at least hindered, her from having the time or resources that other children have to resolve and deal with important tasks associated with their own lives and period of development. Accordingly, her early pattern of "supernormal" behavior can, from this perspective, be seen as laying a possible foundation for later problems (depending, of course, on what happened later in childhood).

Further examining these notions regarding the definition of abnormality in the context of normality, Wakefield (1997) has argued that the task of discriminating disorder from nondisorder during development is more difficult than it appears at first glance. Consistent with the developmental psychopathology perspective, he contends that the study of disorder should focus on (1) underlying processes and mechanisms, not simply symptoms; (2) the relation between an individual's history and the development of symptoms; and (3) interactions between the environment and internal mechanisms. However, the developmental-deviation perspective of disorder, that is, psychopathology as a deviation over time from normality, is seen as incomplete unless the question of whether deviations are disordered is answered. For example, deviations can be normal variations in development, healthy adaptations to deviant environments, or unusual solutions to adaptive challenges, and, therefore, not disorders. Deviations can also be due to true dysfunctions, but if no harm results, Wakefield argues that these deviations are not properly viewed as disorders. Thus, Wakefield asks, "What is the definition that best explains the distinction between the characteristics of nondisorder and disorder?" As a supplement (not an alternative) to the notions of the developmental psychopathology approach regarding this distinction, Wakefield adds a "harmful dysfunction" criterion—that is, "developmental deviations . . . are disorders when and only when they are harmful dysfunctions, where harm is judged by social values, and dysfunction is the failure of some internal mechanism to perform a function for which it was naturally selected" (p. 288).

Wakefield's (1997) analysis thus draws attention to the importance of further examining criteria by which abnormality and normality are compared from a developmental psychopathology perspective. In particular, disorder cannot be easily distinguished from nondisorder simply by making comparisons with so-called normal groups. However, there are also questions that can be raised regarding Wakefield's added criteria. For example:

1. Is a behavior, by being adaptive, automatically precluded from being dysfunctional?
2. Is it possible for a behavior to be harmful but not dysfunctional?

In addition, it is by no means settled how one is, practically, to define what is "harmful according to social values" or how one is to determine when an internal mechanism has failed to perform its evolutionary function (how can one test that proposition prospectively?). These conceptually interesting propositions certainly provide no easy answers to hard questions about which children do, or do not, exhibit disorder.

In any case, while the field may offer a more compelling conceptual definition of psychopathology than that provided by traditional nosological approaches, clearly, the matter of how to define childhood disorder from a developmental psychopathology perspective requires further consideration. We return to the general issue of assessment and classification, in much greater length, in the last section of this book.

EVALUATING CHILDHOOD DISORDERS IN CONTEXT

Another important tenet that merits discussion when considering normal and abnormal processes together is *contextualism*; that is, related to the discussion by Wakefield, one cannot evaluate whether a pattern is disordered or not without evaluating the context in which the pattern occurs. For example, to an outside observer, some behaviors may appear as disordered, but may actually be healthy adaptations from the point of view of individuals in the contexts in which they are living. A related notion is *contextual relativism*; that is, what constitutes optimal or near optimal functioning in one situation or context may be suboptimal or maladaptive in another setting.

For example, parental depression and marital conflict are highly correlated (Cummings & Davies, 1994b). In the context of a maritally distressed relationship, dysphoric reactions of depressed mothers sometimes have the short-term adaptive value of reducing the length of their husbands' bouts of anger. However, in the long run, repeated cycles of dysphoria are associated with increased marital conflict (Biglan et al., 1985; Hops et al., 1987). Thus, dysphoric reactions are maladaptive within the larger context of marital relations because they foster more frequent, explosive bouts of marital conflict in the future (Cummings & Davies, 1994b).

This concept may allow explanation of otherwise puzzling phenomenon. For example, children have been shown to respond with greater distress and anger with repeated exposure to adult or interparental anger (Cummings & Davies, 1994a). Why do they not habituate, that is, get used to the fact that their parents fight a lot and have many intense, disruptive disagreements? Experiencing hyperreactivity is unpleasant in the short term and in the long term may challenge developing emotion regulation systems. However, it may well be adaptive for children to respond in this way in terms of the broader family context. Discordant homes are often characterized by explosive, escalating bouts of anger and aggression that may proliferate to include bystanders, including the children. Lower thresholds for experiencing distress more quickly alert children to these potentially dangerous situations and serve to activate them to be prepared to take prompt action if necessary (e.g., flight, intervention) (Cummings & Davies, 1996; Thompson & Calkins, 1996).

Thus, it is important to recognize that patterns of adaptation cannot be viewed as disordered except in terms of the particular contexts in which they develop (Richters & Cicchetti, 1993). However, incorporating an understanding of contextual influences into investigations of childhood disorder has proven to be challenging to researchers (Richters, 1997), including questions of how to operationalize, conceptualize, and analyze context appropriately (Cicchetti & Aber, 1998). There are many different conceptualizations of context, from those emphasizing the importance of immediate situational or interpersonal influences to those that focus on multiple and nested levels of contexts of human development, for example, micro-, meso-, exo-, and macrosystems (e.g., Bronfenbrenner, 1979). Among the most important, but rarely considered, issues in this regard is culture. For example, as we see in a later chapter, parenting practices may have different meanings in different ethnic groups in the United States. A limitation of much research is that much of it is based on middle-class, Caucasian families. There are also daunting issues regarding appropriate methods for measurement (e.g., quantitative vs. qualitative; Sullivan, 1998), and numerous questions regarding the relative merits of different analytic strategies (Cicchetti & Aber, 1998) that are beyond the scope of this volume. Thus, matters pertaining to how to take context into account when assessing child adjustment are far from resolved, and methodologies are still being developed.

Nonetheless, there are numerous examples that illustrate vividly the importance of context, even beyond the immediate and familial. Thus, Lynch and Cicchetti (1998a) reported that levels of community violence related to rates of child maltreatment, including physical abuse, and that these factors were associated with children's adjustment. Cicchetti, Rogosch, and Toth (1998) reported that contextual risk, that is, risk including marital quality, parenting hassles, social support, perceived stress, and level of conflict in the home, partially accounted for the relation between maternal depression and child adjustment. Furthermore, Kazdin (1997b) has noted that risk factors often come in "packages," so that it is difficult, and can be potentially misleading, to attempt to identify singular and simple risk profiles.

In an important treatment of how to conceptualize and study social–contextual influences on child psychopathology, Boyce and colleagues (1998) offered the following operational definition of social context: "a set of interpersonal conditions, relevant to a particular behavior or disorder and external to, but shaped and interpreted by, the individual child" (p. 143). Moreover, a set of recommendations is offered as guideposts for future research on the relations between social contexts and child adjustment:

> (a) contexts are nested and multidimensional; (b) contexts broaden, differentiate, and deepen with age, becoming more specific in their effects; (c) contexts and children are mutually determining; (d) a context's meaning to the child determines its effects on the child and arises from the context's ability to provide for fundamental needs; and (e) contexts should be selected for assessment in light of specific questions or outcomes. (p. 143)

These notions embody another fundamental aspect of the developmental psychopathology perspective: There are dynamic, transactional relations between individual children and their social contexts, with social contexts figuring quite powerfully into children's risk for development of maladaptations that constitute psychological disorders. Intriguing evidence indicates that social contexts can actually influence children's neurobiological functioning in such a way as to influence their predispositions to disorder.

Thus, social contexts may influence children's risk for disorder not only due to psychological influences on the child, but also as a result of neurobiological effects. Although the evidence is in an early stage of accumulation, Boyce and colleagues (1998) suggest that there may be "the *transduction* of contextual influences into pathways of biological mediation" (p. 143). Such a possibility dramatically brings home the considerable significance of social–contextual factors to the understanding of children's risk for psychopathology.

THE STRESS AND COPING APPROACH: FURTHER ILLUSTRATION OF A PROCESS-ORIENTED PERSPECTIVE

How does one think about functioning at a process-oriented level? This level of conceptualization is somewhat elusive. It is easier to think about "its" or "things" than about a notion of an individual's dynamic, constantly changing adaptations to situations and contexts of family, school, or work. Yet this is the level of analysis at which children adapt to an ever-changing and constantly flowing pattern of events. Change, for good or ill, occurs gradually and in terms of multiple and multidimensional responses to the challenges, exigencies, and demands of daily life. Certainly, sometimes traumatic events may have disproportionate effects, and there may be periods in which change is especially rapid due to the a special convergence of organizations within the individual in transaction with timely or especially significant events. In fact, the direction of nonlinear dynamical systems analyses is concerned with just such events. But such occurrences are relatively rare and, regardless of the rate of change, it is still the case that change is microsocial and, ultimately, involves highly specific patterns of intra- and extraorganismic interactions.

Accordingly, as a means to advance further the presentation of these notions, this chapter closes by considering the metaphor provided by the stress and coping literature as a way of thinking about these matters; that is, returning to issues surrounding the conceptualization of process, the stress and coping approach offers another process-oriented level of analysis. Given the importance of communicating the fundamentals of a process-oriented perspective to an understanding of developmental psychopathology as a discipline, we also consider this example as another illustration of this approach.

As noted, a process-oriented approach reflects a concern with more than charting simple relations between risk factors (e.g., biological, psychological, environmental) and psychopathology. The assumption is that risk factors and child outcomes are interrelated due to the action of underlying mechanisms and processes (e.g., specific behavioral, biological, social response patterns), and that the understanding of causality obtains from articulating how the risk factors set in motion these processes and mechanisms, and, further, how these processes and mechanisms result in diagnoses or classifications of health-related outcomes.

Thus, for example, high exposure to the sun does not immediately cause skin cancer; rather, over time, high exposure to the sun probabilistically increases the likelihood of changes in the action of the skin at a cellular level that ultimately, and in interaction with other factors (e.g., genetic predispositions toward cancer or vulnerability to the sun; social behavior, such as the application of sunblocks), result in cancerous cellular functioning. Similarly, exposure to social environments characterized by high psychosocial stress does not immediately result in mental health disorders. Rather, over time, high exposure to such environments increases the likelihood of behavioral, cognitive, or social dysregulations that ultimately, in interaction with other factors (e.g., genetic predispositions toward depression or aggression; social environments, such as an unsupportive family), result in adjustment problems.

The stress and coping model offers another useful way of thinking about underlying processes and mechanisms that may explain causal relations between risk factors and health-related outcomes. Lazarus and Folkman (1984, p. 19) define stress as "a particular relationship between the person and the environment that is appraised by the person as taxing or exceeding his or her resources or endangering his or her well-being." Coping is conceptualized as a dynamic process; that is, "the changing thoughts and acts that the individual uses to manage the external and/or internal demands of a specific person–environment transaction that is appraised as stressful" (Folkman, 1991, p. 5).

When coping is viewed in this way, emphasis is placed on the *specific* thoughts, acts, biological reactions, and other responses that the individual uses to cope with *specific* contexts, as guided by personal biological, genetic, behavioral, and psychological dispositions (e.g., behavioral habits, cognitive response patterns) or predispositions (e.g., genetic influences). The notion of specificity and precise definition is critical to a process-oriented perspective; for example, it is important to know how much an individual drinks and other multidimensional aspects of functioning (body weight, gender), not simply whether he or she drinks, in order to predict whether consumption of wine will be related to healthy or harmful consequences. Individual differences also figure prominently in outcomes, and it is important in a process-oriented perspective to be as specific as possible about individual-difference factors in attempting to explain or predict outcomes. Individual-difference dimensions include, for example, personal dispositions or habits, biological functioning, family history, age, and gender. Interactions between the individual and specific environmental contexts find expression in multidimensional coping processes and strategies that develop into patterns that contribute over time to health or illness, adjustment or maladjustment.

Put another way, adversity, stress, and exposure to risk factors do not lead directly to diagnoses of psychopathology or other health-related problems. The development of psychopathology, as well as other health-related problems, reflects a series of microsocial processes that occur interactively over time, typically reflecting gradual adaptations by individuals to circumstances, although, in the case of traumatic events, effects may be virtually immediate; that is, the interval of time needed to induce health-related outcomes varies; for example, immediate consequences may occur from serious accidents, whereas effects may be more gradual with some environmental hazards (e.g., smoking). Nonetheless, even a stressor that typically has relatively immediate health-related consequences does so by inducing complex patterns of change at a microsocial level; that is, specificity and multidimensional characterization of response processes remain important to the possibility of causal explanation. In summary, stress and coping processes, responses, and styles that come to occur in specific biopsychoenvironmental contexts account for relations between risk factors on the one hand, and health-related outcomes on the other.

A point meriting emphasis is that relations between risk factors, stress and coping processes, and psychological or physical health may change significantly, or even dramatically, during development. For example, the impact of toxins (e.g., chemical, infectious agents) varies considerably even during the relatively brief period of prenatal development (Kolberg, 1999a). As another example, the long-term implications of bone loss due to dietary inadequacies are particularly significant in adolescent girls (Kolberg, 1999b).

On the other hand, age, per se, is not necessarily the best index of period of development, as individuals develop at different rates, with these differences "fanning out" with age, so that dissimilarity between individuals in aging is considerable, especially in later life (Bergeman & Wallace, 1999). In other words, since aging itself is a process, periods of development are better conceptualized in terms of processes of biopsychological functioning rather than chronological age.

The stress and coping perspective is offered as another useful heuristic for outlining a process-oriented approach. There are many questions, for both this model and for the developmental psychopathology approach, including questions about how best to conceptualize the study of processes and mechanisms, and to describe causality and etiology in multivariate, longitudinal models, including processes that may underlie relations between risk factors and adjustment problems or other health-related outcomes. Some of these issues are examined later in this volume, but other issues, consistent with the notion that developmental psychopathology is a discipline in the making, remain unresolved at this time.

Finally, the example of the stress and coping model underscores an important point: The goal of a process-oriented perspective is more than just a statistical modeling of variables related to child outcomes. The adequate measurement of process variables, and the articulation and demonstration of how and why processes serve as mechanisms for children's adjustment and functioning in specific developmental contexts, are also key elements of process-oriented explanation. The concern of the developmental psychopathology approach with multivariate assessment and taking into account the role of interrelations between complex sets of variables over time reflect the proposition that development is a dynamic, not static, process. Thus, statistical demonstrations in themselves may be regarded as a necessary, but not sufficient, condition for articulating the processes underlying children's development and adjustment over time. While statistical treatments are invaluable for many process-oriented directions, they can shed no more light on the processes underlying children's development than is permitted by the adequacy of the measurement of psychological constructs, particularly with regard to the dynamic nature of specific person–environment transactions over time.

CONCLUSION

This chapter provides an outline of arguments supporting the need to study the processes underlying relations between risk factors and adjustment problems in children. As we have seen, adjustment problems in children must be conceptualized in terms of adaptation and development, that is, patterns of responding to situations in context, while also considering change over time. Processes of change are complex and multidimensional, and pathways of development are dynamic and ever subject to change. Thus, the model presented for understanding the origins and etiology of children's adjustment is a demanding one, both conceptually and empirically. However, the need for a "second generation" of research and theory on children's adjustment problems is very apparent, and the notions offered by developmental psychopathology as a field provide steps toward better understanding children's adjustment problems. In the next several chapters, we further develop the characteristics of this new field as an approach to unraveling these questions.

CHAPTER THREE

Methodological Directions in Developmental Psychopathology Research

We have now seen that the developmental psychopathology tradition makes strong requirements concerning the types of information that are necessary in order to describe human development adequately. The level of understanding that is required to achieve the practice and scientific demands of this approach is thus quite considerable. Traditional approaches to the study of childhood psychopathology have typically not required such a level of information for research and practice. Accordingly, it is incumbent upon developmental psychopathology as an approach to put forth a model for how to advance this level of understanding of childhood psychopathology from a methodological as well as a theoretical perspective.

In response to these concerns, considerable space has been devoted to outlining methodological directions for research in this area (Cicchetti & Cohen, 1995b). While these matters have somewhat different implications for practice than for research, these issues nonetheless also have significant implications for the conduct of clinical practice for childhood psychopathology (e.g., What measures are appropriate for assessment in the context of practice? What conclusions can be drawn for these purposes? What are the limitations? On another front, what conclusions can the clinician legitimately take away from reading published research studies?).

Thus, developmental psychopathology is not just a theory about psychopathology in the abstract sense of, say, Freud, Jung, Klein, or other grand theorists who helped articulate broad psychodynamic principles that for decades defined psychiatry, clinical psychology, and other disciplines concerned with mental health. On the contrary, developmental psychopathology as an approach also forcefully advances a template for the directions of scientific research in these areas that are required for the needed advances in understanding to take place.

METHODOLOGICAL DIVERSITY AND THE ADVOCACY OF METHODOLOGICAL INCLUSIVENESS

A central thesis of the developmental psychopathology tradition is that methodological diversity is key to substantial new advances and the continuing vigor of this field of study. Moreover, the broad scope of this area requires contributions from many different disciplines to study these matters; that is, there is a recognition that multiple disciplines have something to contribute to the unraveling of the complex processes leading to adjustment and maladjustment.

Put another way, the field advocates the use of multiple methods in the study of multiple domains of children's dynamic processes of responding to developmental contexts, as well as the study of the contexts themselves. This is consistent with the assumption is that children's adaptations to contexts of development are complex and occur on many different dimensions of functioning that also vary in response to the multiple contexts that the child encounters on a daily basis. Thus, different methodologies requiring wide-ranging expertise are needed to elucidate fully the processes that underlie development.

The emphasis on the need to study multiple domains of functioning in order to account for the processes that underlie development is consistent with the organizational perspective that is at the heart of the developmental psychopathology approach. As Cicchetti and Cohen (1995a) stated:

> The organizational perspective focuses on the quality of integration within and among the behavioral and biological systems of the individual. This focus on variations in the quality of integration provides the building blocks on which the developmental psychopathologist characterizes developmental status. Further, the organizational perspective specifies how development proceeds. Development occurs as a progression of qualitative reorganizations within and among the biological, social, emotional, cognitive, representational, and linguistic systems proceeding through differentiation and subsequent hierarchical integration and organization. (p. 6)

Importance of Multiple Methods

The importance of multiple and diverse methodologies in the study of childhood psychopathology is a relatively new issue and is at odds perhaps with a traditional tendency for disciplines to be insular rather than expansive toward competing or complementary areas of work. However, times are changing and the developmental psychopathology tradition is at the forefront in advocating this direction.

However, it is not clear that the adoption of rigorous, data-intensive assessment of children's functioning across multiple domains and contexts has taken hold; that is, it is still the case that disciplines concerned with childhood psychopathology rely to a considerable extent upon limited methodologies. For the developmental psychopathologist, it is important to raise the bar a bit higher, at least over time and in the context of a programmatic series of investigations. Thus, Cicchetti and Cohen (1995a) make the following additional points regarding the methodological and measurement requirements of a developmental psychopathology approach:

> An organizational perspective on development highlights the importance of assessing multiple developmental systems concurrently. Although various domains may be studied independently, organizational theorists seek an integrated understanding of the organization of various psychological and biological developmental systems. Psychopathologists who adhere to an organizational view of developmental process must increasingly incorporate age-appropriate assessments of the effects of biological, psychological, and sociocultural factors on the same individuals, in their strivings to uncover the roots of . . . adaptation. Along these lines, the investigation of multiple aspects of the developmental process concurrently can shed light on the nature of the interrelations among various ontogeneic domains. For example, how do cognition, affect, and neurobiological growth relate with one another at various points during ontogeny? When an advance or lag occurs in one system, what are the consequences for other systems? (p. 12)

By contrast, a common direction in the study of risk and children's adjustment is to rely on single methods. Although singular use of any method (e.g., observation, interview, questionnaire) reduces the ability to make firm conclusions in given area of study, we illustrate these limitations in the context of questionnaire research due to their predominant use. Questionnaire construction heavily reflects the psychometrician's own conceptualization and operationalization of key constructs, the significant events or observations that comprise the constructs, and the factor structure of the phenomenon (e.g., how the items or observations hang together). Thus, the practice of solely relying on an established battery of questionnaires has limitations: The measurements may frequently, in fact, not fully capture the constructs that developmental psychopathologists hope to test in their own conceptual models. Moreover, relying heavily on questionnaires in programmatic research lines imposes a narrow, preestablished organization of how the world operates that may miss or obscure new and exciting ways of conceptualizing and assessing constructs. Embracing concepts of diversity, uniqueness, and novelty in contextualism requires constant methodological innovation geared toward exploring alternative constructs and networks of relations between variables.

Further complicating the picture, questionnaires are constrained by well-known problems that affect their interpretability, such as response biases, biases of perception, or memory errors. Memory errors are inherent in retrospective reports, particularly when responding is not immediate, and they are exacerbated when participants are asked to make multiple, detailed, and precise judgments based upon recall across long periods of time in the past. Relatedly, significant domains of functioning may be missed by questionnaires. For example, participants may simply not be aware of their own nonverbal communications or physiological reactions. Thus, sole reliance on batteries of questionnaires may not adequately capture many levels of process, particularly in mapping: (1) the fine-grained unfolding of streams of behaviors (e.g., sequences of appraisals, coping strategies, and emotions in response to stressors), (2) interrelations between physiology and psychological functioning, (3) aspects of functioning that are unconscious or semiconscious. Statistical tests of models, regardless of how well they are conceptualized and how carefully the statistical package is selected, are only as good as the measures used. Even the most sophisticated statistical analyses cannot fix poor or limited data.

This matter merits elaboration because it is a serious problem. Statistical packages are seductively easy to use. Thus, one may encounter in the literature impressive diagrams representing advanced statistical analyses, such as structural equation modeling, and read authoritative-sounding conclusions about causal relations. Consumer of clinical science beware! The reader should know that conclusions, although potentially informative, are limited if the data are entirely based on a single methodology, including self-report methodologies. While advanced statistical analyses may claim to identify the dynamic processes underlying childhood problems, such findings simply lack cogency if based upon inadequate measurement of children's functioning or other key variables (e.g., historical characteristics of family functioning; contexts of current family functioning). Certainly, a logic of causality can be gleaned from such approaches. However, this is not the same as verifying children's specific and multiple response processes (e.g., emotional, cognitive, social, physiological) in the context of specific and meaningful situations that reflect the child's everyday experience. Moreover, while such analyses can be important as a step toward understanding, in the context of a broader, programmatic line of research, the use of other methods and approaches should nonetheless be planned. In particular, the experiment ought to be used far more often to verify and provide stricter tests of causal hypotheses (Cummings, 1995b). Also, from a statistical perspective, when conducting structural equation modeling or other statistical tests of causality, one should include in a model multiple measures of each pertinent construct that are roughly equivalent in their ability to reflect the construct of interest but maximally different in the method used to assess the construct to obtain the most cogent tests of theoretical models.

This is not to question the considerable value and importance of the questionnaire or a related self-report approach, the clinical interview. That is not the point. These methods are potentially very powerful research tools when used appropriately and may sometimes provide the best and most appropriate assessments of certain domains of functioning (e.g., clinical diagnoses of psychopathology). Notably, questionnaires, when meeting stringent tests for psychometric adequacy (e.g., reliability, multiple tests of validity), can be a most informative tool in research. Nor is the point to provide a quick lesson in the interpretation of statistical analyses. However, questionnaires—and this is the key point—or *any single methodology* are best used in combination with other methodologies when the issue is the study of the processes that underlie relations between predictors and child outcomes. Moreover, when claims are made to assess the dynamic processes underlying functioning, the level of analysis of functioning should reflect the dynamic processes as they occur over time as closely as possible and at a sufficient level of complexity to do justice to the phenomenon. Even when multiple methods are used, the perspective on the causal processes influencing development will be limited if analyses are based on cross-sectional research designs; that is, prospective longitudinal research designs are essential to the study of the processes underlying changes in development over time.

The developmental psychopathology approach, then, includes a strong commitment to multimethod research. It is important to recognize that no one method constitutes a royal road to the truth. The questionnaire is highlighted here because it is in such common use and too often is the sole research tool. Such overreliance is not consistent with the methodological goals of a developmental psychopathology approach, or with the broader goal of substantially advancing our understanding of the processes that underlie development. Every methodology has its strengths and weaknesses. Like blind men feeling different parts of an elephant, each may hold an aspect of the truth, but none provides the whole picture.

The Importance of Studying Multiple Domains of Functioning

Just as there is no one way to study the processes that underlie childhood disorders, there is no one response dimension that provides "the truth," and our best approximations of that lofty goal can be obtained only by examining the multiple response domains over time that determine adjustment; that is, children's response processes are best understood by examining the multiplicity of ways they react across a range of salient dimensions of overt behavior and internal states. These responses include emotional, social, cognitive, physiological, and other levels of functioning. In addition, it is important to consider higher organizations of functioning (e.g., patterns of attachment) as well as specific levels of responding in specific situations (e.g., crying in response to separation) (Cummings & Cummings, 1988). Moreover, a complete consideration of all of the relevant influences, processes, and levels of analysis of functioning that contribute to the development of psychopathology may require the consideration of response dispositions and functions that psychologists are not normally trained to examine. Hence, interdisciplinary research collaborations are especially pertinent. For example, Cicchetti and Cohen (1995a) note:

> Many of the internal and external processes implicated in the causes and consequences of maladaptive and/or disordered outcomes tend not to occur in isolation. . . . It is likely that a multitude of rather general factors across the broad domains of biology, psychology, and sociology will be at least indirectly related to the etiology, course, and sequelae of risk conditions and psychopathology. A comprehensive articulation of the processes and mechanisms that have promoted or inhibited the development of competent adaptation over the course of ontogenesis may be more important than specific predictors of the immediate or proximal onset of a psychopathological disorder. (pp. 8–9)

It is not possible in this volume, which aims to provide an accessible primer to the developmental psychopathology approach in a relatively short space, to attempt to provide coverage of the principles and research findings from the numerous disciplines that are relevant to an understanding of the processes underlying childhood psychopathology. Moreover, we, as psychologists, certainly do not have the requisite expertise. Notably, significant space is devoted elsewhere to the contributions of other disciplines. For example, research and methods from psychobiological traditions receive extensive space in the first volume of the *Handbook of Developmental Psychopathology* (Cicchetti & Cohen, 1995b). In addition, special issues (e.g., Fall 1994) of *Development and Psychopathology* (edited by Cicchetti & Nurcombe), as well as occasional articles in that journal, are devoted to psychobiological methodologies and findings.

Nonetheless, we wish to provide an example of how data from another discipline are pertinent to explaining the processes that underlie development. This example is relevant to a classic issue in the development of psychopathology: Is proneness to disorder due to nature or nurture? The matter is often posed as an either–or question. A related assumption is that early appearing biological dispositions reflect the operation of "nurture." However, some research suggests quite persuasively that nurture can influence nature, if one takes fundamental biological dispositions as evidence for nature (which is often assumed).

Thus, for example, Schneider and colleagues (1998) reported findings indicating that brain biogenic amine levels in primates are altered by prenatal stress, with implications for the monkey's behavioral responding in social situations. The responses of infant rhesus monkeys of mothers exposed to mild unpredictable stress (noise bursts) during the prenatal period were compared to the responses of other infant rhesus monkeys whose mothers were not exposed to these stresses. Under conditions of stress (separation), prenatally stressed infants were found to evidence higher levels of neurochemical responding at 8 and 18 months of age, and these differences were persistent over time in stressful situations. Prenatally stressed infant monkeys also showed elevated levels of social behaviors in reunions with other monkeys following the separations (e.g., more time clinging to their surrogates; less time playing and locomoting). Particularly when considering that responses of human infants to reunion following separation have been linked with emotional security, emotion regulation, and proneness to psychopathology (Greenberg, Cicchetti, & Cummings, 1990b), one can make a case that these responses are indicative of greater disturbance and emotional distress among infant monkeys of prenatally stressed mothers.

The particular relevance of this study, and related research, derives from the fact that brain biogenic amine neurotransmitter system function has been implicated in psychopathologies of various types in humans; that is, individuals with psychopathology differ from controls in brain biogenic amine system function; moreover, the use of pharmacological agents has been found to help the treatment of psychopathology (e.g., depression). While genetic factors have been implicated in producing differences in these biological functions and therefore have sometimes been assumed to play a causal role at this level of analysis, there is increasing and converging evidence from studies of human and nonhuman primates that psychosocial stresses can also cause persistent alterations in these functions. Notably, in other studies, postnatal, as well as prenatal, environmental events have been implicated in changes in these biological systems (Cicchetti & Tucker, 1994). Accordingly, Post and Weiss (1997) have argued that while the "basic wiring" of the central nervous system is due to genetics, relatively fine-grained changes, but nonetheless changes potentially significant to emotional experience and psychopathology (e.g., depression), in these functions may occur due to experience throughout the life span. Thus, Post and Weiss hypothesized that experience-based neuroplasticity may occur even at higher levels of neurobiological functioning, and, therefore, experiential influences on neurobiological influences should be considered in both theoretical models of psychopathology and directions for therapeutic interventions for major affective illnesses.

Of course, we are not advocating that biological measures are the "silver bullet" to understanding childhood disorders. In fact, this line of research persuasively makes the case that nonbiological (i.e., environmental) factors weigh importantly even in directions that might be assumed to be the purview of behavioral genetics or biological psychiatry. The point is that multiple methods and directions in assessment are necessary.

THE UTILITY OF MULTIPLE METHODS: DEVELOPMENTAL PSYCHOPATHOLOGY AND FAMILY RESEARCH

Relatedly, there are various levels of analysis to consider when evaluating which research methodologies are most pertinent to an issue regarding the development of psychopathology. Obviously, no one study, or program of research, can include all possible methodologies and all possible responses. It is an overwhelming prospect to have to consider all possibilities and clearly not feasible. Thus, informed decisions must be made; but, at the same time, every effort must be made to extend study beyond a single methodology and a single context. The researcher (and also the clinician, where pertinent) needs to carefully weigh what the methodology can, or cannot, effectively tell one about the processes and dimensions of functioning that are of central concern. Notably, the methodologies that may be useful vary considerably in terms of the measurement methods, sources of information, and contexts in which the information is obtained. These matters of practicality and feasibility also need to be weighed in the conduct of individual studies. As the substantive focus of this volume, family research provides a specific and pertinent context for illustrating these concerns and matters. While it is most desirable to include as many pertinent methodologies as possible, certain substantive considerations, which are outlined here, should be carefully considered in the selection of particular methodologies to address particular questions.

Questionnaires

Given adequate psychometrics, a strength of this methodology is that one can obtain the "big picture" on parental, marital, family, and child functioning and adjustment by means of a mode of data collection that is relatively cheap and easy to use, and can be readily compared across studies and across the results obtained from multiple laboratories. However, there are a number of possible problems: (1) the potential for memory or response-bias errors, (2) limitations on the specificity of dimensions of family or child responses that can be obtained, (3) limitations on the number of response dimensions that can be reliably or sensibly assessed (e.g., physiological responding), and (4) limitations of questionnaires for uncovering new dimensions of responding that are not already thought by investigators to be important at the time of scale construction.

Another problem is that questionnaires may not be particularly engaging and may even be tedious for some individuals to complete. Thus, individuals may not be particularly motivated to give their best answers, or they may not understand the intent of the questions. Questionnaires also require considerable aptitude for language, which limits their utility for some samples. For example, younger children may not be able to complete questionnaires reliably, particularly when the items place considerable load on representational, language, reading, or inferential abilities.

On the other hand, there is often a need for reports from people who have interacted with an individual over long periods of time. Thus, while the reports of trained observers have virtues in relation to some of the limitations of questionnaires completed by parents, teachers, or the children themselves, observers have access only to limited samples of data. Therefore, another virtue of the questionnaire is that the data obtained are often based upon a relatively extensive sampling of the individual's behavior in relation to the data obtained by trained observers (Achenbach, 1997). The following additional issues about the use of questionnaires are considered:

1. *Who is reporting on the child's behavior?* The data that one obtains about children's functioning are affected by who is reporting about the child. One reason for obtaining data from respondents other than children is that the children may not be the most accurate reporters about some matters; that is, at least until adolescence, children are somewhat limited in their capacity to provide psychological information about themselves. Moreover, it is sometimes desirable to seek responses from parents, teachers, and the child. A reason for obtaining data from multiple respondents is that children's behavior may differ across settings, such as the home and school. Their behavior may also differ from one person to another even within a given setting, such as behavior with the father versus the mother in the home. Given that children are likely to behave differently in different settings, obtaining reports from multiple informants is likely to improve the quality of the data on children's functioning. However, even when data are obtained from multiple respondents, it is not the same as collecting different types of data (e.g., observational, questionnaire, biological) on children's functioning. As described earlier, questionnaires have inherent limitations in which dimensions of functioning can be assessed, and in the rigor and precision with which functioning can be measured.

2. *Who is reporting about what aspect of behavior or context?* In deciding which questionnaires to employ, another issue to consider is which individuals are the most appropriate for providing the data of interest. For example, for children's externalizing problems (e.g., conduct disorders, aggression), parents or teachers may provide the most accurate reports (Loeber et al., 1993). Parents and teachers may be more aware of disruptive and aggressive behavior than the child, and also have the cognitive capacities to provide a more complete assessment. Similarly, studies focusing on social competence and adjustment in the peer group often rely on peer nominations and assessments (e.g., Coie et al., 1993). However, for children's internalizing problems (e.g., anxiety, depression), children or adolescents may often be the best reporters. Parents and teachers may simply not be aware, or may be only minimally aware, of the child's internal struggles and anxieties. For example, children's own reports of depressive symptomatology may be more sensitive than parental reports about their children's internal states, because parents may not notice or attend to children's depressive symptomatology, or children may hide or not express such feelings to parents.

In other instances, self-report measures will be most appropriate for a given construct. For example, measures of an individual's attributions or perceptions of others can only be assessed with carefully constructed instruments that are completed by the individual him- or herself. Other persons may be unaware of the individual's thought processes in this regard, or may have only very limited information about these thought processes. Finally, children's appraisals of important events are often best assessed directly, rather than with parents' reports. For example, children's reports of marital conflict may be more closely linked to the impact of marital conflict on the children than parents' reports of their own conflicts (Cummings, Davies, & Simpson, 1994).

3. *What other aspects of functioning are being measured?* As we have seen, a central tenet of the developmental psychopathology approach is that children's functioning is affected by the broader context of development. For example, children's responding may vary as a function of life events, marital functioning, family emotional climate, and so forth. Accordingly, from a developmental psychopathology perspective, it is important to represent contexts of development as fully as possible. Obviously, not all elements of a child's contexts of development (e.g., multiple aspects of parent–child, family, and extrafamilial environments) can be represented in any one study. Thus, it is often necessary to rely upon theory or other informed criteria (e.g., such as the evidence in the scientific literature concerning variables that are related to the domains of interest in the study) as guides to the selection of measures of context. As we have noted, the questionnaire methodology is particularly well-suited for obtaining "big picture" data on domains of functioning, since the procedures are relatively cheap and easy to use, and responses to questionnaires can often reasonably be compared across groups. Thus, questionnaires often offer a valuable means to obtain data on family and other contextual variables that may not be the key interest of the study, and, accordingly, are not targeted in data collection and assessment but nonetheless merit consideration.

4. *How does one compare information about multiple informants?* Given that one has obtained data from multiple informants, how does one combine or otherwise make overall sense of the data? This is a big issue, and an important one, in child psychopathology. On the one hand, for the methodological reasons already described, there are obvious virtues in obtaining data from as many respondents as possible about an individual's functioning. On the other hand, it is not entirely clear how to integrate data from multiple informants, particularly when the respondents disagree.

It should not be a surprise that, in reality, cross-informant agreement is always less than 100%. On the plus side, meta-analyses of cross-informant correlations across numerous studies indicate that the correlations are often statistically significant. Meta-analyses are a statistical means for summarizing the outcomes of different studies, in which each study provides an estimate of the size of an effect, and the meta-analysis produces a statistical result reflecting whether the effect is significant across all of the studies surveyed in the analysis. However, the size of these correlations may be relatively modest, especially when informants play different roles in different contexts with the individuals (e.g., parents and teachers) (Achenbach, 1997). The problem is not necessarily one of poor validity or reliability. The fact is, different informants can provide valid, but somewhat different, characterizations of children's functioning, partly because they may observe children in different settings or situations.

This issue creates problems for clinicians and clinical researchers when it is necessary to judge whether psychopathology in the child is categorically present versus absent. In such cases, discrepancies among informants, even sometimes relatively small discrepancies (e.g., the child's score is just above the cutoff for clinical disorder according to one respondent and just below that cutoff according to the other) may yield quite different judgments about the child's mental health status (i.e., a diagnosis of a disorder is present vs. absent).

Various suggestions have been made to address this problem, but there does not, as yet, appear to be an ideal solution. Achenbach (1997) has recently surveyed some of the possible directions one might take: (a) the "or" rule; that is, if any informant reports a problem, the problem is considered to be present; (b) averaging scores across all raters for each syndrome; (c) classifying individual as deviant or nondeviant on each syndrome for each informant according to clinical cut points, and then using a decision rule as to how many deviant scores across informants are needed to decide that deviance on the syndrome is present; or (d) using a taxonomic decision tree to integrate data from multiple sources in coming to a decision about deviancy. Each of these approaches has advantages but also presents difficulties. For example, with regard to the "or" rule, different informants may have quite different opportunities for observing the behavior of the child, or different criteria for reporting its occurrence, and these difference may vary as a function of the age or gender of the child for different informants. Achenbach has argued in favor of empirically guided approaches (e.g., [d] above), since they avoid making forced choices about normality and provide a systematic, information-based guide for making clinical decisions based on multiple sources of data. However, individual clinicians may want to make decisions based on different assumptions and criteria than are suggested by these approaches, so that they may not find the decision trees or other decision-making templates useful for their clinical goals and purposes.

Interviews

Data from parents, children, and teachers are often collected with structured and semistructured interviews. Structured diagnostic interviews are used in many research studies to obtain standard data about children's symptoms and degree of impairment. The most widely used of the diagnostic interviews, the Diagnostic Interview Schedule for Children (Shaffer, Fisher, Dulcan, & Davies, 1996; Shaffer, Fisher, Piacentini, Schwab-Stone, & Wicks, 1993) and the Children's Assessment Schedule (Hodges, Cools, & McKnew, 1989), were originally developed to assess the symptoms of childhood disorders as delineated in the *Diagnostic and Statistical Manual of Mental Disorders*, third edition (DSM-III, American Psychiatric Association, 1980; see Chapter 10, this volume). These interviews have been revised to accommodate subsequent changes to the diagnostic criteria. By definition, structured interviews have clear guidelines for questioning parents, teachers, and the children themselves about symptoms and dysfunction, for making decisions about the presence or absence of a symptom, and for making diagnoses. Thus, they have added a degree of standardization to what was once a relatively haphazard enterprise based primarily on unstructured clinical inquiry. Data from numerous studies indicate that these diagnostic interviews tend to be reliable and valid indicators of children's distress (Hodges et al., 1989; Shaffer et al., 1996), and they are often used in tandem with questionnaires to describe children's problem behavior (e.g., Pierce, Ewing, & Campbell, 1999).

However, interviews also have their share of problems. As with questionnaires, different respondents will have different perspectives on the child's behavior, and decisions about how to combine data will need to be made (e.g., the "or" rule, discussed in the previous section, may be utilized with interviews as well). In addition, interviews tend to be unreliable with children under 10 (Edelbrock, Costello, Dulcan, Kalas, & Conover, 1985). Furthermore, as with questionnaires, children tend to be better reporters of internalizing problems but seriously underreport externalizing problems that are often the concern of parents and teachers (Edelbrock et al., 1985). Finally, because there are concerns with the coverage and developmental sensitivity of the diagnostic criteria (see Chapter 10, this volume), these interviews may overlook important problem areas and be less contextually based than traditional clinical interviews. For example, because peer relations play only a limited role in the symptoms that define disorders, important aspects of peer relations, friendship patterns, and social skills are assessed only minimally in these interviews. However, it is well known that peer relationships and friendships are important markers of adjustment in children (e.g., Coie, Dodge, & Kupersmidt, 1990; Coie, Terry, Lenox, Lochman, & Hyman, 1995). Still, standard diagnostic interviews are an important component of the multimethod assessment of research participants and they allow for a common metric of problems across studies.

In addition to diagnostic interviews, structured interviews have been developed to assess family functioning, child-rearing practices, developmental milestones, and other aspects of child and family development. However, these have received much less attention and are used less systematically in research, with many investigators developing their own interviews for specific purposes. A comprehensive review of these interviews, therefore, is beyond the scope of this volume.

Observations

Analogue Observations in the Laboratory

Analogue studies, that is, studies in which simulations or other constructed representations of family events (e.g., on videotape or audiotape) are presented to family members to obtain their reactions, are one form of laboratory procedure that can be used to assess children's reactions to family events. An advantage of this approach is that various dimensions of the family event (e.g., marital conflict, parental depressive symptomatology) can be precisely specified and presented in the same way across all participants, and objective recording of responses on multiple dimensions (e.g., cognitive, verbal, emotional, physiological) is possible. These elements make it possible to test hypotheses about causal relations under controlled conditions, and to differentiate effects due to variations in histories of exposure from responses due to the particular characteristics of the present family situations. Another advantage is that such stimuli can be presented in a manner that is lively and engaging, so that even small children may be highly motivated to participate and be responsive to the questions asked of them about the family events. Thus, the data may provide a better reflection of how participants feel or behave than presentation formats that fail to elicit much interest or seem somewhat vague. Contrary to the stereotype of experiments as conservative methods than can only be used to test concepts generated by other procedures, analogue procedures potentially provide a relatively cheap way to explore new questions (Cummings, 1995b). Accordingly, this approach is most useful when the stimuli and responses are specified as precisely as possible, presented in an ecologically valid manner, and include procedures to explore reactions to new dimensions of family situations.

One potential limitation of this methodology concerns generalizability. However, to some extent, this problem is characteristic of all methodologies, including behavioral observation of the family at home (e.g., does the slice of behavior observed in the home represent typical behavior?). Data to support generalizability can be generated for these procedures as well as for other methodologies. For example, there is evidence that children's reactions to analogue presentations of marital conflict are consistent with family histories of marital conflict and children's risk for adjustment problems. Thus, presumably, children's reactions are reflective of significant individual differences in everyday response patterns (Cummings & Davies, 1994a). Moreover, the goal of analogue procedures, as with any laboratory procedure, is not to recreate the exact conditions of the family environment (an impossibility), but to induce the critical response processes, and to investigate the process relations that underlie responding in natural settings, such as the home. Thus, reactions to analogue stimuli are informative if they are meaningfully related to response patterns in the home, whether or not these responses are precisely the reactions that occur in the home. For example, one would not expect children to be as distressed by mild conflicts between strangers in a videotaped presentation format as by actual, and intense, marital conflicts that take place in the home. However, when assessing responses across children, one might expect that the degree and type of responding in one context would be related to the degree and type of responding in the other. Another limitation of analogue methods is that some family situations and issues may not be amenable to presentation in this way, and complex patterns of back-and-forth interaction in family contexts, which may be highly significant to understanding risk for psychopathology or other adjustment problems (e.g., Gottman, 1994), cannot be recorded.

Laboratory Observations: Unstructured and Structured

A virtue of laboratory observation is that one can obtain records of actual behavioral interactions between family members that are not tainted by the various methodological limitations and concerns that are possible problems for self-reported instruments (discussed earlier). For that reason alone, that is, the avoidance of problems inherent in other methods, the laboratory observation methodology is an excellent candidate for multimethod research in the developmental psychopathology area. There is also a significant gain in terms of the richness of the data records obtained. For example, multiple dimensions of behavioral and emotional responding can be assessed, and multidimensional and time-based analyses of interrelations and sequencings of behavior can be analyzed. Thus, there is the opportunity to discover new relationships and patterns in child and family functioning that are not anticipated in the development of the measure. By contrast, questionnaires often begin with the investigator's notions with regard to which variables are important, which may constrain to some extent the outcomes of analyses.

A strength of employing observational methodologies in the laboratory is that considerable rigor in setting up the situation and in coding responses is possible. Coding may include detailed, microanalytic coding of live or videotaped interactions. Another advantage is that actual behaviors are observed, with an assumption that behavioral patterns occurring in the home are to some extent reenacted. Even if responses in the home are not recreated exactly, it is likely that there is a similarity to the process that does occur in the home. However, since interactions are allowed to vary after a context is defined for participants (e.g., a toy play task), one loses some control over the comparability of responses across participants once the task begins; that is, family members are responding to each others' behaviors and not a controlled laboratory context or situation in a traditional experimental sense, if they are allowed to interact freely. On the other hand, the interaction sequences that occur may be inherently interesting in their own right as indices of family relations. For example, the unit of analysis of interest may very well be interactive behavior in a toy play context. There are again concerns about whether responses generalize to everyday situations in the home. Nonetheless, it might be presumed that everyday interactions would be more readily elicited in response to other family members' behaviors than in response to analogue situations, which often involve actors who are strangers to the family.

Laboratory observations can be structured to target certain domains of children's functioning, thereby making it more likely that the behaviors of interest will be observed. There are numerous examples of such tasks. Thus, parents have been asked to play a game with the child (e.g., an Etch-a-Sketch) in order to observe their warmth and other dimensions of the socioemotional communication between parents and children in the context of a task situation presenting certain challenges (e.g., the need to cooperate; Brody, Stoneman, & Burke, 1987). In another example, to assess child management and disciplinary practices, parents have been instructed to request that the child obey certain rules or do certain chores (e.g., cleanup the lab) (Kochanska, 1997; Kochanska, Kuczynski, Radke-Yarrow, & Welsh, 1987). Parents' emotional communication to the child has been manipulated in other studies in order to learn more about how parental emotions affect children. Thus, in the Still Face task, parents are required to withhold (briefly) their emotional responding to the infant's behavior in order to assess the effects of a lack of parental emotional response on children's own affect regulation capacities (Cohn & Tronick, 1983). In each of these instances, the laboratory context is shaped so that investigators can target specific domains of children's functioning, thereby permitting a focus in the data-collection effort on the dimensions of responding of greatest interest to the goals of the study.

In some instances, investigators may simply wish to obtain a representative slice of children's behavior or parent–child interaction. Such procedures have the advantage of not limiting or biasing children's or parents' responding in any way, which has advantages if a goal is to minimize parental and child reactivity to the presence of observers and to maximize the potential generalizability of responding to the home environment. A limitation of such methodologies, however, is that a representative slice of family behavior may not occur unless the observation session is relatively lengthy.

Another advantage of lab observations over analogue procedures is that it may be possible to study even younger children, which typically require verbal reports and, thus, the use of language. For example, the age at which the responses of children to conflict scenarios can be obtained is further reduced when live actors simulate conflicts in the presence of children (e.g., 2-year-olds; Cummings, Iannotti, & Zahn-Waxler, 1985; Cummings, Pellegrini, Notarius, & Cummings, 1989). A variation is to have the mother and an actor engage in a simulated conflict, which has the advantage of providing records of children's responses to conflicts involving a family member (Cummings et al., 1989). Multimethod data collection may also be possible, adding to the richness of the data records. For example, with regard to the previous example, by preschool age, one can enrich the data records based on the observation of children's social and emotional behavioral responding to interadult conflicts with interviews concerning children's covert reactions taken just after the observational session has ended (Cummings, 1987). Moreover, one can make records of children's physiological reactions (heart rate, blood pressure, skin conductance) while the exposure to interadult conflicts is going on (El-Sheikh & Cummings, 1992; El-Sheikh, Cummings, & Goetsch, 1989).

Multimethod assessments may provide more informative characterizations of children's reactions than reliance on any single dimension of responding. For example, it has been found that some children behave as if they do not care about background conflicts between adults during exposure to these events. This result might lead the investigator to assume that the child does not care about the occurrence of background conflict. However, if one interviews the children, one finds that such children report particularly high levels of angry feelings (Cummings, 1987). Thus, the inference supported by multimethod data collection (i.e., children are holding in angry feelings) is quite different from that supported by only observing behavior (i.e., children are unaffected).

Patterns or organizations of children's responding can also be recorded in laboratory observations, which may permit added richness in characterizing the quality of their functioning and make possible a level of characterization of individual functioning that is especially important in assessing risk for psychopathology. The Strange Situation has been a particularly valuable observational methodology for obtaining data on infant's patterns of attachment to their parents (Ainsworth, Blehar, Waters, & Wall, 1978). In this procedure, children's behavior is observed in a laboratory setting in response to a structured series of stressful events (e.g., the parent leaves the child in an unfamiliar room and later reenters). The patterns of infants' responding have been demonstrated to elicit emotional and behavioral responses that are indicative of the quality of their attachments to their parents (Ainsworth et al., 1978). This methodology has been used in a vast number of studies, generating seminal data on children's patterns of attachment their parents and the relation of these patterns to other domains of their social and emotional functioning, including their risk for adjustment problems (Colin, 1996). Notably, the patterns or organizations of children's responding based on behavioral observation records are highly significant with regard to their processes of socioemotional functioning, but early research has indicated that analyses focusing only on single responses in this context (e.g., crying upon separation from the parent in the unfamiliar laboratory context) were neither stable over time nor related to other significant aspects of functioning (Ainsworth et al., 1978). This result supports the importance and relevance of the principle of holism to considerations of methodology; that is, the attachment work suggests that children's functioning within the family is much better informed by considering broader organizations of functioning than by records based upon discrete responses (e.g., crying).

Naturalistic Observations

Naturalistic observations may be obtained in the home, or other settings. The strength of observing behavior in the home or school is that these are often the contexts in which the behaviors of interest to researchers occur, so that questions about validity and generalizability are diminished. However, careful research design is still necessary and concerns about the representativeness, and thus the generalizability of the behaviors, still must be considered. For example, if the assessments are too brief, do not appropriately sample the targeted behaviors, or the responses of those observed are highly reactive to the presence of observers, then the generalizability of the results to the phenomenon of interest may still be questioned. Moreover, naturalistic observations are typically expensive to obtain and their utility is reduced unless proper coding schemes are employed. In fact, the quality and complexity of the data obtained may be overwhelming and difficult to analyze and assess unless effective and appropriate coding schemes can be developed. However, when such data can be obtained, they may prove invaluable, perhaps especially as a support for less expensive and more focused data collection in the laboratory.

For example, the observation of attachment behavior in the home is considered to be the "gold standard" for demonstrating the operation of the attachment behavioral system and for validating other procedures as indices of attachment. Thus, the validity of the Strange Situation procedure for assessing patterns of attachment, which has been used productively in hundreds of studies, ultimately rests on the demonstration of relations with parent–child functioning in the home based upon laborious, long-term home observations (e.g., Ainsworth, Blehar, Waters, & Wall, 1978).

A particular challenge for home observation methodologies is to maintain the rigor of coding and data collection in the face of the variability of everyday home environments and their relative inaccessibility for data collection methods that may preserve the quality and complexity of the behavioral records (e.g., videotaped records). The introduction of data-collection technology may also create reactivity among family members to the procedures, so that the data are not representative of everyday functioning. Moreover, it is inherently difficult to compare across families because the events around which observations may be taken can vary widely (e.g., eating, watching television, and so forth). In an effort to address these problems with conducting naturalistic observations in the home, Zahn-Waxler and Radke-Yarrow (1982) brought the home to the laboratory in an "apartment study"; that is, families were videotaped in a carefully constructed family environment in the laboratory, complete with kitchen, television, sofas, toys, bathroom, and so forth, over a period of several consecutive days at a time. Moreover, the "days" were structured so that the same contexts (e.g., breakfast, watching television) occurred for each family at the same time each day. Finally, advanced, but unobtrusive video-recording technology permitted the family's behavior to be recorded throughout the "days."

Another problem for naturalistic observation in the home is that for some critical family events with particular relevance to children's risk for psychopathology (e.g., marital conflict), the rate of occurrence may be so infrequent that observers are unlikely to be present when they occur. Such events may also be so sensitive to the presence of observers that reactivity can be a severe problem that undermines the potential representativeness of the behaviors. To address this problem for the study of marital conflict and children's reactions to it, Radke-Yarrow and colleagues (Cummings, Zahn-Waxler, & Radke-

Yarrow, 1981, 1984) developed a methodology for training parents to be observers of their own marital conflicts and their own children's responding. Moreover, parents were carefully trained to make behavioral records, just as laboratory staff are trained. The assumption was that the viability of parents as observers is underestimated, since parents rarely receive adequate training. In fact, the results suggested that parents are reliable observers of family events after they have received adequate training in making such records.

Test Measures

A large number of measures might fit comfortably under the rubric of psychological tests. For the purposes of this chapter, we just highlight the range of measures that are often administered to child participants in standardized fashion to assess some aspect of cognitive functioning, academic achievement, personality, social competence, or self-perceptions. In general, when we refer to psychological tests, we mean that a measure has been standardized and normed on a particular group of children and that specific guidelines for administration and scoring are contained in a test manual. Among the most widely used measures are those that assess intelligence, such as the Wechsler Intelligence Scales, as well as academic achievement (e.g., reading, arithmetic) and specific cognitive skills (memory, visual perception for details, sequencing, language processing). Numerous measures exist to assess the many aspects of cognitive functioning considered germane to understanding children's adjustment and competence. The interested reader is referred to Sattler (1992) and Mash and Terdal (1997).

Personality assessment runs the gamut from projective tests, which have come under much criticism, to more standard self-report measures that assess such characteristics as anxiety, positive mood, sociability, negative affect, and so on (Mash & Wolfe, 1999). These more standardized self-report measures are appropriate for school-age children, but they have all the problems already identified in the earlier discussion of questionnaires.

In addition, laboratory measures have been devised to assess other aspects of personality and relationships. These measures provide a more objective indicator of young children's responses to standard stimuli meant to elicit particular types of responses, but their usefulness hinges on how valid they really are for assessing the construct in question. For example, measures of self-regulation have been devised to assess resistance to temptation (e.g., Calkins & Fox, 1992; Campbell, Pierce, March, Ewing, & Szumowski, 1994). These measures determine how well a young child can delay responding in the face of a highly appealing stimulus such as an engaging toy or a tempting food. The underlying assumption is that these tasks relate to other aspects of the child's self-regulatory capacities and have predictive validity for later functioning. Other researchers have developed methods to assess behavioral reactivity and reaction to novelty (e.g., Kochanska, 1997), meant to measure aspects of personality and temperament such as inhibition and fearfulness. Still others have devised puppet stimuli and story stems to assess children's internal working models of relationships and attachment (see, e.g., Bretherton, 1985), self-concept and self-esteem (see, e.g., Eder, 1990), and other aspects of self-understanding (see, e.g., Denham, 1989).

A number of story measures and vignettes have also been developed to assess school-age children's attributions about peer relations and the meaning of other children's aggressive and prosocial responses in the context of every-day situations (e.g., Crick, 1995; Crick & Dodge, 1996; Dodge & Coie, 1987). Research demonstrates that children's attributions about the negative intentions of others and the specific way they respond to others when they are aggressive (e.g., do they just react when provoked, or do they initiate aggres-sion? Is their aggression primarily physical or do they engage in gossip and ex-clusion?) has implications for both concurrent adjustment and later function-ing (Crick, 1995; Dodge & Coie, 1987). Furthermore, negative attributions about the hostile intentions of other children tend to fuel peer conflict and to mediate some of the associations between the quality of children's home envi-ronments and their levels of conflict in the peer group (Dodge, Pettit, & Bates, 1994a; Dodge, Pettit, Bates, & Valente, 1995; see Chapter 11, this volume). Clearly, many measures have been developed, then, to assess children's behav-ior across a range of situations associated with good versus poor adjustment. Many of these are laboratory procedures that have been tailored to answer specific questions about children's personality and the social-cognitive pro-cesses thought to underlie disorder (see Figure 3.1). Because of the many mea-sures that fit into this category, a more detailed discussion is beyond the scope of this book.

Physiological Measures and Other Biological Measures

A fundamental assumption of the developmental psychopathology perspec-tive is that multiple levels of organization, including psychological and bio-logical functioning, are organized and regulated by the individual during development. Moreover, this self-regulation and self-organization, which follow from the notions of holism and active organism, are assumed to be actively integrated at multiple levels, including physiological and biological dimensions of functioning. Thus, while developmental psychopathologists to date have focused on the study of psychological processes and mechanisms, it is inherent in the developmental psychopathology perspective that mature, process-level understanding requires taking into account physiological and biological aspects of normal development and the development of psycho-pathology (Cicchetti & Tucker, 1994). Thus, the assessment and measure-ment of physiological and biological responding, as well as psychological functioning, are consistent with the goals of programmatic research for the developmental psychopathologist. On the other hand, physiological mea-sures do *not* offer the promise of providing a "silver bullet" for understand-ing psychopathology in children and are properly considered, like other individual response dimensions, only in the context of broader domains of responding.

Toward this end, Fox and Card (1999) have provided the following recommendations for incorporating physiological assessments into the larger battery of psychological measures. First, making inferences about the meaning of physiological measures requires simultaneous, synchronized assessments of physiological and psychological responses. Second, using multiple methods, rather than solely relying on physiological data, permits more use of behaviors or other indices of psychological responding as "anchors" from which to interpret the profiles of physiological assessments. Third, most conventional assessments of physiological responses are complex functions of multiple intra- and extraorganismic factors, and typically occur within quick, brief temporal windows. As such, physiological responses do not fully reflect responses to the target stimuli of the research study. However, repeated assessments across time and, if possible, relevant stimuli, may help to increase the stability and psychometric properties of the physiological observations.

The contribution that psychophysiological studies have made to the study of developmental psychopathology has grown exponentially in recent years. Thus, while a technical and exhaustive discussion of this substantial area of developmental psychopathology is beyond the scope of this volume (e.g., skin conductance—Dozier & Kobak, 1992; cognitive brain event-related potentials—Pollack, Cicchetti, Klorman, & Brumaghim, 1997), we selectively outline some of the central and promising domains of psychophysiological assessment for developmental psychopathology.

Cardiovascular Functioning

Cardiovascular functioning is not a unitary construct. Rather, cardiovascular functioning consists of multiple dimensions, including baseline heart rate level, heart rate change in response to stimuli, heart rate variability, vagal tone, changes in vagal tone, systolic blood pressure, diastolic blood pressure, and mean arterial pressure (Boyce, Alkon, Tschann, Chesney, & Alpert, 1995). Even restricting interest to reactivity to stressors yields several options (e.g., heart rate reactivity, suppression of vagal tone, changes in blood pressure) that may reflect different organismic processes and, as such, may have different developmental roots, correlates, and sequelae (Ballard, Cummings, & Larkin, 1993).

For example, heart rate has historically been one of the most commonly used psychophysiological measures. However, the meaning of heart rate is difficult to determine. Heart rate indices are by-products of multiple factors, including multiple regions of the brain, bodily functioning (e.g., respiration), motoric activity, and basal heart rate level. Thus, heart rate may not necessarily reflect psychological states (e.g., Fox & Card, 1999). Mixed findings on the interrelation between heart rate change and children's psychosocial responses and experiences further caution against drawing firm conclusions based only on heart rate (e.g., El-Sheikh & Cummings, 1992; Spangler & Grossmann, 1993). Nevertheless, when appropriately evaluated in the context of a broader pattern of assessments, heart rate acceleration can be a useful index of negative emotional arousal and active coping in the face of stressors; whereas heart rate deceleration may reflect attention and orientation to environmental novelty or challenge (El-Sheikh, 1994; Sroufe & Waters, 1977b). Moreover, links between heart rate deceleration during mood induction and prosocial dispositions suggest that heart rate reductions signify, in part, the ability of children to exhibit other-oriented, empathetic distress (e.g., El-Sheikh, Cummings, & Goestch, 1989; Fabes, Eisenberg, & Eisenbud, 1993).

Other assessments of cardiovascular functioning yield similar conclusions regarding the specificity of cardiovascular indices. Higher baseline heart rates, for example, have been linked to lower externalizing symptoms, empathetic concern, prosocial behavior, and even behavioral inhibition (e.g., El-Sheikh, Ballard, & Cummings, 1994; Kagan, Reznick, & Snidman, 1987; Zahn-Waxler, Cole, Welsh, & Fox, 1995). Recent attempts to isolate the component of the heart rate that is linked to the parasympathetic nervous system (respiratory sinus arrhythmia) has resulted in a type of more specific psychophysiological index: vagal tone and suppression of vagal tone in response to challenge or stress (Fox, 1989; Porges, 1997). High vagal tone is proposed to serve as a marker of greater autonomic system integrity, particularly in terms of responding to environmental stress and restoring physiological and psychological homeostasis (e.g., self-soothing, emotion regulation) (Fox & Card, 1999). Consistent with this hypothesis, high vagal tone in children predicts greater reactivity, social skills, and organized self-regulatory strategies (Gunnar, Porter, Wolf, Rigatuso, & Larson, 1995; Stifter, Fox, & Porges, 1989). Moreover, the suppression of vagal tone in response to environmental demands is theorized to reflect an adaptive process of reallocating physiological resources to attend to and cope with the stressor in an organized way (Katz & Gottman 1997b). There is evidence, although far from definitive, for links between suppression of vagal tone and parental ratings of soothability and lengthier infant attention spans (e.g., Huffman et al., 1998). Also demonstrating the promise of such research, Katz and Gottman (1995a, 1997b) found support for the notion that high vagal tone and the suppression of vagal tone serve as buffers for the risk posed by marital discord to children.

Brain Electrical Activity

The experience, expression, and regulation of emotion are thought partly to be a function of activity in the frontal lobe of the brain. Although the findings are not always consistent, emotional experience appears to be related to the configuration of activity in the left and right hemispheres (see Fox, 1994; Fox & Card, 1999). High left hemispheric activity is linked with approach (e.g., interest) and lower thresholds for experiencing affect (e.g., joy). By contrast, high right hemispheric activity is associated with withdrawal and negative affect (e.g., sadness) (Davidson, Ekman, Saron, & Senulis, 1990; Fox, Calkins, & Bell, 1994).

Recent groundbreaking work has begun to pinpoint the developmental correlates and sequelae of different profiles of brain activity. Individual differences in patterns of frontal brain activity are likely to have a hereditary basis (see Calkins, Fox, & Marshall, 1996). Yet, according to Dawson, Frey, Self, and colleagues (1999), experiential histories also may "sculpt" the configuration of neuronal circuits responsible for the brain activity, particularly in the first few years of life, when brain growth is at its peak. During this proposed sensitive period, adverse social environments (e.g., depressive family contexts) foster negative affect and diminished positive affect, and in the process strengthen the neuronal pathways associated with negative emotion and selectively "prune" the pathways linked with positive emotion (also see Field, Fox, Pickens, & Nawrocki, 1995). If so, early experiences of adverse home environments may contribute to patterns of brain activity that lower thresholds for negative affect and raise thresholds for positive affect (Dawson, Frey, Panagiotides, et al., 1999; Dawson, Frey, Self, et al., 1999).

Adrenocortical Activity

Cortisol is a "hormone of energy" that is released by the hypothalamic–pituitary–adrenocortical (HPA) system in response to a variety of different types of environmental stimulation (Fox & Card, 1999; Stansbury & Gunnar, 1994). It has been particularly valuable as a physiological indicator of stress in developmental psychopathology research. Unlike the majority of other measures of physiological reactivity, elevated cortisol production in response to acute stressors is a by-product of lengthy interplay between organismic events involving psychological stimuli, brain activity (e.g., limbic system, hypothalamus, pituitary), hormones (e.g., cortisol-releasing hormone, vasopressin), and biochemic reactions. Accordingly, rises in cortisol are normally detected between 15 and 30 minutes after the onset of the stressor. The release of cortisol in challenging circumstances plays a substantial role in marshaling physical and psychological resources and maintaining homeostasis through allocation of resources to various biological systems. Psychological manifestations of these functions, which regulate and are regulated by HPA activity, are thought to be evidenced by heightened vigilance and attention to the environment, increased energy and sense of "vitality," and, eventually, predispositions to withdraw and recuperate from the challenges of coping with the stressor (see Stansbury & Gunnar, 1994, for an extensive discussion). Given its broad and profound influence on the integrity of biopsychological systems, efficient onset and termination of the HPA system may be essential for the individual to meet, but not exceed, the demands of context and thus maintain healthy functioning (Trout, de Haan, Campbell, & Gunnar, 1998).

The efficiency with which the HPA system is regulated appears to have significant implications for patterns of adaptation and maladaptation in the children (Hart, Gunnar, & Cicchetti, 1996; Pollack, Cicchetti, & Klorman, 1998). For instance, withdrawal, inhibition, and shyness in the face of novelty is theorized to originate in the amplification of neuronal circuits involved in the experience of stress and thus should be manifested in lower thresholds for cortisol activation (Kagan, Reznick, & Snidman, 1988; Stansbury & Gunnar, 1994). Consistent with this notion, higher baseline levels of cortisol and elevated cortisol reactivity under stressful psychosocial conditions have been associated with greater behavioral inhibition and internalizing symptoms (Kagan, Reznick, & Snidman, 1987; Granger, Weisz, McCracken, Ikeda, & Douglas, 1996). However, conflicting findings are reported across studies. Thus, it is difficult at this time to draw any firm conclusions about the role cortisol plays in the developmental histories and trajectories of children.

QUASI-EXPERIMENTAL DESIGNS: HYBRIDS OF EXPERIMENTAL AND NATURALISTIC DESIGNS

In recent years, there has been a tendency to draw a sharp distinction between laboratory and field research designs, with the advantage of the former being a degree of control over interactional patterns and the latter a measure of ecological validity. In fact, however, varying measures of control and ecological validity may be obtained with each approach, so the distinctions between the two approaches are not nearly as sharp as is sometimes assumed. Moreover, because of the different strengths and weaknesses of the two approaches, neither is likely to be sufficient, and these two approaches frequently work best together toward addressing particular research questions (see Parke, 1979, for an excellent discussion). For example, a multistep strategy is often desirable in the investigation of a particular research question, beginning with observations in the naturalistic setting in the early phases of research and in later phases tests of specific hypotheses emerging from field research by means of a series of laboratory experiments.

The strengths and limitations of field and laboratory designs clearly complement each other. Maximizing ecological validity in field research is often attained at the expense of internal validity. By contrast, laboratory and analogue designs compromise ecological validity in the process of increasing internal validity. Is there a way to integrate these two designs in a way that preserves some degree of internal and ecological validity? Hybrid designs, which incorporate features of both field and laboratory research, afford researchers the potential to achieve some level of internal validity without substantially compromising ecological validity. For example, theories of interparental conflict have postulated that histories of exposure to destructive interparental conflict sensitizes children to subsequent conflict, as evidenced by heightened emotional distress, behavioral dysregulation, and negative appraisals and representations of parents. In support of this proposition, field research has demonstrated that children from high-conflict homes do react more negatively to naturalistic conflicts in the home (Garcia-O'Hearn, Margolin, & John, 1997). Yet these designs, by themselves, cannot determine whether the greater negativity experienced by children of high-conflict homes is due to the sensitizing effects of distal, conflict histories or the destructive nature of the proximal conflict context. Analogue studies, by contrast, can effectively isolate the effects of conflict history on children's subsequent responses to marital conflict. However, they can only ascertain whether exposure to distal histories of adult conflict *can* cause sensitization in children. Whether lengthier histories of conflict between actual parents *do* actually cause sensitization remains unanswered (Davies, Myers, Cummings, & Heindel, 1999; El-Sheikh, Cummings, & Reiter, 1996). Thus, to preserve some level of ecological validity, researchers have obtained reports of actual interparental conflict history from family members. Within the same design, some level of experimental control and, hence, internal validity can be achieved by assessing children's responses to conflicts in standardized, stressful conflict contexts in the laboratory (e.g., audiotaped or videotaped conflicts between adults; "live" simulated conflicts involving the mother and experimenter) rather than the highly variable, naturalistic contexts (e.g., Davies & Cummings, 1998; El-Sheikh, 1997; Grych, 1998; O'Brien, Bahadur, Gee, Balto, & Erber, 1997).

The advantages of these blended designs expand beyond the confines of interparental conflict research. For example, if the goal of the researcher is to understand how family relationship histories may shape how children negotiate the set goal of security in the parent–child relationship, employing naturalistic assessments of both family history and attachment (e.g., attachment Q-sort) still leaves open the possibility that the relationship between family context histories and children's attachment organization is mediated by some proximal variable in the home (e.g., parental caregiving, disorganized home environment). Thus, exercising some level of experimental control or standardization in the assessment of children's emotional security (e.g., Strange Situation) is one effective step toward ruling out the confounding nature of the proximal context. Blended designs, although still rarely used in developmental psychopathology, have also proven to be invaluable tools in further explicating (1) the etiology of coping difficulties in children of depressed parents (e.g., Cohn & Campbell, 1992; Field, 1984), and (2) the parameters of low self-efficacy in parenting (e.g., Bugental & Cortez, 1988; Bugental, Lewis, Lin, Lyon, & Kopeikin, 1999).

OPERATIONALIZING THE MULTIDIMENSIONAL AND MULTILEVEL NATURE OF THE FAMILY

The principle of floating holism dictates that the family can be usefully conceptualized at multiple levels depending on the research question at hand (Magnusson & Cairns, 1996). At the individual level, the family is comprised of multiple family members (e.g., children, mother, father, extended relatives) whose roles in regulating and being regulated by the family system have traditionally been a key focus of research even prior to the emergence of developmental psychopathology (e.g., Boyce et al., 1998). For example, delineating the bidirectional effects of parents and children, which has a rich history in the developmental sciences, has been effectively carried forward by developmental psychopathologists (e.g., Dodge, 1990b; Lytton, 1990; Shaw & Bell, 1993; see also Chapters 5 and 6, this volume).

At the dyadic level, the family is conceptualized as a series of relationships or subsystems that, in the traditional family, may include the marital, coparenting, mother–child, father–child, and sibling relationships. Traditionally, dyadic conceptualizations of the family were typically limited to identifying the individual-level causes (e.g., maternal responsiveness), correlates (e.g., parental depression), and sequelae (e.g., autonomy, agency) of a dyadic-level construct such as parent–child attachment. However, with its underlying roots in contextualism, family systems theory has alerted developmental scientists to the value of conceptualizing the family as a series of interdependent dyadic relationships or subsystems (Cox & Paley, 1997; Minuchin, 1985). Although the development of systems methodologies has lagged behind the acceptance of theory, some significant headway is beginning to be made. Progress in assessing key dimensions of the marital (Kerig, 1996; Lindahl, 1998), coparenting (e.g., Gable, Belsky, & Crnic, 1995), parent–child (e.g., Barber, 1996), and sibling relationships (e.g., Brody, 1998), which traditionally occurred in isolation from the other subsystems, is being increasingly integrated into single studies (e.g., Cowan, Cohn, Cowan, & Pearson, 1996; Dickstein et al., 1998; Hayden et al., 1998; McHale & Rasmussen, 1998). The end result has been exciting new advances in understanding (1) the nature and parameters of interdependencies between the family subsystems (Brody, Stoneman, & Gauger, 1996; Hetherington, Henderson, & Reiss, 1999; McHale, 1995), and (2) children's development and adjustment as part of the mutual interplay among the family subsystems (Conger et al., 1993; O'Connor, Hetherington, & Reiss, 1998; Owen & Cox, 1997).

At a broader, family level of analysis, the family can be usefully conceptualized as a unit or whole in models of developmental psychopathology. This approach is motivated by several considerations. First, because any form of adversity in the family tends to occur in the context of multiple, co-occurring family risk factors (Dickstein et al., 1998; Sameroff, Seifer, Baldwin, & Baldwin, 1993; Shaw & Vondra, 1993), the multicollinearity among the factors obscures the power and precision necessary to understand the predictive specificity of any one factor (Ackerman, Izard, Schoff, Youngstrom, & Kogos, 1999). Second, through the coordination and organization of multiple roles, regulatory processes, and transactions across relationships and subsystems, it is the whole family rather than any single risk factor or relationship that serves important developmental functions, particularly as sources of security, stability, relatedness, socialization, and the internalization of values (Bretherton, Walsh, Lependorf, & Goergeson, 1997; Sroufe & Rutter, 1984). Successful adaptation may thus depend largely on children's collective experiences in the family unit, an accumulation of family stressors and disruptions, and their ability to procure resources in the family as a whole (e.g., Ackerman, Kogos, Youngstrom, Schoff, & Izard, 1999; Forehand et al., 1991; Hetherington, Stanley-Hagan, & Anderson, 1989; Sandler, Wolchik, Braver, & Fogas, 1991). Finally, unlike the study of dyadic relationships (e.g., marital or sibling relationship), conceptualizing the family as the unit of analysis, at least in some forms, affords a certain level of flexibility and generalizability in that the same construct (e.g., family conflict, family instability) can studied simultaneously across different, diverse family forms (e.g., extended family, divorced, single-parent households) (Kurdek, Fine, & Sinclair, 1995). Attesting to the significance of family-level analyses, global family assessments continue to predict parent and child adjustment even after taking into account individual or dyadic (e.g., marital and parent–child relations) measures of family functioning (Dickstein et al., 1998; McHale & Rasmussen, 1998).

As a precautionary note, some forms of family-level composites do run the risk of providing little more information than the popular-press principle that maladaptation tends to run in families (i.e., the old adage that "the apple doesn't fall far from the tree"). Family-level assessment, however, need not compromise rich descriptions of family process within and across dimensions or relationships. Multiple dimensions, such as conflict, instability, cohesion, support, control, and organization, can be precisely assessed and differentiated at the family level (e.g., Ackerman, Izard, Schoff, Youngstrom, & Kogos, 1999; Dickstein et al., 1998). Likewise, new applications of pattern-based analyses permit holistic assessments of family-level organization while still preserving the rich characterizations of the quality (e.g., warmth, control) of each family subsystem (i.e., marital, mother–child, father–child, sibling). For example, cluster-analytic methods of classifying of families (not variables) on the basis of members' profiles or configurations of functioning within and across different relationships is a new methodological tool that has led to promising new advances and directions for developmental psychopathology (O'Connor, Hetherington, & Reiss, 1998). Thus, unlike earlier approaches in which any one family dimension is likely to be "washed out" in some multifactorial composite, the specific characterization of each subsystem maintained its integrity in the pattern-based family variable.

As was the case in the analysis of methods of measurement, no single operationalization of family constitutes the "royal road to truth." Individual, dyadic, and family-level operationalizations of the family are each important parts of the puzzle of developmental psychopathology. Ultimately, the operationalization of the family cannot be guided by some dogmatic absolute standard of what constitutes the best family conceptualization. There is no absolute best! Each has its strengths and weaknesses that become more or less salient within specific studies. Thus, the relative merits of developing a specific operationalization must be guided by the specific research question under investigation and the underlying theoretical foundation of the investigator.

LONGITUDINAL RESEARCH DESIGNS

Longitudinal research consists of the collection of data on participants on multiple occasions over a period of time. Longitudinal data are absolutely essential to addressing many of the questions of greatest concern to the developmental psychopathologist. As we have seen, the developmental psychopathologist is very interested in identifying the *processes* that underlie normal development and the development of deviancy. First, the processes and mechanisms that account for human development *cannot* be identified by cross-sectional data, which can only show that variables covary. Longitudinal data, on the other hand, can show that variable *a* precedes variable *b* (or the other way around). Identifying the temporal ordering between variables in this way, especially when the research design can rule out alternative explanations (see later discussion), gives a much better indication of the causal relations between variables than simply showing that the variables may covary, as in cross-sectional research.

Second, the developmental psychopathologist is concerned with charting pathways of development, including the form, direction, and shape of developmental pathways (for more discussion of these matters, see Chapter 4, this volume). These functions can only be identified with cogency by means of the collection of repeated measurements over time; that is, the pattern of continuity or change in development can only be demonstrated by assessing the functioning of individuals on multiple occasions over a period of time and tracking how individuals change, or remain the same, over that period. Thus, comparing groups of children of different ages in the context of cross-sectional research designs cannot demonstrate the nature and course of developmental pathways, but only that groups of different ages may, or may not, differ. It is important to be aware of this significant limitation of cross-sectional research. Findings of differences between children of different ages are sometimes overinterpreted, that is, are seen as having more meaning regarding developmental continuity and change than is appropriate. Showing group differences for children of different ages simply does not demonstrate individual pathways of development. Cross-sectional studies may provide suggestions about the possible course of development over time, for example, if one assumes that groups of children compared cross-sectionally do not differ in important sampling characteristics. However, such research designs have very limited implications for the confirmation of the nature of pathways of development over time, which is at the heart of the interests of developmental psychology and developmental psychopathology.

Expanding upon these points, van der Kamp and Bijleveld (1998) describe several possible additional goals of longitudinal investigation from a developmental psychopathology perspective:

> First, we may want to describe the subjects' intraindividual and interindividual changes over time; in doing so, we may want to describe both the magnitude of

certain changes as well as the pattern of changes. Secondly, we may want to explain these changes in terms of certain other characteristics. These characteristics can be stable (for instance, randomly assigning interventions in experiments or non-randomly assigning characteristics such as gender and religious affiliation) or unstable (for instance, time-varying characteristics such as medication or mood). Ultimately, we might want to forecast subjects' scores on the variables of interest. (p. 3)

However, given the great importance of this methodology to the domain of developmental psychopathology and its undoubted strength as an approach, it is especially important to place this powerful methodology in an appropriate context; that is, it is important to consider the costs and limitations, as well as the strengths, of this methodology (Magnusson & Cairns, 1996). Similar to the case for physiological and biological assessments, it is not a "silver bullet" for solving the riddles of developmental psychopathology as a stand-alone approach. Moreover, longitudinal research that is not conducted properly, or is conduced prematurely given the status of an area's development, can constitute a significant loss of time and resources, and in some instances, such time and resources may have been more productively put by the investigators into other methodologies at that point in time.

Longitudinal research that compares the functioning of a single group across multiple time points is in many ways inherently more difficult to accomplish than cross-sectional research that compares the functioning of two or more groups at a single point in time. Simply in terms of cost per participant, longitudinal data collection is more expensive than cross-sectional data collection because (1) two, or more, measurement occasions must be completed for each participant, which is obviously more demanding that collecting data for each participant on only one occasion; (2) following participants over time is inherently time-consuming (i.e., one must wait for individuals to age) and often expensive (e.g., it may be necessary to find people who have moved and possibly transport them some distance); and (3) tracking participants, keeping in contact with them, and keeping the research team together are each difficult and often costly tasks to accomplish in their own right (van der Kamp & Bijleveld, 1998).

Care must also be taken in the conduct of longitudinal research. Simply collecting data on participants on multiple occasions does not guarantee that the data will be especially interesting or important. In fact, there are potential pitfalls for the appropriate conduct of longitudinal research. First, it is important to be aware that evidence for causality in longitudinal designs is not the same as in randomized experiments, so that causal conclusions should be stated more tentatively than the findings of a carefully controlled laboratory investigation (Glenn, 1998). On the other hand, longitudinal data provide the best means for identifying potential causal factors in a developmental sense, as opposed to causality in the context of time-limited experimental tests. The point is, it is important to be aware that current procedures for analyzing longitudinal data have some inherent limitations for interpretation (Bradbury, 1998). Second, measures may become outdated before data collection is completed and can be published, weakening the potential importance of the results for the discipline. Third, the design of the research can be such that key questions may not be answerable. For example, if data on important covariates of the target variable are not assessed, or are not assessed on a sufficient number of measurement occasions, one may not be able to rule out cogent "third variable" alternatives to the findings of a study; that is, one may not be able to determine whether the third variable provides a viable alternative explanation to the results that the investigator would want to attribute to the target variable. Thus, there is a need to be aware that correlated variables may potentially account for effects that one wants to attribute to the identified independent variables (Christensen, 1988; Glenn, 1998). Great care in the design of the data collection for longitudinal research is thus essential (of course, this problem also exists for other research designs, and is made even more serious because one cannot assess predictive relations between even those variables that are assessed).

There are also other, more subtle, potential pitfalls and problems. For example, some loss of participants over the years of data collection in long-term longitudinal research is inevitable. However, there is a strong possibility that the loss of subjects will be systematic rather than random. Specifically, the likelihood is that the families lost to the study will most often be those that are the weakest in terms of family functioning, the most unstable, or the most maladjusted—families that are the least likely to (1) have stable residences or parental employment patterns, (2) remain together as families due to the stress and adversity faced by the family, or (3) be able to follow-through on their commitment to the study. These are the very families who are most likely to contain children with adjustment problems, or who are likely to develop adjustment problems. Thus, if the loss of families follows this pattern, there is likely to be an attenuation of effects with regard to the prediction of adjustment problems.

There is also a need to ensure in the research design that the findings will be sufficiently informative. Simply showing that two variables are related over a significant period of time provides limited clues about pathways of development. With regard to this issue, Fincham, Grych, and Osborne (1994) have outlined suggestions for more informative longitudinal research. One direction is to test competing theoretical models rather than merely a theoretical model versus a null model. Even when a test against a null model is successful, questions inevitably remain about whether the theoretical model provides the best possible fit for the data; that is, other models that are not examined may account for children's development over time better than the investigator's hypothesized model. Thus, testing against a reasonable alternative model yields a more definitive test about the viability of the particular theory and may be much more informative about the particular processes and pathways that account for and describe the children's development over time.

Another issue pertinent to the adequate examination of pathways of the development of adjustment problems is to test whether change in a dimension of interest (e.g., quality of attachment or other family variable of interest) predicts *change* in adjustment, rather than adjustment in an absolute sense (Fincham, Grych, & Osborne, 1994). For example, suppose one found that change from secure to insecure attachment between 1 and 5 years of age predicted adjustment problems at age 5. Such a finding would certainly be interesting, but one would not know whether the change in attachment status was responsible for adjustment problems at age 5. The situation would be improved with regard to the demonstration of causality if it were shown that a group that maintained secure attachment across the two time points was better adjusted at age 5 than the group that changed attachment status over that age span. However, the most cogent case would be made if adjustment and attachment data were collected at both ages, and changes in attachment were shown to *vary systematically* with changes in adjustment between ages 1 and 5.

In addition, it is important that the number of data points sampled over time is sufficient, particularly when the data have certain characteristics. In fact, analysis of longitudinal data can sometimes yield misleading results, particularly when a two-wave design is employed and the focal variable is highly stable and highly correlated with the other variable(s) of interest (Bradbury, Cohan, & Karney, 1998). Under these circumstances, common modes of analysis of two-wave longitudinal data (e.g., the difference score method, the partial correlation method, and the semipartial correlation method) have been shown to be vulnerable to yielding inaccurate estimates of the association between variables, even results that are the inverse of predictions (Karney & Bradbury, 1995). In these instances, improvement in prediction results from multiwave assessments (i.e., more than two assessments) in longitudinal research designs and also from the use of certain procedures for data analyses that minimize the likelihood of statistical artifacts (e.g., growth curve modeling).

Another limitation of longitudinal methods pertaining to causal inference merits notation; that is, even when longitudinal studies produce evidence for causal relations between variables, the evidence must be interpreted cautiously with regard to the origins of the effect. In particular, there is always the possibility that causal relations existed before the first observation of the prospective study. For example, one might find evidence in a longitudinal research design for causal relations between marital conflict and depression in a sample of young married adults (see Chapter 9, this volume). Thus, one might conclude that marital conflict caused depression in the adults in this sample. However, if the study did not begin assessment until the individuals were adults, one cannot rule out the possibility that depression had an initial onset before marriage and adulthood in the adults evidencing depression, and that marital conflict therefore was a precipitant, but not a cause, for depression among adults already having a history of proneness for depression.

Finally, it bears emphasizing that while there is no substitute for longitudinal data for the study of pathways of development and the processes that underlie pathways of development, longitudinal research has strengths and limitations, just as do other methodologies. For example, after an analysis of the strengths and weaknesses of the longitudinal research design, Glenn (1998) concluded:

> Although longitudinal . . . research is valuable, maximum understanding of how dysfunction arises . . . will not be achieved solely through more and better panel studies. The greatest need now is to integrate information gathered with a variety of methods and from different disciplinary perspectives. Enthusiasm (for prospective longitudinal research) . . . could be destructive if it should lead researchers to reject or ignore evidence from . . . cross-sectional surveys with large and representative samples, clinical case studies, and so forth. All of these kinds of studies have strengths and limitations, and though it would be folly to attribute equal value to each one, all can contribute to our understanding. . . . (p. 438)

Thus, while longitudinal research is an essential methodology for the developmental psychopathologist, the most desirable strategy for the programmatic investigation of substantial matters in this area over a series of studies is to employ multiple research designs, as well as multiple methods, in the systematic analysis of the issues. A critical point is that methodological diversity and inclusiveness are important for optimal advances in the study of normal development and the development of psychopathology.

STUDYING MULTIPLE SAMPLES AND OTHER SAMPLING ISSUES

A central tenet of the developmental psychopathology approach is that effects and relations pertinent to the development of psychopathology may vary as a function of the samples that are studied. Thus, it cannot be assumed that general rules and principles for a process-oriented understanding of normal development and the development of psychopathology will emerge only from the study of normal samples, or any particular ethnic group (e.g., white, middle-class families). A fully articulated understanding of developmental processes related to childhood adjustment requires studies of diverse clinical and normal samples, and samples that vary in terms of cultural and ethnic backgrounds. Moreover, depending upon how samples are obtained and other aspects of sampling procedures, questions may also be raised about the generalizability of the results for understanding of process.

The Role of Deviant and Normal Samples in the Study of Psychopathology

We have discussed matters pertaining to the fact that the normal and abnormal are not a dichotomy, and that one serves to define and inform understanding of the other (Sroufe, 1990). Studying samples that vary widely in terms of the incidences, types, and risks for childhood disorder across the span of childhood also adds to the understanding of the bases for deviant and normal development. The dynamic processes and broader causal net influencing development may vary substantially as a function of risk group, particular childhood disorder, and developmental context. Accordingly, the developmental pathways and influences associated with the etiology of the various disorders of childhood may vary considerably. For example, problems in the security of attachment relationships may contribute substantially to risk for depression in adolescence and adulthood (Cummings & Cicchetti, 1990) but may be much less significant contributors to other types of psychopathology, or, minimally, may be less salient as factors in relation to other influences (Colin, 1996). Research on psychological phenomena in multiple clinical, at-risk, and nonclinical samples will increase understanding of the processes and pathways that underlie normal development and the development of multiple forms of psychopathology. Thus, process-oriented research on samples varying widely with regard to normalcy is needed to advance understanding of the bases for the broad purview of psychopathology.

Attending to Cultural and Ethnic Variations

Consistent with the propositions of Bronfenbrenner's (1979) ecological perspective, childhood development is best understood as embedded in a variety of social and other ecological contexts, including community, cultural, and ethnic contexts of child development. Each of these factors may exercise important influences on child and family functioning, and may even in some instances change the relative impact of particular family practices on child development. While there is evidence that models explaining the influence of family processes on pathways of child development can sometimes be generalized across ethnic groups (Cowan, Powell, & Cowan, 1998), this is clearly not always the case. For example, as we see later, in Chapter 7, the effects of certain parenting practices and styles on children's functioning vary in some instances as a function of particular cultural and ethnic contexts. Accordingly, there is an urgent need to include more diverse ethnic and cultural groups in research to advance further understanding of the universe of developmental effects, processes, and relations. Neighborhood and community, socioeconomic status, and ethnicity (including generation and acculturation) are among the contextual–ecological influences that may affect the functioning of families and children, including the relative efficacy of different socialization practices (Parke & Buriel, 1998). Thus, it is critical for both tests of theories and clinical interventions that attention be paid to whether the socialization models developed on middle-class Caucasian samples are appropriate to other, often neglected, samples (Cowan et al., 1998). Such directions are also essential toward the fair and appropriate inclusion of multiple ethnic and cultural groups in the potential benefits that accrue for children from the advanced understanding of the influences on their healthy development that may follow from research.

Nationally Representative Samples and Epidemiological Approaches

A related issue regarding the choice of samples is whether the results of research based on relatively small, nonrandom samples can be generalized to national samples. To respond to this concern, Kellam and van Horn (1997) have advanced a developmental epidemiological approach that attempts to integrate notions of developmental science and public health toward the goal of promoting longitudinal research based on integration of life-course developmental orientation and community epidemiology. This approach aims to reduce the selection bias that is inevitably associated with volunteer samples and to increase the representation of ecological contexts by making efforts to ensure that the environment within which samples are studied is well-represented and well-defined. By studying developmental pathways longitudinally within well-defined cohorts, this approach also promises to advance the bases for more effective and targeted prevention approaches. While the implementation of this approach presents obvious practical challenges in terms of costs and logistics, the approach merits serious consideration by developmental psychopathologists as another avenue toward greater generalization of findings and more complete and precise articulation of the developmental pathways and processes underlying the development of childhood disorder.

AN ILLUSTRATION OF A PROCESS-ORIENTED MODEL FOR HUMAN DEVELOPMENT

To this point, we have considered the definition of developmental psychopathology, its relation to other disciplines, and some of the fundamental assumptions about the course of development. As the final task of this chapter, we provide a concrete example or illustration of what a process-oriented model for child development might look like. One final goal is to demonstrate the complexity and sophistication in methodology and research design that should be the goal for adequate directions in the study of pathways of development and the processes and mechanisms that underlie, and account for, pathways of development. We return to this framework frequently in this volume to illustrate the elements of a developmental psychopathology perspective.

A framework for a process-oriented model is presented in Figure 3.1. The left side of the figure outlines the various factors that potentially influence adjustment, and the right side reflects broad categories of psychological adjustment that might be assessed at any point in time. The middle section of the framework outlines the response processes of the individual over time (i.e., psychological functioning) that may mediate relations between influences on development on the one hand, and adjustment-related outcomes on the other.

The significance of period of the life span to processes of development is signified in the lower part of Figure 3.1. Consistent with the assumption of directionality, it is expected that organizations of psychological functioning at one point in time will influence psychological functioning at a later point in time (i.e., time 1 functioning will be a factor in time 2 functioning). In other words, development will reflect the emergence of "pathways" over time rather than a series of discontinuities from infancy to childhood to adolescence to adulthood to older age. However, this does *not* mean that psychological functioning will necessarily be stable, since influences on development, and changing biologically based maturation, also influence psychological functioning and may change over time, possibly causing changes in psychological functioning. On the other hand, instability in the sense of nonsignificant correlations between time 1 and time 2 on some dimension of psychological functioning (e.g., depression) does *not* mean development is discontinuous. The assumption is that development remains "lawful" whether patterns remain the same or change with time in response to individual maturation and changing experiences and circumstances (Egeland & Farber, 1984).

Thus, as illustrated by this framework, individual factors (biological, genetic, psychological), family and other social supports (marital, parent–child, siblings, extrafamilial, peers), and societal and environmental factors (government, financial, community, physical and health environment) each influence psychological "outcomes" (Bronfenbrenner, 1979). It is assumed that these various biopsychoenvironmental influences are interrelated and interdependent, and that quite different patterns of interrelations may occur within a given point in childhood. Moreover, different factors in the model may be more or less important at different points in development. For example, family relations and parent–child interaction are especially important in early childhood, whereas peer group influences increase in salience in middle childhood and may overwhelm family influences by adolescence. However, the arrows of influence do not proceed directly from influence to outcome, but are mediated by multiple, specific psychological processes and patterns reflected in day-to-day functioning (i.e., psychological functioning) in multiple specific contexts (e.g., family, school, peer group, neighborhood); that is, over time, and across periods of development, the various influences are posited to affect day-to-day psychological functioning, and underlie what is summarized (imperfectly and globally) in measures of adjustment, either positive or maladaptive. The critical assumption of the model is that multiple, specific individual processes in response to day-to-day events underlie developmental outcomes. These mediating response processes may be cognitive, social, biological/physiological, and/or emotional.

Moreover, these response processes are seen as dynamic and changing over time, rather than static or fixed, reflecting transactional relations among influences on development, and processes of responding to these influences.

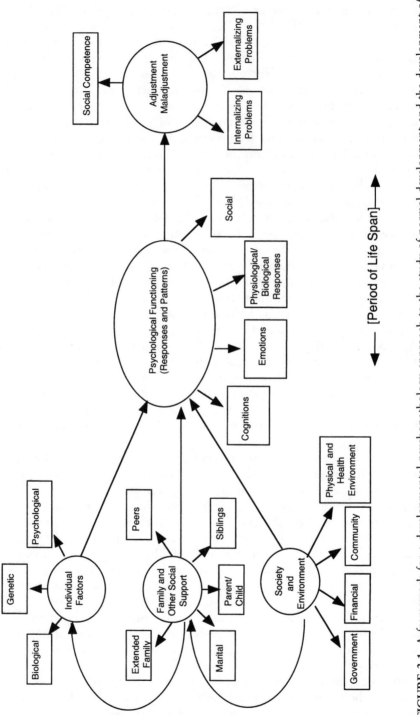

FIGURE 3.1. A framework for a developmental psychopathology approach to the study of normal development and the development of psychopathology. From Cummings (1999). Copyright 1999 by Lawrence Erlbaum Associates, Inc. Adapted by permission.

Furthermore, psychological responses may be organized as patterns, reflecting multiple specific elements of cognitive, emotional, and other domains of functioning. In fact, consistent with the principle of holism, it is expected that higher-order patterns of responding will more fully reflect the individual's reactions to events than will specific, isolated responses.

Finally, responses are expected to vary in terms of the specific, individual contexts in a child's experiences. For example, children react differently to marital conflict, separation from parents, playful interactions with parents, and so forth. On the other hand, again consistent with the principles of holism, these patterns of multiple responses across multiple specific contexts are expected to cohere into meaningful wholes. For example, an emotionally insecure child often evidences emotional insecurity across multiple contexts; that is, a child who is emotionally insecure about family functioning may also evidence greater emotional distress and other indices of dysregulation in reaction to separation from parents, marital conflict, and other family stresses (Davies & Cummings, 1994). In addition, patterns of responding to immediate situations are expected to leave "residues" that may have implications for future functioning. Thus, a child exposed repeatedly to interparental abuse typically will react with high levels of distress, with the "residue" or effect over time being that the child will evidence sensitization (i.e., heightened emotional and behavioral reactivity) to marital conflict in comparison to children from low-conflict family backgrounds (Cummings & Davies, 1994b).

The focus on specifying precise relations in time between predictors and outcomes as mediated by dynamic processes or mechanisms of psychological functioning defines a *process-oriented* perspective on child development. These notions are inherent in conceptualizations of developmental psychopathology (Cicchetti & Cohen, 1995b), developmental science (Cairns, Costello, & Elder, 1996), general systems theory (Sameroff, 1995), and in specific applications to the study of the effects of parental depression (Cummings & Cicchetti, 1990) and marital conflict (Cummings & Cummings, 1988; Cummings & Davies, 1996) on children, and in models for the development of mood disorders in children (Cicchetti & Toth, 1995) and attachment disorders (Carlson & Sroufe, 1995).

Outcomes in this framework are designated by results of diagnostic interviews or other formal assessments of psychological adjustment, consistent with the focus in mental health practice on the importance of nosology as an outcome variable that is very useful for purposes of clinical intervention and treatment. A diagnosis also communicates effectively that significant mental health concerns exist. However, outcomes, of course, are not static, consistent with the assumption of an active organism. The word "outcomes" is marked by quotations to reflect the notion that outcomes are characterized by underlying processes that are in a constant state of flux. Although there may be stability in overall organization, there may also be change, particularly when major changes occur in children's experiences or other contextual influences.

For example, early loss of a parent may have profound implications for a child's later development (Bowlby, 1980), independent of the child's initial level of adjustment to the loss. Thus, diagnostic assessments are no more than snapshots of an individual's psychological status at a given point in time. Moreover, adjustment may be conceptualized in terms of several of the broad dimensional categories typically assessed in psychological research, such as social competency, internalizing problems (e.g., depression, anxiety), and externalizing problems (e.g., aggression, conduct disorder). Psychological assessments may also result in categorical diagnoses (e.g., depression, anxiety disorders, conduct disorder), reflecting disorder in the psychiatric sense. Issues of dimensional and categorical approaches to the classification of children's problems and to the description of outcomes are discussed in a later chapter.

The influences on development also may function as protective factors and sources of resiliency, or risk factors and sources of vulnerability. Moreover, multiple risk factors increase the risk for psychopathology, with multiple risk factors additively, or even multiplicatively, increasing risk for medical and/or psychological disorder (Hauser, Vieyra, Jacobson, & Wertlieb, 1985; Rutter, 1980, 1981). Furthermore, different influences on development may affect the *same* processes in predicting risk for health-related problems (Cummings & Davies, 1994a; Jaffe, Wolfe, & Wilson, 1990). For example, similar disturbances of emotional regulation have been reported in children exposed to parental depression, marital conflict, or physical abuse, respectively, with especially heightened risk for problems in children exposed to two or more of these factors (Cummings & Davies, 1994a; Jaffe, Wolfe, Wilson, & Zak, 1986). In addition, in some instances, variables may act as mediators of psychological outcomes (e.g., depressive cognitions), whereas in other instances, variables may serve as moderators (e.g., gender is a common example). (An extensive treatment of the distinction between mediators and moderators in predicting psychological outcomes is given in Chapter 5.)

The period of the life span, and change across age, are also significant to psychological outcomes (see Figure 3.1). Development can be conceptualized in terms of pathways that emerge over time, with specific pathways *probabilistically*, but not certainly, related to normal development or the development of psychopathology (Cicchetti & Cohen, 1995a; Cicchetti & Richters, 1997; Rutter, 1986; Rutter, Tizard, Yule, Graham, & Whitmore, 1977; Sroufe, 1997; Sroufe & Rutter, 1984).

In other words, as we saw in Chapter 2, disorder can be viewed as a deviation over time, with the possibility of not only multiple pathways leading to the same manifest outcome but also the dispersion of pathways from similar early risk trajectories (Egeland, Pianta, & Ogawa, 1996). Nonetheless, while change is possible at many points in a pathway, change is also constrained by prior adaptation. Earlier structures of the individual's organization are incorporated into later structures; thus, early vulnerability tends to predict later vulnerability. Moreover, there is also an interplay between nature and nurture in development of these structures (Rutter, Tizard, Yule, Graham, & Whitmore, 1977). In other words, development is a series of successive adaptations of persons to their environments, with structural organizations and reorganizations within and between the biological and behavioral systems of the individual underlying developmental continuity and change. We consider these matters in more depth in Chapter 4.

The framework in Figure 3.1 thus provides a general way of conceptualizing multiple pathways of effect between biopsychoenvironmental factors and normal development, and the development of psychopathology. Notably, the model assumes that both past and present influences are related to the current psychological status of an individual. However, while the framework is relatively inclusive, there is no claim that it is exhaustive (i.e., other factors not listed here may also be important). The purpose is to provide a heuristic for thinking about what is meant by a process-oriented perspective, illustrating in terms of a specific model some of the issues already considered, and also laying a foundation for further discussion of related issues in subsequent chapters.

CONCLUSION

We have now outlined the subject matter that a developmental psychopathology perspective aims to address (i.e., uncovering the processes that underlie the development of childhood disorders) and have reviewed the discipline's theoretical and methodological assumptions about how to study development. The developmental psychopathology approach offers the promise of significantly advancing understanding of child development, particularly the development of psychopathology in children. The aim of developmental psychopathology as a field is to elucidate the critical processes underlying psychopathology and its development. As we will see, this approach also offers new avenues for the development of interventions that target more precisely the mechanisms that cause psychopathology and provides new bases for identifying early pathways of risk for psychopathology, allowing for the development of more effective prevention programs that prevent early risk from becoming full-blown disorder. As we have shown, developmental psychopathology is distinct from other disciplines and foci concerned with clinical research and practice in a number of ways that are important, and, accordingly, makes a distinct contribution to the common enterprise of understanding and treating mental health problems. However, there are a variety of other issues pertaining to pathways of development and the interplay of positive and negative influences on development that require further consideration and discussion for a fully developed exposition of the principles of this approach. Thus, we are at a middle point in our discussion of these issues. In Chapters 4 and 5, we further define and develop the particulars of the contributions of this field to principles needed to understand the development of children's adjustment problems.

✵ CHAPTER FOUR

Pathways in Development

To this point, we have considered the various defining elements of the developmental psychopathology perspective in contrast to several other approaches, including past approaches to understanding the development of childhood disorders. We also have considered some of the assumptions that underlie notions about development of disorders in children, but we have not yet systematically examined the perspective on pathways of development that is a fundamental contribution of this approach. Delineating different developmental pathways is especially important for an understanding of childhood disorders, since psychological functioning develops and changes dramatically between infancy and early adolescence.

Moreover, some behaviors that seem normal at one age or appear to be normal reactions to stressful transitions may, over time, become entrenched responses that signify problems. For example, normal separation distress, if it does not abate, or if the child is exposed to frequent, unexpected, or prolonged separations from primary caregivers, may develop into a more serious problems such as separation anxiety disorder. Similarly, the temper tantrums that often occur in toddlerhood may become more stable and persistent over time if they are handled poorly by adults, or if other factors lead to their exacerbation over time. Thus, when considering pathways of development, it is also important to be aware of the specific behaviors of concern and their timing in development. Because studies of adult psychopathology have devoted less attention to processes underlying continuity and discontinuity, this is an area in which developmental psychopathology can make a special contribution. Finally, notions about the psychological processes underlying child development, which we began to consider in previous chapters, must include conceptualizations of how processes change dynamically in time. Consider the following example:

At 1 year of age, Nicole and Lisa, childhood friends, were each securely attached to their parents and came from homes in which the parents were happily married. In third grade, Lisa's mother died and she suffered from feelings of depression and sadness in response to her loss and did poorly in school that year. By contrast, Nicole's family situation remained stable and well-functioning. That year, Nicole and Lisa were assessed by school counselors and had very different psychological profiles, with Lisa diagnosed with an affective disorder. By seventh grade, Nicole had developed difficulties in school and peer relations following a move to another state, and Lisa continued to have problems after her dad remarried. However, by early adulthood, with sensitive and responsive care from their parents and other adults in their lives, and despite the various forms of adversity, both were again well adjusted.

As one can see, Nicole and Lisa started very similarly, diverged in various ways during childhood and adolescence, but then converged again in the sense that both were well adjusted as adults. This example illustrates the dynamic and changing nature of the processes underlying development and the fact that children may move back and forth between good and poor adjustment at different points in time. This example also brings home the point that disorders are not something children "have," as in a disease model of childhood disorder, but reflect patterns of functioning in response to contexts of development that may change because of their own internal responses, changing circumstances, or complex interactions among these factors. In this chapter, we examine how the field of developmental psychopathology has begun to fill gaps in how we can conceptualize these issues.

ASSUMPTIONS ABOUT DEVELOPMENT PATHWAYS

With regard to conceptualizing pathways of development, Sroufe (1990, 1997) has proposed a branching tree as a metaphor for the multiple pathways individuals may follow during the course of development. Bowlby (1973) has proposed an alternative metaphoric representation of continuous, branching tracks in a railway station. We follow the tree metaphor to illustrate notions about pathways of development.

One may think of relatively normal development as reflected by continuous growth at or near the main body or trunk of the tree (see Figure 4.1). Pathways involving large groups of individuals are represented as large branches diverging only slightly from the tree trunk and reflecting approximations of "normality." As development proceeds, the growth of ever smaller branches represents more differentiated pathways of progressively smaller groups of individuals. Abnormality is reflected by a succession of branchings away from the main body of the tree, so that some distance develops between the tree trunk and the branches. When these branches diverge greatly from the tree, they can be seen as representing substantial deviation from common

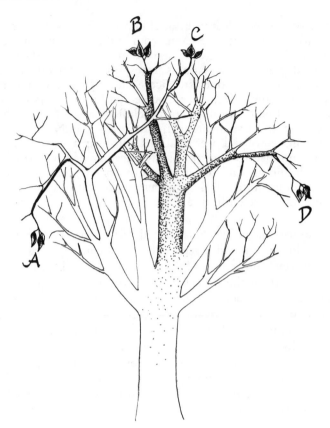

FIGURE 4.1. Pathways of development as a branching tree. From Sroufe (1997). Copyright 1997 by Cambridge University Press. Adapted by permission.

pathways. However, after initial divergence, secondary branches may actually grow closer to its major branch or other major branches, thus representing the potential of individuals to achieve a common outcome despite following different pathways at the outset, as we saw in the cases of Lisa and Nicole. Each nodal point in the tree can be seen as a period of developmental transition, a "turning point," or major life choice.

For example, in Figure 4.1 (adapted from Sroufe, 1997), the pathway denoted as A reflects continuity of maladaptation, resulting in disorder. Pathway B illustrates normal adaptation throughout development, that is, continuity of positive adaptation. Pathway C shows an example of a resilient developmental pathway, that is, early maladaptation followed by positive change later in development. Finally, Pathway D illustrates how early normal development can be followed by subsequent negative changes toward psychopathology.

The notion that there are multiple pathways during development, including multiple avenues toward normality or abnormality, is called *developmental pluralism*; that is, development involves many more possibilities toward normality or abnormality than one, or even a small subset, of trajectories. Development may involve many different starts and stops, directions toward competence or disorder, as the child gets older. Continuing the tree metaphor, trees come in all shapes and sizes, and may grow many, or only a few, branches as they develop. One may think of different trees as reflecting different cohorts or groups of individuals from very different contexts or environments.

Thus, returning to our example, one can see how Lisa and Nicole, who were from similar backgrounds and the same cohort, may follow different developmental pathways, reflected in successive branchings of the tree. At the outset (infancy), both were part of the main trunk of the tree. However, in response to various adversities (e.g., death of a parent, moving), they diverged away from the main body of the tree at various times during their development. On the other hand, with favorable circumstances of development (i.e., nurturance in the transaction between their intraorganismic characteristics and the social contexts of development), their "branches" (i.e., developmental patterns) eventually grew back toward the trunk (i.e., normal or well-adjusted development). Implicit in this example is the notion that most individuals are resilient and actively marshal resources to maintain or return to optimal functioning.

Several assumptions of developmental psychopathology are illustrated by this metaphor. One is that the organism and the context that supports the organism are inseparable, just as the growth of a tree cannot be separated from the environmental circumstances that support (or fail to adequately support) its growth. One cannot consider the individual in isolation from the environment and contexts of development; that is, developmental is a complex function of interrelations between the child and environment over time. Moreover, continuities may be due to stabilities in the organization of the environment over time, or stabilities in the organization within the child (Sameroff, 1995).

In this metaphor, one can also clearly discern that development may also reflect deviation over time; that is, abnormal processes of functioning do not just appear, just as a branch on a tree does not grow separately from the tree. Rather, abnormal growth or development occurs gradually over time as a function of the mutual influences among intra- and extraorganismic factors, building upon the growth (i.e., development) that has occurred before, but also responding continually to present and future conditions. Thus, when childhood disorder occurs, it typically reflects repeated failures to adapt optimally over time (i.e., maladaptation) with respect to the issues facing children during development. Moreover, in positing a living, growing, and changing organism, the tree metaphor also communicates that one must consider interactional, historical, and contextual factors when assessing the pattern of a child's development; that is, the relative normality or abnormality of the child's development is a function of many past, current, and, ultimately, future transactions between the child and the environment. However, any one influence is likely to have a limited effect; that is, it is unlikely that any one factor, in itself, will determine development. Thus, as Sroufe (1997) puts it:

> Pathology generally reflects repeated failure of adaptation. . . . A particular adaptational failure at any point in time is best viewed as placing an individual on a pathway potentially leading to disorder or moving the individual toward such a pathway. Thus, for example, maladaptive patterns in infancy (anxious attachment) are not viewed as psychopathological per se but in terms of developmental risk for disturbance. Pathology involves a succession of deviations away from normative patterns. (pp. 253–254)

Thus, psychopathology results from a continual process of interrelations between the individual and the environment; that is, the development of psychopathology is lawful and occurs over time as a result of repeated transactions (a two-way street) between the individual and the environment. The resulting response processes and patterns that eventuate from these transactions over time produce the organization of internal reactions (e.g., anxiety, sadness) and external behaviors (e.g., aggression, tantrums) that may be labeled as a clinically significant syndrome. Thus, disorders reflect successive and changing patterns of adaptations and maladaptations of persons to their environments.

These concerns are at the heart of the developmental psychopathology perspective; that is, the entire enterprise ultimately is concerned with explaining how complex patterns of influence over time are reflected in diverse pathways, some leading to normal and desirable outcomes, and some to maladjustment and psychopathology. Thus, even the complex patterns of influence, processes, and outcomes outlined in Figure 3.1 are not enough to account for the directions development may take. One must also factor in time, and the possibility of continuity and change over time.

Of course, very severe threats to the growth and survival of a tree can destroy, permanently damage, or otherwise have highly negative and lasting effects. Similarly, during child development, very traumatic events may occur (e.g., a car accident that causes brain damage) that have, in themselves, highly-destructive, even irreversible effects. However, these events are likely to be the exception. In the face of most single events, children have the potential to recover and to return to adaptive functioning. The risk for maladaptation is greatly increased, however, when there are multiple and repeated threats and stresses. In such instances, the increase in risk for psychopathology may be multiplicative rather than merely additive (Rutter, 1981; Rutter & Quinton, 1984). Another limitation of a branching tree metaphor is that it implies that some types of outcomes may be completely impossible for some children; in fact, "improbable" is a more accurate characterization (Sroufe, 1997).

Using the tree metaphor again, another principle of developmental psy-

chopathology is that the same general principles guide both normal development and the development of psychopathology. As the tree grows, each part
of the tree responds similarly to rainfall, sunlight, and so forth, although some
parts of the tree may be exposed to different conditions than others (e.g., sunlight, shade); that is, branches deviating farther from the trunk are not responding to different laws of nature than branches growing closer to trunk.
For children, too, the same general principles or rules of child development
are assumed to guide normal development and the development of psychopathology, although individuals may experience very different circumstances
or have different personal characteristics. Thus, psychopathology is not a special case but is the result of current and prior adaptations in transactions with
current and past situations. Both normal and abnormal development follow
the same rules governing interrelations among contextual influences on development and biological and psychological processes. This is reflected in Figure
3.1, where a range of outcomes is possible.

It follows that understanding abnormal development is enhanced by
studying the course of normal development; the rules for one population are
the same as for the other, and the examination of these principles in a variety
of contexts and situations serves to better define the nature of these influences.
Moreover, the general principles governing development are better understood by examining the range of natural variations in conditions of development. It also follows, given the complexity of transactions between the
individual and developmental context, that the risk for psychopathology developing in individual children, even in the presence of multiple, significant
predictors of psychopathology, is never certain. For example, there may also
be positive and supportive events that help to counteract the impact of negative events. Also, many children have internal and personal resources that allow them to be remarkably adaptive even in the face of adversity, even in the
most difficult and challenging of circumstances (Garmezy, 1985; Garmezy &
Masten, 1991; see Chapter 5, this volume). Thus, even events and circumstances associated with relatively high risk for the development of adjustment
problems (e.g., parental depression, family violence, child abuse) only probabilistically predict later dysfunction. Therefore, there are typically many individual exceptions, even when the prediction of childhood disorder, evident in
comparisons for proband and normal groups, is highly significant statistically
at the level of group differences. As Cicchetti, Rogosch, and Toth (1998) note
"Even in studies that reveal significant differences between children of depressed and nondepressed caregivers, a substantial number of children of depressed caregivers do not evidence dysfunction. Such findings have resulted in
increased attention to the broader social context in which children of depressed mothers develop" (p. 283). Moreover, some individuals subjected to
numerous risk events develop normally. But other individuals confronted with
much less risk, at least as assessed from the perspective of an outside observer,
may nonetheless develop serious adjustment problems.

Both of these types of cases are of great interest to the developmental psychopathologist because exceptions may be particularly helpful for under-standing the principles governing development. In addition, there is always the possibility of change, so that dysfunctional individuals may begin to func-tion more adaptively over time; that is, in terms of the tree metaphor, the branch may grow back toward the main body of the tree. These various possi-ble pathways underscore the notion of childhood disorder as resulting from a continual process of interrelations between the child and the environment. When psychopathology does occur, its emergence is lawful, due to a process of repeated transactions (a two-way street) between the child and the environ-ment. Thus, the possibility of psychopathology resulting from any of the forces and factors impacting upon the child is never more than probabilistic, and a diagnosis of psychopathology is never more than a relatively simplified statement about the nature of the child's functioning at a particular point in time. Following the tree metaphor, a diagnosis of disorder should be seen only as a snapshot of a branch of the tree at a split-second in time. Also, much may be hidden from view; that is, the complex processes underlying individual de-velopment may not always be evident. Thus, the forces that guide the growth of the tree (i.e., adaptive and maladaptive processes) cannot be seen, and the possibility of growth back toward the main body of the tree (i.e., normality) may simply not be evident in the snapshot.

Accordingly, because of the complex interplay of forces that guide devel-opment, change is possible at many points and, moreover, is almost always possible. Just as the branches of a tree may grow in one direction or the other at any time, so the psychological development of the child may become more, or less, adaptive over time. The trajectories of development are not static or fixed, but reflect a constant process of adaptation, so that change from psy-chopathology to normality, or other patterns of change, are always a possibil-ity. As Sroufe (1997) put it:

> Despite early deviation, changes in developmental challenges or other aspects of context may lead the individual back toward a more serviceable pathway. Not only is pathology typically not simply an endogenous given, return to pos-itive functioning often remains possible. It is generally inappropriate to think of maladaptation or disturbance as something a child either "has" or "does not have" in the sense of a permanent condition. (p. 254)

On the other hand, the possibilities for change are not unlimited and only a function of current circumstances; change is constrained by past organiza-tions and structures of the individual during development. Just as a tree's fu-ture growth is constrained by past growth, so the future development of the child is to some extent limited by what has previously occurred during devel-opment. Thus one can see clearly the assumptions of the developmental psy-chopathology approach of active organism, directionality, and holism; that is, there is an active forward movement of the child adapting in transaction with social experience, but there is also an interplay between the organizations of the system (i.e., holism) and present circumstances as development moves forward (i.e., directionality). Thus, while change is always to some extent possible, the organizational adaptations resulting from past transactions between the individual and contexts of development have an influence on future possibilities for development. Earlier structures of the child's psychological functioning are incorporated into later structures, referred to as *floating holism*. Sroufe (1997) elaborates on this point:

> The longer a maladaptive pathway has been followed (especially in the sense of going across phases of development), the less likely it is that the person will reclaim positive adaptation. . . . This is consistent with the "active child" principle. By creating negative experiences in an ongoing way, failing to engage positive opportunities, and interpreting even benign experiences as malevolent (which are often core features of maladaptation), the child's adaptation may make positive change less likely. (p. 254)

The metaphor of the tree, which is a complex, constantly growing and changing organism, also aptly reflects the concern of developmental psychopathology with charting the diversity and multiplicity of developmental trajectories—the opposite of a "one size fits all" metaphor. This perspective on the life course contrasts with other models of human development. For example, some developmental models have focused on charting a single, normative developmental pathway. Strong "growth" models define development as being restricted to a universal sequence of irreversible changes impelled or guided by a final end state (Baltes, Reese, & Lipsitt, 1980). A corresponding empirical focus is concerned with charting mean levels of behaviors over age periods on the assumption that there is an underlying expected or "normal" pathway for development. Deviations from the average, that is, diversity in developmental course, are treated as beyond the scope of analysis or even as methodological "noise" (i.e., measurement error) that statistically dilutes the power to detect developmental change. Similarly, nosological or classificatory systems in psychiatric models may be based on static, dichotomous frameworks that conceptualize individuals as either having the "disease" or being healthy. Classification proceeds by a narrow focus on searching for a single pathway that characterized the "jump" from risk status to the actual disease (Cicchetti, 1984). Pathways from risk to outcome are conceptualized as simple, direct, and nearly instantaneous (Zucker, 1994; Zucker, Fitzgerald, & Moses, 1995).

A focus on the multidirectionality of development reflects more than a different set of assumptions about the number of possible pathways of development; it also reflects a correspondingly different conceptualization of the causes of development. For example, unidirectional disease, or "magic bullet" models found in biological psychiatry proceed on the assumption that there is a single proximal cause to each disorder that is so overpowering and robust that factors preceding, accompanying, or following the cause have only negligible effect on the disease.

Traditional approaches in psychiatric research toward examining the etiology of disorder inflate support for relatively straightforward etiological models. In particular, retrospective designs have commonly been used in the study of the causal influences on the development of psychopathology. However, the logic that supports causal conclusions based upon retrospective designs is seriously flawed. Thus, in such designs, participants are often identified based on the presence of diagnosed disorders (e.g., aggression, depression) and then past records are examined for the earlier incidence of the disorder. Such research designs may yield seemingly impressive support for the continuity of particular syndromes. However, even if the present disorder is frequently preceded by the same disorder in the past, it is erroneous to draw inferences about causal conclusions, or even necessarily high levels of association, from such studies. Notably, when looking forward prospectively from the early to the later time points, one often finds much weaker links between the variables, for example, the particular childhood disorder may, in fact, lead to many different outcomes (including normalcy). In addition, other sources of error are associated with retrospective designs. For example, when looking backwards, one will tend to find some type of confirmatory evidence for continuity, but may inadvertently ignore or fail to appreciate much else about the evidence pertinent to etiology, such as co-morbidity of the supposed causal agent with other problems that also contribute to risk.

Thus, there are numerous limitations with regard to making causal inferences from retrospective follow-back designs in psychological or psychiatric research. Thus, Cowan, Cowan, and Schulz (1996) have warned:

> Even with good data about parents' psychiatric status from prior records, retrospective studies beginning with samples of diagnosed individuals provide a distorted estimate of risk. Suppose all of the schizophrenic children were found to have at least one schizophrenic parent (decidedly not the case). Researchers would still not be able to conclude that parental pathology was a risk factor in the development of schizophrenia. If the study had started prospectively with parents, researchers would find that most schizophrenic parents do not have schizophrenic children. In logic, the fact that A (schizophrenic children) implies B (schizophrenic parents) do not mean that B implies A. Although concurrent and retrospective research designs can be useful in generating hypotheses about antecedents of psychopathology, these hypotheses must be tested in prospective studies that start with an identified risk and follow subjects forward over time. (p. 6)

These problems with retrospective designs have led developmental psychopathologists to regard prospective longitudinal designs as an essential tool in the search for the etiology of disorder. These research directions have supported the existence of far more complex, dynamic, and pluralistic pathways of development. The pluralistic models that characterize the developmental psychopathology approach emphasize that different outcomes and pathways are the by-product of dynamic, bidirectional relations between contextual factors (e.g., psychosocial factors) and the organism (e.g., genetic, biological, constitutional factors) over time (Lerner, 1996). Diversity is assumed to be further accentuated by the fact that influences differ in terms of their onset, duration, temporal ordering, and co-occurrence (e.g., Windle & Tubman, 1999). Thus, the developmental psychopathology approach places emphasis on processes of initiation, change, and continuity of adaptation and maladaptation (Sroufe, 1997).

Other assumptions about the nature of human development that derive from the developmental psychopathology perspective, which we noted briefly earlier, follow from pluralistic notions of development. Thus, multiple, diverse causes and developmental courses can lead to the same developmental outcome, that is, equifinality. Put another way, a given form of psychopathology does not result from a single cause or causal chain of events but can be the result of various different pathways followed during the course of development. For example, for some individuals, the development of depression may be heavily influenced by genetic risk, whereas for others, traumatic historical experiences (e.g., loss of a parent, maltreatment) may have primary importance; that is, contributors to the development of psychopathology may vary among individuals who have the same disorder.

Returning to the example of Nicole and Lisa, these two individuals had very different developmental courses but ended up indistinguishable as adults in the sense that both became well-functioning. While the example is fictional, one can speculate that following an active organism assumption, these two individuals constantly sought to maintain adaptive functioning and had sufficient intra- and extraorganismic resources eventually to achieve that outcome. However, the fact that, as young adults, these two women were well-adjusted does *not* mean that their functioning was precisely the same as adults; that is, the *manifest* outcomes were the same, but it remains possible that many aspects of internal functioning differed. Again, Sroufe (1997) provides an apt statement:

> When development is viewed in terms of a succession of branchings, it follows that individuals beginning on different pathways may nonetheless converge towards similar patterns of adaptation. [However, a] ... pattern of maladaptation with many different features in common (e.g., lack of social engagement, depressed mood, low self-esteem) may be the result of distinctly different developmental pathways. ... Whether such phenotypically similar individuals differ in terms of "prognosis," subsequent outcome, or effective intervention become key research questions. ... (p. 254)

Expanding on the notion of multifinality, a single cause or developmental pathway may lead to a number of different outcomes (Cicchetti & Rogosch, 1996); that is, the fact that two different individuals are following a similar pathway in some sense at a given point in time does not mean the later end result will be the same. Thus, two children may evidence insecure attachment at a given point in time, but only one may develop later psychopathology. Similarly, in the instance of two preschoolers who are extremely hard-to-manage as very young children, showing defiance and aggression toward peers may have different outcomes based on child and family characteristics and their transactions over time (e.g., Campbell, 1997; Campbell, Pierce, Moore, Marakovitz, & Newby, 1996). Thus, any one component during development may function differently depending on the organizational system in which it operates, with the result being quite different outcomes later in development. Moreover, even assuming that two individuals might evidence several similar characteristics at one point in time, the events that follow may well result in very different later outcomes if these subsequent events are quite different. Again, this reflects the concept of multifinality. Thus, traditional notions of a single cause leading to a single outcome are replaced by the notions that (1) many causes can lead to the same effect, and (2) a single cause may have many different effects.

Further developing the model shown in Figure 4.1, consider the following example:

> At age 5, both Bill and Mike evidenced clinical levels of depressive symptomatology, but Mike also fought a lot with his classmates, whereas Bill was quite and withdrawn. Throughout the school years, Mike was aggressive toward others and developed problems with delinquency. But Bill remained shy and insecure in social interactions. Moreover, the level of depressive symptomatology declined, whereas aggressivity increased, for Mike as he got older. By contrast, Bill's depressive symptomatology slowly became more serious. As adults, Mike evidenced significant problems of aggressivity and hostility in interpersonal situations, whereas Bill was diagnosed with clinical depression.

This example illustrates how two children with some similar symptoms but with different disorders based upon a multicomponent analysis of their functioning evidenced consistently different pathways during development; that is, while an assessment only of depression in early childhood would have suggested that these children started out at a similar place and thus might be expected based on a "disease model" to evidence a similar trajectory of maladaptation from childhood to adolescence, a more comprehensive assessment would indicate that these boys evidenced quite different pathways from the outset and that this different pattern of development continued throughout childhood.

These notions are illustrated by the pattern of findings on developmental pathways of depression based on epidemiological studies involving thousands of children and families conducted over the last 30 years at the Institute of Psychiatry in London (Harrington, Rutter, & Fombonne, 1996). A particular advantage of this work for illustrating pathways of depression is that assessments of depression were first made in childhood, before the onset of puberty. At this early point, a syndrome of depression could be identified and was found to be linked with increased risk for depression in adulthood. Moreover, depression was more likely to be found in first- and second-degree relatives of individuals diagnosed with childhood depression than among others. Thus, at first glance, these data would seem to support a "disease model" of depression and a single pathway of the development of depression. However, the broader pattern of analyses conducted on these children and families over the years tell a very different story.

First, childhood depression was often found to be associated with a variety of other disorders in childhood such as conduct problems; it was not a neat, well-defined "disease entity." Moreover, different patterns of functioning associated with childhood depression predicted very different adult outcomes, consistent with the notion of holism; that is, the overall patterns of functioning, rather than a specific symptom an individual "has," is critical to the course of development over time. Specifically, children who were diagnosed for both depression *and* conduct disorder were *not* at increased risk for major depression in adulthood (although they were at increased risk for other serious disorders in adulthood), whereas risk of adult depression was elevated among those diagnosed with depression but *not* conduct disorder. Thus, there was a multifinality of outcomes at time 2 (adulthood) based on the presence of depression at time 1 (childhood), but these directions were not arbitrary. They reflected overall psychological functioning.

Furthermore, those persons with childhood depressive symptomatology based only on chart ratings of observed *symptoms* were less likely to develop adult depression than children diagnosed with childhood depression based on intensive psychiatric interviews. This suggests that the severity of depression in childhood increased the probability of developing depression in adulthood, since the criteria used to assess depressive symptomatology were generally less stringent than those used to make a formal diagnosis of depression. Thus, the processes associated with depression severity appear to be important to later outcomes, not whether the individual "has" or "does not have" an "entity" of childhood depression.

On the other hand, childhood depression is not a narrow and prerequisite pathway to the occurrence of adult depression. In fact, most adults diagnosed with depression are not diagnosed as depressed in childhood (Harrington, Rutter, & Fombonne, 1996). Using the tree metaphor, these data suggest that there are various, different "successive branchings" that may lead to adult depression, illustrating again the notion of equifinality. On the other hand, childhood depression may be a particularly common nascent branch of the tree of development for predicting this outcome, and this branch may lead more often than most others to adult depression (Kovacs, 1998).

As another example, much research has been conducted on pathways from early aggression and noncompliance to later outcomes (e.g., Campbell, Pierce, Moore, Marakovitz, & Newby, 1996; Moffitt, 1990, 1992; Patterson, DeBaryshe, & Ramsey, 1989; Shaw, Owens, Vondra, Keenan, & Winslow, 1996). For example, Campbell (1990) has suggested that children with early emerging aggression, tantrums, defiance, and overreactivity in the preschool period are at risk for continuing problems. However, only a small proportion of children with early emerging oppositional behavior will have serious problems later (Moffitt, 1990; Moffitt, Caspi, Belsky, & Silva, 1992) and whether they do or not appears to be partly a function of the severity and variety of their difficulties, as well as their family context (Belsky, Hsieh, & Crnic, 1998; Loeber & Stouthamer-Loeber, 1998a; Moffitt, 1990). Again, using Sroufe's tree metaphor, some children with early tantrums and noncompliance will be on that pathway or branch only briefly, suggesting that their difficult behavior reflects age-related developmental transition (the terrible twos and threes; Belsky et al., 1998). Other children showing this symptom picture in early childhood may continue along that branch until school entry, when they show positive adaptation to new developmental challenges and expectations, and the branch diverges. A small proportion of problem children will continue on a negative pathway from early oppositional behavior to conduct problems in middle childhood or adolescence, to antisocial problems in early adulthood (Moffitt et al., 1992). These examples illustrate developmental pathways and continuity–discontinuity in aggressive and defiant behavior.

CONTINUITY AND DISCONTINUITY IN PATHWAYS OF DEVELOPMENT

Thus, as we have seen, a central notion of the developmental psychopathology perspective is that development follows pathways reflecting dynamic transactions between the individual and contexts of development. However, a variety of other, specific issues merit further consideration as we move toward a fuller account of the developmental psychopathology perspective on pathways of development.

Continuity

The issue of continuity in development is not as easy one, because the ideal level of analysis has to do with processes of functioning over time rather than any relatively simple judgment of categories of outcome at discrete points in time. Main effects models traditionally have attributed continuity to genetic factors or environment (Sameroff, 1995), whereas the new models increasingly view it as product of reciprocal interactions between both a robust, genetically mediated constitution and a stable environment (Cicchetti & Toth, 1995; Cummings & Davies, 1999; Moffitt, 1993a; Rutter, 1992; Sroufe & Egeland, 1991); that is, it is an oversimplification of the developmental model to focus on whether the manifest behaviors reflecting a disposition or trait (e.g., aggression) remain stable versus not stable, or continuous versus discontinuous. Nonetheless, following the tree metaphor, there may be *relative* stability in the direction followed by successive branchings of the tree as it grows, that is, in patterns of processes underlying development, and notions of stability and continuity have heuristic value for students of child development. Accordingly, continuity in processes of development may be conceptualized at several different levels of analysis; for example, aggression, irritability, and anger may be different manifestations of negative mood, and one or another may be more salient at different points in development. We next consider some of the concepts pertinent to notions of continuity over time.

Homotypic Continuity

The most easily conceptualized type of continuity, called homotypic continuity, refers to the expression of similar behaviors or attributes in individuals at different periods of development. For example, there is evidence that some preschool children who exhibit aggressive behaviors tend to exhibit aggressive behaviors in middle childhood, preadolescence, adolescence, and even adulthood (Campbell, 1990, 1995; Cicchetti & Toth, 1991). For example, Loeber (1991a, 1991b) has demonstrated that early onset disruptive behavior, more varied problems, and more chronic problems greatly increase the likelihood that children will follow a persistent behavioral problem pathway (e.g., aggression). Furthermore, Loeber and colleagues (1993) provide preliminary data to support three pathways in development of conduct disorders in children: (1) an early conflict with authority pathway (e.g., defiance, stubbornness), (2) a covert pathway (e.g., lying, shoplifting), and (3) an overt pathway (e.g., aggression, violence). Moreover, there is overlap across the pathways, with boys evidencing characteristics of all three pathways most likely to commit later serious acts of delinquency (e.g., violence).

Similarly, Campbell, Pierce, Moore, Marakovitz, and Newby (1996) reported high levels of continuity of externalizing problems in a sample of hard-to-manage boys assessed at 4, 6, and 9 years of age. However, although there was a high level of continuity, there were also environmental factors that systematically affected continuity. In particular, even controlling for earlier levels of symptoms, maternal control at age 4 predicted externalizing problems at age 9. Moreover, problems were more likely to continue when there was chronic family stress, including marital dissatisfaction, maternal depressive symptoms, and negative life events. At age 9, diagnoses of oppositional defiant disorder and/or attention deficit disorder were linked with each of these factors (i.e., earlier symptom levels, family stress, and maternal control). These results demonstrate that even in instances of homotypic continuity, there may be lawful relations with family events and other factors predicting the extent to which problems persist.

However, even in this instance, continuity is unlikely to reflect the same rates and types of behaviors found in an individual across development. Instead, developmental changes in the form and frequency of behaviors may be found; continuity may mean that an individual's relative problems in terms of a given class of behaviors remain stable in relation to other individuals. For example, aggression among boys tends to remain highly stable during child-hood, but the forms and frequencies of particular aggressive acts may change considerably (Cummings, Iannotti, & Zahn-Waxler, 1989; Loeber, 1984; Olweus, 1979). In addition, it is important to trace developmental pathways from a point prior to the onset of disturbance, that is, patterns of adaptation, weaknesses and strengths, that precede the actual identification of a manifest disorder, and that reflect the full network of causal influences that contribute to developmental pathways (Sroufe, 1997). For example, Shaw, Owens, Vondra, Keenan, and Winslow (1996) reported that a variety of risk factors assessed at 12 months (i.e., infant disorganized attachment status, marital disagreements about child rearing, maternal maladjustment) predicted clinically elevated aggression at 5 years of age. Thus, conceptualizing trajectories of development beginning only at the point at which disturbance is first formally identified misses important earlier influences on development that are likely to continue to be important.

Heterotypic Continuity

Continuity also may be found in the underlying organization, function, and meaning of the behaviors, rather than overt behaviors (Sroufe & Rutter, 1984). This form of continuity, which is termed heterotypic continuity (Caspi & Moffitt, 1995; Rutter, 1996), moves beyond simply documenting similarities in the overt expression of behaviors over time (i.e., homotypic continuity) by stressing coherence at a conceptual level of the underlying meaning and organization of psychological functioning.

For example, Finnegan, Hodges, and Perry (1996) examined school adjustment correlates of children's preoccupied and avoidant ways of relating to parents. Preoccupied children expressed upset, emotional dysregulation, and temper tantrums during stressful periods of the mother–child relationship. Avoidant children withdrew and minimized the overt expression of distress. Narrowly focusing on homotypic continuity may lead to the hypothesis that preoccupied children are at risk for externalizing symptoms (e.g., aggression, conduct problems) by virtue of their earlier lack of emotional and behavioral control, while avoidant children are at risk for internalizing symptoms (e.g., social withdrawal, depression) due to their dispositions to withdraw and internalize their distress. In fact, the results of this study show an opposite pattern of relations; avoidant coping predicted externalizing symptoms, whereas preoccupied coping predicted internalizing symptoms.

While these results may initially be puzzling, the hypotheses of Finnegan and colleagues were actually consistent with the results. This was because they focused on coherence and continuity at a deeper level, based on the meaning and function of the behaviors. Specifically, in underscoring heterotypic continuity, they reasoned that the devaluation of social relationships, lack of regard for others, and social disengagement underlying avoidant coping renders children particularly vulnerable to externalizing symptoms. Conversely, pre-occupied coping styles, which are theorized to reflect excessive fears and inhibit mastery of the environment, may increase children's risk for anxiety problems, helplessness, and depressive symptoms (Cummings & Davies, 1995). Thus, continuity was found at the level of the fundamental organization and meaning of behavioral patterns, rather than at the level of the surface or manifest behaviors.

Hierarchical Motility

Continuity may also result from hierarchical motility, whereby old psychological organizations are carried over in qualitatively new systems. However, given the new level of organization, perfect, one-to-one correspondence between the old and new ways of functioning is not expected. Hence, *some* of characteristics and features of old psychological structures can be found within the backdrop of a progressive change toward new levels of functioning (Cicchetti & Cohen, 1995a).

Returning to the living cell example, brain and skin cells continue to have common characteristics and structures (e.g., nucleus) despite their different developmental trajectories, organizations, and ways of functioning. Within developmental psychopathology, similar kinds of continuity are also found in the context of change. The study of emotion regulation provides a vivid illustration of continuity at both a normative (i.e., group) and individual-difference level. At a group level, both newborns and 1-year-olds reduce distress by non-nutritive sucking (e.g., finger and thumb sucking). However, while this illustrates a carryover in a sense, the organization of non-nutritive sucking is qualitatively different in the two periods. Among newborns, it is a preadapted involuntary reflex. Conversely, among older infants, it is part of a conscious, purposeful coping repertoire for regulating affect (e.g., reducing distress) (see Kopp, 1989).

A commonsense expectation is that while continuity may be found in certain dispositions in certain groups (e.g., aggression in boys), the extent to which continuity is observed will inevitably decline with age. However, as has been pointed out by a number of theorists, this is not necessarily the case. One reason is that canalization may occur. The concept of canalization specifies how previous development limits the probability, degree, and nature of future change in adaptation (Waddington, 1957). The rule of thumb is that "the longer an individual continues along a maladaptive ontogenetic pathway, the more difficult it is to reclaim a normal developmental trajectory" (Cicchetti & Cohen, 1995a, p. 7). This rule also applies to adaptive developmental trajectories; that is, individuals experiencing lengthier histories of adaptive pathways can withstand greater challenges to their psychological adjustment. Thus, shallow and wide "behavioral canals" that characterize early development become much deeper and more narrow as development proceeds. Accordingly, plasticity and change in psychological systems (e.g., room to "navigate" within the canals or "jump the banks" of the canal) become progressively more limited with development (Gottlieb, 1991a).

It follows from this notion that clinicians and mental health workers should target early stages of the life span in attempts to treat or prevent psychological disorders. If problems are caught early in their developmental course, navigating psychological change toward adaptive trajectories is much more efficient and successful (Ramey & Ramey, 1998). In fact, a number of directions in intervention and prevention (e.g., intervention for problem aggression) have been guided by this notion (Reid, 1993). For example, Greenberg, Speltz, and colleagues have proposed that early interventions in the parent–child attachment relationship meant to foster greater security of attachment may serve as an intervention to reduce risk for later disruptive behavior problems (Greenberg, Speltz, & DeKlyen, 1993; Speltz, Greenberg, & DeKlyen, 1990).

On the other hand, actual demonstrations of canalization are relatively uncommon, although some examples can be found: Zucker, Fitzgerald, and Moses (1995) reviewed studies on the development of alcohol and associated adjustment problems, which, pooled together, provided compelling support for increasing stability of maladaptive behavior over time (see also Turkheimer & Gottesman, 1991). Alcohol problems among individuals who had been relatively free of psychological problems in earlier stages of the life span were more temporary and unstable (Zucker, 1994; Zucker et al., 1995). Similarly, longer spans of conduct problems (e.g., aggression) during childhood placed individuals on increasingly stable and crystallized pathways of deviance, including delinquency, criminal activity, alcohol problems, and substance use (Loeber, 1991a, 1991b) in early adulthood. Moffitt, Caspi, Dickson, Silva, and Stanton (1996) reported that life-course-persistent (LCP; ages 3–18) and adolescent-limited (AL) antisocial behavior appeared *on the surface* to be indistinguishable at late adolescence in terms of contemporary information about levels of antisocial behavior. On the other hand, closer inspection revealed that the overall personality profiles of the AL boys were not nearly as pathological as the profiles for LCP boys; that is, they had closer relationships with families, were not extreme on aggressiveness, had some desirable leadership qualities, and appeared to be largely ensnared in a "rebellious" posture toward traditional values. Thus, their prognosis was judged to be much more optimistic than that for LCP boys. LCP boys were typified by persistent antisocial behavior across multiple areas: individual, family, school, peer, and justice system, reflecting "the many years of accumulated maldevelopment of personality structure" (p. 422). Thus, the results were interpreted to support very early detection and intervention (before age 3) to avoid the establishment of childhood-onset patterns (i.e., LCP patterns), another example of crystallized patterns of functioning.

However, even here the evidence is not without other possible interpretations. Thus, as a counterpoint to the notion that continuity of alcohol problems systematically increases with age, some maintain that these problems exhibit more plasticity during early (e.g., adolescence, young adulthood) and later stages of the life span (i.e., old age) than middle adulthood (Fillmore, 1985; Fillmore & Midanik, 1984). As another example reflecting the complexity of the issues with regard to antisocial behavior, some children with early onset aggression outgrow their difficulties by middle childhood, although others appear to be on a more lethal developmental trajectory toward serious problems in adolescence (e.g., Campbell, Pierce, Moore, Marakovitz, & Newby, 1996; Moffitt, 1993a).

Theoretically, hierarchical motility may also foster increasing stability of behavioral traits or phenotypes within individuals over time. Specifically, successive changes in behavioral traits are influenced by the incorporation of old traits into the new phenotypes. As the influence of old traits in the new phenotypes continues to accumulate as development proceeds, the by-product may be greater behavioral stability and resistance to change (Turkheimer & Gottesman, 1991).

Although early conceptualizations of increasing continuity with age emphasized that this sequence was caused by a predetermined genetic program that was insulated from experience, new models no longer pit nature (i.e., genes) and against nurture (i.e., environment) in accounting for the processes underlying canalization (Cairns, 1991; Gottlieb, 1991a; Greenough, 1991). Instead, it is now widely accepted that this phenomenon, when it occurs, is the result of complex interactions and coactions between genetic substrates and experience.

In summary, there are various forms and ways in which continuity may be exhibited aside from a simple one-to-one correspondence between earlier and later behavior. Accordingly, failing to find continuity at one level of analysis does not mean that it does not exist at another level. The degree and levels of organization of continuity may be highly variable and it thus behooves the investigator or clinician to think broadly, and in terms of multiple possible levels of analysis, about how continuity might be manifested. Moreover, even these terms for various forms of continuity (homotypic, heterotypic, hierarchical motility) are no more than heuristics and are likely to oversimplify matters if taken too seriously; that is, continuity is not likely to be heterotypic to the exclusion of homotypic, for example, which means that both constructs may to a degree be relevant to conceptualizing development. These are not either–or matters, but the discussion of these constructs is meant to illustrate some of the different ways in which development may proceed.

Discontinuity

There are also emerging notions for how to conceptualize discontinuity in development, although, as we have seen, from a developmental psychopathology perspective, pathways of development at a process level are rarely truly "discontinuous." Discontinuity is in some sense primarily a reflection of the exercise of comparing "outcomes" at different discrete points in time. Thinking about development in this way contradicts some of the assumptions of the developmental psychopathology perspective (e.g., coherence); that is, underlying processes of everyday functioning are assumed to move forward systematically, reflecting progressive adaptations and maladaptations of the individual in transaction with the environment: Development does not proceed in the abrupt, categorical manner implied by the term "discontinuous." However, as a practical matter, the concept of discontinuity has meaning and importance, even though, in a sense, it is a shorthand for far more complex processes of development.

Compas, Hinden, and Gerhardt (1995) provide an example of a heuristic model that grapples with how to characterize discontinuity in relation to continuity. Some individuals may manifest stable adaptive and maladaptive trajectories in functioning from childhood through young adulthood. However, other individuals may experience discontinuity in various patterns and stages of development. Attempts to understand discontinuity in trajectories must not only incorporate the possible role of simultaneous or cumulative psychosocial processes, but also the role of genetic and constitutional factors. Drastic changes from adaptive to maladaptive behavior during adolescence may be the result of interacting influences of (1) certain genes that become particularly pronounced around puberty (e.g., Cairns, Gariepy, & Hood, 1990); and (2) the peak accumulation of stressors during early to middle adolescence (e.g., early timing of puberty, transition to a secondary school) (Graber & Brooks-Gunn, 1996; see also Compas et al., 1995).

However, it cannot be assumed that the same causal processes necessarily underlie all discontinuous trajectories. In the "turnaround or recovery" pathway, the transition from early and persistent maladaptation to subsequent adaptation during later adolescence or early adulthood may be largely explained by a positive chain of processes brought about by life events such as entry into the military (e.g., discipline, broadening job skills and opportunities) or carefully planned marriage (e.g., spousal support, warmth) (Rutter, 1989b). Yet another pathway, characterized as a transient period of experimentation with problem behavior during adolescence (e.g., heavy drinking, delinquency), may reflect a combination of peer pressure and frustration with societal rules. Thus, the interplay of forces that influence discontinuity in development are complex and multidimensional.

More concrete and elaborate forms of this generic framework are evident in a number of substantive areas in developmental psychopathology. As another example, in the study of antisocial behavior, Moffitt (1993a) has proposed that to conclude that antisocial behavior is "stable" may obscure fine-grained differences. She posits at least two developmental trajectories of antisocial behavior. The first trajectory, called LCP antisocial behavior, consists of a small group of individuals who exhibit high, persistent levels of antisocial behavior from early childhood through adolescence and adulthood. Thus, this group explains, in large part, the often-reported stability of antisocial behavior (e.g., Olweus, 1979). According to Moffitt (1993a), the origins of LCP antisocial behavior are likely to be rooted in a transactional interplay between early neuropsychological vulnerabilities and adverse home environments (e.g., neglect, discord).

However, a second trajectory, which is called AL antisocial behavior, consists of individuals who exhibit a sharp increase in antisocial behavior during adolescence that is preceded and followed by an absence of antisocial problems in childhood and adulthood. This group may explain why antisocial behavior also manifests considerable change across development. AL youths are thought to mimic or model the deviant behavior of LCP youths during adolescence because they view them as successfully overcoming the frustrating gap between biological maturity (e.g., sexual and cognitive maturity) and the numerous restrictions imposed by society (e.g., financial dependency, societal pressure to delay sex, increasingly older drinking age).

The study of alcoholism also offers promising, trajectory-based frameworks (Zucker, Ellis, Fitzgerald, Bingham, & Sanford, 1996). Zucker's (1986, 1994) alcoholism model distinguishes smong four different developmental trajectories for alcoholism: (1) antisocial, (2) developmentally cumulative, (3) developmentally limited, and (4) negative affect. The different trajectories of alcoholism, which vary both in developmental onset and course of disorder, are hypothesized to have distinct etiological histories, co-occurring problems, and sequelae.

In summary, there is likely to be discontinuity as well as continuity to development. However, in an important sense, there is not discontinuity in development if there are simply systematic changes in response to circumstances during development. Interpreting such "lawful" changes as evidence for discontinuity makes the error of assuming that developmental organizations are static "entities" that either stay the same or become different entities. Referring back to the tree metaphor outlined earlier in this chapter, that model of development may be consistent with traditional psychiatric views of development, but it is not consistent with a developmental psychopathology perspective. Another common error is to assume that a failure to find statistically significant evidence for continuity means that there is discontinuity. In fact, weak measurement or inappropriate level of analysis, insufficient statistical power to detect effects, and a variety of other alternative interpretations are typically also possible. In other words, it is an error to accept the null hypothesis; that is, assume that lack of positive evidence for continuity means that there is discontinuity. Such conclusions may make for dramatic reading in discussion sections of research articles (e.g., "Our results show that temperament is discontinuous"), but may be more a matter of shedding heat than light on the issues. Of course, developmental progressions are not always slow and methodical, proceeding step-by-step in equal intervals of change over time. In some instances, and under certain circumstances, change can be more dramatic than would be predicted by past changes. This state of events does not necessarily mean change is unlawful and, in fact, such circumstances may sometimes be predictable, as has been indicated by certain nonlinear dynamic mathematical models for the influence processes in marriages and due to peers.

PERSON- AND PATTERN-BASED APPROACHES

Developmental study has typically been concerned with evaluating "average" effects. In extending the science of averages to risk models, even the most elegant explanatory proposals have considered "average" effects (Cicchetti & Rogosch, 1996). However, there are problems with examining group averages in order to define pathways of development. Patterns of adaptation and maladaptation occur at the level of the individual, not the group. Group averages may miss some of the most important interrelations among processes underlying developmental pathways. In fact, averaged results may typify not a single individual! Thus, exclusively studying development in terms of population averages at best only provides an approximation with regard to elucidating the patterns and processes of individual differences in intraindividual change (Cicchetti & Rogosch, 1996). A shift is needed in research direction, that is, a shift from treating individual differences in within-individual change as "noise" or error variance toward more concern about identifying individual differences in developmental trajectories, and patterns of individual differences in within-individual change (Magnusson & Cairns, 1996). The developmental psychopathology perspective is at the forefront in advocating this different view of the appropriate level of analysis of developmental pathways.

The pertinence of examining development from a person-oriented, rather than variable-oriented (i.e., "averaged" effects) perspective, follows from the holistic model of human functioning and development that is posited by the developmental psychopathology tradition (Bergman & Magnusson, 1997); that is, individuals are seen to function as organized wholes, developing as a totality, not as a set of separate, independently operating response dispositions (Magnusson & Cairns, 1996). Much of the discussion thus far has served to develop this point, which is hardly a new one in developmental science. The problem is that a person-oriented level of analysis is inherently difficult to achieve because it subsumes all possible variables and requires separate tests for every person, since every person is ultimately unique if measurement is entirely comprehensive. Moreover, the most familiar statistical and measurement approaches provide a variable-oriented level of analysis, rather than a person-oriented level of analysis. A partial solution is to move to the level of study of specific patterns of operating factors, as opposed to isolated variables. As progress toward this ideal, Bergman and Magnusson (1997) emphasize the importance of multivariate measurement, assessing the dimensionality of indicators, classificatory approaches to analysis (e.g., cluster analysis), studying function at the level of complex dynamic systems, and other approaches that focus on patterns of operating factors. However, they also conclude that currently available methodologies for a person-oriented level of analysis are not as sophisticated as variable-oriented approaches for comprehensively testing theoretical models or for handling measurement error, and also place higher demands on sample size and quality of measurement (e.g., measurement must be more comprehensive). Nonetheless, person-oriented approaches, even in approximations to the ideal, provide more realistic assessments of the complex, holistic processes of functioning that characterize the course of the individual's development. Obviously, however, the achievement of the measurement and statistical requirements dictated by a holistic view of development remains a goal rather than an accomplishment.

INTERPLAY BETWEEN NATURE AND NURTURE

Another fundamental question is the extent to which pathways of development can be attributed to nature and nurture. Returning to the tree metaphor, one might ask how much the growth of a tree depends upon its genetic inheritance and environmental conditions, such as soil, water, and sunlight. How much of continuity in development is due to genetic influence and how much is due to environment? In fact, the evidence suggests that genetics and environment both have ubiquitous influence on developmental processes, and support for these effects is overwhelming (Rutter et al., 1997). Behavioral genetics research, in particular, has demonstrated genetic effects on normal development and the development of psychopathology in childhood for a surprising number of traits (e.g., attitudes and beliefs, exposure to life events and experiences; Plomin, 1994a, 1995b). On the other hand, behavioral genetics research has moved beyond documenting how much population variance is due to genetics, or environment, toward elucidating the causal processes by which such influences operate. For example, while 20–60% of population variance in almost all aspects of child behavior can be attributed to genetics (Rutter et al., 1997), this does not inform us about how such influences work. Genetic, or environmental, effects do not operate in isolation, so efforts to partition the effects due to genetics, or environment, inevitably oversimplify the processes that underlie pathways of development. Thus, returning to our metaphor, there is a constant transaction between these factors during successive branchings of the limbs of the tree during development.

What do we know about genetic and environmental influences with regard to continuities and discontinuities of pathways of development? Rutter and colleagues (1997) discuss some of the current lacunae in current theory and research. First, effects are likely to be at the level of general, rather than very specific, response processes. In particular, individuals differ in their reactivity to the environment, and this has been identified as accounting for many behavioral features that underlie risk for childhood disorders (e.g., behavioral and autonomic responsivity to stress). For example, behavioral and emotional overreactivity in the face of marital conflict (e.g., increased aggressiveness) have been linked with children's adjustment problems (Davis, Hops, Alpert,

& Sheeber, 1998). On the one hand, overreactivity to marital conflict, which can take many forms (e.g., heightened emotional distress, intervention in parental disputes), has been associated with a history of marital conflict (Cummings, Zahn-Waxler, & Radke-Yarrow, 1981). On the other hand, there is also evidence of stability over time in these responses (Cummings, Iannotti, & Zahn-Waxler, 1985; Cummings, Zahn-Waxler, & Radke-Yarrow, 1984), which suggests a temperamental contribution. Second, the interplay between individuals and their environment is continual and two way. Thus, it may be assumed that biological measures reflect genetic influences, but, in fact, autonomic and other responses may be changed due to environmental events (e.g., high stress). Similarly, a common assumption is that environmental or psychological measures reflect environmental influence. However, children's difficulties (e.g., learning to read) may also be due to underlying response dispositions that are biological in origin (e.g., problems in maintaining attention to learning tasks). Moreover, the interplay of environmental experience (e.g., reduced exposure to reading material) and biological dispositions (e.g., difficulties attending) may, over time, exacerbate children's problems. A third point is that the interplay between environment and genetics must be considered within the larger, ecological context of development. For example, poverty and other social disadvantage may increase difficulties associated with family discord and other family problems, both making family problems more likely and adding to any effects of these stressors on children. Fourth, consistent with the active organism assumption of the developmental psychopathology approach, children respond at a process level to the interplay of nature and nurture; that is, they are not just passive recipients of experience. It follows that understanding the course of development needs to be addressed at a process level of analysis, beyond simply charting associations between experiential and individual characteristics. Fifth, individuals act on their environment, as well as react to it, during their development. Thus, experiential histories of risk (e.g., negative life events) are due to some individuals seeking out these experiences (i.e., nature). It follows that the effects of personal dispositions may increase, rather than decrease, with development, as individuals increasingly seek out experiences that suit their personal dispositions.

Rutter and colleagues (1997) also consider some of the main findings of research in this area, many of which are by no means obvious. For example, childhood disorders are multifactorial and involve multiple genes, not just one. Moreover, so-called genetic effects may be due to particular environmental circumstances that may be missed if environment is not measured with adequate rigor and sophistication. In addition, risk due to genetics may not present itself as a specific disease, but as a dimensional risk factor (e.g., reactivity to stress), this is a continuously distributed dimension of vulnerability. Thus, the transmission of risk across generations, and continuities in pathways of development, cannot simply be attributed to a main effect of genetics. For example, when risk is associated with problems with parents, the risk for disorder in children is nonspecific; that is, disorders in children may, or may not, be the same as the parent's problems. Thus, children of depressed parents are at greater risk for the development of broadband adjustment problems, including depression, but also a variety of other disorders (Fendrich, Warner, & Weissman, 1990). In addition, risk for disorder associated with parental psychopathology, despite a genetic component, may also be environmentally mediated. For example, parental depression may cause parents to be emotionally unavailable or otherwise to exercise less-than-optimal parenting (NICHD Early Child Care Research Network, 1999), which may increase the risk for later disorder by inducing emotional, social, and cognitive problems associated with insecure attachment (Cummings & Cicchetti, 1990; Radke-Yarrow, Cummings, Kuczynski, & Chapman, 1985; Teti, Gelfand, & Pompa, 1990). Another implication of a dimensional perspective is that risk due to genetic diathesis in many individuals may become manifest at a subclinical level (e.g., reactivity to stress with sadness and poor self-concept) rather than as a disease category. Similarly, multiple environmental events may increase risk for any particular outcome, and there may be genetic contributions to so-called environmental effects that are missed if genetic contributions are not adequately assessed.

However, the bottom line is that the evidence suggests that a complex transaction characterizes the interplay between genetics and environmental conditions during child development, and many questions remain about how to conceptualize the processes underlying person–environment interactions in normal development and the development of psychopathology, which is the level of analysis ultimately of greatest concern to the developmental psychopathologist; that is, surprisingly little is known at a process-oriented level of analysis about the causal mechanisms that describe interrelations between genetic and environmental effects. As Rutter and colleagues (1997) state:

> With regard to genetic effects . . . although there was excellent evidence that they were operative, very little was known about *which* genes were influential and *how* they were operative. Exactly the same applies to environmental factors. Very little is known on which aspects of the environment carry the risk for different types of psychopathology or what they do to the organism. (p. 343)

PERIODS AND STAGES OF DEVELOPMENT

As we have seen, the etiology of childhood disorders can be quite gradual and can be characterized in terms of stages as patterns of maladaptation unfold over time. These stages, for heuristic purposes, can be divided into periods of onset, maintenance, remission, recurrence, and termination. Of value in making these distinctions is that each of these periods may be associated with different constellations of influences, etiological mechanisms, and sequelae. For example, causes for the onset, maintenance, and remission of a disorder may be different than the causes of recurrence and termination. For example, family conflict may play an etiological role in the *onset* of conduct disorders, but peers and teachers may *maintain* or further *intensify* the problems even in the face of marked reductions in family conflict (Fincham, Grych, & Osborne, 1994; Patterson, DeBarshe, & Ramsey, 1989). However, there has been relatively little emphasis on differentiating between the processes leading to onset, maintenance, remission, and termination of maladaptive functioning or psychological disorder.

Individuals also vary in their susceptibility to maladaptation as a function of developmental period. As a case in point, children may be most vulnerable to parental depression during the periods of infancy and adolescence (Burbach & Borduin, 1986; Campbell & Cohn, 1997; Cummings & Davies, 1994b; Gelfand & Teti, 1990; LaRoche, 1989). However, cataloging age differences is a relatively imprecise step toward disentangling the developmental processes that may lead to changing risk across the course of development. Age does not explain or cause psychological continuity or change; rather, it is a global marker variable for several specific developmental processes that involve maturational, cohort, and experiential influences. Since specific developmental processes commonly interact or offset the effects of one another, focusing on age differences or changes may even mask or obscure a complex constellation of developmental processes (Rutter, 1989a).

Age differences may reflect, in part, variations in exposure to experiential influences over the life cycle. For example, adolescents of depressed parents may exhibit particularly high rates of psychopathology largely because, on average, they have been exposed to depression for a longer period of time than their younger counterparts (Cummings & Davies, 1994b). In a similar vein, infants of depressed parents may exhibit more adjustment problems than older children due to exposure to more severe stressors (e.g., increased marital distress and conflict) that arise from especially difficult family changes new parents must face (e.g., greater role demands, fatigue, less leisure time; Belsky & Rovine, 1990). Finally, another perspective on developmental pathways is a life-course view in which one considers the multiple developmental trajectories in which developmental paths of adults and children interact (Parke, 1988). In this view, multiple classes of events and transitions need to be distinguished from both the adults' and children's perspectives in examining pathways of development, including normative and non-normative events, and transitions that directly affect the child (e.g., school entry) and those that are dictated by adults (e.g., divorce, loss).

Cohort effects or secular trends may also contribute to age differences in risk (Baltes, Reese, & Nesselroade, 1988; Rutter, 1989b); that is, age differences in risk may be partly due to new sociohistorical contexts each successive generation experiences. For instance, over the last half of the century, new generations (e.g., "baby-boomers," "generation X") have had to cope with increasing rates of problems in many public health domains, ranging from depression and suicide to crime, drugs, and violence (Rutter, 1996, 1997).

Explaining this larger web of secular changes, its interplay with other developmental processes (e.g., experiential influences), and its effect on psychological functioning is a critical but alarmingly neglected task of developmental psychopathology.

Age differences may also be explained by the operation of sensitive periods, a process in which specific environmental influences become particularly salient within certain windows of development (Cicchetti, 1993). Thus, some researchers have speculated that the stress of living with a depressed parent may more easily overwhelm adolescents who, by virtue of their unique developmental status (1) are more sensitive to family distress, (2) face a number of challenging developmental tasks (e.g., career decisions, independence from parents, establishment of romantic relationships), and (3) must cope with the peak occurrence of stressful life events (Davies, Dumenci, & Windle, 1999; Davies & Windle, 1997). Nevertheless, demonstrating the existence of sensitive developmental periods is a challenging conceptual issue to say the least. Multiple domains of functioning change across developmental periods in such a way that some changes serve to protect against increasing vulnerability in other domains. Adolescents' more effective coping repertoire and extensive support networks (e.g., friends, schools, peers) may offset their developmentally linked vulnerabilities (Cummings & Davies, 1994b).

Individuals may be differentially susceptible to various forms of maladaptation across development. Whereas infants and young children are more likely to respond to stressors with temper tantrums, aggression, and oppositional behavior, older children increasingly exhibit psychological distress through dysphoria and passivity (Cummings & Davies, 1994b). This proclivity toward depressive profiles is accompanied by a greater tendency to develop negative self-cognitions and depressive disorders, particularly as children progress through adolescence (Angold & Rutter, 1992; Compas, Hinden, & Gerhardt, 1995). Similarly, rates of delinquency rise and peak during middle adolescence (Moffitt, 1993a).

Another perspective on pathways of development is that individuals face stage-salient challenges, and their relative success or failure in overcoming these tasks at the appropriate points in development is significant in determining whether problems develop or development proceeds normally. This view has a long history in psychology (Freud, Erickson), and continues to have influential adherents within the developmental psychopathology tradition (Sroufe, 1979; Sroufe & Rutter, 1984). Thus, individuals are assessed in terms of their progress in coping with stage-salient tasks. Stage-salient frameworks conceptualize development as a series of challenges that become prominent at a given period and remain important throughout an individual's lifetime (Cicchetti, 1993). These developmental challenges constitute a period of normative transition for most, if not all, individuals and require significant reorganization in functioning (Graber & Brooks-Gunn, 1996). As a result, some level of change or discontinuity is expected by definition. For example, the common task of achieving an intimate, romantic relationship in young adulthood is associated with marked declines in drug use and alcohol problems (Bachman, Johnston, O'Malley, & Schulenberg, 1996; Miller-Tutzhauer, Leonard, & Windle, 1991).

At each developmental stage, individuals are faced with resolving a number of significant tasks across several domains of functioning (e.g., social, emotional, cognitive, physiological). Since these tasks are already challenging in themselves, their successful resolution may be particularly sensitive to the effects of risk and protective factors. For example, working from the presupposition that the acquisition of affect regulation skills is a central developmental task in the toddler years, Zahn-Waxler and colleagues demonstrated that children of parents with bipolar depression exhibited more problems with affect regulation than children of nondepressed parents (Zahn-Waxler, Cummings, McKnew, & Radke-Yarrow, 1984). Affect regulation problems in toddlerhood, in turn, predicted subsequent childhood problems (e.g., school, peer, and self-image) only in offspring of depressed mothers (Zahn-Waxler, Iannotti, Cummings, & Denham, 1990). The larger promise of integrating developmental challenges in risk models has been explicitly highlighted by Graber and Brooks-Gunn (1996) in their notion of *transition-linked turning points*. Specifically, they posit that turning points, or significant life events, that occur within challenging transitional periods may have the most lasting impact on subsequent development.

In accordance with the orthogenetic principle, successful negotiation of each newly emerging developmental task is thought to depend on adequate differentiation and integration of earlier stage-salient tasks (Cicchetti, 1993). The stage termination hypothesis, which builds upon this principle, specifically proposes that earlier developmental status shapes, in large part, the way individuals cope with developmental challenges (Graber & Brooks-Gunn, 1996). For example, in order to achieve the key stage-salient task of interpersonal intimacy and caring, adolescents must draw upon and combine the increasingly diverse developmental tools forged in the process of dealing with previous (e.g., empathy, self-control, and social agency) and current (e.g., perspective taking, moral reasoning, autonomy, and relatedness) developmental challenges (Chase-Lansdale, Wakschlag, & Brooks-Gunn, 1995).

The proposed interplay among developmental tasks provides a rich breeding ground for more specific predictions about lawful process relations in the form of heterotypic continuity (Cicchetti & Toth, 1991; Waters & Sroufe, 1983). Thus, although homotypic continuity may be demonstrated by stability in the quality of friendship relations from childhood to adolescence, stage-salient frameworks also call for more hypotheses about continuity at the deeper level of the meaning and function of the behaviors. For example, successfully establishing a close, same-sex friendship in childhood may foster involvement in romantic relationships in adolescence by providing a means to address relevant stage-salient tasks such as learning about intimacy, social understanding, and perspective taking (Connolly & Johnson, 1996; Furman & Wehner, 1994). Over the long run, successful negotiation of developmental challenges at any given stage is thought to guide individuals toward progressively more adaptive developmental trajectories. Conversely, failure to resolve these tasks steers individuals toward increasingly maladaptive courses of development.

As a whole, then, the progressive accumulation of success, or failure, in coping with stage-salient tasks or developmental transitions may be a key mechanism for the process of canalization in which individuals become "stuck" in increasingly stable, diverging trajectories over the life span. Thus, proposals espousing significant discontinuity and change during developmental transitions must be balanced by the recognition that individual dispositions and unique patterns of adaptation and maladaptation may also become increasingly pronounced when people are faced with stressful developmental transitions (Graber & Brooks-Gunn, 1996). As a clear-cut illustration of this process, Caspi and Moffitt (1991) reported that facing the transition of early menarche actually "accentuated" individual differences in behavioral problems among adolescent girls.

By the same token, it is assumed that relations among developmental challenges and the development of psychopathology are probabilistic rather than deterministic in nature. Failing to resolve stage-salient tasks does not necessarily damn individuals to a life of suffering and psychopathology; nor does successfully negotiating the tasks guarantee a life of psychological health and happiness. For example, children who exhibited difficulties resolving stage-salient challenges during the preschool period (e.g., impairments in self-control, initiative, mastery, and self-reliance) were considerably more likely to "rebound" and manifest competence (i.e., peer and emotional adjustment) during the elementary school years if they successfully negotiated developmental tasks in infancy (i.e., attachment) and toddlerhood (e.g., emotion regulation, autonomy, compliance) (Sroufe, Egeland, & Kreutzer, 1990).

The prognosis during the school-age period for children who had problems resolving developmental tasks across the infancy, toddler, and preschool years was much poorer. As the Sroufe, Egeland, and Kreutzer (1990) study illustrates, charting individuals along these tasks yields multiple, diverse trajectories rather than a single, universal pathway. In keeping with the assumption of equifinality described at the outset, children may vary in the number and kind of developmental tasks they resolve and still exhibit similar profiles of competence or psychopathology, as reflected in the preschool assessment of the Sroufe and colleagues study. Conversely, as is implicit in the assumption of multifinality, children who reveal similar levels of competence (or vulnerability) in navigating their way through given developmental tasks may nonetheless develop diverse profiles of adjustment, as did the children between the preschool and childhood stages of the Sroufe and colleagues study. Are different temporal patterns of family stress responsible, in part, for different developmental trajectories? Do early histories of competence allow some poorly functioning preschoolers to rebound during childhood by actively seeking out and taking better advantage of opportunities in the school setting? Understanding the pattern and timing of etiological processes that shape these diverse developmental trajectories remains a critical task for future research from the developmental psychopathology perspective (Sroufe & Egeland, 1991; Sroufe & Jacobitz, 1989).

Finally, the temporal duration of influences may be important. Cicchetti and colleagues have offered a generic conceptual distinction between transient and enduring influences that may be usefully applied to a number of areas in developmental psychopathology (Cicchetti, 1989; Cicchetti & Toth, 1995). Enduring factors, which have a relatively long life span, may be constitutional (e.g., difficult or easy temperament), psychosocial (e.g., secure vs. insecure attachment patterns), or ecological (e.g., dangerous or close-knit neighborhoods and schools). As short-term, temporary "states," transient factors also fall within a range of domains, including constitutional (e.g., physical illness or health), psychosocial (e.g., marital discord or harmony), and ecological (e.g., school transitions). However, enduring factors are not inherently more powerful than transient factors in predicting the development of psychopathology. For example, transient bouts of severe stress may have a more profound impact on an individual's development than some enduring factors.

CONCLUSION

Developmental psychopathology is concerned with charting the causes, processes, and pathways of normal and abnormal development across the life span. Thus, the focus on deviations from the normal course of development differentiates developmental psychopathology from developmental psychology. At the same time, the focus on the course and mechanisms involved in the developmental transitions from (1) normal to abnormal development and (2) abnormal to normal development differentiates it from the primary concern of abnormality within clinical psychology and psychiatry. These concerns are pertinent to directions that focus on both genetic (Rende & Plomin, 1990) and environmental contributions to continuities and discontinuities in development; ideally, of course, research will come to consider both genetic and environmental causes, and their interplay, within integrative research designs (Rutter et al., 1997).

With regard to pathways of development, developmental psychopathology has been influenced in large part by the contextualistic philosophy that likens normal and abnormal development to a living organism. As we have seen, the branching tree metaphor described by Sroufe offers a useful way of thinking about development from an contextualistic perspective. From this viewpoint, individuals are viewed as actively contributing to their own development in the sense that they construct their knowledge and interpretations, and seek out and modify the contexts in which they live. Developmental pathways can be thought of in terms of the successive branchings toward or away from the trunk, with the trunk serving to represent normative development. Development is thus holistic and can only be truly understood within the larger intra-, inter-, and extrapersonal contexts in which it occurs (i.e., the entire tree and the environment that supports its growth). According to the orthogenetic principle, psychological systems move from relatively simple, global organizations to more complex, interrelated systems consisting of multiple dimensions, levels, and hierarchies. Through this process, development can take the form of quantitative (e.g., increases or decreases in preexistent functioning) or qualitative (e.g., emergence of novel forms of functioning) change. The principle of developmental pluralism posits that multiple, reciprocal causes guide individuals along multiple trajectories that become more diverse as development progresses. Studying age differences in risk only constitutes the "tip of the iceberg" because they only identify marker variables indexing a number of developmental processes such as different experiential histories, secular trends, sensitive periods of development, and the progression of new "stage-salient" tasks or developmental challenges. Moreover, one of the most essential directions of research for the future is to develop person- or patterned-based approaches that emphasize individual differences in developmental pathways.

The primary goal of theories and conceptual models in this field is to translate these abstract themes into concrete ways of understanding topical areas in developmental psychopathology. Obviously, process-oriented research on pathways of development is at a relatively early stage. However, even the beginning conceptual and empirical ground that has been won constitutes heartening progress. In the next chapter, we consider additional principles from the developmental psychopathology (Cicchetti & Cohen, 1995b) and related (e.g., developmental science; Cairns, Elder, & Costello, 1996) traditions, specifically the even more sophisticated model of development introduced by the constructs of resiliency and protective factors, and more toward an even fuller development of how to think about and study the etiology of childhood disorder.

❖ CHAPTER FIVE

Complex Patterns of Influence: Risk and Protective Factors

*T*he model of human development that is espoused by the developmental psychopathology tradition is quite sophisticated and proposes new ways of thinking about clinical problems in human development. The assumptions and propositions of this approach demand much more of the clinical researcher and practitioner than traditional approaches to the science and practice of psychopathology as guided by the medical model. For example, causal models have traditionally been assumed to be linear, that is, moving in a relatively straightforward fashion from cause to effect, with emphasis placed on the search for single causal agents that can account for discrete diagnostic outcomes. By contrast, the developmental psychopathologist is concerned with the search for the dynamic mediating processes that account for patterns of adaptation and maladaptation over time. Moreover, causal models are not linear, but transactional, with bidirectional or reciprocal patterns of effect among the multiple elements of the model accounting for children's functioning over time (Cowan, Cowan, & Schulz, 1996).

Given the complexity of the issues, a restatement of where we are at this point in the formulation of the principles of developmental psychopathology merits consideration. To recap, a developmental psychopathology perspective emphasizes dynamic processes of interaction between multiple intra- and extraorganismic factors. Relatedly, as illustrated in Figure 3.1, the study of process is assumed to require the examination of multiple domains and responses (e.g., cognitive, emotional, physiological) that may mediate relations between influences on development and child outcomes. One implication is that clinical research is required to do more than paper-and-pencil assessments or even clinical interviews; that is, observational and laboratory research are needed. Ultimately, the study of process can be no more cogent than the appropriateness and rigor of the measurement of the variables that are entered into statistical equations. Moreover, while new, advanced statistical methodologies invoke language that suggests that causality is established, the "logic that supports causal inferences should not be confused with the controlled, experimental study so familiar to psychologists" (Fincham, 1994, p. 125).

Contextual factors associated with person–environment interactions are also assumed to underlie process. While mapping the complex pattern of influences on development is a step in the right direction (see Figure 3.1), even this level of analysis is not sufficient, since children's reactions may depend more upon their perceptions and cognitions about events than upon "objective" events themselves. For example, the meaning and interpretation that children ascribe to marital conflict and violence in the broader context of the family is at least as significant as the occurrence of particular interparental behaviors (Cummings, 1998a, 1998b; Fincham, 1998). Moreover, the pattern of events, rather than which specific events occur, may also be important, reflecting the role of mediating cognitive processes. Thus, children may evidence few negative effects from exposure to high levels of marital conflict even if parents are very expressive and emotional during conflicts, but usually resolve their disagreements (Davies & Cummings, 1994). On the other hand, children may have great difficulty adjusting when parents rarely fight openly, but the occurrence of conflict seems to carry serious implications for the future intactness of the family, for example, when conflicts include parental threats to leave (Laumakis, Margolin, & John, 1998).

As we have noted, emphasis is also placed on the study of developmental processes underlying both normal development and the development of adjustment problems, with the assumption that a focus only on extremes provides a limited window into mediating processes. Again, taking the example of marital conflict, specific types and intensities of conflict have been shown to elicit very different responses from children (Cummings & Davies, 1994). Thus, a focus on one element of conflict (e.g., overt violence) yields limited information about the effects of conflict and violence on children, and a potentially narrow, even misleading, perspective on key mediating processes and developmental sequelae. Thus, it is important to examine a continuum of effects; studies of harmonious and adverse family contexts are expected to be mutually informative and essential to the understanding of processes underlying the effects of marital conflict on children.

Finally, the developmental psychopathology approach emphasizes thinking about development in terms of pathways rather than end points. Put another way, individual development is conceptualized in terms of moving pictures rather than static snaphots, the clear implication being that individuals may potentially move in an out of diagnostic classifications over time (Cowan, Cowan, & Schulz, 1996). Accordingly, clinical diagnoses become no more than a useful shorthand for characterizing a child's status at one point in time and may or may not be informative as to the child's clinical status in the future; that is, some clinically significant effects that emerge over time may not be evident as clinically significant early in development (i.e., "sleeper" effects). For example, a young child exposed to marital violence may appear to be functioning well, even extraordinarily well. Thus, it is not uncommon for children from high-conflict homes to act as "caretakers" for their parents, comforting them following conflicts, acting as confidants, and taking care of household chores. These behaviors and the role played by children within the family may give the appearance to an outside observer that the child is functioning exceptionally well. However, the role of caretaker is likely to place undue burdens on children and may contribute to the development of problems that emerge later, even much later, in development. Thus, children's mediation in parental conflict has been linked with later adjustment problems (Cummings & Davies, 1994), illustrating "sleeper" effects.

However, the developmental psychopathology approach emphasizes the need for even more complexity in conceptualizing processes underlying normal development and the development of psychopathology than we have already described. Traditional research on psychopathology and clinical practice focused on risk, stress, and adversity but neglected positive processes and events. The developmental psychopathology perspective also calls attention to the significance of positive events to understanding development in adverse family circumstances. The concepts of resiliency, compensatory factors, and protective factors, in particular, are important for understanding the role of positive processes in children's functioning. Furthermore, from the standpoint of understanding process, children who do not develop problems despite growing up in high-risk environments are just as interesting as those who do; that is, there may be "good" outcomes from apparently "bad" environments. What protective factors, or personal or environmental sources of resiliency, account for children's adaptive outcomes in very adverse circumstances?

On the other hand, children from apparently "good" environments may develop "bad" outcomes. Understanding developmental processes among these children is also necessary and may shed light on processes underlying the development of maladjustment. What stress factors or personal or environmental sources of vulnerability explain why some children have difficulty when most children living in similar environments, even siblings in the same family, do not? As with other elements of the developmental psychopathology model, resiliency is conceptualized as a dynamic process that unfolds over time and in the course of development, as opposed to a static trait. Cicchetti and Garmezy (1993) summarized this perspective in the following way:

> By uncovering the mechanisms and processes that lead to competent adaptation despite the presence of adversity, our understanding of both normal development and psychopathology is enhanced. Within this context, it is important that neither adaptive, maladaptive, nor resilient functioning be viewed as a static condition but, rather, as being in dynamic transaction with intra- and extra-organismic forces. (p. 499)

However, a question here needs to be addressed: How much do we need to recast the model in Figure 3.1 to take into account protective factors? Is "resilience" a special case that needs special elaboration, or is it merely a type of outcome that can be incorporated somehow within a general model of process-oriented development? Both conceptual and statistical issues are raised by these questions. In this chapter, we explore these matters concerning concepts of risk, vulnerability, and protective factors, and take a position on a somewhat controversial issue: How special is the "special case" of resilience?

RESILIENCE

Theoretical Definition

A long-standing challenge in the study of developmental psychopathology has been the translation of abstract concepts into empirically testable theories and hypotheses. In a special section of *Developmental Psychology* devoted to dialogue on the implications of developmental themes for research, Robert Cairns (1991) succinctly diagnosed the problem by stating that "the revolutionary implications of the developmental perspective have been blurred by weak metaphors and trivialized by vague statements of 'interaction' and 'organization'" (p. 23). As a consequence, explaining how these themes influence the development of theory and hypotheses in substantive areas of developmental psychopathology sometimes has become lost in the shuffle. Thus, it is not surprising that developmental scientists have issued calls to "go beyond the metatheoretical framework to a more precise theoretical exposition that applies to human development" (Gottlieb, 1991b, p. 33). Cicchetti and Garmezy (1993) underscore this point:

> Perhaps first and foremost, researchers must clearly operationalize their definition of resilience. At present, various researchers employ different definitions of resilience that can range from the absence of psychopathology to the recovery of a brain-injured patient. Definitional diversity results in sometimes disparate profiles of competent adaptation as well as different estimates of rates of resilience among similar risk groups. Depending on how broad or conservative the definition of resilience is, vastly different conclusions can be drawn. (p. 499)

There is a consensus that resilience is about children functioning well in the face of adversity. Thus, Masten, Best, and Garmezy (1990) state that "resilience refers to the process of, capacity for, or outcome of successful adaptation despite challenging or threatening circumstances" (p. 425). However, the question arises as to whether resilience is limited only to individuals under high risk and how that is defined. As Egeland, Carlson, and Sroufe (1993) put the matter, "Resilience is often conceptualized as the positive end of the distribution of developmental outcomes in a sample of high-risk individuals

(Rutter, 1990). While these definitions are accepted by researchers of risk and resilience, factors defining risk samples and definitions of adaptation and competence vary widely across studies" (p. 517). If it is accepted that psychological development is generally resilient, then why should resilience be limited to only certain groups?

Fitting Resilience into Process Models

Process models or theories may provide a key to tying the abstract metatheoretical themes such as resilience to more concrete, substantive models of developmental psychopathology. An assessment should be made of how varying concepts of resilience fit into standard process-oriented models and statistical methodologies used to analyze these models. In particular, it is important to move away from the romantic view of resilience as akin to "invulnerability," that is, a static, trait-like construct that identifies those individuals capable of function adaptively, or even in a superior fashion, in the face of all odds. Resilience is not unidimensional, nor is it an all-or-none phenomenon (Luthar, Doernberger, & Zigler, 1993).

In attempting to conceptualize how matters fit into a broader scheme at the level at which analyses of mediating processes can be conducted, one may be able to come to some decisions about how these matters may be addressed. Process models underscore the view that a specified set of factors leads to a particular developmental course and a given outcome. The goal of these models, then, is to help guide the study of developmental pathways to maladaptive and adaptive outcomes. In developmental psychopathology, the most useful and promising process models typically take the form of transactional models (Sameroff, 1995). Rather than conceptualizing the development of psychopathology as simple, additive relationships among factors, transactional models underscore the fact that maladaptive and adaptive trajectories of development are the result of dynamic (i.e., changing), bidirectional relations between experiential (e.g., quality of family context, peer relations) and organismic factors (e.g., temperament, genetic and constitutional makeup). Accordingly, notions of risk, protective factors, and resilience need to be considered in terms of such models. We consider each of these elements in turn in the context of the notion of process models.

THE CONCEPTUALIZATION OF RISK

Multivariate Matrix of Risk and Process

Simply conceptualizing links between a particular risk factor or a combination of risk factors and child outcomes is only the first step among many in formulating transactional risk models (Fincham, 1994; Rutter, 1994). Concepts of holism and developmental pluralism underscore the view that any risk factor or group of risk factors must be considered in a larger biopsychosocial context. Moreover, a complex myriad of risk and protective factors operates over time in human development, with the etiology of disorder an outcome of a combination of risk and protective factors of diverse sorts. Thus, as Cowan, Cowan, and Schulz (1996) note:

> Risks predispose individuals and populations (identifiable as groups of people) to specific negative or undesirable outcomes. . . . The magnitude of risk is measured as the probability of a specific negative outcome in a population when the risk is present, compared with the probability when it is absent, or as a correlation between risk and outcomes measured as continuous rather than categorical variables. . . . Traditionally, risk was conceived in static terms as a marker, a stressor, or a "factor" predicting undesirable outcomes. . . . Risks should be thought of as process. The active ingredients of a risk do not lie in the variable itself, but in the set of processes that flow from the variable, linking specific risk conditions with specific dysfunctional outcomes. (p. 9)

For example, children exposed to parental psychopathology (e.g., parent depression, alcoholism) do not experience this risk in a psychological vacuum. Instead, parental psychopathology is probabilistically linked with the co-occurrence of numerous familial (e.g., parenting impairments, disturbances in parent–child relations, marital discord), sociocultural (e.g., poverty, community isolation, poor social support networks), and biological and constitutional factors (e.g., genetic diathesis, birth complications, difficult temperament) (Cummings & Davies, 1994b, 1999). These factors, in turn, may add to or account for the risk of children growing up in depressive or alcoholic families.

Process models are also geared toward unraveling the multidimensional complexities of risk factors that may appear on the surface to be homogeneous. For example, representing parental depression as a single risk factor in theoretical models does not mean it is unidimensional. The diagnosis itself can vary considerably in terms of form (e.g., bipolar, unipolar, postpartum), frequency, severity, duration, time of onset, and recurrence. With all else being equal, different manifestations of psychologically significant symptoms (e.g., dysphoria, vegetative symptoms, interpersonal problems, lack of motivation) can underlie identical clinical diagnoses. The manifestations of depression differ and the experience of children also differs as a function of timing in development, parental behavior, and child characteristics. Variations in the underlying organization of multidimensional risk factors such as depression have been shown have different implications for developmental outcome (Campbell, Cohn, & Meyers, 1995; NICHD Early Child Care Research Network, 1999; Radke-Yarrow, Nottleman, Belmont, & Welsh, 1993; Seifer, 1995).

In a similar vein, many of the conceptualizations of environmental influences on development simply compare or contrast children along molar dimensions of geography, ethnicity, family structure (e.g., single parents), and social background (e.g., poverty) (Bronfenbrenner, 1986). While these models provide us with a general "social address," they tell us little in terms of the more precise, proximal characteristics and conditions of interpersonal contexts that influence development (e.g., family processes, peer relations).

This is not to say that researchers who study inter- and intrapersonal processes are any more immune to the traps of "social address" thinking than those studying community- or cultural-level variables. Prototypes of "social address" thinking are found at all levels of developmental psychopathology. In the substantive area of family psychology, many so-called family process models fail to make distinctions between the very different experiences each family member has while living under the same roof (Pike, McGuire, Hetherington, Reiss, & Plomin, 1996; Wachs, 1996). As such, they tend to address the experiences shared by family members rather than nonshared aspects of the familial environment. However, even siblings who are close in age may have diverse family experiences that have quite powerful effects on their development (McGue, Sharma, & Benson, 1996). For example, research has shown that parents do treat their children differently. With the exception of twins, siblings may have different experiences in the family because they (1) entered and progressed through the family at different times (i.e., cohort effects), or (2) possess different sensitivities, skills, and coping repertoires by virtue of their different developmental levels or dispositions (e.g., temperament) (Wachs, 1996). Boys and girls also experience family events differently.

In summary, a better understanding of the factors and processes that might account for risk requires both (1) a broad focus on mapping the multivariate nature of risk contexts, and (2) a fine-grained focus on distinguishing between diverse constellations of risk processes. However, the co-occurrence of risk and protective factors often makes the task of disentangling underlying influences on outcomes difficult.

The Conceptual Ordering of Risk Process

Exposure to risk does not predetermine the occurrence of psychopathology; that is, risk will not necessarily be translated into a specific maladaptive outcome for children. Heterogeneity of developmental outcomes is the rule even with exposure to some of the most robust risk factors. For example, although parental depression is considered a robust risk factor, children of depressed parents exhibit a wide range of both adaptive and maladaptive outcomes (e.g., internalizing symptomatology, externalizing problems, academic impairments). The demonstration of multifinality across several types of risk contexts underscores the significance of the next major component in building process models: accounting for when, how, and why only some children exposed to risk develop problems. Instead, children exposed to similar constellations of risk factors develop along multiple trajectories ranging from extreme maladaptation to adaptation and competence. Since risk factors vary in the nature and extent of their causal relations to developmental outcomes, specification of process requires imposing some conceptual or etiological order to the catalog of risk factors in the multivariate web.

MEDIATORS AND MODERATORS: TESTING NOTIONS OF RESILIENCE IN PROCESS MODELS

Mediational Pathways: The "How" and "Why" of Developmental Psychopathology

Mediational models provide answers to the question of "how" and "why" risk conditions lead to maladaptive outcomes. Mediators are the "generative mechanism" by which an independent variable (e.g., parental depression) influences outcomes (e.g., child adjustment) (Baron & Kenny, 1986). Mediators, by definition, are conceptualized as explaining, at least in part, how and why risk factors (e.g., parental depression) lead to maladaptive outcomes (e.g., adjustment problems). In other words, the fundamental aim is to delineate the processes that account for the linkage between a particular risk factor (or set of risk factors) and psychological problems (Baron & Kenny, 1986). Rather than searching for a single causal mechanism that accounts for the impact of a risk factor, a major assumption in developmental psychopathology is that *multiple* causal mechanisms may be operating in complex chains (see Figure 3.1).

Returning to the example of parental depression, the goal would be to describe precisely the mechanisms by which parental depression leads to child behavior problems. The key here is the word *precisely*: Taking notions of holism and developmental pluralism to the extreme leads to loose, uninformative conclusions that "everything relates to everything else." Narrowing the scope (i.e., the range of psychological events explained) of the model is thus necessary to achieve greater precision in explaining mediating processes. For example, Cummings and Davies (1994b, 1999) acknowledged the important role of biological and genetic processes underlying the risk of parental depression, but narrowed the scope of their model to address interpersonal mechanisms that mediate links between parental depression and children's functioning.

Figure 5.1 illustrates their interpersonal model of parental depression, providing a framework for a process-oriented conceptualization of risk applied to the specific case of the effects of parental depression on children. The first relevant component of the model is the risk factor itself (i.e., parental depression). Within interpersonal models, parental depression may be directly experienced by children; that is, children may be influenced by exposure to the characteristics of depression in parents (i.e., their depressive symptomatology) (Cohn & Tronick, 1983, 1989; Field, 1992), but this influence is only one of many possible influences on child outcomes. The goal then is to delineate the interpersonal pathways by which parental depression leads to child outcomes. The risk factor in the mediational models, then, is more precisely referred to as the *distal, marker,* or *exogenous* variable to denote that it is farthest from the dependent or outcome variable in the etiological matrix.

The second component of interest is the class of mediating events. Mediators, by definition, are conceptualized as explaining (at least in part) precisely how and why distal variables increase children's risk for psychopathology. In Figure 5.1, expressions of family discord (e.g., parental characteristics, par-

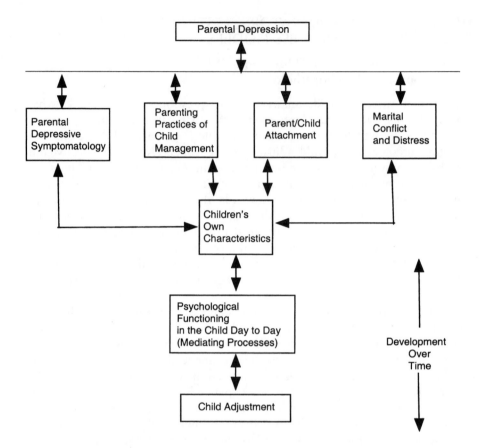

FIGURE 5.1. A developmental psychopathology framework for the multiple interpersonal and intrapersonal mediators of the effects of parental depression on children within the family.

ent–child relations, marital functioning) and child characteristics (e.g., temperament) constitute types of mediating events. More specifically, parental depression is hypothesized to be associated with characteristics of family discord in complex, reciprocal ways. By virtue of this co-occurrence, children's exposure to family discord, in turn, is posited to directly compromise children's psychological health and thus account for risk in children with depressed parents. However, these events are still relatively distal from the processes that characterize children's functioning; that is, we are still at the level of characterizing important groupings or classes of influence, but not at the level of specifying the response processes in children that ultimately lead to adaptive or maladaptive outcomes.

As Figure 5.1 illustrates, multiple, rather than single, mediator models are being enlisted increasingly to characterize the multiplicity of pathways and chains of influence in substantive areas of developmental psychopathology (Windle & Davies, 1999). Thus, although single mediator models may be especially valuable as exploratory tools in discovering the potential significance of family processes, such models must ultimately be embedded in the larger ecological and constitutional context of development. For example, although early research on family contexts of parental depression were invaluable in underscoring the potential relevance of marital discord as a mediator of the risk posed by parental depression to children, the focus on single, specific mediational pathways limited conclusions about the conceptual placement of marital conflict in models of depression (Downey & Coyne, 1990). In integrating this chain of processes within larger ecological, familial, and developmental models, the move to more complex mediational models has permitted a more fine-grained account of the direct and indirect pathways of parental depression and marital discord in the development of adaptation and maladaptation (e.g., Conger et al., 1992; Davies & Windle, 1997).

While increases in the theoretical precision and detail of mediational models accrue by narrowing the scope of inquiry, advances in precision must always be kept "in check," with an eye toward the bigger theoretical picture. Principles of floating holism and developmental pluralism dictate that conceptualizations of cause, process, and effect are relative and often interchangeable depending on the scope and purpose of the mediational model (e.g., Emery, Fincham, & Cummings, 1992). For example, a myopic focus on interpersonal models can lead to the conclusion that mediating events or classes of events linking parental psychopathology to child outcome only reflect environmental processes (e.g., parenting, family conflict) despite compelling support for the mutual influence of genetic substrates as key mediators in offspring risk (Rende & Plomin, 1993), particularly in the example of parental depression (Harrington et al., 1993). Genetic influences affect both risk for psychopathology and interactional processes within the family.

Even within the same conceptual model, conceptual roles of key mediating constructs are not independent and may be multidetermined. Thus, different familial processes may each affect children's specific processes of adaptation to family events. However, the level of children's responding in the context of daily events and situations is the most proximal level of analysis for characterizing their patterns of adaptation or maladaptation (see Figures 3.1 and 5.1). For example, children's attributions of responsibility for parental functioning may be affected by multiple aspects of the elements of family functioning outlined in Figure 5.1, and (hypothetically) these response patterns are ultimately what account for children's adjustment problems. Thus, at a different level of analysis, developmental psychopathologists may strive to account for the role of attributions of personal responsibility as a process mediating relations between family discord and the development of psychopathology in children (e.g., Cummings & Davies, 1995). It may be that children's overresponsibility for others' distress mediates the effects of family discord on their adjustment, even without considering reactions to parental depression.

On the other hand, parental depression may also influence children's perceptions of personal responsibility for their parents' functioning. Studying either pathway in itself may provide a useful explanation in terms of models of mediating processes, although considering both sets of pathways together is likely ultimately to provide a more powerful prediction. However, as a practical concern, it may not be possible to examine both pathways of influence on adjustment in the same study, or even in the same set of studies. On the other hand, over time, more complex models for adjustment via these attributions may be derived as increasingly complex sets of influences are added to the conceptual model. As a result, embedding the evaluation of specific models in holistic theories that recognize the complex, time-varying, and transactional nature of causality is an essential task in developmental psychopathology. But the bottom line is that one needs to define and characterize how children's adaptive functioning in daily contexts is affected (e.g., recall the stress and coping metaphor for processes of responding to daily events). Thus, marital conflict, parenting, and other factors are classes of events in a chain that ultimately accounts for children's functioning, but do not actually mediate that functioning in a process-oriented sense. Later, we review evidence suggesting that children's emotional security is one type of process mediator that is multiply affected by family events associated with parental depression. However, we save that topic for a later discussion.

Moderator Pathways: "Who" Is at Risk and "When" Does It Occur?

Moderator models work from the assumption that the nature and degree of any risk–child psychopathology relationship is not necessarily uniform across different conditions or people. Moderators specify the strength and/or direction of relations between an independent variable (e.g., parental depression) and an outcome (e.g., child adjustment) (Baron & Kenny, 1986; Holmbeck, 1997). Moderators reflect the fact that the nature and degree of risk is not necessarily uniform across different conditions and people. For example, children's gender may serve as moderators of relations between family functioning associated with parental depression and child adjustment. In addition to specifying "who" is at risk, moderator models may also reflect "when" risk occurs. For example, risk for adjustment problems in children of depressed parents may be disproportionately greater when multiple family systems are dysfunctional (e.g., marital and parent–child relations) than when only one system is deviant. Thus, like mediating pathways, moderator models move beyond simply documenting bivariate relations with the goal of specifying the conditions under which risk factors most powerfully predict children's developmental outcomes (Baron & Kenny, 1986). Two of the most common moderator models in developmental psychopathology consist of (1) the synergistic or multiplicative effects model and (2) the organism–environment interaction model (e.g., Rutter, 1983).

Toward the goal of identifying "when," or more specifically, under what conditions, risk factors have their most powerful effects, synergistic models specify that the co-occurrence of two or more factors incurs a greater deleterious impact than the sum of the factors considered in isolation from each other (e.g., Pellegrini, 1990; Rae-Grant, Thomas, Offord, & Boyle, 1989; Rutter, 1983). As a result, one factor, or a set of factors, may potentiate or exponentially increase the risk of another factor. In a classic demonstration of this model, Rutter, Tizard, Yule, Graham, and Whitmore (1977) found that risk for psychopathology in children exposed to any one of six family risk factors (e.g., family discord, maternal psychiatric disorder, family dissolution) in isolation was comparable to risk for children who experienced no risk factors. However, experiencing two or three risk factors increased the incidence of children's psychiatric disturbance threefold (6% vs. 2%), with still another exponential increase in disturbance with exposure of four risk factors (20%).

Since synergistic models do not take a single, uniform pattern, a critical task of risk research is to specify the exact nature of the synergistic effect (Rutter & Pickles, 1991). Whereas the Rutter and colleagues (1977) study showed that none of the six family problems could be considered risk factors by themselves, other models of developmental psychopathology may be best described as interactions between "provoking agents" that have a direct, precipitating impact on the development of psychopathology even by themselves, and "vulnerability factors" that pose no direct risk on their own but catalyze the deleterious effects of provoking agents (Brown & Harris, 1978; Goodyer, 1990; Rutter, 1983). For example, lack of a confiding relationship has been shown to be a vulnerability factor in the development of depression in adult females; while posing no risk in and of itself, it seems to catalyze the already potent impact of stressful life events (Goodyer, 1990).

As another class of moderator models, organism–environment interaction or diathesis–stress frameworks seek to answer the question of who is specifically at risk. The organism component consists of vulnerable, personological characteristics such as personality differences, attributional patterns, or coping patterns (Wachs, 1991a; Windle & Tubman, 1999). However, just because organismic factors are within the person does not mean they are equivalent to constitutional or genetic effects; rather, they are more appropriately considered as inextricable by-products of transactions between environmental and genetic forces (Sroufe & Egeland, 1991; Wachs, 1991b).

The stress or environmental component, by contrast, reflects exposure to stressful events in the environment. When integrated together, such models posit that individuals with certain intrapersonal attributes respond differently, or more specifically, with greater maladaptation, to similar environmental contexts. For example, models focusing on the link between depressed parents and child outcomes have proposed that children with difficult temperamental styles (i.e., diathesis) may exhibit greater vulnerability in depressive family contexts (i.e., the stress) than children with easy temperamental styles by virtue, in part, of their greater reactivity to negative family characteristics

(Cummings & Davies, 1994b, 1999). As a complement to these organismic specificity models (Thompson, 1986; Wachs & Gandour, 1983), "goodness of fit" models provide another useful subset of organismic–environment interactions. Specifically, they suggest that certain personological characteristics become particularly potent risk factors when they are inconsistent with the expectations, demands, or pressures of the context (Lerner, 1983; Windle et al., 1986). For example, greater discrepancies between children's behavioral styles (e.g., negative mood, withdrawal) and parental expectations for behavior have been linked with teacher reports of lower levels of social and academic adjustment (Lerner & Lerner, 1989).

Multiple moderator models have also proven useful in incorporating principles of contextual and ecological relativism in substantive areas of research. In alcohol conceptualizations, protective factors, such as a good parent–adolescent relationship, have been tacitly treated as if they were static "traits" that retained their buffering power across contexts (Hawkins, Catalano, & Miller, 1992). More dynamic, contextual models, however, underscore that the nature of the moderating effect of any factor depends on the larger ecological context. For example, in a recent study, Andrews, Hops, and Duncan (1997) found that adolescents who had a good relationship with their parents were more likely to model parent alcohol and substance use. Thus, in alcoholic or drug-using families, strong bonds between parents and adolescents may increase, not decrease, their vulnerability, at least in certain domains of functioning such as drug use.

In life-span conceptualizations of the processes underlying alcoholism in old age, the revised tension reduction hypothesis suggests that the moderating role of alcohol consumption in the link between stressful life events and psychological distress among older adults varies as a complex function of the perceived value of the social domain or role. Thus, recent work suggests that the way in which alcohol consumption affects the strength of the relationship between stressful life events and psychological distress (i.e., the nature of the moderating effect) depends on the larger social context, or what is termed a "hierarchical moderator." One hypothesis is that alcohol, as a means of escape, is effective in coping with stressors that are less threatening to self-identity (i.e., less salient), but when stressors are threatening to self (i.e., salient role), alcohol consumption hinders the direct use of problem-solving strategies necessary to alter the stressor and its negative effects. Consistent with this "double moderator" proposition, recent results suggest that (1) the deleterious impact of salient role stressors on emotional adjustment in the elderly is exacerbated under conditions of high alcohol consumption; and, in contrast, (2) high alcohol consumption serves as a buffer or protector factor by lessening the impact of nonsalient stressors on emotional adjustment in elderly populations (Krause, 1995). Therefore, alcohol use in an elderly sample is not a fixed, static protective or risk factor, but is best conceptualized as dynamic, with the risk or protective value of alcohol gaining meaning from the larger context.

Mediated Moderation and Moderated Mediation: Why Are People Vulnerable Only under Certain Conditions?

Thus, because moderator models tackle the question of "who is at risk" and "when is the risk most potent," they are potentially useful in providing a basis for the study of process. However, to examine response processes as a function of groups, another step is needed; that is, notions of moderator and mediator models need to be integrated into the same model. In such instances, moderator models serve as a foundation for answering the mediator question of why people possessing certain characteristics or experiencing certain conditions are more vulnerable to disorder (Rutter, 1983; Rutter & Pickles, 1991). This process of integrating moderator and mediator models has been termed "mediated moderation" and "moderated mediation" (Baron & Kenny, 1986). Notably, for the present discussion, assessment of moderations in statistical models in this way can determine whether certain groups are more, or less, affected by a family event or other influences in the prediction of adjustment as a function of specific, or classes of, response processes. In other words, analyses of grouping variables (e.g., maltreated vs. nonmaltreated children) can permit a determination of differential risk, or differential protection, in the context of a process-oriented model (e.g., Figure 3.1).

For example, Barrera, Li, and Chassin (1995) first identified ethnicity and parental alcoholism status as moderators of the relationship between stressful life events and adolescent psychological functioning. These findings specifically indicated that (1) adolescent children of alcoholics (COAs) exhibited greater vulnerability to stressful life events than non-COAs, and (2) Caucasian adolescents were at greater risk for developing problems in the face of stressful life events than Hispanic adolescents. However, moving a step further, they attempted to account for why these groups were at greater risk. Illustrating moderated mediation, a model was supported whereby the greater vulnerability of COAs to stressful life events could not be explained by greater risk of accompanying family conflict. On the other hand, in this case, Caucasian adolescents appeared to be more susceptible to stress than Hispanic adolescents by virtue of the stronger association between stressful life events and family conflict. Because the explanatory mechanisms for the moderation took place at the beginning of the process chain, this illustrated mediated moderation (see Baron & Kenny, 1986).

Although these two models are likely to prove quite useful in elucidating the specificity of pathways among risk, process, and outcome, they certainly do not exhaust the number of possible ways to conceptualize the integration of mediator and moderator models in developmental psychopathology. For example, while studies have consistently shown that maternal depressive symptoms predict psychological maladjustment for girls, but not boys, during adolescence (Hops, 1995, in press), simply ending inquiry at the conclusion that gender is a moderator of maternal depressive symptoms is inherently unsatisfying without an understanding of why. In the search for process explanations for this result, Davies and Windle (1997) found that adolescent girls' greater vulnerability to family discord may account for (or mediate) the gender-specific effects of maternal depressive symptoms on their psychological adjustment. However, even when complex forms of mediated moderation are indicated, they only constitute an initial foray as the principle of floating holism, then move the search for mechanisms toward explaining why, for example, girls are more sensitive to family discord. Key questions posed might then include the following: Is this vulnerability due to the observation that the origins of girls' self-esteem are more heavily grounded in close interpersonal relationships (Josephs, Markus, & Tafarodi, 1992)? Could the mechanisms lie in adolescent girls' tendencies to ruminate over negative family events, feel "caught" in family problems, or become enmeshed in problems of other family members (Chase-Lansdale, Wakschlag, & Brooks-Gunn, 1995; Josephs, Markus, & Tafarodi, 1992)? These questions highlight the various levels of complexity inherent in these models.

PROTECTIVE FACTORS AND THE "SPECIAL CASE" OF RESILIENCE

The previous discussion provides a basis for testing models of differential risk for different groups as a function of processes of responding to events. The groundwork is also laid by this discussion for a consideration of differential protection, which in the case of high-risk groups is interpreted as evidence for resilience.

Resilience and Competence

While mediator and moderator models of risk are critical aspects of transactional models, they hold only one key to unraveling the mysteries of developmental psychopathology. Risk, by definition, reflects the notion that children experiencing a particular risk factor have an increased probability of experiencing psychological problems; it does not denote that all or most children at risk will develop psychopathology. For example, as already discussed, even though children of depressed parents are two to five times more likely to develop behavior problems than children of nondepressed parents, the majority of them develop along normal, adaptive developmental trajectories (Cummings & Davies, 1994b). As we have noted, a complex myriad of risk and protective factors operates over time in the course of human development, with many children developing adaptively despite exposure to conditions of risk. Thus, a focus on risk is logically complemented by a study of resilience in order to understand why many children develop competently and adapt successfully to life's challenges under highly adverse conditions (Egeland, Carlson, & Sroufe, 1993; Masten & Coatsworth, 1995; Windle, 1999). But the question remains: Is resilience only a special case for certain groups?

Risk: A Prerequisite of Resilience?

Since resilience, by definition, cannot occur without some appreciable risk, the occurrence of resilience first requires careful documentation of the presence of risk. Thus, the primary challenge is to distinguish between two general groups of competent children: (1) relatively "normal" children, who after careful investigation were found to have actually experienced minimal or no adverse conditions, and (2) resilient children, who developed relatively normally in the face of considerable risk (Garmezy, 1985; Luthar, 1993; Masten, Best, & Garmezy, 1990). Actually, it is not a simple matter to determine who has experienced "considerable risk." For example, it cannot merely be assumed that children of depressed parents who develop along adaptive trajectories are resilient (Cicchetti & Garmezy, 1993). Many of these competent children may, in fact, be experiencing benign or even healthy contexts of development characterized by parental warmth, effective child management techniques (e.g., consistent discipline, close supervision), safe and supportive neighborhoods, and high-quality schools. This is just one of the problems with a "considerable risk" criterion for the demonstration of resiliency.

This problem of determining "considerable risk" is equally relevant to genetic and organismic factors (see Rende & Plomin, 1993). Offspring of parents with psychopathology are often genetically vulnerable to disorders, but the absence of psychopathology in these individuals may be due to the absence of risk (not the presence of resilience), because even offspring from the same biological parents may vary considerably in the degree of genetic risk. Moreover, the notion of resilience from a developmental psychopathology perspective implies processes that result in functioning that is as good or better in the face of adversity as in the absence of adversity; that is, resilient individuals, rather than simply avoiding negative outcomes associated with adversity, demonstrate adequate or more than adequate adaptation when faced with challenge or stress (Cowan, Cowan, & Schulz, 1996). Thus, it cannot be assumed that children of parents with major disorders have met the criteria of "considerable risk"; therefore, it cannot be assumed that such children are evidencing resilience when they exhibit adaptive functioning.

Resilience: A Dynamic, Multidimensional Construct

Conceptual frameworks must also be sensitive to the notion that resilience is best characterized as a dynamic, multidimensional construct; that is, it is not a simple yes–no proposition even when considerable risk is clearly present. First, whereas early conceptualizations often characterized resilience as a relatively static "trait" over time (i.e., exhibiting considerable continuity over time), the observation that resilient children may experience bouts of considerable problems over time underscores the developmental notion that resilience often resembles a dynamic "state" (Luthar, 1991, 1995; Luthar, Doernberger, & Zigler, 1993). With this recognition, terms such as "resilience" or "profiles of resilience" have replaced early unconditional labels such as "invincible" or "invulnerable" (Pellegrini, 1990; Rutter, 1985).

Second, until recently, researchers implicitly assumed that resilience was homogeneous; that is, if individuals exhibited competence in one domain (e.g., social), then they must be competent in other domains (e.g., emotional). However, programmatic work by Luthar and colleagues has compellingly shown that resilience is multidimensional (Luthar & Cushing, 1999; Luthar & Ziegler, 1993). For example, at-risk individuals exhibiting adaptive functioning or competence in one or two domains may demonstrate high levels of psychopathology in other domains of functioning, particularly with respect to depressive symptoms and anxiety (Kaufman, Cook, Arny, Jones, & Pittinsky, 1994; Luthar, 1991). Similarly, more stringent criteria for resilience that require demonstration of adaptation across many areas of functioning have yielded more pessimistic outlooks for high-risk children, with some studies revealing that *no* children evidenced global positive adaptation under highly adverse conditions (Egeland, Carlson, & Sroufe, 1993; Farber & Egeland, 1987). Consequently, calls have been issued for a new conceptual order in resilience models that more precisely specify the nature of resilience within and across multiple domains of functioning (e.g., academic, social, emotional, behavioral).

Third, conceptualizations of resilience must also be sensitive to the possibility that the meaning of "competence" and "resilience" may change across contexts and people. For instance, within predominantly low-risk, white samples of children (e.g., Dishion, 1990), peer ratings of child popularity and social competence have been associated with greater academic (e.g., better grades) and behavioral competence (e.g., low levels of aggression). By contrast, as reported by teachers, high-risk inner-city adolescents who were popular among their peers exhibited more conduct problems and lower academic achievement. In this same sample, academic competence was part of a larger constellation of social risk characterized by low popularity and isolation from peers, and high levels of self-reported internalizing symptoms. Thus, under certain contextual conditions (e.g., high-risk subcultures), ratings of competence are relative and may depend specifically on the eye of the beholder (e.g., peers vs. teachers), the domain of competence under investigation (e.g., peer vs. academic competence), and the developmental stage of individuals (e.g., children vs. adolescents). Consistent with the organizational perspective, these findings not only highlight the utility of capturing resiliency status across multiple domains of functioning, but they also underscore the point that conceptual advances in understanding risk and resilience may require broader, pattern-based *constellations* or *profiles* of resilience (e.g., high academic but low social and emotional competence).

Factors and Processes Underlying Resilience

Once scientists achieve the thorny goal of identifying people who meet criteria for exhibiting resilience, the next step is to delineate the *protective factors* and *processes* that account for their adaptation under adverse conditions (Garmezy, 1985). Unfortunately, the study of "when" and "why" people are resilient has its own set of problems revolving around the considerable debate about what constitutes a protective factor (Windle, 1999). Initial taxonomies of resilience primarily distinguished between protective (also called buffers) and compensatory factors (Garmezy, Masten, & Tellegen, 1984; Masten et al., 1988; Rutter, 1987). A factor was designated as protective only if two requirements as a moderator or interaction were met: the potential protective factor must reduce the deleterious impact of a stressor while having a negligible link to adaptation among people experiencing low risk. By contrast, the term "compensatory" was reserved for a "main effects model," in which the factor in question predicted greater psychological adjustment regardless of whether individuals experienced risk (Downey & Walker, 1989).

Illustrating the utility of this taxonomy, Forehand and colleagues (1991) found that a good father–adolescent relationship within depressive family climates changed roles as a compensatory and protective factor across different forms of adolescent maladjustment. Whereas adolescent appraisals of positive father–child relations were associated with lower risk for externalizing symptoms regardless of the degree of family stress experienced (compensatory model), these same appraisals are particularly salient in reducing risk for internalizing symptoms under conditions of considerable family stress (buffering or protective model).

Accompanying the initial success of this taxonomy was also considerable confusion. For example, some researchers have used the term "protective factor" more broadly to denote factors that differentiate between high-risk children who exhibit positive versus negative adjustment, without comparable consideration of children at low risk (see Luthar, 1993), while others have expressed dissatisfaction with limiting conceptualization of protective factors to interactive models (e.g., Zucker, Fitzgerald, & Moses, 1995). In order for resilience to remain a viable concept and a fruitful area of study, it is crucial that researchers achieve some consensus on a classification scheme for protective factors (Windle, 1999). If one removes the "considerable risk" criterion, one simply needs to demonstrate that a factor fostered positive adaptation in the face of adversity.

Another avenue is to make more distinctions. Luthar (1993) has developed a promising new taxonomy (see Figure 5.2). In this model, one can see that the influence of an attribute on competence varies as a function of the level of risk. Thus, the attribute is consistently "protective" for all groups (i.e., regardless of risk status, all groups do better than when the attribute is absent), but distinctions are made in terms of the level and type of protection that occurs as a function of the level of risk. Guided by a focus on process, the taxonomy makes a fine-grained distinction among interactive models of protection and risk. Briefly, three types of interaction are distinguished: (1) *protective–stabilizing effects*—the protective factor fosters comparable levels of competence across levels of risk (Figure 5.2A); (2) *protective–enhancing ef-*

fects—the protective factor facilitates better coping in the face of adversity and thus serves to increase competence as risk increases (Figure 5.2B); and (3) *protective–reactive effects*—the protective factor fosters competence across levels of risk but is particularly effective under low levels of risk (Figure 5.2C). Finally, Figure 5.2D shows the attribute operating as a protective factor in a "main effect" fashion; that is, similar levels of protection are provided, regardless of level of risk. Thus, Figure 5.2D illustrates the traditionally viewed compensatory factor as a subset of protective factors. Thus, unlike many previous taxonomies that implicitly treat compensatory effects as different from and secondary to protective effects, this conceptualization expands the scope of the conceptualization of protective and compensatory effects. On the other hand, while the specification of possible relations between these variables is quite useful, one might wonder whether this level of complexity regarding the conceptualization of whether factors are compensatory or protective is really necessary; that is, does it make sense for the developmental psychopathologist to single out for special attention the factor's special advantages for the subgroup of children at highest risk when all children are faced with adversity,

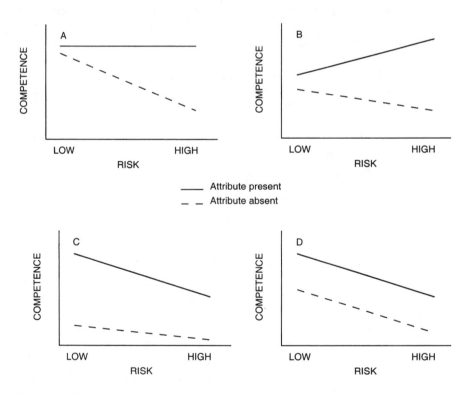

FIGURE 5.2. A taxonomy of protective factors. From Luthar (1993). Copyright 1993 by the *Journal of Child Psychology and Psychiatry*, Cambridge University Press. Adapted by permission.

and all children are at some level of risk for the development of psychopathology? We return to this question and its implications for the conceptualization of resilience.

While the selection of protective factors often varies depending on the orientation of the investigator and the research area, Garmezy (1985) has offered a tripartite framework of protective factors that has proved helpful in organizing conceptual models across topical areas (e.g., Luthar & Ziegler, 1993; Pellegrini, 1990; Rutter, 1987): (1) *dispositional attributes within the child*, including temperament, personality traits, gender, coping styles, locus of control, and self-esteem; (2) *family characteristics*, including family cohesion and warmth, positive parent–child relationships, and harmonious interparental relations; and (3) *domains of extrafamilial contexts*, including the availability of a positive adult figure (e.g., teachers), positive school experiences academically and socially, and safe, supportive neighborhoods.

Much of the search for protective factors has proceeded as if the concept were synonymous with inherently positive characteristics. Protective factors, however, are not necessarily intrinsically pleasant or desirable; in fact, they are often considered to be adverse and stressful. Epitomizing the old adage "With adversity comes growth," *challenge models* specify that stressful conditions, especially in small or moderate doses, may actually have "steeling effects" that serve to enhance coping and adjustment, and inoculate individuals against subsequent psychological insult (Garmezy, Masten, & Tellegen, 1984; Rutter, 1985, 1987). Incorporating this model into the study of the effects of parental depression, Cummings and Davies (1994b) proposed that children may learn adaptive skills of interpersonal sensitivity and empathy through exposure to moderate expressions of negative affect in some depressive family contexts. However, in spite of their inherent appeal in the lay community and robust analogues in medicine (e.g., vaccinations), only a handful of projects have attempted to investigate steeling effects (see Compas, Hinden, & Gerhardt, 1995; Petersen, Sarigiani, & Kennedy, 1991).

Concepts of holism and contextual relativism also underscore the notion that protective effects may be confined to specific contexts or domains of functioning. For example, social anxiety and inhibition may protect or buffer adolescents from involvement with deviant peers, alcohol and substance use, and delinquency; however, by the same token, the common occurrence of peer neglect may serve to increase loneliness, depression, and withdrawal (Tubman, Windle, & Windle, 1996; Windle & Windle, 1993). Similarly, while authoritarian styles of parenting characterized by strict control have been associated with greater psychological problems in low-risk community samples, some evidence suggests that they may actually promote adaptation in dangerous contexts of disadvantaged communities (Baldwin et al., 1993; Luthar, 1993).

Identifying protective factors and the form taken by their effects across contexts and domains of functioning is useful primarily in the sense that they are indirect markers for the ultimate pursuit of understanding the processes that lead to resilience. While many researchers have used the terms inter-changeably, the distinction between "protective factors" and "protective pro-cesses" (or mechanisms) is critical. Like risk factors, protective factors only fo-cus on the characteristics of contexts (i.e., when) and individuals (i.e., who) that may promote adaptation in the face of adversity. While answers to the "when" and "who" questions of resilience may provide clues about underly-ing protective processes, they do not, by any means, directly address the ulti-mate process or mechanism question of "why" and "how" these protective factors promote resilience (Rutter, 1993; Rutter & Pickles, 1991).

There are a variety of circumstances in which resilience may be demon-strated. For example, Masten, Best, and Garmezy (1990) discuss three types of circumstances in which resilience may be observed: (1) resilience as overcom-ing the odds (i.e., good outcomes despite high-risk status), (2) sustained com-petence under adversity (i.e., stress resistance), and (3) recovery from trauma (i.e., recovery). With regard to the first circumstance of resilience, Egeland, Carlson, and Sroufe (1993) discuss the instance of poverty, which has been found to have a pervasive negative effect on children's adaptation. Thus, chil-dren who do well despite poverty may seen as demonstrating resilience. Pro-tective factors suggested by research include effective schooling, good parent-ing, high intellectual skills, and church membership. Another example are children of HIV-infected mothers, who are reported to have elevated levels of difficulties in multiple domains of psychosocial functioning (i.e., externalizing and internalizing problems) compared to children from similar sociodemo-graphic backgrounds whose mothers are not HIV-infected (Forehand et al., 1998). The only significant protective factor in this instance was the parent–child relationship. Specifically, high levels of monitoring combined with a highly positive parent–child relationship were associated with the highest resiliency score (Kotchick, Forehand, Brody et al., 1997). Resilience as sus-tained competence under adversity may be found in divorce, which does not pose the same high odds for poor adjustment as poverty but is associated, nev-ertheless, with increased risk for adjustment problems, most notably in the years just after divorce. Protective factors identified in research in this case in-clude a good parent–child relationship, authoritative parenting, self-confi-dence and self-efficacy, and low interparental conflict (Hetherington & Clingempeel, 1992). An example of resilience as recovery from trauma is chil-dren's development after physical maltreatment. Protective factors implicated by research include later improvements in environment, physical attractive-ness, positive school experiences, and later development of a good relation-ship with a spouse (Masten, Best, & Garmezy, 1990).

Since resilience is an ongoing, dynamic developmental construct rather than a static trait, it is optimal to study resilience over time. Cicchetti and Rogosch (1997) examined the adaptation of maltreated and nonmaltreated school-age children from socioeconomically disadvantaged backgrounds over three consecutive years as assessed in a summer camp program. As expected, they found that a higher percentage of maltreated than nonmaltreated children were consistently in the lower adaptive range (i.e., lower levels of ego resiliency, higher levels of ego undercontrol, less adaptive relationships with their camp counselors). Particularly interesting with regard to the present discussion was the finding that different predictors of resilience exist among maltreated and nonmaltreated children. Relationship variables were particularly strong predictors of adaptive functioning across the 3 years for nonmaltreated children from disadvantaged economic backgrounds. The relationship achieved with the camp counselor, ego resiliency, perceived emotional closeness with the mother, and intelligence were all significant predictors. Intriguingly, individual characteristics (ego overcontrol, self-esteem, ego resiliency) were the significant predictors of 3-year adaptive functioning for maltreated children. Thus, for the group that faced the greatest adversity, personal reliance on the self appeared particularly important in achieving adaptive outcomes in the face of significant odds.

One may also examine protective factors in terms of the processes that account for their effects. The processes by which protective factors may lead to resilient outcomes include (1) mitigating the riskiness of the stressor; (2) reducing exposure to the stressor; (3) breaking adverse cycles or chains of misfortune brought about by a stressor; (4) fostering positive appraisals of the self (e.g., self-esteem, confidence); (5) increasing the range of positive opportunities and options in life; and (6) facilitating coping and emotion regulation skills (Rutter, 1993). Thus, simply identifying a protective factor (e.g., warm father–child relationship) is only a beginning step that must be followed by a search for why it leads to resilience.

Resilience as Process: Identifying Resilience within a Process-Oriented Framework

As we mentioned at the outset of this chapter, Cicchetti and Garmezy (1993) note that the popularity of resilience as a construct far surpasses the extent to which it has been subjected to systematic research and study. Accordingly, as a popular trend, there is danger that the concept will lose scientific credibility without further, systematic exploration. We return to the point that it is important to be able to place this relatively elusive construct into a process-oriented framework for human development. The question is: How does one conceptualize resilience in terms of a higher-order model of influences on development? In the spirit of furthering the discussion of definition, we now consider the place of resilience in our process-oriented framework for human development (Figure 3.1). How does one think about resilience as part of the "big picture" of a process-oriented model for human development? While there is no marker for resilience as a special category in this model, the construct of resilience can be developed in terms of this model.

Resilience is currently used in two ways that specifically reflect different usages of the construct. First, resilience refers to positive psychological outcomes in the face of adversity. In this sense, resilience can be seen as the extent to which "diagnostic outcomes" of greater social competence and fewer adjustment problems (e.g., internalizing disorders, externalizing disorders) are found despite negative influences on development (e.g., poverty, parental illness). This definition reflects a "static" notion of resilience. In this view, protective factors are those influences on development that foster "resilient" outcomes. While a static notion of resilience is not consistent with cutting-edge conceptualizations in the developmental psychopathology tradition, nonetheless, this usage remains relatively prevalent.

On the other hand, at a process level of analysis, resilience refers to those dynamic processes of "psychological functioning" that foster greater positive, and reduced negative, outcomes in the face of relative adversity, both at the present time and in the future (see Figure 5.1). Thus, while resilience is defined, in part, relative to psychological influences on development and developmental outcomes, it ultimately refers to those psychological processes in context that lead to relatively positive, and not negative, outcomes. In this sense, protective factors refer to those various intra- and extraorganismic factors that foster processes of resilience. More precisely, protective factors are those compensatory processes that serve to promote adaptation in children.

It is this usage of the concept of resilience typifying the notion of "resilience as process" that is advocated by core theorists in the developmental psychopathology tradition. Thus, Egeland, Pianta, and O'Brien (1993) note that resilience is "the capacity for successful adaptation, positive functioning, or competence despite high risk status" (p. 517). Similarly, Masten, Best, and Garmezy (1990) contend that resilience is "the process of, capacity for, or outcome of successful adaptation despite challenging circumstances" (p. 425).

However, given these considerations, one is forced again to return to the question of whether resilience is appropriately viewed as a "special case" that only characterizes individuals facing greater adversity and does not apply to those facing lesser adversity, or whether it typifies some individuals and not others in situations of adversity; that is, adversity is not an either–or proposition. Adversity is relative, and multifaceted, with every individual facing some, or many, sources of adversity. Where does one draw the line? To some extent, if one does draw such a line, one is necessarily relying on marker variables (e.g., comparing children of depressed and nondepressed parents, when, in some cases, closer inspection would reveal that the latter face more adversity than the former). Moreover, the great majority of people show some or many processes of resilience, at least in some contexts, and also fail to some extent to evidence resilience in other contexts (Luthar, Doernberger, & Ziegler, 1993). Thus, resilience as a process is not confined to any one group or subgroup, but, logically, must be regarded as a general phenomenon of coping with stress and adversity (see the earlier discussion of Luthar's distinctions among protective and compensatory factors). Children who qualify as coming from high-risk environments (e.g., children of depressed parents) may be of particular interest to clinicians and developmental psychopathologists, but that is a different proposition than the notion that resiliency as a process is confined to such groups. Cowan, Cowan, and Schulz (1996) makes this point forcefully:

> It would be tragic if the real difficulties families face as they attempt to raise young children were to be ignored on the assumption that help is needed only by those in more traditionally high-risk samples. We believe that the frequency of distress in non-clinical families is (unfortunately) large enough to justify concerted attempts to apply risk paradigms to studies of normal family adaptation. (p. 31)

Viewed from this perspective, resilience refers to psychological processes that operate in opposition to processes of vulnerability to adversity. Since every individual faces adversity, every individual is likely to evidence processes of resilience, although more is required for adaptive functioning among those exposed to high adversity. Similarly, every individual is likely to evidence some vulnerability to adversity, at least in some contexts. It is the balance between processes of resilience and vulnerability to adversity in contexts of development that determine whether psychopathology or normal development is the outcome at a given point in time.

Accordingly, from this perspective, the goal of developmental psychopathology is to develop theories about psychological processes of resilience or vulnerability to adversity, with no sharp line drawn between individuals from high- and low-risk environments. While more personal resources of resilience are surely needed among individuals from high-risk environments for adaptive development across the life course, and these cases are of particular interest to clinical scientists, in an important sense, the issues are the same for individuals from a variety of contexts of low and high risk. Moreover, it is important to understand individuals from apparently low-risk environments who may nonetheless develop psychopathology, especially the reasons for their low levels of resilience, both from the perspective of clinical science and clinical practice.

This view of resilience, therefore, places the construct at the center of understanding processes that underlie normal development and the development of psychopathology. Specifically, resilience refers to those processes within the category of "psychological functioning" in Figure 3.1 that allow the individual to overcome adversity and evidence adaptive developmental outcomes. Given that most individuals do develop normally (Masten, Best, & Garmezy, 1990), resilience is not a "special case" or a minority outcome, but constitutes a central class of processes underlying human development.

In summary, the notion of protective factors calls attention to the importance of considering positive factors as well as risk factors in developmental models. The construct of resilience highlights that the fact that individuals at risk may function adaptively, or develop adaptive functioning patterns over time (e.g., recall the examples of Lisa and Nicole in Chapter 4). Moreover, for the child clinical psychologist or others with an interest in practice issues, factors that promote adaptive functioning in samples at risk for adjustment problems are more interesting than factors that generally promote adaptive versus maladaptive outcomes. However, it is the contention here that it is not necessary for scientific models to limit the study of these matters to certain groups and, in fact, the domain of positive and negative processes (i.e., classes of mediators) during development is of general interest. While it is certainly important to define groups in analyses, one need not assume that only certain groups are potentially capable of being resilient. Put another way, it makes sense to consider the normal and abnormal together with regard to protective factors and resilience, as in other matters of developmental trajectories and adaptive and maladaptive functioning. Moreover, the concern with how responses vary as a function of contexts and periods of development can be dealt with by testing whether groups constitute one or another class of moderators of development. A virtue of this perspective is that mainstream multivariate statistical procedures (e.g., structural equation modeling, hierarchical linear analysis, or growth curve analyses) can then be readily applied to the questions at hand, without the need to consider provisions for "special cases" of individuals facing adversity. The point does not in any way diminish the importance of the distinctions, issues, and nuances that we described earlier. The chief gain is a form of conceptual clarity about the matters at hand. Next, we turn to a consideration of some of the approaches that are available to test statistically pathways and trajectories implicated by process-oriented models, such as the framework outlined in Figure 3.1.

APPROPRIATE STATISTICAL APPROACHES TO ANALYZING PROCESS-ORIENTED MODELS

Another element of moving forward with process-oriented tests of protective factors and resilience is to consider directions toward analyzing such models. While only the briefest of treatments is possible here, consistent with the emphasis of the developmental psychopathology approach on methodology as well as theory, some brief consideration of such matters is appropriate. Issues of feasibility and practicality are important for researchers grappling with cutting-edge, complex issues in child clinical and developmental science. Practitioners also should be familiar with these matters from their perspective as consumers of available clinical science. Among the pertinent questions are the following: Is it possible to test models such as the one depicted in Figure 3.1? What statistical approaches might be used?

Obviously, one must do more than simply show correlations between predictor and outcome variables, or some variation in demonstrating that predictor and outcomes, or various marker variables, are interrelated. These are important matters, but such issues can be described as matters for the "first generation" of research on childhood disorders, and in many areas of study, researchers are prepared to move beyond that. For example, we know that marital hostility is linked probabilistically with an increase in children's adjustment problems. The questions now are why (i.e., what are the mediating processes?), and what groups are particularly affected (i.e., moderators) by exposure to marital conflict? Moreover, consistent with the goals of the present chapter, one might also ask why some groups are more or less vulnerable or resilient than others (i.e., mediated moderation).

The matter of moving one step beyond showing correlations between predictors and childhood psychopathology, that is, demonstrating mediators in process models, is relatively straightforward statistically. Tests for whether particular processes mediate relations between predictors (e.g., parental depression) and outcomes (e.g., childhood disorders) have to meet several criteria, that is, demonstrations of significant relations between (1) the predictor and outcome, (2) the predictor and the process, and (3) the process and the outcome. Another criterion is that the relation between the predictor and outcome becomes nonsignificant, or is reduced significantly, when the process is factored into the analysis (Baron & Kenny, 1986). Testing simple process models at this level of analysis can be successfully accomplished with well-known, long-standing (e.g., regression analyses) statistical methods.

However, as we have seen, testing questions about resilience requires taking into account groups moderating relations between variables, and processes mediating outcomes, which means that moderators and mediators must be considered in the same model. Moreover, one is typically interested in multiple predictors, multiple mediators, and multiple outcomes, as in Figure 3.1. More advanced statistical approaches are needed for such purposes.

Structural Equation Modeling

In order to accomplish the conceptual goals for developmental models proposed by the developmental psychopathology approach, the challenge is to go beyond examining simple relationships between variables, toward understanding the complex processes underlying these relationships and their moderators. Structural equation modeling (SEM), that is, causal modeling, provides the researcher with a statistical methodology for testing more advanced theoretical models (Biddle & Martin, 1987). This methodology uses the correlations among all of the measures assessed in a study to estimate the specific pathways predicted by the hypotheses of a theory. A "good fit" between a model and a theory means that the pathways predicted by the theory do not differ from the pathways derived from the observed correlations. Using this method, it is also possible to compare the proposed model with alternative models that add or remove relationships among the constructs. When used appropriately, this approach can provide a better estimate of true scores by statistically removing measurement error and also determining how well different purported measures of a psychological variable relate to an underlying construct. SEM can be adapted to address the issues raised by mediational models (e.g., mediating processes), longitudinal models (i.e., developmental models), and group differences (i.e., moderational models), and can include all of these matters at the same time in a comprehensive test of theory. However,

SEM does not provide a shortcut for measurement issues, which we considered at length in Chapter 3. One must be very careful in evaluating the measurement quality and characteristics of research before accepting conclusions based on SEM or any other analytic technique. Tests of models can only be as good as the measures, and multiple measures of each construct are needed for optimal representation. Moreover, relatively large sample sizes are required to meet the statistical requirements of this technique. Thus, a tension inevitably results for those aiming to apply this procedure to test advanced models of theories about development for at-risk and normal groups of children. Rigorous and extensive measurement of the variables pertinent to advanced theory is expensive and time-consuming, which tends to limit the sample sizes that can be included in research. However, the statistical requirements of SEM demand relatively large sample sizes.

Growth Curve Modeling

Growth curve modeling (hierarchical linear modeling, or HLM) can address issues in longitudinal research concerning change over time that cannot be readily addressed by other means (Bryk & Raudenbush, 1987). Given the concern of developmental psychopathologists with pathways of development, this procedure merits particular consideration. Specifically, this approach can be used to examine interindividual differences in intraindividual change. By contrast, multivariate approaches to repeated measures are limited to examining average intraindividual change across participants in a study (Maxwell & Delaney, 1990). Clearly, the matters that can be addressed by HLM are pertinent to the person-oriented level of analysis that is of particular interest to the developmental psychopathologist (Sroufe & Rutter, 1984). For example, suppose one assessed relations between marital conflict and children's adjustment over a 5-year period, with assessments being conducted each year. By applying HLM to longitudinal data, one would be able to investigate interindividual differences in the developmental trajectories of children exposed to marital conflict over the 5-year period. Using this technique, one could also potentially investigate the effects of changes in marital conflict on changes in the degree of a child's behavior problems. However, as with SEM, there are demanding requirements for the appropriate use of this procedure, that is, the simultaneous need for both the rigorous measurement of psychological variables and relatively large sample sizes. In addition, of course, one must collect data for all participants across multiple occasions; that is, longitudinal data must be collected, and this is also expensive in terms of both time and resources.

Soft Modeling

As we have noted, the stringent requirement for relatively large sample sizes in these advanced statistical approaches based upon maximum likelihood estimation presents inherent challenges for conducting process-oriented studies that are essential to cutting-edge research in this area; that is, time and resource costs for obtaining the extensive and rigorous data sets needed to adequately assess and represent the variables in process models for developmental psychopathology inevitably reduce the feasibility of obtaining data on large samples. This problem is particularly significant for research in early phases of the articulation of process models from a developmental psychopathology perspective; that is, some initial assessments of models are inevitably necessary in the early phases of research to assess fundamental viability, or to improve or perfect conceptual models prior to undertaking the much more costly (in terms of time and resources), more cogent theory testing.

An alternative form of structural equation modeling procedure that may address this gap is the latent variable path analysis with partial least squares estimation procedure (LVPLS), or soft modeling, procedure (Falk & Miller, 1992). This approach, which can examine hypothesized relations between variables without imposing certain of the restrictive assumptions required by the previous statistical approaches to modeling, can therefore be employed with relatively small sample sizes and sizable numbers of manifest and latent variables in the exploratory tests of process-oriented models (see Cowan, Cohn, Cowan, & Peason, 1996; Davies & Cummings, 1998). LVPLS does not calculate standard errors; thus, the adequacy of specific parts of the structural model cannot be evaluated by means of formal significance tests. On the other hand, it provides guidelines for whether meaningful amounts of variance in children's functioning are accounted for by pathways and, thus, a form of assessment of the adequacy of models. Thus, LVPLS is particularly appropriate for initial stages of theory testing or for exploratory directions in research, but it does not provide tests of theoretical models with the same level of statistical rigor as the approaches mentioned earlier.

CONCLUSION

The developmental psychopathology approach holds up lofty goals for the clinical researcher. Advanced statistical, theoretical, and measurement concerns must be met for adequate process-oriented understanding of the trajectories of development that lead to normal functioning or the development of psychopathology over time. In Part II, we consider the application of these issues to the area of families and children, and examine how far we have advanced toward a process-oriented understanding of children's normal development and development of psychopathology in the context of family environments.

◈ PART II

Research

Thus far, we have been concerned with describing the basic principles of the developmental psychopathology approach. However, despite the consideration of examples, matters are abstract at this level of analysis. Accordingly, questions remain about precisely how these issues might be applied to research. Part II of this volume considers the application of these notions to the study of children and families. It is intended to illustrate the applicability of these principles to research directions concerned with the development of psychopathology in children.

The developmental psychopathology approach is especially pertinent to the study of children and families because it incorporates the inherent complexity of patterns of influence in these environments; that is, many different aspects of family environments influence children's development, and a sophisticated model is required to account for these influences. One is limited in understanding children's development in families in terms of any single family process or subsystem. Moreover, each factor is inherently complex in its influence on children.

In a seminal contribution, Belsky (1984) called attention to the fact that parenting influences on children's socialization are a product of processes affected by multiple intra- and extrafamilial determinants, including the effects of the children on the parents.

This perspective is contrasted with a traditional view that a single causal arrow from parental behavior to child outcomes might suffice, as shown in the model in Figure II.1.

Current research suggests that this framework can be expanded to include ethnic, cultural, and other ecological contexts beyond social networks and work. However, in many respects, the framework was prescient in highlighting directions for research that have since become well-developed, espe-

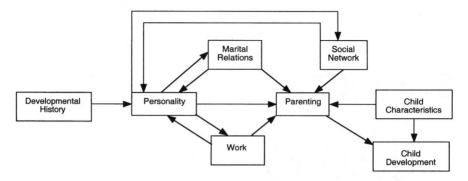

FIGURE II.1. A process model of the determinants of parenting. From Belsky (1984). Copyright 1984 by the Society for Research in Child Development. Reprinted by permission.

cially the findings of close interrelations between marital relations and parenting, although the need for a causal arrow *directly* from marital relations to child development is also now indicated. Moreover, as Belsky argued, parental personalities, including parental adjustment problems, have also emerged as significant influences on the family processes that affect children's development, and these dispositions may have roots in parents' own developmental histories. Interestingly, Belsky highlighted parental depression especially as a potentially significant influence as a function of parental personality. Certainly, the evidence of the past 15 years has borne out that hypothesis.

On the other hand, while Belsky's propositions with regard to family determinants of children's socialization were groundbreaking, subsequent research has indicated that even more inclusive ecological models are required. Recently, Parke and Buriel (1998) called attention to the emergence of an increasing diversity of family forms, and the significance of the cultural and ethnic variations in the family, and other ecological contexts in which family socialization takes place. For example, the extended family is particularly important in the African American family. However, relatively little is known about the distinctive socialization practices of many ethnic groups, including Asian American and Latino families. Changes in families over the past several decades are also associated with increasing rates of teenage pregnancy, the high rates of divorce, and the many variations in custody arrangements following divorce (Emery, 1994). Moreover, other agents play a role in the socialization of the family, including schools, peers, and the media, and these influences may interact in their effects on family socialization.

At the same time, recent research indicates the need to look more closely at patterns of functioning within families. Consistent with the holistic and organizational assumptions of the developmental psychopathology approach, it is important to consider influences in terms of broader family patterns. Cox and Paley (1997) have recently provided an excellent discussion of the importance of understanding the functioning of families as an organized whole. From this perspective, multiple family subsystems are seen as organized within the larger family system in their operation. The family, in turn, is embedded in larger, extrafamily systems in its functioning. While each family subsystem has a degree of integrity as an influence on children's functioning, there are also patterns of influence across larger organizations within the family (e.g., interrelations between individual, parent–child, and marital relations). One might also examine larger family units than the subsystem, such as whole family dynamics (McHale & Rasmussen, 1998). Cox and Paley provide an insightful analysis of the operation of families that is quite consistent with the developmental psychopathology perspective on the functioning of individuals; that is, families, like the individuals within families, are portrayed as engaging in continual efforts to adapt to stress and challenges. Moreover, families are seen as relatively resilient and as responding dynamically and continually to threats, stresses, and other challenges to their organization and functioning.

On the other hand, while it is important to recognize this diversity and complexity of family forms, influences, and levels of analysis, it is beyond the scope of this volume to treat the entire range of family-related influences on socialization in an exhaustive fashion. Moreover, unfortunately, relatively little is known about these emerging issues. Accordingly, to illustrate the applicability of the developmental psychopathology approach in the in-depth fashion that this discipline requires, several of the most significant family subsystems that affect children's socialization are the focus, including those family subsystems or conceptualizations of the influence of family subsystems that have been studied is greatest depth and about which the most is known at this point. Moreover, while it is recognized that families are optimally seen as reflecting integrated wholes, research has focused on individual family subsystems and their effects on individuals for heuristic reasons. Accordingly, we follow that pattern in reviewing both appropriate research on the effects of families on children, while acknowledging that families reflect larger organizations and patterns of relationships and interrelationships, and evidence pertinent to these matters.

Thus, returning to the groundbreaking framework offered by Belsky (1984), we focus on (1) the parent–child subsystem (Chapters 6 and 7), and (2) the marital subsystem and children (Chapter 8). To accomplish some consistency in treatment across topics, we consider (1) prediction of children's adjustment problems, including results for normal and abnormal samples; (2) what is known about the dimensions of risk and protection; (3) relations between the family variable and other aspects of family functioning; (4) evidence concerning pathways of development based on studies of the family variable; and (5) theories or models about the processes underlying relations between the family influence and child outcomes, including the consideration of possible moderators of childhood disorder.

This coverage is intended to highlight the themes that we reviewed in the section on principles, including the focus on identifying dynamic processes that mediate development; the study of the abnormal in the context of the normal; the pertinence of the theoretical (holism, active organism, directionality, coherence, and organizational perspectives) and methodological assumptions (use of multiple methods and the study of multiple domains of responding); the value of charting complex pathways of developmental deviance and normality; and the need to consider protective factors and resilience in the face of adversity as well as risk factors and the incidence of childhood disorders.

In closing, we consider the effects of a particularly important dimension of parental personality on child development, that is, parental depression (see Figure II.1; see also Chapter 9, this volume). As another means of providing a broader, more integrated perspective on the developmental psychopathology of family environments, this concluding chapter pulls together different threads of evidence illustrating the operation of multiple family factors in the prediction of outcomes for a particular group of children at relatively high risk for adjustment problems, that is, children of depressed parents. Because a variety of family factors have been related to the adjustment of children of depressed parents in a relatively large body of studies, research on this risk group provides a particularly pertinent familywide perspective on family factors related to children's adjustment from a developmental psychopathology perspective.

CHAPTER SIX

Child Development and the Parent–Child Subsystem

*P*arenting has long been known to have a profound impact on the socialization of children in the family. The legacy of parenting research is rich and highly informative (Maccoby, 1992). Despite some controversy (Harris, 1995), the overwhelming evidence suggests that parenting justifiably occupies a central role in any understanding of the normal and abnormal development of children. Thus, from a developmental psychopathology perspective, it follows that consideration of the effects of parental behavior is an essential component of any model of the effects of families on children.

Despite the salience of parenting in research in both normal and abnormal child development, as well as the importance of parenting in clinical practice, we are far from knowing all of the answers about parenting practices and child development (Maccoby & Martin, 1983). This fact, in part, reflects the complex nature of the phenomenon. There are no simple answers to the question of how to parent, and no optimal parenting style exists for all children of all ages in all situations. Moreover, even when parenting dimensions are consistently associated with desirable (e.g., parental sensitivity; De Wolff & van IJzendoorn, 1997) or undesirable (e.g., harsh and inconsistent parenting; Patterson, DeBaryshe, & Ramsey, 1989) child outcomes, the extent to which differences in children's outcomes are explained by any single parenting dimension is often modest. Given the complexity of both the parenting construct and familial, extrafamilial, and other contextual influences (e.g., genetic) on parenting, no single dimension or conceptualization of parenting can, or probably ever will, provide a complete account of the effects of parent–child relations on child development. Adding to this complexity, the effects of parenting are often properly understood by their interaction or transaction over time with multiple other factors (e.g., marital relations, genetics, child characteristics) in predicting children's outcomes. In short, understanding the effects of parenting requires a sophisticated conceptualization of parenting, and of the relations between parenting and contextual influences, that affect the pathways and processes of child development. The developmental psychopathology approach offers promise to this daunting challenge: As applied to this topic, it would seem to provide precisely the types of heuristics needed to articulate more sophisticated developmental models of the effects of parenting on normal development and on the development of psychopathology.

The tendency to seek simple answers to complex questions about parenting, in part, reflects the understandably popular interest in finding relatively simple solutions to the problems that parents face in raising children. However, the way that social scientists have traditionally conceptualized parenting and conducted parenting research has also fostered overly simple perspectives on parenting, and the developmental psychopathology perspective offers a specific antidote to these limitations of family science. Problematic past directions include (1) the analysis of differences in child functioning as a function of a single parenting variable (i.e., univariate research designs); (2) examination of relations between parenting and child functioning at a single time point (i.e., *unitemporal* measurement; Clarke-Stewart, 1988); (3) samples based almost exclusively upon white, intact, middle-class families (i.e., *uniformity* of research samples across studies; Holmbeck, 1996; Smetana, 1995); and (4) the assumption that parents influence children but children do not affect parenting (i.e., *unidirectional* pathways of influence; Darling & Steinberg, 1993). As a consequence of following these research practices, researchers have tended to ignore the possible effects of unmeasured "third variables" on parenting (e.g., marital conflict; see Chapter 7) and to make questionable assumptions about the simplicity of the nature and direction of causality (Emery, Fincham, & Cummings, 1992) and the supposed generalizability of effects from white, middle-class families to other ethnic or cultural groups.

An illustration is provided by social bonding theory (Hirschi, 1969), which proposes that the bond between the parent and the child predicts child and adolescent delinquency. Obviously, many other variables factor into delinquency! Moreover, the bond only referred to a single parental trait of caring versus indifference. As we will see, current notions of the organizational nature of parent–child attachment presuppose far more complex bases and characteristics of emotional bonds. These bonds were assumed to have a unidirectional, rather than reciprocal, influence on the child, although the problem with that assumption is well known (Bell, 1968)! Finally, all but ignored were the underlying processes that led to delinquency in the child, the everchanging interplay between parent and child over time, and the interplay among family, intrachild, and ecological changes in influencing pathways of development (Shaw & Bell, 1993). This way of viewing parenting influences is not unique to social bonding theory, but it provides a concrete illustration of a more general problem. Consider the following examples:

Dawn's family lived in an affluent suburb of a major city. Dawn went to the best schools and also had many special opportunities, including trips to Europe and vacations to exotic places. Although her parents both had careers that demanded much of their time, they doted over her publicly when they were with her and gave her every material thing that she wanted. However, entering school, she had many problems relating to peers and created discipline problems. Upon entering adolescence, Dawn became involved with a popular but risk-taking crowd and developed problems with alcohol and drugs. In addition, her already mediocre performance in school further declined. Her parents were puzzled, because they had always given her what she wanted and had never closely monitored her behavior or presented unpleasant consequences to her. Thus, why was she not happy and successful?

Missy came from a middle-class family. Her very strict parents constantly monitored her behavior. Punishment for misdeeds was severe, and Missy felt that it was often unfair and about matters that she could not control or that were not her fault. As she entered school, Missy had many problems relating, and was unpopular and rejected by her peers. Upon entering adolescence, Missy became involved with an unpopular, risk-taking group and developed problems with alcohol and drugs. In addition, her already mediocre performance in school further declined. Her parents were puzzled, because they had always kept a close eye on her behavior and frequently presented unpleasant consequences to her. Thus, why was she not happy and successful?

These relatively simple examples of some of the pitfalls of parenting illustrate the difficulty of being a good parent. Both Missy's and Dawn's parents felt they were doing the right thing and were, in fact, doing some things that experts would agree were desirable parenting behaviors. However, the children had developed problems growing up. As we will see, these outcomes would, in fact, be expected given the parenting behaviors described. Moreover, as illustrated in Chapters 7 and 8, the matter of being a good parent subsumes many issues and concerns that are considerably more complex than even the ones described here.

TOWARD MORE SOPHISTICATED CONCEPTUALIZATIONS OF PARENTING AND CHILD DEVELOPMENT

As we will see, the developmental psychopathology approach provides concepts that foster more sophisticated conceptualizations of parenting influences on children's development. Moreover, it is consistent with an emerging consensus among parenting experts that the next generation of parenting research requires a move from the "family address model of parenting" to a family process model of parenting (e.g., Darling & Steinberg, 1993; Holmbeck, 1996). A family process conceptualization seeks to elucidate the precise process relations and direction of effects between dimensions of parenting and children's outcomes, in order to articulate the intervening processes underlying these interrelations. Such an approach also requires differentiating the multiple dimensions of parenting that are significant to the various phases of children's development.

Figure 3.1 provided an outline of the multivariate factors pertinent to a general model of the developmental psychopathology approach. In applying this model to the study of parenting, we can see that the process-oriented study of parenting must be embedded within a larger multivariate, developmental framework (Darling & Steinberg, 1993; see Figure 3.1). To illustrate one point of this model, following the principle of holism, parenting should also be considered in terms of the larger ecological context (e.g., family system, neighborhood, subculture, developmental period). Focusing on this particular relationship, as shown in Figure 6.1, the arrow running from the ecological context to the arrow that runs between parenting and child adjustment shows how ecological context may moderate the relation between parenting and child adjustment; that is, the effectiveness of some methods of raising children may vary across particular family systems, developmental contexts, and domains of functioning (e.g., academic vs. social competence). More broadly, differences or changes in the biopsychosocial matrix of development can be seen in Figure 3.1 potentially to affect the efficacy of methods for raising children.

In this chapter and the next, we illustrate how the developmental psychopathology approach provides useful heuristic tools for changing the research landscape on parenting from relatively simplistic and inevitably limited models to more adequate parenting models, underscoring, for example, the role of pluralism and multiplicity in influences, developmental pathways, and ecological contexts. As Clarke-Stewart (1988) put it, "We no longer assume that parents' effects on children's development are simple, one-sided, or powerful. . . . We have opened up a complexity by demonstrating the contributions of the child and context to development by tapping into an apparent myriad of factors in each of the three categories—parent, child, and context" (p. 65). In particular, a developmental psychopathology perspective posits that (1) the interplay between parenting and child functioning reflects a reciprocal process unfolding over time that cannot be reduced to the actions of a single participant (i.e., the *transactional principle*); (2) change is basic (e.g., intrachild maturational changes, family change, and extrafamilial and ecological change, such as school) and ultimately affects and is affected by parenting in different ways, which inevitably leads to rejecting the assumption that parenting practices have uniform, persistent influences across development (the *transformational or epigenetic* theme); (3) assigning primacy to a single parenting dimension is woefully inadequate, as there are multiple dimensions of parenting, and any parenting characteristic and its effects are influenced by and dependent upon the larger matrix of parenting, family, ecological, and other contextual variables (the *multivariate principle*).

Given the abundance of research and theory on parenting, we have no

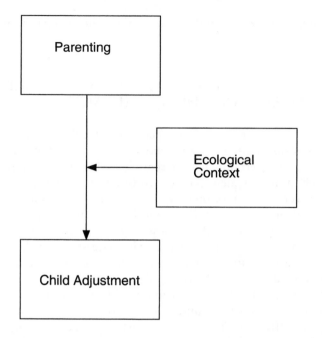

FIGURE 6.1. Ecological context as a moderator of relations between parenting and child adjustment.

choice but to provide selective, rather than exhaustive, illustrations of the utility of a developmental psychopathology approach to a more complete understanding of the effects of parenting on child development. As a means to manage the presentation of the material in this chapter, we loosely divide the consideration of parenting practices into two parts: (1) *control*—parenting as behavioral or psychological control and child management, and (2) *emotional relationship*—parenting as emotionality, sensitivity, and emotional bonds or attachments. We describe this division as "loose" because some conceptualizations give considerable weight to both parts (e.g., Baumrind, 1971), and many of the major directions in theory and research at least recognize the importance of each. Moreover, matters with regard to attachment concern the emotional bond between the parent and child rather than parenting practices per se. Issues pertaining to mediating processes are a particular concern (i.e., a process-oriented perspective), but we consider certain other themes pertinent to a developmental psychopathology approach (e.g., treating parenting as a multidimensional rather than a global construct). Moreover, in this chapter, we focus on these matters primarily as they pertain to *specific* parenting practices and styles. In Chapter 7, we broaden the discussion and provide a more integrative treatment of the developmental psychopathology approach as it relates to general issue of parenting, including application of the developmental psychopathology perspective to the study of the abnormal parenting behaviors of maltreatment.

TWO BROAD DIMENSIONS OF PARENTING PRACTICE: DIFFERING EFFECTS ON CHILD ADJUSTMENT

Thus, social scientists from various theoretical traditions have reached remarkable consensus in differentiating between these broad dimensions of parenting practice, one pertaining to parenting as behavioral or psychological control and child management (i.e., control), and the other loosely related to parenting as acceptance, emotional availability, sensitivity, and a parent–child emotional bond or attachment (i.e., emotional relationship) (Barber, 1997; Cummings & Davies, 1995). Awareness of the distinct nature of these two parenting dimensions has led to advances in understanding the influences of specific parenting behaviors on child outcomes. For example, although each of these parenting dimensions shares significant variance in predicting individual differences in children's externalizing problems, internalizing symptoms, and competence, each also has unique effects on child adjustment even after considering the effects of the other dimensions (e.g., Herman, Dornbusch, Herron, & Herting, 1997). Child internalizing symptoms are the most consistent sequella of high levels of parental psychological control, whereas high parental behavioral control (e.g., consistent monitoring, firm discipline) is related, most commonly, to lower levels of externalizing symptoms (Barber, 1996, 1997; Barber, Olsen, & Shagle, 1994; Herman et al., 1997); harsh and inconsistent control are often associated with conduct problems (e.g., Patterson, DeBaryshe, & Ramsey, 1989). Dimensions pertaining to the parent–child emotional relationship have also been found to predict a wide range of adjustment problems.

PARENTING AS CONTROL

Controlling and managing children's behaviors and development are important facets of socialization and child rearing (Cole & Zahn-Waxler, 1992; Hetherington & Martin, 1986; Maccoby & Martin, 1983). Behavioral control, for example, consists of multiple dimensions of parental behavior, characterized by communication of a set of rules, enforcement of the rules, monitoring and supervision of children's whereabouts, and the use of inductive discipline techniques that stress the consequences of children's actions on others (Barber, 1996; Cummings & Davies, 1995; Maccoby & Martin, 1983). These parenting behaviors are significant mechanisms in inculcating behaviors and values in children related to conformity to and eventual acceptance of rules and regulations that promote social order and harmony. Thus, even though, as we will see, parental warmth or emotional availability provides groundwork for healthy development, particularly in domains reflecting successful interpersonal connectedness and autonomy (e.g., high self-esteem, self-confidence), parents who exercise lax or inconsistent patterns of behavioral control nonetheless run the risk of raising children with significant psychological problems, despite their efforts to foster a positive emotional relationship with their children (Barber, 1996; Baumrind, 1971; Steinberg, 1990).

At least among white, middle-class families, close supervision, strict enforcement of family rules, and a democratic recognition of children's viewpoints are associated with desirable child outcomes across broad windows of the life span (Maccoby & Martin, 1983; Radke-Yarrow, Zahn-Waxler, & Chapman, 1983). For example, parents of well-functioning preschoolers are not only warm but are also consistent in monitoring their children, clearly setting and enforcing rules, and stressing the consequences of children's actions in relation to others (Denham, Renwick, & Holt, 1991; Maccoby, 1992; Zahn-Waxler, Radke-Yarrow, & King, 1979). Likewise, even after taking the effects of parental psychological control and the parent–child emotional relationship into account, high levels of behavioral control predict better child adjustment, for example, declines in delinquency and substance use involvement over a 1-year period (Herman, Dornbusch, Herron, & Herting, 1997). It is also sometimes reported, albeit less consistently, that children whose parents exert behavioral control are at lower risk for developing internalizing symptoms (e.g., Barber, 1996). Thus, appropriate levels of behavioral control are consistently associated with lower levels of behavior problems, particularly with regard to delinquency, externalizing symptoms, and affiliation with deviant peers. This fact is well established and a systematic review of the evidence for these relations would be redundant given the numerous, much more extensive, published accounts (Conduct Problems Prevention Research Group, 1992; Maccoby & Martin, 1983; Patterson, 1982; Patterson & Yoerger, 1997). The goal for the next stage of research, consistent with the developmental psychopathology perspective, is to understand the multidimensional bases for these relations at a more precise level of analysis, including the processes that mediate these effects. We next highlight some of the issues that emerge from a developmental psycholopathology perspective on behavioral control.

Multiple Strategies for Behavioral Control

One direction espoused by the developmental psychopathology perspective is more precise differentiation of the phenomena affecting children's development. The effects of behavioral control are not uniform across all of the strategies employed. In particular, two dimensions of behavioral control have been differentiated: (1) monitoring—the degree to which parents supervise and track the activities and whereabouts of children; (2) discipline—the consistency of enforcement and the specific strategies parents use to enforce rules and inculcate values in children. Moreover, specific behavioral control strategies may vary as a function of the manner in which they are employed (e.g., consistency, severity) and the developmental level of the child (e.g., developmental changes in limit setting and control).

For example, in adolescents, parental monitoring predicts concurrent and subsequent lower levels of externalizing symptoms (e.g., fighting, delinquency, drug use) (Loeber & Dishion, 1984, McCord, 1979, Patterson & Stouthamer-Loeber, 1984), even after taking into account other aspects of behavioral control or regulation (e.g., Herman, Dornbusch, Herron, & Herting, 1997). Thus, Patterson and Stouthamer-Loeber (1984) reported that poor monitoring predicted at least 250% more variance in adolescent delinquency relative to other measures of parenting skill (i.e., consistency of discipline, problem solving, reinforcement) and was the only measure of parenting skill to differentiate chronic and moderate offenders of the law.

However, increased parental control does not necessarily have the desired effects; outcomes depend to some extent on how control is exerted. Whereas parental disciplinary inconsistency and chronic failure to enforce rules predict children's problems in regulating behavior (e.g., aggression, delinquency, impulsivity), unqualified use of power-assertive disciplinary techniques (e.g., excessive reliance on direct commands, threats, deprivation, and physical force) across multiple disciplinary situations (e.g., not simply situations that present danger to the welfare of the child) does not have an opposite, and desirable, effect. In fact, such practices predict an even wider range of maladjustment than inconsistency, including both internalizing and externalizing symptoms (e.g., Hoffman, 1960). By contrast, induction techniques of disciplining children, which focus on underscoring the painful consequences of the child's transgression for others, have been associated with greater competence, empathy, and prosocial behavior (Hoffman & Saltzstein, 1967).

Relatedly, increasing the rate of parental control does not necessarily increase its beneficial effects. Thus, some researchers have hypothesized that behavioral control by parents is curvilinear in relation to adolescent adjustment. One model posits that moderate levels of parental power and control are a more effective parenting practice than either very high or very low levels. Thus, adolescent well-being is compromised when the balance of power is tipped heavily toward the child (i.e., low behavioral control or permissiveness) or the parent (i.e., high behavioral control or authoritarian control) (Baumrind, 1991; Kurdek & Fine, 1994). Low behavioral control fails to provide guidelines for children to effectively regulate their own behavior, whereas extremely high levels of behavioral control excessively restrict children's developing autonomy and sense of identity.

A second model proposes that behavioral control fosters better adjustment in adolescents incrementally, but only to a certain point or threshold; thereafter, progressively higher levels of behavioral control do little in the way of either promoting or inhibiting adolescent mental health. For example, Kurdek and Fine (1994) reported that the "threshold model" explains, in part, the development of adolescent self-regulation (i.e., low drug experimentation and externalizing symptoms, and high academic grades); that is, behavioral control predicts successively higher levels of self-regulation at the low end of the continuum (i.e., different degrees of laxness); thereafter, at moderate or high levels, its power in predicting self-regulation drastically diminishes. Notably, both of these models linking the degree of control to children's adjustment suggest that too much behavioral control by parents is not advantageous, and may be disadvantageous. However, given findings of inconsistencies across samples and outcome measures, our understanding of these more complex, nonlinear models of relations between parental control and child adjustment is at an early stage of articulation.

Processes Mediating Effects and More on Multiple Control Strategies

What processes are set in motion by behavioral control strategies that can account for child outcomes? As we have seen, this question is a crucial one from a developmental psychopathology perspective. Over the years, various process-oriented conceptual frameworks have been proposed to provide a detailed account of the mechanisms through which different behavioral control strategies influence children's developmental trajectories. These conceptual frameworks are often derived from broader theoretical perspectives (i.e., social learning theory, psychoanalytic and affective–motivational theories, information-processing theory). None yields a complete explanation; rather, each is best regarded as a midlevel theory that provides a detailed, but only partial, explanation for the effects of parental discipline on children's functioning. On the other hand, the models complement each other. Furthermore, when considered together rather than in isolation, they may provide a more comprehensive account of why disciplinary techniques differ in their effectiveness. Notably, these theoretical accounts of processes mediating the effects of parental control strategies also suggest the importance of additional distinctions between these strategies and their degree of use; research associated with each theory provides support for these further distinctions in parental control strategies.

Social Learning Theory

Different strategies of behavioral control, or their failure, may set in motion interpersonal and intrachild processes that increase the probability of developmental trajectories of adjustment or maladjustment. For example, reflecting the transactional interplay between parent and child in the development of antisocial trajectories, Patterson identified a three-step coercive process in parent–child disciplinary encounters. In the first step, parents issue to the child a directive to refrain from continuing a certain behaviors (e.g., temper tantrum) or to initiate certain behaviors (e.g., cleaning up room). Alternatively, the parents resist performing an action that the child demands of them. In the second step, the child escalates his or her level of misbehavior. Parents may continue to request compliance to their own demands. However, as the child continues to escalate misbehavior, the parent may surrender to the child's demands and, in the process, negatively reinforce the child's misbehavior; that is, the child's escalating misbehavior is negatively reinforced because he or she has successfully found a way to escape the parents' aversive demands (Cummings & Davies, 1995; Pettit, 1997). This sequence of coercive processes fosters particularly aversive, overt forms of symptomatology, characterized by aggression, noncompliance, and conduct problems. Children's use of coercive techniques may subsequently generalize to other contexts (e.g., school, peers) and crystallize into a stable set of antisocial traits.

A failure to be consistent in parental control is also expected to lead to problems in children's adjustment from other variations in the social learning perspective (Wahler & Dumas, 1986). Working from the assumption that children value predictability in interpersonal situations, children experiencing relatively unpredictable patterns of parental control would be expected to increase their levels of misbehavior further in an effort to increase the negative, but more predictable and coherent, responses from parents (Pettit, 1997). Consistent with this view, in comparison to nonaggressive children, aggressive children experienced more positive and fewer negative consequences for misbehavior, and fewer positive and more negative consequences for positive behavior.

As we have seen, specifying the dynamic, day-to-day processes that underlie children's adaptation and maladaptation over time is a central aim of the developmental psychopathology approach. Thus, the concern with how the microprocesses become macroprocesses is an extremely interesting direction of the social learning tradition from a developmental psychopathology perspective. In general, social learning theory approaches implicate the day-to-day interchanges between parents and children around limit setting and control in establishing habitual patterns of negative or positive interaction (Patterson & Yoerger, 1997). Thus, attention is directed to the ways in which moment-to-moment interactions over time are gradually consolidated into general styles. The effects of family experiences on children are assumed at the most microscopic level of analysis to reflect the occurrence of small, frequently subtle, changes in interpersonal and social behavior emerging over time in response to the occurrence of daily stressors or positive experiences (Davis, Hops, Alpert, & Sheeber, 1998; Repetti, McGrath, & Ishikawa, 1995). Articulating this perspective, Repetti and Wood (1997) have commented:

> Finding a way to capture that phenomenon—the process by which persistent demands or strains gradually infiltrate and change an individual's life—is a special challenge facing researchers. We approach that challenge by noting that when even small amounts of variance are explained in particular situations, the underlying processes can account for important long-term outcomes if situations recur and the effects accumulate. Chronic stress, by definition, re-

curs, and the effects certainly accumulate. One way to study this process of cumulation, then, is by examining acute responses to short-term increases in common daily stressors. (p. 191)

Affective–Motivational Models

Aside from the effects of behavioral contingencies due to parental control strategies, the children's perspective on the meaning of the disciplinary encounter may have an influence on the effectiveness of a disciplinary practice (Hoffman, 1960). Direct commands, threats, and physical force used by power-assertive parents engender frustration, hostility, and tension, and work against instilling empathy as a precursor of prosocial behavior and interpersonal compassion. Motivated by fear for their well-being, children may temporarily and overtly comply with the threats. However, they may have difficulty accepting and internalizing the moral message and accepting it as their own values. The arousal and fear for their own well-being may disrupt their cognitive attempts to understand the consequences of the transgression. Furthermore, appraisals of threat may serve to redirect their attention and psychological resources away from the transgression itself toward the more significant goal of preserving their own well-being. In the long run, parental threat and the accumulating hostility and tension toward the parent may increase the likelihood that children reject parental and societal values, and direct their hostility toward less powerful scapegoats (e.g., peers) (Grusec & Goodnow, 1994a, 1994b; Hoffman, 1994; Hoffman & Saltzstein, 1967).

On the other hand, as a parental control strategy, induction may promote moral and prosocial development. By directing children's processing of events to the negative interpersonal consequences of their actions, induction techniques serve the dual social-cognitive purpose of highlighting the pain of another and showing children that they are the cause of the pain. Directing children to understand that they are the cause of another's distress is likely to capitalize on their inherent ability to respond empathetically. Empathy resulting from witnessing the pain of another, in combination with stimulating self-awareness that the child was the cause of the pain, is proposed to promote empathy-based guilt and children's critical evaluation of their own behavior. Unlike the overwhelming levels of arousal theorized to be experienced by children of power-assertive parents, the mild distress resulting from parental disapproval may serve to motivate children to attend to and repair their transgressions as a way of regaining love and approval from the parent. By the same token, the mild disapproval expressed by parents desensitizes children to the source of the message (the parent) and, in the process, children internalize and accept the moral value as their own, along with the accompanying feelings of empathy and interpersonal sensitivity (Hoffman, 1983, 1994). Various direct tests of these notions in the context of mediational models have provided support for empathy as a mechanism that accounts, in part, for the relationship between parental use of inductive discipline and children's prosocial behavior (Krevans & Gibbs, 1996).

Falling between these two extremes, the psychological distress of children who commonly experience withdrawal of love as a disciplinary technique is thought to direct children's attention to the painful consequences the transgression holds for their own well-being. Thus, children may be motivated to repair the transgression as a way of regaining parental approval. Yet in failing to direct children's attention to the feelings of others, withdrawal of love is less effective in promoting interpersonal sensitivity, empathy, and guilt over specific actions than induction techniques. In the absence of any specific parental reference to the interpersonal consequences of child misbehavior, experiences of overwhelming guilt and anxiety resulting from parental withdrawal of love may disrupt children's ability to understand the specific source of their distress (Grusec & Goodnow, 1994a, 1994b). Thus, although withdrawal of love has been theorized to fall between power-assertion and induction in terms of its effectiveness, overwhelming, undifferentiated guilt and distress may be prominent forerunners of internalizing symptomatology (Hoffman, 1994; Hoffman & Saltzstein, 1967).

In the spirit of process-oriented research, these affective–motivational theories are continually being refined. Thus, despite initial theoretical predictions that parental disappointment is best considered a form of withdrawal of love (e.g., Maccoby & Martin, 1983), recent empirical findings indicate that it more closely resembles inductive disciplinary techniques in its association with a constellation of more optimal parenting variables (e.g., low reliance on power assertion, high nurturance) and its prediction of high levels of child empathy. Yet while other-oriented induction and parental disappointment to some extent set in motion similar processes that stimulate child empathy, newly revised models posit that when parents express confidence in their child's capacity for competence and prosocial behavior, they may also foster positive child outcomes associated with expressions of disappointment in disciplinary situations. Moreover, unlike the relatively negative effects of inductive techniques on children's self-appraisals, the resulting high expectations for child behavior are hypothesized to enhance children's self-esteem, a prosocial self-concept, and, ultimately, prosocial behavior (Krevans & Gibbs, 1996).

Social Information Processing Models

Complementing the social learning and affective–motivational models for the effects of parental control on child adjustment, Grusec and Goodnow (1994b) have underscored the primacy of children's social-cognitive processes in mediating the effects of parental disciplinary techniques on their internalization of values. Of particular interest from a process-oriented perspective is their focus on more precisely evaluating the effectiveness of specific disciplinary techniques in relation to the particular contextual variables, including the (1) specific misdeed, (2) nature of parental reaction (e.g., arousal of empathy vs. insecurity), (3) nature of the child (e.g., mood, temperament, history of discipline experiences), and (4) parental characteristics (e.g., warmth, disciplinary style). For example, parents cannot easily be classified as using one predominant disciplinary technique. Retaining flexibility by selecting specific disciplinary techniques that are sensitive to the child's transgression may play a key role in promoting optimal development. Transgressions characterized by a failure to show concern for others are commonly handled by using induction techniques, whereas responses to conduct problems may be commonly handled by using power assertion and, in some cases, inductive or reasoning techniques (e.g., Grusec, Dix, & Mills, 1982; Trickett & Kuczynski, 1986). According to their model, the interplay among the contextual characteristics of the discipline encounter affects the probability that children will internalize values by effecting how accurately they perceive the socialization message underlying the parental discipline and the degree to which they accept the message.

Psychological Control by Parents

Another strategy for controlling children's behavior is psychological control, that is, ways of controlling the child by negatively manipulating the parent–child relationship (e.g., Barber, 1992, 1996; Barber, Olsen, & Shagle, 1994). Psychological control consists of parenting strategies that "inhibit or intrude upon the psychological development through manipulation and exploitation of the parent–child bond (e.g., love withdrawal and guilt induction), negative affect-laden expressions and criticisms (e.g., disappointment and shame), and excessive personal control (e.g., possessiveness, protectiveness)" (Barber, 1996, p. 3297). By exercising control over children's psychological world, psychologically controlling parents are theorized to hinder the development of psychological autonomy and the attainment by children of a clear, purposeful sense of identity and appraisal of the self as agentic and competent.

Psychological and behavioral control strategies may have quite different effects, with psychological control setting in motion a different set of processes than behavioral control. Thus, recent research suggests that parental psychological control predicts unique variance in children's adjustment even after taking into account the predictive power of parental behavioral control (e.g., Barber, 1996; Barber, Olsen, & Shagle, 1994). Psychological control appears to be a consistent predictor of internalizing symptoms, although parenting practices indicative of psychological control have been associated with a broad array of adjustment problems, spanning internalizing symptoms (e.g., depression, eating disorders, loneliness), externalizing problems (e.g., delinquency), low academic achievement and expectancies, substance use, and somatic symptoms (e.g., Allen, Hauser, Eickholt, Bell, & O'Connor, 1994; Barber et al., 1994; Fauber, Forehand, Thomas, & Wierson, 1990; Herman, Dornbusch, Herron, & Herting, 1997). Controlling for earlier levels of psychological adjustment, psychological control nonetheless still predicts subsequent increases in adolescent somatic symptoms (Herman et al., 1997), even when simultaneously considering the effects of parental involvement and monitoring. According to recent theory, chronic love withdrawal, over-protection, guilt induction, and discounting the children's perspective and feelings instill (1) negative self-appraisals, particularly in terms of poor self-worth, helplessness, and low self-confidence; (2) prolonged bouts of self-blame, guilt, and excessive worry about the self and family; and (3) coping processes indicative of dependence, inhibition, and submissiveness. These evolving response patterns, in turn, are thought to be precursors of subsequent internalizing problems that become stable across time and context (Barber, 1996). The next challenge is to use theory as a guide toward testing more directly the processes underlying developmental trajectories of children exposed to varying levels of psychological control.

PARENTAL CONTROL AND PARENT–CHILD EMOTIONAL RELATIONSHIPS

An advantage of controlling the effects of other parenting variables is that it provides a way of understanding the specific, unique contributions of a specific parenting construct. The disadvantage from the perspective of fully understanding parenting effects on children is that controlling for "extraneous" parenting variables does not account for the multivariate interplay between the parenting dimensions in affecting child development. A tenet of the organizational perspective of developmental psychopathology is that it is children's holistic experiences with the wider spectrum of specific parenting characteristics (e.g., warmth, behavioral control, psychological control) that ultimately influence trajectories of development. Co-occurring sets of parenting or psychosocial characteristics may be responsible, in part, for child outcomes (Darling & Steinberg, 1993). For example, Grusec and Goodnow (1994a) have examined the influence of disciplinary methods on children's internalization of values and found evidence for the importance of parental warmth and sensitivity to children in facilitating the efficacy of disciplinary techniques and children's internalization of values and moral development. Thus, children's adjustment is not simply a function of additive, unique combinations of specific parenting characteristics; rather, it is a function, in part, of children's experiences with different patterns or profiles of parenting characteristics.

At the outset of this chapter, we proposed that parental control and the parent–child relationship are the two broad dimensions of parenting that have been identified in research as significant to child adjustment. One way of examining interrelationships between parenting characteristics and child adjustment is to consider how interrelations between these two broad dimensions of parenting affect child adjustment. Before providing an in-depth treatment of the effects of parent–child emotional relationships on children's functioning, we next examine directions that consider how broad profiles that combine these factors predict child adjustment.

Classification Systems for Profiles of Parenting

Tripartite Classification

Baumrind (1967, 1971) proposed that neither parent–child emotional relationships (e.g., responsiveness, warmth, availability) nor parental controls (e.g., demandingness, monitoring, consistent discipline) alone are sufficient for healthy child development, because both are important for parents to achieve child-rearing goals. Whereas the former fosters individuality, including autonomy, self-worth, and self-regulation in the children, the latter encourages the development of the child as a contributing member of society (Baumrind, 1991; Darling & Steinberg, 1993). Working from these assumptions, Baumrind developed a seminal classification scheme that distinguished among three qualitatively different types of parenting styles.

Authoritative parents utilize firm, consistent control centered around integrating the child into the family and society, and insisting that the child meet increasing standards of maturity as he or she gets older. Communication styles with children are characterized by warmth, clarity, reciprocality, and verbal give-and-take between parent and child. Thus, control (i.e., high behavioral control) takes place in the context of warmth (i.e., positive parent–child emotional relationship) and encouragement of the child's autonomy and individuality (i.e., low psychological control). Children of authoritative parents are most likely to exhibit a healthy balance between high levels of agency (i.e., achievement-oriented, high self-esteem, independent) and communion (i.e., sociable, interpersonally cooperative, friendly) (Baumrind, 1967, 1971). Although the efficacy of authoritative parenting varies somewhat across ecological contexts (see Chapter 7), the positive effects of authoritative parenting are remarkably consistent across developmental periods from preschool through adolescence (e.g., Baumrind, 1991; Lamborn, Mounts, Steinberg, & Dornbusch, 1991; Steinberg, Elmen, & Mounts, 1989) and across socialization contexts of ethnicity, socioeconomic status, and family structure (e.g., Dornbusch, Ritter, Leiderman, Roberts, & Fraleigh, 1987; Steinberg, Mounts, Lamborn, & Dornbusch, 1991).

Authoritarian parents are also firm in their control practices. However, their control strategies differ qualitatively from those of authoritative parents. Strict, unquestioned obedience to parental authority is expected, with any assertion of individuality by the child met with swift and severe punishment. Thus, although children may learn to understand societal rules through their strict emphasis and enforcement by parents, the relative absence of inductive disciplinary techniques (e.g., reasoning, explanations for rules) does not foster children's internalization of the values of family and society. Furthermore, authoritarian parents' detachment, lack of warmth, and discouragement of au-

tonomy deter children from achieving a sense of personal integrity and efficacy. While children exposed to higher levels of restrictive control and
authoritarian parenting styles are less likely to engage in externalizing symptoms, delinquency, sexual promiscuity, and drug use (e.g., Baumrind, 1991),
conformity to the will of convention carries the cost of compromising individuality and agency. Thus, these children are at greater risk for internalizing
symptoms, self-devaluation, social submissiveness, low self-efficacy, and diminished autonomy (Baumrind, 1967, 1971, 1991).

Permissive parents are indulgent in their child-rearing styles, as evidenced
by their acceptance and tolerance for nearly every behavior of their children.
While this accepting attitude is associated with frequent expressions of warmth
and affection by parents, it also translates into a high tolerance for children's
impulsive and disruptive behavior, and reluctance to enforce any rules or impose
any authority. This laxness in monitoring and discipline means that children are
left to regulate their own behavior and make decisions concerning their own actions (e.g., bedtime, meals) (Maccoby & Martin, 1983). The lack of balance between warmth and control, and demandingness for maturity promotes high levels of agency and individual development at the expense of the development of
communion (Baumrind, 1991). Accordingly, children of permissive parents exhibit high levels of self-worth and self-esteem but impairments in maturity, impulse control, social responsibility, and achievement.

Fourfold Classification

Extending Baumrind's work, Maccoby and Martin (1983) proposed that parenting styles can be defined in terms of two parenting characteristics ordered
along linear continua: (1) demandingness and (2) responsiveness. Three parenting styles (authoritative, authoritarian, indulgent) that emerged from cross-
ing these two dimensions were similar to those of Baumrind (authoritative,
authoritarian, permissive). Of primary significance, however, was the emergence of an *indifferent–uninvolved* parenting style. This style is characterized
by emotional uninvolvement with the child, the strategy being to expend as
little energy as possible in caretaking. While not necessarily classifiable as maltreatment, neglect is the rule, and little thought or energy is put toward children's long-range development. Interactions with children, considered an in-
convenience, are dealt with in the way that most quickly and effortlessly
terminates the interaction (Maccoby & Martin, 1983). Failing to facilitate either communion or agency, this style predicts the most maladaptive outcomes
of the various parenting styles (Baumrind, 1991). Children experiencing histories of uninvolved parenting were not only at highest risk for evidencing low
levels of social and academic competence, but they also were prone to a number of forms of antisocial and impulsive behavior, including delinquency, alcohol problems, drug use, criminal acts, and sexual promiscuity (Block, 1971;
Lamborn, Mounts, Steinberg, & Dornbusch, 1991; Patterson, DeBaryshe, &
Ramsey, 1989).

However, despite the apparent similarities, the theoretical assumptions underlying the tripartite and quadratic classification schemes differ in significant ways that have implications for the comparability of the two systems. Maccoby and Martin's (1983) classification system is heavily influenced by a behavioral or social learning perspective. Consequently, responsiveness in this framework refers not to warmth and affection, but rather to the frequency of behavioral contingencies that shape desired behaviors and extinguish or reduce undesired behaviors. Such an approach does not capture the qualitative differences between the parenting styles proposed by Baumrind (1991). For example, linear or quantitative models conceptualize authoritarian and authoritative parents as using comparable, high levels of behavioral control. Yet in Baumrind's (1971) framework, the two styles of parenting reflect very different types of control (e.g., physical punishment vs. explanation). Authoritarian parents exhibit high levels of restrictiveness or psychological control, whereas authoritative parents exhibit high levels of behavioral control (Darling & Steinberg, 1993).

Classifications of Parenting Styles and Parenting Practices

The study of relations between classification of parenting styles and child outcomes leaves open many questions that, we have argued, are critical from a developmental psychopathology perspective for understanding children's development, including (1) the specific parenting behaviors, cognitions, and other practices that occur in association with parenting styles; (2) the associated processes set in motion in the child by parenting styles; and (3) the transactional relations over time between parenting and other factors that ultimately influence pathways of development in the children (Darling & Steinberg, 1993; Lewis, 1981; see Figure 3.1). Thus, while the study of parenting styles as influences on children's socialization has led to important advances, from a process-oriented perspective, just part of the puzzle is addressed by examining only relations between classifications of parenting and child outcomes. Directions in the study of parenting practices are targeted to this more precise analysis of process.

Parenting Practices in Specific Domains

Research on parenting practices and parenting styles has tended to focus on relatively broad aspects of parenting. Studies now need to tease apart these more global constructs in order to understand process better and to highlight specific features of parental behavior for prevention and intervention (see Chapter 11). Thus, one valuable distinction made in parenting practices research is that global parental involvement is distinguished from parental involvement in specific domains of functioning. For example, Maccoby and Martin (1983) defined parental involvement as the extent to which a parent is "committed to his or her role as a parent and to fostering optimal child development" (p. 48), whereas in parenting practices, research parental involvement is defined as "the dedication of resources by a parent to the child *within a given domain*" (emphasis added, Grolnick & Slowiaczek, 1994, p. 238). The point is that even parents who are highly involved at a stylistic or global level may not necessarily be heavily involved in dedicating resources to all domains of child socialization (e.g., emotion regulation, social skills and peer popularity, empathy and prosocial orientation, athleticism, academics). The reverse also holds true: Parents who are relatively uninvolved at a stylistic level may still be involved in promoting specific socialization goals (e.g., academics).

For example, with regard to academic functioning, Grolnick and Slowiaczek (1994) examined the specific resources and means by which parents become involved in promoting (or inhibiting) children's academic achievement. They found evidence for several different types of parental involvement: (1) behavioral involvement (e.g., participation in school events), (2) personal involvement (e.g., affective communication of enthusiasm regarding academic events), and (3) cognitive involvement (e.g., structuring and organizing intellectually stimulating activities). Moreover, they examined the intrachild motivational processes that mediated the relationship between types of parental involvement and children's academic achievement. Illustrating the notion that multiple pathways can lead to the same outcome, they found that maternal behavioral and cognitive involvement each predicted greater school achievement by promoting children's perceived competence in academic activities. On the other hand, illustrating that sometimes a specific pathway is found, children's understanding of the means to achieve academic success emerged as the only mediator of the link between parental behavioral involvement in schooling and child academic success.

Thus, one can see how more focused study of parents' behavior in specific contexts can advance understanding of the processes mediating adjustment, consistent with the types of questions raised by a developmental psychopathology perspective on family influences in children's adjustment. Unfortunately, specific parenting practices and styles are sometimes treated as competitive rather than complementary models (Darling & Steinberg, 1993). The examination of the adaptive (or maladaptive) value of specific parenting behaviors in the context of well-defined socialization settings is useful for elucidating the intrachild mechanisms that mediate parenting effects (Lollis & Kuczynski, 1997). This research, however, has typically ignored the larger constellation of potentially influential parenting characteristics (e.g., quality of parent–child emotional relationships, coparenting relationships, family ecology variables), which can result in potentially misleading conclusions about process. By contrast, the classification of parenting styles does capture constellations of parenting characteristics, including features of limit-setting and affective experience. On the other hand, as we have seen, global conceptualizations of parenting do not illuminate the nature of specific parenting characteristics and the mediating processes that influence child outcomes.

Given the complementary strengths and limitations of these two levels of analysis of parenting, a challenging question is: Can we integrate both more general and specific models into a single cohesive framework? Consistent with the developmental psychopathology perspective, multivariate models assessing the role of significant categories of mediational processes and moderating conditions are required to map adequately the several different levels of conceptualization and analysis (e.g., parenting styles, parenting practices in the context of socialization goals and settings, intrachild processes, child adjustment). We next turn to research directed toward a more integrative study of different levels of analysis of parenting.

Parenting Practices as Mediators of Parenting Styles

Parenting styles may influence child development by shaping parenting practices in specific socialization contexts. For example, recent work indicates that authoritative parenting leads to increases in school success over time (Steinberg, Lamborn, Dornbusch, & Darling, 1992). Moreover, tracing the specific channels by which authoritative parenting is expressed in the context of school- or achievement-related activities, Steinberg and colleagues (1992) found that parental school involvement mediated the pathway between authoritative parenting and improvements in school performance. Beyond this exemplary study, however, surprisingly little research has explored the mediational interplay between parenting styles and specific parenting practices in predicting children's functioning within specific domains such as empathy and prosocial behavior, coping styles, emotional expressiveness, self-control, agency, and school engagement.

Another relevant direction is Gerald Patterson's (1997) distinction between macroparenting and microparenting in understanding children's social development. According to this model, the link between macroparenting variables—characterized by discipline, monitoring, and problem-solving—and children's conduct problems is mediated by microparenting practices that arise in specific disciplinary situations. More specifically, it is hypothesized that underlying ineffective discipline and lax monitoring, a set of behavioral contingencies (e.g., escape conditioning, intermittent positive reinforcement) more directly shape children's aggressive dispositions that eventually generalize across settings. Support has also begun to emerge for this characterization of relations between two levels of analysis of parenting (e.g., Snyder, 1991; Snyder, Schrepferman, & St. Peter, 1997).

Parenting Styles as Moderators of Parenting Practices

In addition, Darling and Steinberg (1993) have postulated that the full impact of parenting styles on child development cannot simply be explained through a mediational model of parenting practices. Parenting style may also be moderator of the effects of specific parenting practices on child outcomes; that is, parenting style is conceptualized as a contextual variable that modifies the link between parenting practices and child outcomes in two ways. First, the parenting style may shape the effectiveness of the specific parenting practice. For example, authoritative parents may be more effective with children in certain socialization contexts (e.g., academic) by virtue of their use of explanation and encouragement of children (especially adolescents) to participate actively in decision making. Thus, the parenting style may enhance or diminish parental practices directed toward helping children achieve socialization goals. Second, parenting style may influence the child's personality or, more specifically, openness to parental guidance, which, in turn, may modify the influence of parenting practices on child's outcomes. Authoritative parenting may foster children's respect for parents, thereby increasing their desire to follow parental advice, and instill parental pride by achieving parental socialization goals expressed in specific parenting contexts (Grusec & Goodnow, 1994). In accordance with these postulations, Steinberg, Lamborn, Dornbusch, and Darling (1992) found that authoritative parenting style did act as a moderator of the specific association between parental involvement in schooling and children's academic performance. Specifically, the magnitude of relations between parental involvement and children's academic success was substantially stronger when children reported experiencing higher levels of authoritative parenting.

EMOTIONAL RELATIONSHIPS BETWEEN PARENTS AND CHILDREN

The discussion thus far has examined parenting in terms of practices for controlling children's behavior, or, more broadly, relations between parental emotional behavior and strategies for controlling children's behavior, which, in turn, predict children's adjustment. Despite some overlap in themes across the various sections of this chapter, the focus thus far has been decidedly on parenting as behaviors and emotions, and children's perspectives on these control techniques. We have focused less on the emotional qualities of the parent–child relationship, or the importance of the emotional bond that forms between parents and children as another important dimension of parenting. However, as we will see, a quite considerable literature supports the importance of examining the emotional qualities of parent–child relationships as being significant to children's adjustment. It is to this topic that we turn next.

Parental Acceptance and Emotional Availability

Although complexity and diversity in operational definitions of "acceptance" or "emotional availability" are appreciable (Biringen & Robinson, 1991), many, if not most, conceptualizations refer to a common set of parenting characteristics, including parental support, expressions of warmth or positive emotional tone, sensitivity to children's psychological states, and responsivity to children's psychosocial needs. As a result of this long history, especially within psychoanalytic theoretical traditions (Darling & Steinberg, 1993; Ladd, 1992; Maccoby & Martin, 1983), a rich foundation of research has long demonstrated that parental acceptance and responsiveness predict positive child development outcomes, including greater sociability (Clarke-Stewart, 1973), self-regulation (Stayton, Hogan, & Ainsworth, 1971), prosocial behavior (Rothbaum, 1988), self-esteem (Loeb, Horst, & Horton, 1980), and constructive play (Alessandri, 1992). Parental behaviors indicative of a lack of responsivity or availability, by contrast, have been prospectively linked with a variety of maladaptive outcomes, including social withdrawal (Bakeman & Brown, 1980; Egeland, Pianta, & O'Brien, 1993), aggression (Egeland, Carlson, & Sroufe, 1993; Pettit & Bates, 1989), and attention deficit disorder (Jacobvitz & Sroufe, 1987). However, consistent with a central theme of the developmental psychopathology perspective (see Chapter 2), simply documenting bivariate associations between a predictor (i.e., parental emotional availability) and children's developmental outcomes is only the starting point toward a process-oriented understanding of how a predictor influences pathways of development (see Chapter 4).

A Multidimensional Construct

As we have seen, one important theme of the developmental psychopathology perspective is that global predictors of child adjustment are frequently markers for multiple underlying dimensions that uniquely and differentially predict child adjustment. It follows that an understanding of influences on development is blurred, at best, when predictors that yield quite different outcomes are lumped together (e.g., constructive and destructive marital conflict styles; see Chapter 8). Thus, an important direction in family research, as in other areas of research within the developmental psychopathology tradition, is to determine which of the multiple dimensions that underlie global predictors of child adjustment are most significant to distinguish, and then to examine their particular effects on child outcomes.

Thus, it is consistent with the developmental psychopathology tradition that researchers be challenged to more carefully specify the substance and content of key constructs such as parental emotional availability and support. While these notions are often discussed as if they were unidimensional constructs, they, in fact, refer to a complex constellation of dimensions. Even the long-held assumption that manifestations of parental support tend to co-occur or "hang together" does not necessarily hold. Recent research indicates that parental support dimensions (e.g., warmth, involvement, calm discussion of disagreements, proactive teaching), which do not even fully encompass the range of parenting strategies comprising parental acceptance, are generally unrelated to one another (Pettit, Bates, & Dodge, 1997). In fact, Pettit and colleagues (1997) present findings to indicate that parental support dimensions differentially predict various forms of functioning (e.g., externalizing symptoms, social skillfulness, academic performance). Moreover, Parke and Ladd (1992) have hypothesized that parental expressions of warmth or acceptance to children may be expressed in many ways or contexts and still promote healthy child development. These findings suggest that relying only on unidimensional assessments of parental warmth or acceptance, or assessments made only in one context of parenting, may obscure the precise nature of socialization pathways.

Treating parent–child emotionality as a multidimensional construct also advances the practice implications of research. For example, the knowledge that parental emotional warmth, broadly construed, is a significant ingredient in successful child rearing is minimally useful for the practitioner, especially given that forms of emotional warmth vary widely, and are comprised of multiple elements that determine their effectiveness in specific contexts, and that optimal types may vary depending on the age of the child. It is more valuable to provide precise information about the quite specific skills and response patterns that comprise optimal patterns of emotional availability, and to provide this information in the context of specific developmental periods of childhood. Maccoby and Martin (1983), for example, have underscored that parental sensitivity, a particular dimension underlying parental warmth, reflects parents' accuracy in interpreting the symptoms and the causes of distress in children, especially among infants who are incapable of articulating their problems. According to their conceptualization, any particular act of sensitivity must be considered as a process in itself, consisting of three stages: (1) assessing the problem, (2) taking action consistent with the assessment, (3) evaluating the consequences of the intervention. Even very sensitive parents are not always effective in their first attempt at intervention, so oftentimes, the process is continually reenacted until an effective solution is reached. Adding further complexity, each cycle consists of specific behaviors that may be evaluated as more or less "sensitive" depending on the specific goal of the parent and the context. For example, the timing and pacing of specific parental behaviors are essential to promoting ongoing parent–child interactions, particularly among young infants who rely on parents to structure and synchronize interactions effectively. Sensitive and responsive parents encourage the social bids of infants through contingent social stimulation that specifically consists of smiling, making dramatic faces, and otherwise responding positively. As infants withdraw in an effort to regulate the increasing bouts of emotional and physiological arousal, sensitive parents appropriately recognize their signals and aid in the regulation process by waiting patiently for the infants to reinitiate social interactions (Cohn & Tronick, 1983, 1989; Tronick, 1989).

Processes Mediating Effects

Consistent with a developmental psychopathology perspective, even at a specific level of definition, the assessment of dimensions of parent–child emotionality provides only a first step toward understanding effects. A next step is to determine the processes set in motion in the child by experiences with a particular parenting behavior.

A variety of strategies may be employed to elucidate the processes mediating the effects of parent–child emotionality on children's development. Observing interactional bouts between parents and children provides one method for understanding the processes that parenting practices induce in children, influencing adaptive or maladaptive developmental pathways. For example, children have been found to exhibit different coping behaviors following exposure to different forms of parental negativity. Whereas parental withdrawal and unresponsiveness has been shown to elicit infant protest, distress, and wariness, children commonly react to parental intrusiveness and hostility by withdrawing and disengaging (Cohn & Tronick, 1989). In the former case, infant protest may hold short-term adaptational value in increasing emotional responsivity in inattentive parents. In the latter case, disengagement may be one of the only means of successfully reducing contact with the source of stress, thereby reducing physiological and affective arousal (Cummings & Davies, 1995).

Acknowledging the multiplicity of pathways and processes leading to developmental outcomes requires the use of multiple, rather than single, mediator models. Parke, Cassidy, Burks, Carson, and Boyum (1992), for example, have proposed a tripartite mediator model whereby children's various affect management skills mediate relations between parenting style and children's developmental functioning. Specifically, different styles of parenting (e.g., stimulation, responsiveness) result in individual differences in children's emotion regulation, interpersonal information processing (e.g., encoding, decoding) in social–emotional contexts, and understanding of emotion (e.g., ability to recognize and produce emotional expressions, understanding of the causes and meaning of emotion, understanding one's own history of emotional experiences and other's emotional displays), which, in turn, impair or improve their ability to function competently in other interpersonal contexts (e.g., with peers, in friendship groups) (Denham, Renwick, & Holt, 1991; MacDonald, 1987; Parke, Cassidy, Burks, Carson, & Boyum, 1992).

Although we are presently focusing on emotional conceptualizations of mediators within the child, as we have seen, a common theme irrespective of substantive focus is the necessity of mediational models to characterize process. In fact, the interdisciplinary diversity of developmental psychopathology is a call for the consideration of multiple mediating processes from different theoretical perspectives (see Chapter 2). A particularly promising research direction in this regard is the identification of social information-processing patterns as explanatory processes in the link between negative parent–child emotionality and children's adjustment. For example, theory and empirical work have suggested that adverse parenting may foster negative attribution styles about parent–child relations that are subsequently used as a blueprint or lens for processing peer events and relationships (Dodge, Pettit, Bates, & Valente,

1995; Weiss, Dodge, Bates, & Pettit, 1992). Proclivities toward hostile evaluations and response tendencies, in turn, have been proposed to increase children's susceptibility to poor peer relationships, aggression, social isolation,
and depression (e.g., Quiggle, Garber, Panak, & Dodge, 1992; see also Crick
& Dodge, 1994, for a review). Notably, explorations of social information-
processing "steps" as mediators of parenting have largely been confined to
more negative parenting practices. Thus, a gap exists in research concerning
the exploration of these social-cognitive processes as possible mediators between positive parenting practices and positive child adjustment (Crick &
Dodge, 1994; Dodge et al., 1995; Weiss et al., 1992).

Despite differences in conceptual emphasis across these different theories,
both emotion regulation and information-processing models bear remarkable
similarity to some of the central mechanisms proposed to mediate parent–
child emotionality (e.g., acceptance and availability). In the aggregate, these
models converge to support the notion that parental availability promotes interpersonal connectedness among children, equips them with social skills necessary to further increase the quality of interpersonal relations, and fosters a
general view of the social world as a safe, secure place (Barber, 1997).

Parental Responses to Children's Emotional Expression

Another dimension of parent–child emotionality is parental responses to children's emotional expressions. While this is a subset of parental sensitivity and
responsivity to children's signals, evidence suggests that parental responses to
children's emotionality merit consideration as a distinct dimension of parenting related to the quality of the emotional relationship between the parent and
child. Different parenting responses in this regard are clearly illustrated in an
example by Gottman, Katz, and Hooven (1997) on the importance of meta-
emotion philosophy to children's emotional functioning:

> Suppose a parent is driving on a hot summer day with a child, and gets caught
> in unrelenting bumper-to-bumper traffic. The child says, "Dad, I want some
> cold milk." Dad says very sweetly, "Honey, there's nothing I can do until we
> get home. Then I'll get you some milk." Not mollified, the child repeats the re-
> quest more insistently: "I want some cold milk now!" Dad repeats himself, ex-
> plaining why he cannot get the milk now. This exchange continues, with the
> child escalating, adding whining and crying as the exchange continues. . . . All
> this . . . might have been avoided if the father had originally said something
> like, "Yeah, cold milk sounds great. I wish I had some myself right now." The
> child, whose feelings are understood, would have said, "Yeah," and the father
> might have added, "Some ice cream would be nice too," and the child might
> have continued, "Yeah, an ice cream sundae." Dad: "Yum." (p. 20)

Notably, the father's actual response in this vignette is characterized by
warmth, patience, responsivity to the child's bids, and use of explanations,
and appears to be consistent with a parental acceptance and warmth. Despite

this, his response is not the most optimal way to respond in terms of the emotional relationship between father and child, because the father's reaction fails to communicate that he understands his child's specific experiences with negative affect (Gottman, Katz, & Hooven, 1996, 1997). The study of parental meta-emotion philosophies further underscores the utility of contextualizing the multidimensional framework of specific socialization practices and emotions within the larger organization of underlying parenting beliefs and philosophies (Gottman et al., 1996, 1997). Meta-emotion philosophy refers to the constellation of feelings, thoughts, beliefs, and goals regarding the regulation and function of one's own, and one's child's, emotions. Thus, this work stresses not only the importance that parental efforts be warmly responsive to children's bids, but also that parents respond appropriately in terms of the social signals and demands of the broader socioemotional context.

Unlike the hypotheses supported in other areas of the research on parent–child emotional relationship indicating that greater warmth and acceptance are related to greater child competence, the study of parenting in the context of children's negative emotionality suggests that parental encouragement of emotional expression may be related to child adjustment in a curvilinear way. Fabes, Eisenberg, Smith, and Murphy (1996) have hypothesized that children may display the most constructive ways of regulating and expressing negative emotion when parents show moderate, rather than high or low, encouragement of emotional expression. Although more work is needed to examine this hypothesis systematically, the results do indicate that, at least for girls, moderate encouragement of emotional expression by parents is related to the highest levels of prosocial behavior.

Yet within the larger process model, parental encouragement of emotional expression is regarded as only one component of a multidimensional constellation of techniques parents may use in responding to their children's emotions (Eisenberg, 1996). Additional dimensions such as parental distress, dismissing children's emotions, comforting, and encouraging and helping children to solve the problem that is the source of their distress have been shown to have unique implications and consequences for children's development that cannot be captured by any global characterization of how parents respond and behave (Eisenberg, 1996; Eisenberg & Fabes, 1994; Eisenberg et al., 1996). This fine-grained process orientation has been particularly valuable in (1) outlining the constructive and destructive dimensions of parental reactions to child distress and (2) generating hypotheses regarding the underlying intrachild mechanisms that mediate the link between these parenting practices and child adjustment (e.g., Eisenberg, 1996).

Emotional Bonds and Parent–Child Attachment

The effects of parental behavior on children's adjustment are not just a matter of the behaviors that parents direct toward their children, or even the emotional intensity of interactions, but they reflect the quality of the relationship between parents and children; that is, interactions between parents and children are not just "a kind of intellectual exchange" (Hoffman, 1994, p. 26) but are influenced by their history, especially the emotional bond or attachment that has formed between them. Thus, in deciding how to behave, children respond not only to the behaviors directed at them by parents, but also to their emotional relationships with parents.

John Bowlby and Mary Ainsworth's attachment theory provides the most influential conceptualization of the nature of the emotional bonds between parents and children (Ainsworth, Blehar, Waters, & Wall, 1978; Bowlby, 1969). Moreover, the attachment theory tradition provides considerable empirical support for the significance of attachments to children's (and adults') adjustment (e.g., Bretherton, 1985; Carlson & Sroufe, 1995; Colin, 1996; Hazan & Shaver, 1990), although variability in the stability of attachment over time, and in the prediction of later behavior based upon earlier attachment, is evident in the literature (Belsky, Campbell, Cohn, & Moore, 1996; Belsky & Cassidy, 1994; Thompson, 2000). In the last part of this chapter, we consider the evidence for emotional bonds between parents and children as an element of parenting that contributes to normal development and risk for the development of psychopathology in children. Given the extensiveness of this literature, we cannot provide more than selective coverage of some of the key themes.

Historical Overview

The notion that the early emotional bonds between parents and children are significant to later development can be traced to psychoanalytic notions of object relations and, later, the learning theory concept of dependency (Ainsworth, 1969). However, these notions about the importance of early parent–child emotional bonds to later development characterized these relations as immature and reflecting the lack of adequate development. The close emotional bond between parent and child in early childhood was viewed as a state of affairs to be outgrown, so that it followed that it was in some sense undesirable and problematic for relations with such immature response dimensions to continue beyond infancy. Moreover, the relationship was seen as evolving out of the parents' role in the satisfaction of primary needs, such a hunger, thirst, and so on, rather than as having developmental significance in its own right.

However, subsequent research showed that the satisfaction of primary needs was not essential (e.g., Schaffer & Emerson, 1964); rather, parent–child emotional bonds developed out of the particular quality of the interactions between parents and children (Ainsworth, 1967). Moreover, a body of clinical research on the effects on children of long-term separations, deprivation of care, and loss on children provided vivid evidence for the desirability of close relationships between parents and children for children's long-term adjustment (Ainsworth, 1962; Bowlby, 1951, 1969). The conclusion was that the formation and maintenance of emotional bonds between parents and children were a highly desirable state of affairs that predicted positive qualities of children's adjustment. Accordingly, Bowlby (1958) coined the term "attachment" to distinguish the new, positive view of parent–child emotional relationships for children's adjustment from the earlier, somewhat pejorative characterizations of the nature and developmental implications of these relationships. Based on research with nonhuman primates (Harlow, 1958) and other species, Bowlby (1969) also argued for the developmental primacy and biological bases of parent–child emotional bonds in their own right, and for their importance to species survival from an evolutionary perspective, particularly in the early origins of the species (i.e., in the "environment of evolutionary adaptiveness"). Finally, rather than being a developmental stage to be outgrown, attachments were viewed as providing influential initial models for later, close relationships, and as being formed and having positive implications for adjustment throughout the life span; that is, attachment was seen as significant to an understanding of normal functioning and risk for psychopathology from infancy to old age. Thus, the formation of early close emotional bonds or attachments was seen as normal and desirable, and not a source of deviancy or dependency, with their function being to provide the individual with a sense of security, particularly in times of stress.

An Organizational Construct

Given the emphasis thus far on parenting practices as behaviors, it merits emphasis that the essential element of attachment is the emotional bond, not specific behaviors. The bond is seen as not simply the sum of the behaviors; rather, it serves as the source of a higher-order goal or plan around which behaviors are organized and directed. In this sense, attachment is an organizational construct that motivates and directs a relatively complex and sophisticated behavioral control system in response to the contextual demands of situations faced by the child. Moreover, the behaviors in the service of attachment are flexible and interchangeable based on the moment-to-moment needs of the dyad in the context of the attachment relationship (Sroufe & Waters, 1977a). Thus, attachment behaviors are properly interpreted in terms of the meaning they have for the quality of the underlying bond in a situational context, rather than in isolation from the broader patterning and context of behavior. For example, an infant can indicate a secure response to reunion with the mother after a brief separation by greeting her across a distance, or alternatively, by running up to her and giving her a hug. While on the surface these behaviors are different, in terms of a holistic interpretation of the implications of the behaviors for the quality of attachment they may have precisely the same meaning. Notably, attachment behaviors have stability and predictability for children's functioning and adjustment when interpreted from a holistic and organizational perspective with regard to their meaning for the quality of the emotional bond between parent and child (i.e., attachment security). On the other hand, when scored only as individual behaviors outside of an organizational perspective, such behaviors do not evidence stability over even very short periods of time (Masters & Wellman, 1974; Waters, 1978). Finally, attachments are seen as specific to individual relationships between parents and children rather than being generalized traits (Bowlby, 1973).

Interdisciplinary Perspectives

As we have seen, the developmental psychopathology approach also fosters interdisciplinary study of developmental phenomena (Chapter 1). The commitment to an interdisciplinary approach is embodied in Bowlby's formulation of attachment theory, in which he accomplished the laudable feat of cogently integrating concepts from such diverse disciplines as psychiatry (discussed earlier), ethology, control systems theory, cognitive psychology, and developmental psychology (Bowlby, 1969).

Ethology and the Observation of Parenting in Naturalistic Settings. A particular emphasis in attachment theory is on the detailed behavioral observation of parent–child interactions in naturalistic environments (i.e., the home), which originated in the European tradition of ethology that stressed the importance of careful observation of animal behavior in natural habitats. The concern with intensive data collection in naturalistic settings was consistent with Bowlby's formulation that attachments are shaped by experience and that understanding the development of attachment relationships is informed by the day-to-day experience of interactions between parents and children. Remarkably, this emphasis on behavioral observation ran counter to the much greater significance accorded by psychoanalysis to intrapsychic influences that were not necessarily of experiential origin and decidedly were not categorized as observable behavior. Thus, Ainsworth's original formulations of the secure-base function of parent–child attachments were based upon lengthy and meticulous observations of mother–child interactions in natural settings in Uganda (Ainsworth, 1967) and Baltimore (Ainsworth, Blehar, Waters, & Wall, 1978). Subsequent investigators have continued this tradition of naturalistic observation of mother–child interaction over substantial periods of time in the home (e.g., Belsky, Rovine, & Taylor, 1984; Egeland & Farber, 1984; Grossmann, Grossmann, Spangler, Suess, & Unzner, 1985). Moreover, the observation of attachment relationships in the natural environment (i.e., the home) is viewed as an essential point of comparison for attachment research, since the ultimate goal of that research is to understand the functioning of parent–child relationships in real life. Thus, strong emphasis is placed on uncovering the nature of daily experience and its relations to the development of attachment and the operation of the attachment system in the provision of emotional security (Cicchetti, Cummings, Greenberg, & Marvin, 1990; Cummings, 1990). Relatedly, in reaction to the methodological flaws of retrospective reports identified by Ainsworth (1962) and Bowlby (1951) in their early, seminal reviews of the importance of the parent–child emotional bond as indicated by retrospective clinical studies on the highly negative impact of the absence of these relationships (i.e., research on the effects of "maternal deprivation"), attachment theory from the beginning strongly emphasized the scientific merits of prospective, longitudinal research designs, which we have seen are essential to a process-oriented approach (Chapter 3).

Control Systems Theory: Contextualizing Attachment Behavior. Another valuable direction, also consistent with principles of the developmental psychopathology approach, is the importance of *context* in understanding and interpreting children's functioning. In articulating the role of context in the operation of the attachment behavioral system, Bowlby was influenced by control systems theory, which conceptualizes how complex behaviors and systems are organized and directed around fixed set-points or goals of the individual. Thus, the infant's attachment behavioral system is not in a state of constant activation, but only becomes activated (i.e., the infant seeks proximity to the mother) when intra- (e.g, illness) or extraorganismic (e.g., external dangers) factors pose a threat, as appraised by the infant, to the infant's felt security. Such appraisals cause the infant's sense of security to be reduced below the desirable set point. As a consequence, the attachment behavioral system becomes activated, and the child engages in behaviors (e.g., seeks proximity to the mother) that seek to increase his or her appraised sense of security, ideally to again achieve the desired set point of felt security (Sroufe & Waters, 1977a). This formulation allowed Bowlby to explain how attachment behavior and relationships were ascendant in children's functioning during some situations but not others. Thus, during many situations, especially when stress, danger, illness, or other threats were not present, the infant could feel free to explore, feed, play, or engage in other behaviors not related to attachment, although the attachment relationship might still be seen to support these other behaviors (i.e., serve as a secure base from which to explore).

Process-Oriented Directions

Thus, the attachment theory tradition is also consistent with a developmental psychopathology approach in its concern with accounting for the processes mediating relations between family experiences and child outcomes. Bowlby's formulation of attachment theory is a theory of process rather than outcome (Sroufe, Egeland, & Carlson, 1999). Various themes in attachment theory and research reflect process-oriented themes.

Specificity in the Study of Process. The attachment bond is not conceptualized as explaining the totality of functioning related to the parent–child relationship, but is concerned specifically with the function of close emotional relationships as related to secure base behavior and support (Waters & Cummings, 2000). Thus, it follows that other aspects of parenting may be more significant for other dimensions of children's functioning, and that the emotional relationship between parents and children may be about numerous matters other than emotional security. For example, self-determination theory postulates that the humanistic goal of preserving felt security is a lower-order goal, subsumed under a larger set of psychological needs for relatedness; relatedness, in turn, is one of three higher-order goals centering on the intrinsic motivation for competence and autonomy (e.g., Ryan, Deci, & Grolnick, 1995). Attachment theorists, of course, may disagree with relegating felt security to a lower-order goal under the need for relatedness, especially with the emphasis on the protective function of the attachment system and the need to distinguish it from affiliative systems (Ainsworth, Blehar, Waters, & Wall, 1978). Nevertheless, attachment theory does acknowledge that the goal of felt security in the attachment system must be distinguished from other goal-corrected systems such as affiliation, competence, and autonomy (Sroufe & Waters, 1977a; Waters & Cummings, 2000). The attention to precision in describing process relations among family, child, and circumstance, as opposed to the presumption of making global claims, is another element of the attachment theory tradition consistent with the developmental psychopathology approach.

Underscoring this point, Waters and Cummings (2000) have stressed that the secure base control system, with emotional security as its set goal, is central to the conceptualization of the functioning of the parent–child attachment relationship. While the attachment behavioral system, like other fundamental psychological processes, has biological bases, attachment control systems as an expression of the personal relationship between a parent and child are constructed through experience, not prewired, and are theorized to play a role in the organization of behavior and emotion in the relationship between the parent and child. Thus, the child's attachment to his or her mother is reflected in the operating characteristics of an underlying control system that takes into account information about the child's state, the state of the environment, and past and current experiences with the caregiver.

Self-Regulatory Processes. Another process-oriented direction described by Bowlby was the role of self-regulatory processes, including children's emotional and cognitive appraisals of situational and contextual challenges and threats influencing emotional and behavioral responding. In particular, emotional reactions reflecting children's evaluations of events were conceptualized as playing a role in organizing and motivating children's responses to these events, a point made by Bowlby and subsequently expanded by later theorists (Carlson & Sroufe, 1995; Sroufe & Waters, 1977a). Over time, these emotionally based self-regulatory patterns, which reflected the relative security or insecurity afforded by children's experiential histories with parents in multiple situations, were seen as characterizing their functioning in response to current experiences. Thus, such responses were one class of processes derived from day-to-day experiences with the parents, reflecting their success in providing security for children in stressful situations, and over time, they served to mediate relations between experiential history and child outcomes; that is, these processes reflected internal self-regulatory structures derived from experience that served to guide current responding. As articulated by Carlson and Sroufe (1995):

> From a developmental perspective, these self-regulatory structures and mechanisms are viewed as characteristic modes of affect regulation and associated expectations, attitudes, and beliefs internalized from patterns of dyadic interaction. . . . These processes, or internalized "models" (Bowlby, 1980), serve not as static traits, but as guides to ongoing social interaction, supporting the maintenance of existing patterns of adaptation. What is incorporated from the caregiving experience are not specific behavioral features, but the quality and patterning of relationships, as mediated by affect. . . . Such processes are of great theoretical and practical importance, not only because they may explain continuity in individual development but also because they may lead to an understanding of pathogenesis itself. (p. 594)

This direction in attachment research and theory is consistent with other research and theory that demonstrates that self-regulatory processes may mediate relations between children's emotional experiences with the parents and developmental outcomes (e.g., Campos, Campos, & Barrett, 1989; Cole, Michel, & Teti, 1994; Thompson, 1994). For example, Eisenberg and her colleagues have stressed the role of children's regulatory capacities in accounting for relations between familial experiences (e.g., parents' positive or negative emotional expressivity toward the child), children's temperament, social competence, and risk for adjustment problems (Eisenberg et al., 1996, Eisenberg, Spinrad, & Cumberland, 1998; see also Rothbart, Ahadi, & Hershey, 1994; Thompson & Calkins, 1996). Relatedly, there is increasing evidence that children's self-regulatory capacities are influenced by their relationships with parents (Gottman, Katz, & Hooven, 1997; Kochanska, Murray, & Coy, 1997). Consistent with the developmental psychopathology perspective, these results from attachment and other parenting research and theory underscore the active role of children in directing their own development.

Internal Working Models. Another process-oriented direction given even more emphasis by Bowlby involves the cognitive processes or "internal working models" that mediate relations between experiential histories with caregivers and child outcomes. This direction reflects the impact of cognitive psychology as another of the eclectic influences on Bowlby's development of attachment theory (Colin, 1996). The issue is how children represent and organize their cognitions about themselves and their relationships with others as a function of experience with parents and other attachment figures, particularly in times of stress, and how expectancies about the availability and responsivity of parents and others affect their ongoing functioning. Bowlby's (1969, 1973) hypothesis was that early relationship experiences with parents would over time lead to generalized expectations about the self, the world, and others. While these "internal working models" were expected to emerge in some form very early in development, these representations were expected to continue to evolve as a function of attachment-related experiences throughout development.

Accumulating evidence suggests the promise of this characterization of cognitions that result from children's experiences with attachment figures as another direction toward understanding the mediating processes that underlie children's socioemotional development (Main, Kaplan, & Cassidy, 1985; Oppenheim, Emde, & Warren, 1997). Internal representations may mediate the impact of stable family circumstances on the continuity of developmental trajectories, or, alternatively, changing internal representation due to altered family circumstances may mediate discontinuity in developmental pathways. For example, while attachment may tend to be stable over time, early attachment would not be expected to predict later attachment if family circumstances, and consequently internal representations, changed over time (Sroufe, Carlson, Levy, & Egeland, 1999). However, research on this topic is in a relatively early phase of development. Recently, Thompson (2000) identified several key questions for future research: (1) What are the relations between children's development of episodic memory, event representation, social cognition, and other cognitive capacities and change over time in internal working models? (2) During development, when are internal working models most susceptible to emergence or change as a function of attachment experiences? (3) How do other developing systems of thought (e.g., personal beliefs related to ability and competence) affect the development of internal working models of attachment relationships?

Toward Further Articulating the Processes Mediating Development. Thus, consistent with the process-oriented model for the study of developmental psychopathology outlined in Chapter 2, Bowlby proposed that attachment develops as a function of a dynamic process of daily person x environment interactions whose effects accumulate over time. Moreover, as we have seen, emotional regulatory and cognitive representational processes arising from parent–child interactions in the context of the attachment relationship were posited to generalize over time to affect functioning in other contexts. Cummings and Davies (1996) have provided a further explication of the emotional, behavioral, and cognitive regulatory and representational processes that mediate relations between attachment and other family relationships, and child outcomes over time. However, although a theoretical foundation is in place, to this point there have been few direct tests of elaborated developmental models, including the explicit consideration of multiple mediators and moderators of children's functioning (see Figure 3.1), although the importance of this issue as a next step in attachment research is widely recognized (Sroufe, Carlson, Levy, & Egeland, 1999; Waters, Weinfield, & Hamilton, in press).

A Holistic Level of Analysis of Parenting

A theme stressed in the developmental psychopathology tradition is the importance of understanding children's functioning at the level of complex patterns of responses occurring in specific contexts. Such a holistic or higher-order level of analysis provides an integrative and therefore potentially more informative characterization of the meaning of parenting. The concept of attachment reflects these themes. Attachment, like parenting, is neither defined as simply a set of observable behaviors at a microscopic level of analysis nor as a global trait. Rather, attachment is an organizational construct, that is, goals or plans that serve to organize and motivate behavior that emerges from the functioning of the attachment behavioral system. Moreover, this system functions in a manner that is highly sensitive to context, including the past history of the relationship (e.g., the perceived availability and sensitive responsiveness of the parent) and the circumstances of the immediate situation (e.g., the appraisal of threat to emotional security). Accordingly, while attachment is conceptualized as reflecting an emotional bond, it is also seen as continually sensitive to transactions between the child and the environment, and therefore possibly subject to change over time, especially if the appraisals of past and present context (e.g., perceived reduced availability and responsiveness of the parent) change. Thus, it is a dynamic system that is responsive to experience in an ongoing pattern of organization and reorganization rather than a static trait.

Thus, assessment of the quality of attachment requires analysis at an organizational level of the meaning of *patterns* of behavior between children and parents as functions of the contexts of observation. While methods have been developed to assess attachment patterns throughout the life span (including attachments in the context of other, close emotional relationships, such as romantic or marital relationships; e.g., Hazan & Shaver, 1990), for the purpose of illustration, we focus on how attachment patterns have been assessed in infancy, which was the starting point for the assessment of patterns of attachment and remains the most heavily researched age period.

Individual differences in patterns of attachment are assessed in infancy based on the Strange Situation (Ainsworth, Blehar, Waters, & Wall, 1978), which consists of a sequence of eight brief (about 3 minutes each) contexts for observing the infant's functioning in relation to the parent's presence, absence, and return (and certain other conditions, including the presence of a strange adult) in an environment that is unfamiliar (i.e., "strange") to the child. Consistent with theory about the function of attachment as a provision of felt security, patterns of attachment are classified to distinguish parent–child relationships in terms of the relative effectiveness of the infant in deriving security from the parent in these various contexts, and the parent's effectiveness in providing security after brief separations from the infant. Separations are typically the most stressful of the various contexts for the child; thus, parent–child interactions upon reunion are potentially most informative with regard to the functioning of the attachment system. Four major classifications (one secure classification and three main types of insecure classification) have been distinguished (and a number of subcategories within each, which we will not discuss here), based on infant behavior across all eight episodes, with an emphasis on the infant's apparent goal of achieving felt security upon reunion with the attachment figure.

Classification of Attachment Security

The organization of children with *secure* attachments reflects optimal use of the attachment figure as a secure base and support in the context of the attachment relationship. The child thus demonstrates a coherent strategy for using the parent as a source of security. For example, upon the return of the parent after separation, the child readily makes an emotional connection with the parent by physically seeking contact, closer physical proximity, or through effective signaling of the parent across a distance (e.g., greeting the parent). Moreover, the recovery from an overly aroused or distressed state due to separation from the parent is smooth and readily carried to completion; that is, after making connection with the parent, the child rather quickly returns to a nondistressed state and to exploration or play. This pattern is associated with greater responsivity and warmth by parents toward the children in the home, consistent with the theoretical proposition that such parent–child interactions foster a secure attachment relationship.

The behavioral pattern exhibited by children with *avoidant* attachments indicates less than optimal secure base use and support in the context of the attachment relationship. Avoidant infants use the particular strategy of diverting their attention from anything that would activate attachment behavior, and, therefore, do not appear to rely upon the attachment figure in times of stress. Thus, upon reunion, the child conspicuously avoids proximity or contact with the parent. Avoidant infants are not responsive to parental attempts at interaction, may quite demonstratively turn or look away from the parent, and fail to proactively initiate interaction with the parents (Ainsworth, Blehar, Waters, & Wall, 1978). Evidence suggests that these children are more fussy and readily distressed by separation in the home, and may have more difficulty with arousal control at a physiological level in the Strange Situation. Thus, it is inferred that these children are not comfortable turning to the parent for security in the relatively threatening and stressful context of the Strange Situation. Such an interpretation is supported by evidence that parents of avoidant children are more rejecting, tense and irritable, and avoidant of close bodily contact with the children in day-to-day interaction in the home, thereby fostering less confidence in the child about the parents as a reliable source of security. Other evidence suggests that mothers of avoidant infants are more intrusive and overstimulating (Belsky, Rovine, & Taylor, 1984). Among adults, the pattern of attachment is characterized as "dismissing" (Main & Goldwyn, 1984).

The organization of *anxious/resistant* attachment also reflects the infant's relatively ineffective use of the parent as a source of security in times of stress, and the particular strategy of extreme dependence. Prior to separation, these infants are often clingy and uninterested in toys. Upon reunion, resistant children may mix angry behavior (e.g., struggling when held, stiffness, hitting or pushing away) with excessive contact and proximity seeking. Children are not readily reassured by the parents' presence or comforting (e.g., continued fussing and crying) and have considerable difficulty settling and returning to well-regulated emotional functioning. These attachment patterns are also associated with problematic histories of parent–child interaction in the home, including parenting that is relatively inept or inconsistent. This pattern is characterized as "enmeshed" among adults (Main & Goldwyn, 1984).

On the other hand, in an important sense, each of these three patterns is indicative of a coherent or organized strategy on the child's part for coping with stress and using the attachment relationship as a source of security in these situations. In a final pattern termed *disorganized/disoriented* (Main & Solomon, 1990), children have failed to develop a coherent strategy. Thus, these children may exhibit a variety of behaviors indicative of disturbance and lack of organization during reunion with the parent, including unusual sequences of behavior, both avoidant and resistant reactions in the context of the same reunion, and/or highly apprehensive or depressive behavior. Such patterns are thought to reflect relatively extreme problems in the attachment relationship, in which the child derives ineffective support from the parent. Disorganized attachments have been found to be particularly evident among maltreated children and children of parents with psychopathology (e.g., depression); that is, such patterns appear to be associated with parent–child relationships that are relatively deviant.

In summary, one contribution of attachment research has been to provide classification systems that accomplish holistic analyses of complex patterns of interactions between parents and children that also take into account the contexts of these interactions. Moreover, the body of research in this area has successfully demonstrated that such characterizations of parenting are related to past histories of parent–child interactions and statistically to other aspects of concurrent and later functioning in children, including their adjustment (Colin, 1996).

Attachment Is More than Parental Acceptance and Emotional Availability

As we have noted, parental behaviors reflecting acceptance and emotional availability have been shown to predict children's functioning, without the need to invoke the notion of a persisting emotional bond between parent and child. Thus, the question arises: Is it necessary to posit the existence of an emotional bond between parent and child in order to account for children's relationships? From a purely scientific perspective, it would be more parsimonious not to invoke such a construct, if it were not necessary.

Constructs pertaining to parental acceptance and emotional availability are correlated with attachment, and, in fact, have been shown to predict the development of later attachment in a number of studies using prospective longitudinal research designs, which adds to the credibility of positing a causal relationship between these variables (e.g., Ainsworth, Blehar, Waters, & Wall, 1978; see Chapter 3, this volume). However, a core prediction of attachment theory from its initial formulation was that the child's sense of emotional security would derive from the sensitive responsiveness, warmth, and emotional availability of the parent; thus, this finding is hardly surprising, entirely expected, and would, in fact, be troublesome if it were not found (Bowlby, 1973). Notably, dozens of published studies have reported that constructs reflecting maternal sensitivity and emotional availability are related to the quality of attachment. A recent meta-analysis suggests that the support for this relationship is much more than convincing from a statistical perspective (De Wolff & van IJzendoorn, 1997). On the other hand, prediction of attachment from indices of parental acceptance and warmth is modest, with a great deal of the variability in the quality of parent–child attachment *not* accounted for by parental acceptance and emotional availability. It follows that only a relatively limited portion of the prediction of child outcomes that has been demonstrated in attachment research as due to the quality of parent–child attachment can possibly be ascribed to the greater parental acceptance and emotional availability that is likely to characterize secure parent–child relationships. Even when parents are trained to be more sensitive and responsive to infants, and these response dimensions are shown to predict positive outcomes later in development, the quality of parent–child attachment continues to be an independent predictor of positive aspects of later socioemotional functioning (van den Boom, 1994). Thus, the emotionality of the parent–child relationship and the quality of the attachment relationship are not redundant predictors of child outcomes.

Furthermore, the effects on individuals of breaking emotional bonds are pronounced and painful. It is a commonplace (and well documented; see Bowlby, 1973, 1980) experience of the human condition that loss of a relationship characterized by a close emotional bond is painful and distressing, sometimes with persisting and long-lasting effects on an individual's adjustment, whether the loss occurs due to death, departure, or other circumstances. It is difficult to quarrel with the importance of close emotional bonds to human functioning based on everyday experience (as well as the research literature). The effects of relationships with others on current functioning are not simply a matter of the conditions of immediate interaction, especially when close relationships are involved (e.g., parents, children, spouses, very close friends). On the other hand, context matters in this situation as well as others, so that the availability of alternative attachment figures, and other conditions of the situation, importantly affect adjustment outcomes for the individual when loss occurs (Bowlby, 1980).

Thus, given the importance of both immediate parenting behavior related to emotionality and the formation of close emotional bonds, it is of interest to study the processes by which the various dimensions of parenting as emotionality are interrelated. For example, since infant short-term reactions of withdrawal or disengagement in disrupted parent—child interactions do not necessarily crystallize into more stable patterns of coping, fully capturing the unfolding process underlying the parent—child outcome link also requires a complementary focus on the emergence of more stable response patterns and coping styles. Thus, if we consider a pathway whereby parenting practices lead to child outcomes, we need to delineate the process by which short-term, relatively unstable response patterns (e.g., infant withdrawal in a specific parent—child interaction) eventually coalesce into more stable response patterns (e.g., dismissing or "avoidant" styles of coping across time and context) that, in turn, steer individuals toward certain developmental trajectories. Accordingly, early interactional response patterns of disengagement, protest, or engagement bear remarkable similarities to linkages between forms of parental negativity and the more stable coping and attachment patterns of children in the context of parent—child relations (Ainsworth, Blehar, Waters, & Wall, 1978).

Disengagement in interactional bouts during early infancy may reflect the rudimentary development of representational scripts and coping patterns that probabilistically coalesce into more organized forms of avoidant or dismissing attachment patterns characterized by the masking of negative affect, withdrawal, and representations of the attachment figure as unavailable (Crittenden, 1988). In support of the hypothesis that withdrawal reactions and dismissing or avoidant coping reflect different parts of a chain of processes, research indicates that children exhibiting these patterns of functioning commonly experience histories of parental intrusiveness and rejection (Belsky, Rovine, & Taylor, 1984; Crittenden, 1988; Egeland & Farber, 1984; Isabella, Belsky, & von Eye, 1989; Kobak & Sceery, 1988; Lamb, 1987; Lyons-Ruth, Connell, Zoll, & Stall, 1987). Conversely, bouts of infant protest and tantrums in parent—child interactions may lay an early foundation for the development of resistant or preoccupied ways of relating to parents, characterized by more stable patterns of overdependence, frustration, helplessness, anger, and representations of the self as unworthy of love (Cummings & Davies, 1995). The conceptualization of these two response patterns as different phases in an unfolding process of development is supported by research findings indicating that each appears to originate from experiences with inattentive or unresponsive caregivers (Belsky et al., 1984; Isabella et al., 1989; Sroufe, 1985).

Finally, attachment should not, of course, be regarded as an independent dimension of parenting. Not only does the evidence suggest that attachment is influenced by other dimensions of parent—child relations (e.g., sensitive responsiveness) but also relations are reported between attachment and a wider range of parenting behaviors that have been implicated in the development of attachment. Thus, attachment security may have positive influence on other dimensions of parenting, including the likelihood that parental control techniques will be effective in obtaining compliance. For example, Londerville and Main (1981) reported that toddlers who were securely attached to their parents were more compliant to their parent's disciplinary directives. Lay, Waters, and Parke (1989) found that parental warmth elicited positive affect in children, and positive affect, in turn, heightened compliance in comparison with children experiencing negative emotions. Moreover, clinical data from families of preschoolers with conduct problems suggest that parent training is more effective if steps are taken to improve the quality of the parent–child attachment relationship as well as the effectiveness of the parents' disciplinary strategies (e.g., Speltz, 1990). Other lines of research also indicate that when the quality of the emotional relationship between the parent and child is positive, there is an increased likelihood that parental disciplinary techniques will be effective (Grusec & Goodnow, 1994a). This is consistent, in broad outline, with some models of parental control techniques (discussed earlier).

Pathways of Development

The notion that children's development is best conceptualized in terms of pathways of development was clearly articulated by Bowlby (1969, 1973), and his concepts have served as a seminal influence on the developmental psychopathology tradition (Chapter 4, in this volume). Bowlby's emphasis on the importance of early parent–child attachments is sometimes mistaken to mean that he viewed early attachments as fixed prototypes influencing later development in a manner similar to that of a personality trait. On the contrary, as we have shown, attachment theory and research posit a model for the influence of attachment as a dynamic process over the course of development, which may be characterized by either continuity or change as a function of ongoing and continuing processes of interaction between the individual and context. Thus, Bowlby (1973) wrote that the development of the child "turns at each and every stage of the journey on an interaction between the organism as it has developed up to the moment and the environment in which it finds itself" (p. 364). While it is expected that existing structures and organizations of children's functioning, particularly the initial organizations upon which later development is built (i.e., infant attachment), will tend to persist (Main, Kaplan, & Cassidy, 1985), it is also posited that the child will reorganize functioning when confronted with persistent or significant challenges to current organizations. For example, a child with a secure attachment to the parent may later develop an insecure attachment if significant changes occur in the interactional relations between parent and child (e.g., the parent becomes increasingly unavailable emotionally due to the onset of chronic depression).

Emerging evidence indicates that attachments can have substantial continuity during development (Main et al., 1985; Waters, 1978), but other studies suggest that change in the security of attachment relationships may also occur over time (Belsky & Cassidy, 1994; Thompson, 2000). However, as we have indicated, change per se does not contradict attachment theory. Consistent with the notion that the quality of attachment relationships reflects a constant, dynamic interplay between the individual and the environment, continuity can only be firmly predicted when there is considerable stability in living conditions, especially as they relate to the quality of interaction between parents and children. On the other hand, discontinuity would not be unexpected if the child were faced with significant qualitative changes in living circumstances. The key matter from the attachment theory perspective is whether continuity, or change, can be shown to occur as a systematic function of stability or change in family circumstances (if not, *that* would be a disconfirmation of the theory). In fact, some evidence has emerged to support these predictions regarding continuity and change in attachment security as a function of continuity and changes in living conditions and family stresses (Teti, Sakin, Kucera, & Corns, 1996; Vaughn, Egeland, Sroufe, & Waters, 1979), although, overall, the evidence is mixed with regard to whether changes in attachment security over time are always lawful (Thompson, 2000).

Moreover, until recently, most tests of this framework for pathways of development were based upon longitudinal studies conducted over a relatively short period of time and typically limited to early childhood. Tests of this framework based upon long-term, prospective longitudinal research designs constitute an exciting new direction. Thus, recent studies of the development of attachment over the *span* of childhood indicate that attachment may show both continuity and discontinuity from infancy to adulthood, with some evidence, consistent with attachment theory, suggesting that the continuity versus change in family circumstances is systematically related to adult outcomes. For example, Waters, Merrick, Treboux, Crowell, and Albersheim (in press) reported that security of attachment measured in infancy is significantly related to the security of attachment in adulthood. Moreover, negative life events (i.e., parental divorce, parental psychopathology, loss of parent, life-threatening illness of parent or child, abuse) are important predictors when change in attachment classification occurs. Thus, 56% of the children whose mothers reported significant negative life events during their childhood evidenced changes in attachment classifications from infancy to early adulthood. On the other hand, only 28% of those not reporting such events changed classifications (similar findings were reported by Hamilton, in press). By contrast, in a prospective, longitudinal study based upon a sample initially chosen because of high family adversity (e.g., poverty, high risk for poor developmental outcome), Weinfield, Sroufe, and Egeland (in press) reported no evidence of significant continuity in attachment security between infancy and adulthood. However, further analyses revealed evidence for *lawful discontinuity*, that is, changes in attachments were linked with difficulties in family circumstances (i.e., maternal depression, problems in family functioning in early adolescence, child maltreatment). Given that many of the individuals changed from secure to insecure attachment classifications over the span of this study and faced adverse family environments, the results also support the notion that persistently chaotic and difficult life experiences significantly undermine the possibility of secure attachment.

Moreover, while several recent studies support the outline of pathways of development as hypothesized by attachment theory, these studies only begin to address other elements of this complex framework. In particular, these initial longitudinal studies focused primarily on the assessment of attachment at the endpoints of infancy and adulthood, and on family and life circumstances assessed at a relatively global level of analysis. Thus, we are left with many questions to ponder about the specific *processes* (e.g., emotional or other regulatory processes; cognitive processes of representation) that mediate continuity or change in pathways of development across childhood. As we saw in Chapter 2, a process-level explanation is essential to understanding the bases for the course of normal development and the development of psychopathology. In addition, the results of these and other studies increasingly call attention to the importance of family variables other than parent–child interactions to child outcomes (e.g., Davies & Cummings, 1994; see also Chapters 8 and 9, this volume). Thus, it is increasingly evident that it is necessary to examine *family functioning* in order to account more fully for attachment as an important aspect of parenting.

Attachment and Family Functioning

A cornerstone of modern developmental theory is that children's functioning, including dyadic relationships, is nested within broader contexts, one of the most significant being the family (Belsky, 1984; Bronfenbrenner, 1986). Notably, Bowlby (1949) was one of the first researchers to call attention to the need to consider the family in understanding children's distress and security. Notably, these influences may affect children directly or through their effects on parenting. For example, numerous studies indicate that marital conflict may have directs effects on children's functioning and also affect multiple aspects of parenting, including attachment (Davies & Cummings, 1994). Owen and Cox (1997) recently provided a particularly cogent demonstration of the effects of marital conflict on parenting by documenting negative effects of high marital conflict on both parental behaviors that influence the development of attachment over time (e.g., sensitivity) and direct effects of exposure to frightening parental conflict behaviors on the incidence of disorganized/disoriented attachment, independent of effects on specific parenting practices. In particular, the pervasive direct and indirect effects of the quality of marital relations on children's functioning, as well as on attachment and other dimensions of parenting, indicate that the parents' involvement in marital (or other interpartner) conflict or more positive relations merits consideration as another dimension of parenting (Cummings, Goeke-Morey, & Graham, 1999).

Thus, the evidence supports the need to consider broader aspects of family functioning to account for the development of attachment over time. A recent, long-term prospective study of the course of attachment from infancy to adult-hood adds support to this perspective. Lewis, Feiring, and Rosenthal (in press) examined not only attachment patterns at 12 months and 18 years of age but also other aspects of child and family not only functioning in the period in 1 and 18 years. Lewis and colleagues reported no continuity in quality of attachment over this time span, although quality of attachment at 18 years was related to adjustment at 18 years. On the other hand, divorce, which might be expected to influence the quality of family functioning and parent–child relations (see Chapter 8), was significantly related to insecure attachment status at 18 years, as was the relative positivity versus negativity of childhood recollections recorded at 13 years of age. These results thus underscore the potential significance of broader family relations, particularly marital relations (see Chapter 8) to quality of attachment as well as other aspects of children's functioning.

It also appears necessary to broaden the construct of security itself to re-flect emotional security due to other aspects of family functioning (e.g., mari-tal relations; Davies & Cummings, 1994), thus presenting a familywide per-spective on children's emotional security, taking into account security due to parent–child attachment, the quality of marital relations, and other family fac-tors (see Cummings & Davies, 1996). Byng-Hall (1999) also posited an exten-sion of the notion of emotional security to the family as a whole. Thus, he stressed the importance of a reliable family network and a secure family base, with a shared awareness among family members that attachments should be protected and not undermined. Based on the tenets of attachment theory, Davies and Cummings proposed that emotional reactivity, behavioral regula-tion (i.e., especially efforts to regulate parent's behavior to increase their own sense of security), and representations of family relations were subprocesses that served to define a higher-order construct of emotional security and ex-plicit classes of processes that mediated relations between family functioning (including attachment) and child adjustment. In a preliminary test of this model, Davies and Cummings (1998) reported evidence to support emotional reactivity and representations of family relations as mediators of children's adjustment.

Normal and Abnormal Development

From the outset, Bowlby, as a practicing psychiatrist, was interested in attach-ment theory in terms of the development of psychopathology and as a perti-nence to normal development (Sroufe, Carlson, Levy, & Egeland, 1999). Cer-tainly, a substantial body of research has emerged to indicate relations between insecure attachment and increased probability of children's adjust-ment problems (Carlson & Sroufe, 1995). However, attachment classification is not a classification of psychopathology, and is not meant to be regarded as such. Parent–child attachment is but one of the family factors that may con-tribute in concert with a wide range of other factors to an increased risk for the development of psychopathology (see Figure 3.1). Given the demonstrated significance of early attachments to children's functioning, problems in attachment may well lay a foundation for dysfunctions in developmental processes that can result in psychopathology. For example, in a particularly impressive demonstrative given the prospective longitudinal design and the multiple time points of assessments, Carlson (1998) recently reported that disorganized/disoriented attachments in infancy were related to mother–child relationship quality in early childhood, behavior problems throughout childhood, and dimensions of psychopathology in adolescence and adulthood. Furthermore, analyses indicated that attachment disorganization mediated relations between problems in early caretaking and later psychopathology. As another example, Cummings and Cicchetti (1990) traced numerous lines of research and theory that supported the proposition that disturbances in attachment might be expected to increase the probability of the development of later depression. However, it is entirely inconsistent with the developmental psychopathology perspective that underlies much of attachment theory to equate attachment dysfunction with adjustment problems. Thus, Sroufe, Carlson, Levy, and Egeland (1999) have contended:

> In this perspective early attachment variations generally are not viewed as pathology or even directly causing pathology. Rather, varying patterns of attachment represent "initiating conditions" in systems terms. In this regard, they do play a dynamic role in pathological development because of the way in which environmental engagement is framed by established tendencies and expectations. (pp. 10–11)

Attachment and Normal Development and the Development of Psychopathology

A substantial literature has emerged to support the substantial impact of attachment on child development. Thus, the quality of attachment observed in the laboratory has been related to past histories of parental behavior toward children in the home, especially with regard to the sensitive responsiveness of the parent (De Wolff & van IJzendoorn, 1997), in ways that are predicted by attachment theory. Interventions deriving from the principles of attachment theory (e.g., increase responsiveness to infant's signals) that teach parents to alter behaviors toward their infants have also been shown to improve children's socioemotional functioning (van den Boom, 1994). Quality of attachment has also been related to children's socioemotional functioning, including behavior with parents, siblings, peers, teachers, and strangers, and risk for adjustment problems, both concurrently and in subsequent years, with the prediction of later behavior sometimes spanning the course of many years (e.g., Carlson, 1998). Finally, evidence from both normal samples and samples characterized by adjustment problems has emerged across cultures to support the importance of variations in children's attachment security in understanding children's functioning (see Colin, 1996). The success of attachment theory in adding to our knowledge of child development is unquestionable, prompting one prominent scholar recently to note that "attachment has become the dominant approach to understanding early socioemotional and personality development during the past quarter-century of research" (Thompson, 2000). As we have seen, attachment theory also embodies many of the principles of a developmental psychopathology perspective on development. Notably, researchers and theorists in the attachment theory tradition have been at the forefront in the conceptualization of the developmental psychopathology approach (e.g., Cicchetti, Sroufe). However, surprisingly few tests of relations between attachment as parenting and other conceptualizations of the parent–child subsystem are evident in the literature. In Chapter 7, we suggest how a broader, more complete study of relations between parenting practices and child development can emerge from and inform a developmental psychopathology perspective.

CHAPTER SEVEN

New Directions in the Study of Parenting and Child Development

*I*n this chapter, we move beyond process-oriented analyses of the multiple individual dimensions of parenting and their interplay to consider themes for the next generation of research studies on how parenting affects children's development over time. The identification of the dimensions of parenting and their underlying processes are essential components of a developmental psychopathology model of parenting. Using these components as building blocks, however, developmental psychopathology moves to the higher-order level of contextualizing parenting.

Rather than viewing parenting as a unidimensional shaper of child outcomes, developmental psychopathology conceptualizes parenting as a part of a transactional, developmental process that not only regulates child development but is also regulated by the developing child. Since the evolving parent–child subsystem is also embedded in intrapersonal (i.e., parent and child characteristics), family, and ecological spheres, developmental psychopathology also seeks to explicate the network of multivariate risk and protective factors that may maintain, or alter, children's developmental pathways (Belsky, 1984; see Figure II.1).

The purpose of this chapter is to explicate and illustrate the essential elements of this more complex perspective concerning parental influences on child development, consistent with the model outlined in Figure 3.1. Thus, issues and themes to guide a more informative, next generation of studies on relations between parenting and child development are outlined. The promise is not only a better understanding of parenting from the standpoint of family research, but also a firmer foundation for clinical practice with children and families, which inevitably involves concerns about relations between parenting and child development.

CONTEXTUALIZING PARENTING

Parent–child interactions do not affect children's development in isolation from other influences. Rather, the impact of parenting practices is dependent on the biopsychosocial context within which they are embedded (see Figure 3.1 and Figure II.1). Addressing the flip side of the coin, parenting practices are also components of a biopsychosocial framework that influences pathways between other factors and child development. Thus, a more complete picture of relations between parenting practices and child development requires placing these influences within this larger context.

Conceptualizing parenting in this way may help explain how pathways of child development may be similar, or different, when such outcomes would not be expected simply in terms of parenting practices. First, such models may account for why children exhibit different outcomes even when they share similar experiential histories of parenting (i.e., multifinality). To take one example, children with easy temperaments may react more adaptively to parenting disturbances than children with more vulnerable temperaments, who, under similar conditions, may exhibit behaviors indicative of psychological disturbance. Second, such models may also explain why children who are exposed to different parenting practices may follow similar developmental trajectories (i.e., equifinality). Using the same example, children with easy temperaments may experience considerable parenting disturbances but develop along adaptive trajectories, therefore appearing similar to children with more average temperaments, who do not experience parenting disturbances. Third, parenting factors may also serve to weaken or strengthen the effects of other biopsychosocial factors. For example, children with secure attachments to parents may be less vulnerable to the effects of exposure to marital discord within the family (see Chapter 8) than children with insecure attachments (Emery, 1982). We consider various elements essential for adequately contextualizing the influences of parenting on child development.

Intraindividual Characteristics

The importance of the characteristics of the individual child has been neglected in parenting research despite the obvious fact that the child is 50% of the immediate interpersonal context in many parent–child encounters. Thus, the need to factor the individual child into the parenting equation merits consideration as a first issue in the contextualization of parenting. Although the study of intraindividual characteristics as moderators of child development is still in a relatively early stage, evidence suggests that examining temperamental dispositions, gender, and personality styles as moderators of child outcomes is a promising direction if we are to understand the complexity of relations between parenting practices and child development (Belsky, Hsieh, & Crnic, 1998). Take the following example of 2-year-old toddlers with very different temperaments and parental socialization experiences:

From an early age, Lisa, Josh, and Evan showed evidence of inhibited temperaments, including substantial fearfulness in unfamiliar and mildly stressful situations. For example, at the circus, all showed considerable fear and withdrawal in the face of clowns, strange people, and unfamiliar objects. Whereas the children exhibited similar temperaments, they experienced quite different parenting practices. Lisa's parents primarily relied on gentle explanations for transgressions in disciplinary situations. Emphasis was thus placed on communicating the socialization messages underlying the transgression rather than scolding or asserting power. In contrast, Josh's parents became visibly upset in disciplinary contexts and expressed their distress through raised voices, threats, and mild physical punishment in a conscious effort to teach Josh important "lessons of life." Evan's parents approached socialization in a different way, choosing to strengthen the emotional relationship with him as a way of promoting his motivation to comply and, eventually, internalize important socialization messages.

Which of these parenting practices is the most effective in facilitating adjustment? For example, with regard to a particular child outcome of interest to most parents, which parenting practice would be most likely to promote the development of conscience? In fact, the research suggests that the development of conscience depends upon the temperamental dispositions of the child (Kochanska, 1995, 1997; Kochanska & Thompson, 1997). The research specifically suggests that the gentle forms of discipline used by Lisa's parents would be the more effective in promoting the internalization of values in inhibited children than the techniques of power assertion (i.e., Josh's parents) or building dyadic cooperation (i.e., Evan's parents). In particular, power-assertive techniques would tend to create overwhelming levels of discomfort and external attributions in inhibited children, compromising their understanding and acceptance of the socialization message as their own. Gentle disciplinary techniques would capitalize on the children's natural tendencies to experience discomfort and foster their processing and acceptance of the socialization message. On the other hand, simply strengthening the bond between the parent and child might not effectively communicate the parents' perspectives on social values. However, evidence suggests that the effects of disciplinary practices on child development are not invariant, but depend on the characteristics of the child. Consider the next example:

Gina and Shane had very uninhibited temperaments. Novel, unfamiliar, and mildly stressful situations failed to evoke significant fear or withdrawal. These children were generally hyporesponsive physiologically and behaviorally to potential or real negative consequences of their actions. Because danger was not in their experiential vocabulary, parental prohibitions with regard to household objects were generally brushed aside for more salient and exciting exploratory pursuits. In reaction, Gina's parents thought that making their socialization messages even more salient would be best achieved by increasing power-assertive discipline (i.e., threats, raised voices, mild physical punishment). Shane's parents, in contrast, chose another socialization route by concentrating on building a solid emotional relationship with their uninhibited child as a way of trying to increase the chances he would comply with and accept their socialization efforts.

Which socialization practice would be most effective in this case? A very different socialization technique appears to be more effective with uninhibited children than inhibited children. Again, we consider the common parental goal of developing conscience in the child. In this case, the best approach appears to involve building and strengthening a cooperative, emotional bond with the child. Uninhibited children's prime motive for accepting the message lies in their desire to identify with and emulate their cooperative, emotionally available parent. Parental strategies based on the notion that one should establish the desire to internalize the message as a way of avoiding subsequent anxiety are much less effective with uninhibited that with inhibited children. Because induction and power-assertive disciplinary techniques hinge to some extent on generating some level of discomfort and anxiety, both techniques are relatively less effective with children who are relatively fearless (i.e., have very high thresholds for experiencing anxiety).

Figure 7.1 translates this conceptualization into a model, illustrating that the relationship between parenting styles and affective and motivational processes underlying the internalization of socialization messages is moderated by child temperament.

Thus, for uninhibited children, cooperative parenting practices promote motives to identify with the parent, which, in turn, are thought to facilitate the development of conscience. Identifying with the parent is conceptualized as mediating the link between parental socialization strategy and the building blocks of conscience (i.e., understanding, accepting, and internalizing messages). For inhibited children, gentle, reason-oriented, disciplinary styles are hypothesized to be associated with moderate levels of distress, which, in turn, are posited to predict understanding and acceptance of the message (i.e., development of conscience). Thus, children with different temperamental styles may follow two different mediational routes to the same outcome of optimal conscience development (i.e., equifinality).

The "Active" Child

An important assumption of the developmental psychopathology approach is that children are active agents in influencing their own development (see Chapter 1). This notion holds for the effects of parenting on children's development as well as for other areas of the influence of experience on children's functioning. At a theoretical level, the reciprocity between parental and child behavior in parent–child interaction has long been recognized (e.g., Bell, 1968; Dodge, 1990a; Lytton, 1990). However, the assumption of unidirec-

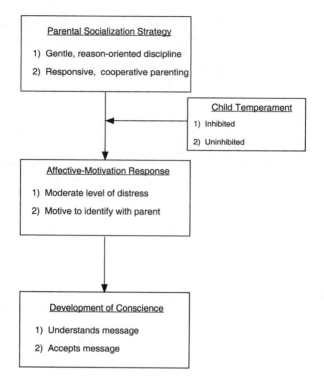

FIGURE 7.1. Child temperament as a moderator of relations between parenting styles, affective–motivational processes, and child socialization.

tional, mechanistic-oriented conceptualizations of parenting still looms large in parenting research. Take, for example, the explicit presuppositions underlying Darling and Steinberg's (1993) influential and informative model of parenting:

> Although some writers have treated parenting style as if it were a developmental process, we disagree. A developmental process is defined by interactions between the developing person and his or her environment. Parenting style is a characteristic of the parent (i.e., it is a feature of the child's social environment), independent of characteristics of the developing person. (p. 487)

The theme of isolating components of parenting and searching for unidirectional pathways among parenting dimensions, mechanisms, and child outcomes remains influential, as reflected in some directions in current research on parenting, including some of the best exemplars of such research. Thus, in the context of discussing individual differences in children as a context for parenting, the notion of the child as an active agent merits discussion and further development as a core theme and central assumption of the developmental psychopathology perspective on children's development in families.

The view of parenting as a characteristic of the parent does have heuristic value as a strategy for advancing understanding, particularly given some limitations in the methodologies appropriate for cogently examining the children as active agents in their own development. However, in terms of the ideal for the next generation of research on parenting in context, it is still only one dimension of a more complex, three-dimensional puzzle of socialization (Belsky, 1984). Accepting the organismic assumption of interdependency among parts of any socialization system means that the origins, sequelae, and adaptive value of parenting cannot be examined exclusively in isolation from the child in developmental and ecological contexts. The most basic step, then, is to embed parenting within a more dynamic, bidirectional model that views the child as an active agent in the process of renegotiating relations with parents over time.

Control systems theory (Bell, 1968) was among the first to begin to sketch a transactional model of parenting. Parents and children are each assumed to have comfort zones or thresholds of tolerance for the others' behaviors. When displays of excessive behavior (e.g., aggression, tantrums, activity) by children challenge the upper thresholds for parental tolerance of child behavior, parents are thought to respond by trying to use control strategies that reduce behavioral excess within some acceptable, comfortable range. Conversely, when children's inhibited and withdrawn behaviors challenge lower limits of parental tolerance, parents respond by engaging in control tactics that increase child involvement (e.g., coaching, supporting). In the same way, children are thought to have upper and lower limits of tolerance for parental behavior that partly shape their responses and functioning (e.g., Lytton, 1990). However, while these models provide a firm foundation for more articulate theories, they typically fail to address how interindividual differences in pathways and outcomes develop (e.g., Maccoby & Martin, 1983).

In addressing this limitation for the particular problem of understanding the bases for the development of aggression in children, the early starter model has proposed that at least one of two family ingredients is necessary to set in motion an escalating, bidirectional spiral of negativity and distress in the parent–child subsystem in early childhood: (1) a troublesome, aversive child (e.g., hyperactivity, difficult temperament), or (2) a parent who lacks effective, consistent discipline techniques (Patterson, DeBarsyshe, & Ramsey, 1989). Moreover, the interplay of a difficult child and an ineffective, lax parent is thought to pose an enhanced risk for the early development of coercive cycles of interactions between parents and children. In support of this model, Martin (1981) reported that an interaction between maternal lack of responsiveness and infant demandingness in infancy predicted subsequent coercive child behavior during the preschool years. The highest rates of coerciveness occurred between unresponsive mothers and demanding infants at 10 months.

Furthermore, the early starter model presents an even more dynamic view of these processes than this type of moderator model. For example, in the risk scenario involving a lax parent and difficult child, the parent responds to child misbehavior with aversive or hostile behavior. In reaction, the child, in turn, maintains or escalates the negative behavior. Sometimes during this escalating cycle of negativity, the lax parent eventually exhibits neutral or positive behavior toward the child as a means of escaping the aversive interaction. However, in the course of ending the negative parent–child interaction, the parent inadvertently reinforces (i.e., negative reinforcement) the child's increasing negativity. As these cycles become more routinized in daily interactions, these behavior patterns become increasingly crystallized in children's behavioral repertoires both in and outside the family, leading to conduct problems, aggression, and delinquency. Thus, in line with a developmental psychopathology perspective, the model not only specifies the parenting and child characteristics that increase risk for psychopathology at a detailed, precise level, but it also regards this process as transactional; that is, a reciprocal interplay between parent and child behaviors that lead to dynamic, evolving changes at both dyadic (i.e., parent–child relationship) and individual (i.e., child, parent) levels of analysis.

Although this theoretical perspective posits that children play a role in shaping their own development and caregiving contexts, they also remain passive agents in their own development in some respects; that is, the model assumes that (1) exposure to a series of behavioral conditioning (e.g., escape conditioning, positive reinforcement, punishment) experiences has an overriding influence, and (2) these critical chains of experiences and their implications are not actively processed by the child. The children are thus considered to be blind to the causes, correlates, and consequences of experiences importantly affecting their own development. Thus, even though it is postulated that children actively seek out interpersonal niches (e.g., aggressive children are attracted to deviant peer groups), they are considered to be *drawn* to various contexts on the basis of overlearned, unconscious behavioral habits developing out of contingencies rather than through the formation of active appraisals, decisions, or choices.

So what may be the next step toward the development of a theory that truly portrays children as playing an active role in forging individual differences in developmental trajectories? One promising solution is to integrate several key theories in a way that builds a detailed, dynamic model of the interplay between parent and child in development. Some examples of the different developmental challenges faced by children and caregivers at different points in the life span are shown in Table 7.1.

The integrative developmental theory of parenting proposed by Shaw and Bell (1993) maintains that individual differences in the pathways blazed by children depend on a complex, reciprocal interplay between how each member of the parent–child dyad adjusts reactions to newly emerging developmental tasks. As in the early starter model, children's risk may begin with aversive behavior by either member of the dyad (i.e., parental insensitivity, temperamentally difficult child) that eventually develops into cycles of increasing negativity and distress in the relationship. The difference, however, is that children's emerging social, cognitive, and motor capacities are thought to

TABLE 7.1. Developmental Challenges Faced by Children and Caregivers from Infancy through Adolescence

Developmental level	Issues	Caregiver role
Infant	Physiological regulation Attachment Interactional synchrony	Sensitivity and responsiveness Availability
Toddler	Exploration of world Sense of mastery Individuation Autonomous self Sense of right and wrong	Secure base Clear, realistic expections for child Consistent discipline Direct, persistent supervision Use of internal-state language Emotion regulation
Preschooler	Self-control Cooperation Sex-role identification Peer relations	Clear roles and values Organize/support peer interactions Flexible management
School-age child	Self-confidence Peer group membership Close friendship School adaptation	Open communication Acceptance Indirect monitoring
Adolescent	Heterosexual peer relations Dating Autonomy Occupational plans Identity formation Romantic relationships	Psychological autonomy granting Indirect monitoring (especially early) Involvement and support

challenge parents continually to develop and reorganize their parenting skills (see the section on *stage-salient tasks* for more details on developmental reorganization). Furthermore, children not only actively influence parenting skills at each new level of development but they also actively process family events in terms of the meaning they hold for social relationships and their own well-being and perceived worthiness. The development of these internal working models, in turn, is used as a guide in developing future predictions and interpretations of social relationships and, hence, play an active role in shaping the nature of close relationships, especially with caregivers (Lynch & Cicchetti, 1998b; Shaw & Bell, 1993).

These transactional theories of the role of children in their own development have profound implications for the interpretation and conceptualization of parenting. Well-established relations between parenting styles and children's outcomes, which were once assumed largely to reflect the impact of parenting styles on children, are now being more critically evaluated. Lewis (1981) was among the first to suggest that different parenting profiles (e.g., authoritative) may be a consequence as a well as an antecedent of differences in children's patterns of functioning. Thus, children who initially showed reasonable, competent, and good behavior are likely to elicit greater warmth from parents and increase the effectiveness of behavioral control and inductive discipline. By contrast, in keeping with control systems theory, children with early, stable behavior problems may test the upper limits of tolerance of even the most authoritative parents. These parents may initially respond with authoritarian methods characterized by increased anger, control, and strictness. Since these efforts are often met with increased resistance on the part of children with conduct problems (Lytton, 1990; Patterson, 1997), repeated experiences with uncontrollable children may eventually cause distressed parents to raise their tolerance levels for misbehavior and, in the process, hopelessly surrender their roles as disciplinarians in a way that closely resembles the uninvolved style of parenting (Stice & Barrera, 1995).

Even though these newer models and hypotheses must still be systematically explored, they remain very promising and interesting in light of the (1) rather modest magnitude of relations between parenting styles and subsequent changes in adolescent adjustment (e.g., Steinberg, Lamborn, Darling, Mounts, & Dornbusch, 1994) and (2) accumulating evidence from experimental (e.g., Anderson, Lytton, & Romney, 1986; Bugental, Caporael, & Shennum, 1980; Pelham & Lang, 1993), intervention (e.g., Barkley, Karlsson, Pollard, & Murphy, 1985), and autoregressive longitudinal designs (e.g., Eisenberg et al., 1999; Stice & Barrera, 1995), which find that children do, in fact, influence parental adjustment and caregiving practices in the short and long term. However, another goal for future research must be the development of new methodologies and statistical procedures that allow researchers to assess transactional relations between parental and child influences on the pathways of child development. This goal is consistent with the emphasis on the use of multiple methodologies and the continual innovation of new methodologies in order to address issues of developmental process in research (see Chapter 3). Such methodological advances are essential for future empirical advances, and for research to catch up with theory in viewing children as active agents in their own development.

Family Characteristics

Relatively few studies have examined family moderators of the link between parenting and child development, but the results have been promising. For example, relationships with siblings may factor in the impact of parenting practices on children. The effects of sibling relationships on children's other relationships within families are an intriguing but little understood issue. McHale and Pawletko (1992), for example, found that children who experience differential treatment in the form of greater relationship involvement between their parents and their sibling, and more power-assertive discipline directed at them in comparison to their sibling, reported the most positive sibling relationships if their siblings were disabled, whereas children with nondisabled siblings experiencing the same type of differential treatment reported the least positive sibling relationships. Thus, although differential treatment may evoke feelings of neglect and loneliness among children across a wide variety of family contexts, in the context of an integrated model of broader family influences, the meaning that children derive from larger family dynamics (e.g., having a disabled vs. nondisabled sibling) may ultimately alter the effects of parenting practices (see Figure 7.2). Children who receive more discipline than their nondisabled sibling may specifically perceive themselves as the scapegoat or problem child of the family. Children with disabled siblings may perceive the same differential treatment as legitimate, understandable attempts by their parents to address the special needs of their sibling. In summary, appraisals of legitimacy may act as a mediator that accounts for why the effects of differential parental treatment on sibling relationship quality are moderated by family context (McHale & Crouter, 1996). Similar models may be useful in understanding how and why other family characteristics, such as parental alcoholism, family cohesion, and parental emotional expressiveness, may moderate the effects of parenting, including the effects of parenting on children's adjustment over time.

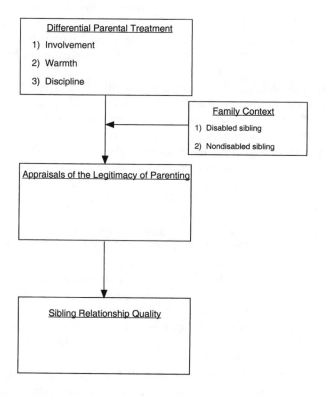

FIGURE 7.2. The disabled versus nondisabled sibling as a moderator of the effects on sibling relationships of differential treatment of children by the parents.

Siblings and the Nonshared Parenting Environment

Much of the parenting research, especially outside the discipline of developmental psychopathology, is implicitly guided by the notion that the relationship between parental socialization practices and child adjustment is generalizable across children and, in particular, siblings. However, although siblings may share some similarities in functioning, recent research, particularly analyses from the behavioral genetics tradition, has underscored the rather large magnitude of differences that exist between siblings in their adjustment (e.g., Dunn & Plomin, 1990; Stocker, 1995).

The notion of nonshared parenting environments suggests limitations of certain research traditions on parenting effects; that is, traditional "social address" models of parenting conceptualize parenting practices as "traits" that operate similarly across different siblings. Thus, these models cannot explain the appreciable differences between sibling that are reported on numerous dimensions of functioning. By contrast, nonshared family environment models, which conceptualize parenting and the biopsychosocial characteristics of siblings as dynamic contexts (i.e., fluctuating across time, individual, and relationship), are in a much better position to account for the origins of sibling diversity. Although the unique interplay between parenting processes and the biopsychosocial characteristics of each sibling can be manifested in myriad ways, three primary effects of nonshared parenting environment have been the focus of research to this point.

In the first model, which we call the "socialization effects" pathway, exposure to different parenting practices (e.g., differential parental treatment) is posited to play a primary role in the development of sibling differences in adjustment. Parental socialization pathways can be further subdivided into the (1) caregiving practices parents use with each child individually (i.e., direct effects) and (2) differential parental treatment, or the discrepancy in parenting, toward the siblings (Brody, Stoneman, & McCoy, 1992). In a second, complementary model, which depicts a "child effects" pathway, differences in exposure to parenting and nonshared family environment are hypothesized to be products, in part, of differences in children's functioning and adjustment (e.g., Dunn & Plomin, 1990; Dunn & Stocker, 1989). For example, children who exhibit higher levels of conduct problems relative to their siblings may evoke more negative control, hostility, and rejection by parents (Campbell, Pierce, March, & Ewing, 1991). In the final model, which we call the "organismic specificity" pathway (O'Connor, Hetherington, & Reiss, 1998; Wachs & Gandour, 1983), siblings may be differentially sensitive to similar or even identical parenting practices by virtue of their unique intraindividual characteristics (e.g., temperament).

Some findings pertinent to these models have been reported. For example, direct parenting influences on individual siblings and differential parental treatment have been shown independently to predict poor sibling relationship quality both concurrently and prospectively (Brody, Stoneman, & McCoy,

1992). Other studies report that differential parental treatment predicts subsequent increases in "less favored" children's externalizing problems after controlling for prior levels of adjustment, while failing to find evidence for a child effects pathway whereby prior levels of adjustment problems predict subsequent increases in differential parental treatment (Conger & Conger, 1994; McGuire, Dunn, & Plomin, 1995). More systematical tests of all three models (e.g., organismic specificity pathway) are an important direction for future research.

As more evidence accumulates in support of these various pathways, another important direction for research in this area involves building and testing more contextual process models. For example, researchers have begun to tackle the question of when differential parental treatment is associated with poor adjustment; that is, the relationship between parental differential treatment and psychological adjustment among siblings may vary depending on (1) the form of differential parental treatment (e.g., discipline vs. positive involvement; see Volling & Elins, 1998), (2) the domain of children's developmental functioning (e.g., sibling relationship quality, behavior problems, emotional adjustment; McGuire, Dunn, & Plomin, 1995), (3) the age and developmental level of the siblings (e.g., sibling age × developmental disability; McHale & Pawletko, 1992; Quittner & Opipari, 1994), and (4) the pattern of functioning in the larger family system (e.g., effects of negative differential treatment may weaken under conditions of discordant parent–sibling relations; O'Connor, Hetherington, & Reiss, 1998; Reiss et al., 1995).

These efforts to increase the specificity of the models may also help further to inform explanatory (i.e., mediator) models geared toward understanding "why" differential treatment may affect sibling functioning differently (i.e., mediator models). For example, Volling and Elins (1998) evaluated the family and child correlates of three systemic profiles of father and mother differential discipline of older siblings: (1) Mother disciplines older sibling more, while father disciplines siblings equally; (2) father disciplines older sibling more, while mother disciplines siblings equally; and (3) both parents discipline older sibling more. The results indicated that when fathers assume a greater role as disciplinarian for the older sibling, families are characterized by the lowest levels of psychological maladjustment and marital conflict, and the highest levels of sibling harmony. On the other hand, when both parents discipline older siblings more than the younger siblings, older siblings exhibit the highest levels of externalizing problems, internalizing symptoms, and negative interactions with younger siblings. Thus, mutual parental efforts to discipline the older sibling more frequently are interpreted as corresponding to a "detouring" family pattern in which parents distract themselves from their own marital problems by focusing their concerns on the difficulties of the older sibling who, in the process, assumes the role of scapegoat (see also O'Connor, Hetherington, & Reiss, 1998). By explicating the specific patterning and correlates of parental treatment, this study advanced understanding of how and when differential treatment of siblings is associated with problems in children and also the relations between specific patterns of differential treatment and broader patterns of family functioning. From a developmental psychopathology perspective, a logical next step would be to specify the intrachild processes that the family-level patterns set in motion within siblings that can account for their differences in risk for psychopathology.

Fathering and Coparenting in Families

Despite the calls for more research on fathers as parents over the past two and a half decades, much of the research has focused on parenting from the perspective of the mother–child dyad. However, fathering accounts for variance in child adjustment that is not captured by mother–child variables, and mother–child and father–child relationships may have independent effects on children's developmental trajectories over time (Phares & Compas, 1992). Fathers may play a particularly significant role in the socialization of children's emotions (Parke & Buriel, 1998). On the other hand, the father's influence on children cannot be adequately conceptualized only in terms of father–child interactions but must be understood in terms of a broader family context. Fathers affect multiple dimensions of family functioning and, in turn, are themselves influenced by multiple factors outside of their relationships with their children (Lamb, 1976; 1997; Parke, 1996). For example, marital quality at the same time is a product of the father's influence and affects his fathers' functioning in the family (Belsky, 1984).

Thus, a systemic, familywide perspective is pertinent for new directions toward understanding influences on father–child relationships and the processes by which fathering relates to children's adjustment and maladjustment in the context of family relationships. Moreover, the father–child relationship may be particularly affected by family context. For example, the evidence to date suggests that the father–child relationship is more affected by the quality of the marital relationship than is the mother–child relationship (Cummings & O'Reilly, 1997). Thus, lower marital quality has more negative impact on the father–child than on the mother–child relationship (Amato & Keith, 1991; Belsky, Rovine, & Fish, 1989; Booth & Amato, 1994). As another example, Lamb and Elster (1985) reported that social support and mother–father engagement is a significant predictor of the degree of involvement and engagement for fathers but not for mothers. Moreover, in instances of high marital conflict and divorce, more negative outcomes are found with particular consistency for father–child relationships than for mother–child relationships (Amato & Booth, 1991). Thus, while divorce is linked with poorer parent–child relationships in the case of both parents, effects sizes are usually reported to be greater for fathers than for mothers (Amato & Keith, 1991).

However, the bases for the greater effects on fathering than mothering of marital quality are not well understood and thus constitute an intriguing direction for future research. One possibility is that mothers may be better at compartmentalizing the parent and spouse roles, so that there is less carryover from the quality of marital relations to the quality of parent–child relations for mothers. Another possibility is that mothers serve as "gatekeepers" concerning the father's role in relations with children and either fail to promote or act increasingly to inhibit relations of fathers with children as marital relations worsen. A third hypothesis is that parental and husband roles are more fused for fathers, whereas parenthood is a more fundamental role for mothers than fathers. Accordingly, mother–child relations may be less susceptible to variations in the quality of other relationships within the family (Cummings & O'Reilly, 1997).

Problems in the mother–father relationship may also interfere with how well the mother and father work together as parents; that is, such problems may interfere with the quality of coparenting. Thus, Parke and Buriel (1998) raise the intriguing possibility that the tendency of fathers to withdraw in the face of marital conflict may also be reflected in fathers' reduced involvement in coparenting as marital relations worsen; that is, withdrawal from worsening marital relations may also have the effect of reducing the father's involvement in triadic relationships between mothers, fathers, and children. By contrast, in the marital relationship, women have been reported to be more likely to engage and confront in the context of high marital distress. Accordingly, the level of involvement of women in the family may not be nearly as affected as that for fathers in instances of high marital discord.

Coparenting may also be a significant issue in the case of single parents if one takes into account the role of extended family members. As we have noted, a developmental psychopathology perspective proposes that the larger ecological context should be considered in evaluating child and family functioning. In this regard, coparenting may involve adults other than the mother and father, particularly in the ecological contexts of families in particular cultural and ethnic groups. For example, the influence and importance of grandmothers and other extended family members as coparents may be considerable in African American families. Family researchers need to be sensitive to the fact that the organization and utilization of social networks (e.g., two-parent families; multigenerational households) may vary significantly across ethnic and cultural groups. In particular, a relative gap in research is understanding the functioning of extended families in the coparenting role (Parke & Buriel, 1998).

Finally, while study of the role of fathers in families has lagged behind investigation of the role of mothers for normal development, this deficiency is even greater with regard to the research pertinent to the development of psychopathology in children. Phares (1997) has suggested that the reasons for the relative neglect of fathers in clinical research include (1) the inappropriate tendency toward mother-blaming in clinical practice and research, (2) the assumption that there are insurmountable practical problems associated with recruiting fathers as research participants, and (3) the tendency to focus on instances of maternal rather than paternal occurrences of disorders in studies concerned with the development of children of parents with clinical disorders.

For example, with regard to this last point, a vast literature has emerged on the effects of maternal depression on children, but little or no attention has been paid to the impact of paternal depression (Downey & Coyne, 1990). Nonetheless, the relatively few studies that have been conducted provide cogent evidence that depression in fathers also serves as a risk factor for psychopathology in the children. More generally, the literature indicates that fathers' as well as mothers' effects are potentially significant contributors to various forms of psychopathology in children, and that the unwillingness of fathers to participate in research has been overestimated (Phares, 1997). Accordingly, and consistent with the themes of this volume, Phares and Compas (1992) have urged that more attention be paid to distinguishing between maternal and paternal effects in the context of more sophisticated developmental models toward identifying the risk and protective factors accounting for children's patterns of adaptation or maladaptation over time.

Thus, this area of research raises many intriguing questions for future research, and a developmental perspective is an especially timely approach toward answering these questions. As we have noted, a developmental psychopathology perspective focuses attention on the importance of understanding the dynamic processes and developmental pathways that underlie relationships within family functioning. Next steps and new directions for research are to focus on precisely such issues with regard to fathering, coparenting, and related directions pertinent to the development of psychopathology in children.

Ecological and Cultural Characteristics

Larger ecological contexts in the form of culture, neighborhood quality, school climate, and friendship and peer relations may also alter the nature and magnitude of pathways between parenting practices and child adjustment. For example, considerable differences are found between ethnic groups in the extent to which children come from two-parent or one-parent homes (Emery & Kitzmann, 1995). Ethnicity, which is a rough proxy for cultural, community, peer, and neighborhood differences, provides an excellent illustration of how ecological factors may moderate the effects of parenting practices. Whereas high levels of authoritative parenting styles or characteristics (e.g., warmth, democratically firm control, granting psychological autonomy) have been associated with greater psychosocial adjustment among white and Hispanic children and adolescents, African American and Asian American students of authoritative parents often fare no better, or sometimes worse, than their same-ethnic-group counterparts from authoritarian (e.g., strict discipline, negative, physical control, criticism) homes (Baldwin et al., 1993; Baumrind, 1997; Chao, 1994; Deater-Deckard & Dodge, 1997a; Speiker, Larson, Lewis, Keller, & Gilchrist, 1999; Steinberg, Dornbusch, & Brown, 1992). Although there is a growing empirical consistency in the finding that the effects of parenting practices differ by ethnicity, the search for the underlying cultural and ecological variables that more precisely mediate or account for the moderating effects of ethnicity is a rich area of study that is far from resolved.

Figure 7.3 is a statistical model illustrating how moderator models of ethnicity (or any other proxy for an ecological characteristic) must move to the level of understanding what ecological processes account for the ethnic differences. Adequate tests, again, require complex integrations of mediator and moderator models. Some conceptual models do provide some important research directions. In an attempt to understand the weak relationship between authoritative parenting style and adjustment in Asian American youth, Steinberg, Dornbusch, and Brown (1992) theorized that the substantial peer support for academic achievement reported by these students may buffer or dilute the deleterious effects of nonauthoritative parenting. Chao (1994), in contrast, provides compelling data that the same behaviors (e.g., strict control) comprising authoritarian parenting may be part of a unique parenting profile that may have a different meanings and underlying motives in Asian American culture. Strict control connotes negative meaning in white America because it appears largely to reflect an underlying motive of "breaking the will" and "beat-

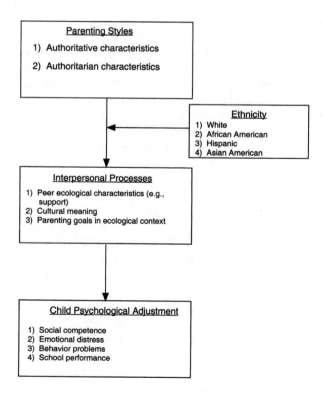

FIGURE 7.3. Ethnicity as a moderator of relations between parenting practices and child adjustment.

ing the devil out" of the child that is directly at odds with the corresponding American ideal of individualism. However, strict control in Asian subcultures has a positive connotation, as it is part of a larger training philosophy and configuration of parenting characteristics that involve "training" or being heavily involved in concern and care for the children. Thus, the apparently weak and counterintuitive effects of parenting styles for Asian American children may reflect a failure to capture the constellation of parenting behaviors that have a distinct meaning for Asian American children derived from a unique cultural history.

Examination of mediating processes having to do with the meaning for children of parental behaviors, rather than simply their surface characteristics, may also explain why African American children with authoritative parents do not fare as well as their white counterparts. First, some evidence suggests that African American families (e.g., mothers) are more likely than white mothers to view physical punishment as one of the most appropriate and effective disciplinary techniques (Deater-Deckard & Dodge, 1997; Deater-Deckard, Dodge, Bates, & Pettit, 1996). Thus, mild physical discipline may hold a different meaning for these African American families and children, such that it may be interpreted and accepted as a sign of involved, caring, and effective parenting (Baumrind, 1997). Second, given the relatively high proportion of African American families living in dangerous, violent communities, tough enforcement of rules and strict demands for unquestioned obedience that characterize authoritarian parenting styles may actually be adaptive in protecting the physical and psychological well-being of children from external dangers they do not yet comprehend (Baldwin et al., 1993; Baumrind, 1972, 1997). In fact, recent studies have reported that higher levels of parental control predict greater adjustment among children in high-risk community or peer environments, whereas lower levels of control are associated with greater adjustment among children from low-risk environments (Baldwin, Baldwin, & Cole, 1990; Mason, Cauce, Gonzales, & Hiraga, 1996). Third, at least in domains of academic achievement, characteristics of the peer ecology may override the beneficial effects of authoritative parenting styles for minority youth. Although authoritative parenting appears to exert an indirect effect on school performance among white students through its effect on promoting adolescent peer affiliations that are supportive of academic pursuits (i.e., peer affiliation as a mediator), there appears to be no relationship among African American children between authoritative parenting and affiliation with peers that support academic achievement. Steinberg and colleagues (1992) have further hypothesized that a relative lack of support for academic pursuits in African American peer groups may sap any constructive effects of authoritative parenting and place African American youth in a more salient dilemma of choosing between academic excellence and peer popularity. Underscoring the controversy in this area, other research suggests that peer support among African American adolescents is, in fact, associated with greater academic performance, although this beneficial effect is greatly diminished under conditions of high neighborhood risk (Gonzales, Cauce, Friedman, & Mason, 1996). However, on balance, we still know very little about the complex matrix of risk and protective factors that underlies ethnicity, ecology, and culture. Thus, while recent findings in this area are intriguing, understanding how cultural and ecological factors may moderate the effects of parenting must be seen as a crucial goal on the agenda for future developmental psychopathology research.

As another example, cultural context may also play a role in understanding the etiology, sequelae, and meaning of parent–child attachment patterns. In an effort to delineate the precise ways in which the development of psychopathology may vary across cultures, Grossmann and Grossmann (1990) draw a distinction between phylogenetic and ontogenetic adaptation. Whereas phylogenetic adaptation is defined as "survival advantage in general" (p. 35), ontogenetic adaptation "refers to adjustment to the environment in the course of development" (p. 35). Drawing from an ethological perspective, phylogenetic adaptation in the attachment system refers to the interplay between caretaking behaviors by the caregiver and proximity-seeking behaviors by the infant, ensuring adequate protection and survival of offspring (Bowlby, 1969; Colin, 1996). Thus, it follows, at least in a phylogenic sense, that the presence and range of attachment behaviors should be universal across cultures. Although more research is needed to test this hypothesis definitively (see Heinicke, 1995), recent research in this area does support the universality of attachment behaviors (e.g., Posada et al., 1995).

On the other hand, with regard to ontogenetic adaptation, ecological systems theories underscore that differences in the definition, meaning, and implications of attachment strategies may vary across subcultural and cultural contexts (Bronfenbrenner, 1979; Grossmann & Grossmann, 1990; Jackson, 1993). In addressing the distribution of attachment strategies, researchers have identified cross-cultural variations in the distribution of attachment using conventional methodologies (i.e., the Strange Situation). Thus, on the one hand, the distribution of secure and insecure infants is relatively similar across cultures, with the majority of infants in Japan, Great Britain, Germany, and the United States being classified as secure. On the other hand, appreciable variations appear to exist in the distributions of the types of insecure attachments (Grossmann & Grossmann, 1990; van IJzendoorn & Kroonenberg, 1988). For example, relative to the United States, Japanese and Israeli samples exhibit higher proportions of resistant attachment, while German samples display higher proportions of avoidant attachment.

Even though the distribution of secure and insecure attachment is relatively comparable across these cultures, cultural differences in the expression of insecure attachment patterns have raised questions about whether the validity and meaning of the attachment classifications may vary across the cultures. For example, consistent with the common philosophy that it is the parents' responsibility to protect children from any experience of stress, Japanese caregivers rarely, if ever, separate from their young children, especially relative to American infants, who commonly experience myriad separations from their caregivers. Because separations are highly unusual for Japanese infants, they may cause far more overt stress, inconsolable crying, tantrums, and clinginess—which are defining features of the anxious/resistant attachment pattern (Takahashi, 1990). Furthermore, Japanese culture generally places greater emphasis on interpersonal communion, affiliation, and harmony relative to the U.S. emphasis on individuality and autonomy. Thus, important features of resistant attachment patterns, such as inconsolable distress, may largely be the result of infants' internalizing the significance of affiliation and union with family members.

On the other hand, Waters and Cummings (2000) have contended that the distribution of Strange Situation classifications in itself has little to say about the pertinence of attachment theory across cultures. Their premise is that the secure base function of attachment is at the heart of the definition of attachment. It follows that attachment theory makes assumptions about relations of caregiver behavior to the organization of secure base behavior. On the other hand, since caregiver behavior may vary across cultures, no assumptions are made about the distributions of attachment classifications across cultures. Thus, Waters and Cummings argued:

> For Bowlby, the function of secure base behavior is always to support competence and promote safety. . . . Attachment theory *does* assume sensitivity to infant signals, cooperative interaction, availability, and responsiveness play a role in attachment development. It *does not* assume that these are equally prevalent in every culture or community or that the distribution of Strange Situation classifications would be similar across cultures. (original emphasis)

Furthermore, because cross-cultural research has predominantly focused on the comparisons of distributions of attachment patterns across cultures, little is known about the role that cultural contexts play in the relationship between attachment and developmental outcomes. Nevertheless, cultural theory and research may provide a breeding ground for the development of hypotheses. For example, the clinginess, desire for closeness, and preoccupation with close relationships evidenced in insecure/resistant attachment patterns may be more tolerated by caregivers and socialization agents in cultures that emphasize collectivism and interpersonal harmony (e.g., Japan) than individualism and agency (e.g., Germany, United States). By contrast, relative to cultures that emphasize collectivism, socialization agents in individualistic-oriented cultures may be more tolerant of insecure/avoidant children who display little or no proximity seeking, dependency, or clinginess. Culture-specific tolerance for certain types of insecure attachment may result in exposure to more optimal caregiving patterns or socialization practices that may help to offset the risk associated with insecure attachment relationships. Testing this hypothesis would first require examining culture as a moderator of the association between attachment patterns and subsequent psychological adaptation. Yet, as we have tried to emphasize throughout the book, specifying the relationship between risk (e.g., attachment insecurity) and developmental outcomes is only the first task in the second generation of research. The next task consists of identifying the processes that explain why culture alters the effects of attachment (e.g., Waters & Cummings, 2000). Thus, testing the prediction that differences in exposure to optimal caregiver patterns or socialization practices partly account for the moderating effects of culture will require more complex, but feasible, integrations of mediator and moderator models (e.g., Baron & Kenny, 1986).

Another important direction for research on the developmental psychopathology of attachment consists of more specifically casting the study of attachment within subcultures. Thus, although the origins, organization, and sequelae of attachment strategies have demonstrated remarkable consistency across a diverse set of economic conditions (e.g., Valenzuela, 1990, 1997), the same parameters and principles of attachment theory, which were developed within a small subset of subcultures, cannot be assumed to be universal without detailed investigation of attachment within the specific subculture of interest. This is perhaps best illustrated by the difficulties researchers faced in attempting to apply the tripartite attachment classification scheme developed in white, middle-class samples (i.e., secure, avoidant, resistant) to high-risk populations experiencing high levels of environmental or family adversity. These difficulties led to new conceptualizations of attachment strategies that incorporated the disorganized attachment pattern.

Falling more squarely within the rubric of subculture, Jackson (1993) has maintained that some principles in attachment theory may not necessarily apply to African American families. For example, the concept of monotropism assumes that children form a primary attachment to a single caregiver that is hierarchically stronger and more significant relative to attachments to other caregivers (e.g., Bowlby, 1969). Montropism may be the norm in subcultures of white, middle-class America, where children are primarily reared by a single caregiver. However, the responsibility of raising children is much more likely to be more evenly shared among multiple caregivers in African American families in light of (1) the greater value placed on extended family and extensive extrafamilial support networks and (2) the economic disadvantage that necessitates that multiple adults in a family be employed. Thus, the organization, origins, and sequelae of attachment relationships may be different across European and African American subcultures. Thus, although preliminary data have failed to uncover different etiological pathways to attachment across subculture (e.g., Barnett, Kidwell, & Leung, 1998; Speiker & Bensley, 1994), Jackson's (1993) compelling hypotheses still require systematic, rigorous empirical testing. Furthermore, this does not necessarily rule out the possibility that attachment relationships in the tradition of Bowlby and Ainsworth might not be as relevant for understanding the social and emotional development of black children in America (Barnett et al., 1998); that is, it does not rule out the possibility that subcultural contexts may moderate the relationship between attachment quality and socioemotional sequelae.

On the other hand, Waters and Cummings (2000) have contended that variations across cultures in the use of multiple caregivers, or in how availability and responsiveness are communicated, are not at all inconsistent with attachment theory if one focuses on the secure base function of attachment rather than on the distributions or identities of attachment figures per se as central to the construct of attachment. Thus, studies of attachments across cultures may also serve to advance and refine the conceptual definition of attachment, as well as broaden understanding of the nature and function of attachment relationships in different contexts.

While acknowledging that little is known about these aspects of the family relative to other areas that we have considered, there is the possibility that the goals and consequences of parenting may be quite different across different cultural contexts. Thus, some have speculated that there are several different hierarchical goals that parents have for their children: (1) survival goal—preserve the health and survival of the child in such a way that he or she lives long enough to reproduce, (2) economic goal—inculcate skills and knowledge necessary for children to become economically self-sufficient adults, and (3) self-actualization goal—promote the achievement of higher-order needs, including the need for relatedness, autonomy, morality, and competence. Since the goals are hierarchical, the lower-order goals or tasks have to be resolved before negotiating subsequent goals (Levine, 1974, as cited in Shaffer, 1994). As an illustration that may serve to stimulate future research and theory on these matters, it is interesting to speculate about how ecological or subcultural contexts may have implications for the goals of parenting and the effectiveness of parenting styles. The examples that follow are intended to draw attention to some of these issues.

For example, among middle-class families, it may be that the economic and educational resources of the families, community, and neighborhood can be marshaled by the parents so that both the survival and economic goals (e.g., safe neighborhood, good schools, supportive peer relations) can be effectively and easily achieved. Thus, the most salient task for parents is to foster skills, habits, and knowledge in their children that effectively promote the development of personal satisfaction, sense of accomplishment, autonomy, achievement, and wealth.

On the other hand, while working-class families (e.g., the father works shifts on the assembly line at the local automobile plant) may meet the survival goal relatively well, they may not have the family and community resources (e.g., safe, but less than optimal, schools) to easily meet the economic goal. The relative lack of resources of parents from these backgrounds may prevent their children from having the benefits of more advantaged, middle-class children, including the economic and personal resources necessary to secure entry into top colleges and, in a broader sense, to achieve the goal of self-actualization. The task of parents, then, is to prepare children to be economically self-sufficient within the working class. Successful employment in the working class may require values of obedience, respect, and neatness (e.g., respect for authority and maintaining a neat, orderly work area are key aspects in factory jobs). Outgrowths of authoritative parenting, which include independence, sociability, creativity, agency, and autonomy, may be at odds with the skills and characteristics individuals need to be economically self-sufficient in working-class contexts. Rather, with the emphasis placed on obedience and orderliness, authoritarian parenting may be among the most effective ways of promoting self-sufficiency in these contexts.

Finally, in poverty-ridden, dangerous ecological contexts (e.g., urban ghettos in contemporary America), parents are likely to be faced with a very different child-rearing goal that may require a different set of child-rearing practices than that of other ecological groups in America. For example, if you were to ask children in these contexts their most important goal or aspiration, sadly, some (or many) might say staying alive or physically surviving. There is so much danger and chaos, and so few resources, that parents have no choice but to concentrate on simply ensuring that their child survives or lives through all the many threats (e.g., violence, drugs, gang activity). The firm, unquestioned obedience demanded by authoritarian parents may be the most effective way of ensuring that the child is adequately protected from these dangers. Reasoning, explanations, and negotiations characteristic of authoritarian parents are likely to be ineffective with many of the children because they fail to have a true understanding of the implications that community violence and disorganization have for their own welfare.

Parenting and Multiple Layers of Context

Relatedly, consistent with ecological and systems theories, it is important to recognize that family dynamics do not simply operate in isolation from societal and community contexts. Rather, the family itself is part of a larger system of interdependent forces in the larger community and cultural contexts that, in turn, are further defined and bounded by the historical period (Bronfenbrenner, 1979). Studying the community and family together can thus be mutually informative.

As an illustration of how an understanding of community characteristics can be advanced by incorporating family process, consider the study of a specific characteristic at the community level: economic hardship and poverty. Whether poverty is studied in the context of the widespread economic Depression of 1930s, the Midwestern agricultural crisis of the 1980s, or the contemporary urban ghettos, families and children who have experienced historical cycles of economic hard times are at appreciable risk for developing psychosocial difficulties (e.g., Conger et al., 1990; Conger, Elder, Melby, Simons, & Conger, 1991; Elder, 1974; McLoyd, 1990; 1998). However, it is important to realize that the effects of poverty and low socioeconomic status are multiply determined and are most appropriately conceptualized in terms of effects of socioeconomic status on processes of child and family functioning over time rather than as a static trait (Parke & Buriel, 1998).

A key research direction is understanding how and why economic adversity increases psychosocial vulnerability (Parke & Buriel, 1998). The family, in this regard, may play a key role in at least two primary pathways. The first pathway hypothesizes that disruptions in the socialization functions of the family may accompany economic hardship and, hence, directly compromise child development. Standing as a conceptual and methodological benchmark project in this area, research conducted by members of the Iowa Youth and Families Project have gathered considerable (albeit not definitive) empirical support for a model in which the burdens and pressures of economic hardship, which are specifically characterized by employment loss and instability, overwhelming financial debt, property foreclosure, and reduced wages and income, demoralize parents and, hence, compromise their emotional well-being. The resulting depression, in turn, is thought to create reverberations in the family that are manifested in marital difficulties and diminished parenting. As the final part of this process chain, children's adjustment is compromised by the disturbances in caregiving of the stressed parents (e.g., Conger et al., 1992, 1993; Conger, Ge, Elder, Lorenz, & Simons, 1994).

Yet disruptions in family socialization practices commonly explain only part of the links between economic hardship and children's socioemotional functioning (Dodge, Pettit, & Bates, 1994a). Thus, as a second pathway, the limited financial and social network resources that accompany the families experiencing poverty, especially urban families, constrain the breadth and quality of children's opportunities to participate in activities that promise social, emotional, and cognitive growth (Huston, McLoyd, & Garcia Coll, 1994). For example, whereas middle- and upper-class families have the resources to send their children to high-quality private schools or relocate to suburban schools, parents faced with economic hardship in urban settings must, in many cases, resign themselves to sending their children to the relatively disorganized, poor-quality public schools in their poor communities (Black & Krishnakumar, 1998). Furthermore, even with subsidized day care, children of poor families still endure poorer quality day care relative to children of middle- or high-income families (Philips, Voran, Kisker, Howes, & Whitebrook, 1994).

Tracing transactions between indicators of community characteristics and family and child functioning, however, is complicated by the fact that even specific constructs such as poverty are illusive in their heterogeneity, multidimensionality, and association with larger network of risk factors. Precise specification of the contextual dimensions of poverty will thus be critical in making further progress on the interplay between economic and family processes. For example, families and children may face very different circumstances and challenges depending on the geographic locus of poverty along the urban–rural continuum (Huston, McLoyd, & Garcia Coll, 1994). Differences in family structure, the nature and quality of kin support networks, ethnicity, access to community and neighborhood resources, and exposure to neighborhood violence are likely to differ as a function of whether poverty occurs in urban or rural settings. Because these various factors may moderate (e.g., access to community resources) or mediate (e.g., exposure to family violence) the risk that poverty poses for family and child well-being, the interplay among economic hardship, family process, and child development may differ widely across these contexts (Brody, Flor, & Gibson, 1999; Huston et al., 1994; Tickamyer & Duncan, 1990). Even focusing more narrowly on the neighborhood context (rather than the broader construct of geographical location) of family economic hardship underscores the multiplicity of influences and pathways between ecological and family characteristics. For example, the multiple structural (e.g., neighborhood socioeconomic status, residential mobility, family disruption, dilapidated housing) and process (e.g., social isolation, gangs, public drunkenness, street harassment, drug trade, noise) dimensions of the neighborhood may play different roles as mediators and moderators of poverty and family risk (Klebanov, Brooks-Gunn, McCarton, & McCormick, 1998; Wandersman & Nation, 1998).

To illustrate how the study of family dynamics can be informed by a larger appreciation of the community and ecological context, consider how divorce and family dissolution increase children's psychosocial risk. The higher incidence of adjustment problems of children who experienced divorce or family dissolution is mediated by disruptions in family process (e.g., Amato & Keith, 1991; Hetherington, Bridges, & Isabella, 1998). Thus, diminished caregiver emotional availability, poor child management techniques, parental emotional distress, and interparental conflict surrounding divorce account, in part, for the risk posed by divorce (e.g., Buchanan, Maccoby, & Dornbusch, 1991; Emery & Forehand, 1994; Hetherington, 1989; Maccoby, Buchanan, Mnookin, & Dornbush, 1993). Yet, at the same time, family processes cannot fully account for the heterogeneity of outcomes experienced by children of divorce. Likewise, the psychosocial risk incurred by the experience of divorce is modest to moderate at best.

A broader view of the context of divorce reveals that divorce is part of a larger, reciprocal network of unstable familial and extrafamilial events and stressors. The psychological burdens carried by adults who experience adversity in the community (e.g., occupational stress, job loss, and impoverishment) are thought to precipitate interparental discord and relationship instability (Conger et al., 1990). Conversely, the instability and dissolution of the interparental relationship is also likely to trigger instability in the form of declines in economic well-being, quality of life, and the community context within which the family is embedded (Hetherington, Bridges, & Insabella, 1998). As a result, conceptualizations of divorce as a discrete event are increasingly being complemented by divorce process models that more broadly capture children's collective experiences with familial (e.g., interparental arguments, parental distress) and ecological (e.g., moving, loss of material possessions) stressors surrounding divorce (e.g., Emery, Waldron, Kitzmann, &

Aaron, 1999; Sandler, Tein, & West, 1994; Sandler, Wolchik, Braver, & Fogas, 1991). Assessments of these cumulative, divorce-related, stressful events and the unfolding meaning, appraisals, and coping strategies children form from these experiences have led to valuable insights into why some children of divorce experience greater adjustment difficulties (e.g., Sandler et al., 1994; Sheets, Sandler, & West, 1996).

New advances in conceptualization of family context have also benefited from understanding the specific circumstances faced by economically disadvantaged families. For example, researchers are beginning to reconceptualize the boundaries in the conventional differentiation between family-level and ecological-contextual factors in the study of family instability. Although serving as a source of continuity, cohesiveness, and predictability in the lives of children is a primary function of the family (Bowlby, 1969; Popenoe, 1994), the higher frequency and diversity of disruptions and stressors inside (e.g., death of family member, caregiver turnover, changes in caregiver romantic relationships) and outside (e.g., caregiver job loss or change, residential mobility) economically disadvantaged families may lead to a great deal of variability in family instability or breakdown in the ability of the families to provide a safe, cohesive haven for children. Results of this groundbreaking research indicated the family instability continues to predict children's concurrent and subsequent adjustment difficulties even in the context of family process variables (i.e., family conflict, family cohesion, caregiver distress) (Ackerman, Kogos, Youngstrom, Schoff, & Izard, 1999; see also Ackerman, Izard, Schoff, Youngstrom, & Kogos, 1999). Although more research is warranted before any firm conclusions can be made, the results are consistent with earlier studies (e.g., Conger et al., 1992) suggesting that the family burdens and upheavals associated with economic adversity are mediated, in part, by family discord and impairments in caregiving practices. More significantly, though, the findings suggest that family instability may directly affect children's intrapsychic processes that compromise their adjustment. For example, family instability may challenge children's sense of security, overwhelm emotion regulation capacities, diminish their sense of agency, and foster hostile family appraisals (Davies & Cummings, 1994; Fogas, Wolchik, Braver, Freedom, & Bay, 1992; Kim, Sandler, & Tein, 1997).

Parenting as a Moderator

As we have seen, it is important in a process-oriented perspective on the effects of parenting on children to determine when other factors serve as moderators. On the other hand, it is also informative in a process-oriented analysis to understand when parenting moderates the impact of other factors; that is, parenting practices may help to clarify when the relationship between other family and ecological variables and child developmental outcomes are strongest or weakest. For example, Grych (1998) reported that the relationship between destructive interparental conflict and children's perceptions of threat and poor coping efficacy in conflict situations was most pronounced when children experienced high levels of paternal aggression. Emphasizing the protective side of parenting, research and theoretical work has also underscored the fact that constructive parenting may buffer children from risk contexts (e.g., Cooper, Peirce, & Tidwell, 1995; Werner, 1986). For example, researchers have hypothesized that the risk posed by parental alcoholism to children's adjustment may be substantially reduced when at least one of the parents exhibits high levels of behavioral control, warmth, and responsiveness (e.g., Curran & Chassin, 1996; Hussong & Chassin, 1997; Sher, 1991).

Some alcohol conceptualizations, however, have tacitly treated good parenting or parent–child relationships as if they were static "traits" that retain their buffering power across contexts (e.g., Hawkins, Catalano, & Miller, 1992). More dynamic, contextual models of developmental psychopathology eschew these assumptions in favor of exploring the possibility of moderating effects that interact with context. For example, the effects of parent–child relations may be further moderated by other contextual factors. Thus, caregiver support and responsiveness may buffer children from the effects of paternal drinking problems (Cooper, Peirce, & Tidwell, 1995). However, this may only apply if the supportive caregiver does not exhibit alcohol problems. In fact, parental substance use has been shown to predict adolescent substance use if the adolescent has a good or supportive relationship with the parent (Andrews, Hops, & Duncan, 1997).

Parenting practices have also been conceptualized as moderators in links between child characteristics (e.g., coping styles, personality traits, temperament, ways of approaching developmental milestones) and child adjustment (e.g., Bates, Pettit, Dodge, & Ridge, 1998; Fuhrman & Holmbeck, 1995; Lamborn & Steinberg, 1993; Mangelsdorf, Gunnar, Kestenbaum, Lang, & Andreas, 1990). For example, according to the "emotional fit" hypothesis, the adaptational value of achieving emotional autonomy, or the process by which "adolescents relinquish childish dependencies on, and conceptions of, their parents" (Lamborn & Steinberg, 1993, p. 483) depends on the larger parenting context (Fuhrman & Holmbeck, 1995). When adolescents are exposed to low levels of parental warmth and high conflict, greater emotional autonomy, indicative of detachment from parents, is actually associated with better adolescent psychological adjustment (e.g., social competence, academic achievement, low externalizing symptoms). By contrast, greater emotional autonomy predicted poorer psychological adjustment when adolescents experienced high levels of warmth and low conflict (Fuhrman & Holmbeck, 1995). Interpreted within the "emotional fit" hypothesis, these results suggest that emotional distancing in the context of a disturbed parent–child subsystem may actually hold short-term adaptational value by reducing children's exposure to family stress and preserving their psychological well-being. Underscoring that development is a process, these investigators also noted that these strategies of emotional detachment from parents may not bode well for subsequent adjustment, particularly in the realm of interpersonal relationship development

(Fuhrman & Holmbeck, 1995; see also Sroufe, 1988). Furthermore, one might predict different results (e.g., psychological adjustment) in younger children, especially in the absence of another involved adult, indicating that the moderating effects of parenting may vary with the child's developmental level.

CASTING PARENTING MODELS IN A DEVELOPMENTAL FRAMEWORK

Thus far, we have focused on demonstrating the value for understanding the effects of parenting on child development and contextualizing parenting in terms of a broader model of the effects of intrachild, familial, and extrafamilial influences on child adjustment. However, the demonstration thus far has been adevelopmental; that is, the issues for the most part could just as readily apply to cross-sectional as longitudinal tests of influences on children's functioning. As illustrated in Figure 4.1, continuity or change in development, and the nature and course of pathways of development, are also essential components of a developmental psychopathology perspective of the influences of parenting on child development.

Moschell (1991) provides some levity while, at the same time, cogently making clear the importance of such considerations:

> Wanted: Parent of Infant. Must be able to function without sufficient sleep for long periods of time. Must be able to walk the equivalent of ten miles a night without leaving the bedroom. Must put social life and sex life on hold while tending to the needs of a totally dependent, demanding, unreasonable, and very tiny boss. If this is a first-born, must have photography skills; less essential for later borns. Must be proficient at interpreting commands in ear-piercing shrieks. Must enjoy, or at least tolerate, highly repetitive tasks: diapering, feeding, burping, diapering, feeding, burping. . . .
>
> Wanted: Parent of Two-Year-Old. Must have extraordinary degree of patience. Must have ability to handle the demands of an unpredictable, negative, stubborn subordinate with delusions of grandeur. Negotiating abilities essential. . . .
>
> Wanted: Parent of Preschoolers. Must be omniscient, able to answer any "Why?" question while performing tasks such as driving through heavy traffic, cooking, showering, or making love. Depending on child's ability to nap you may have to relinquish all coffee breaks. Mechanical skills needed to assemble trikes, wagons, and associated plastic toys, usually without the instructions. . . .
>
> Wanted: Parents of Elementary School-Aged Child. Chauffer's license essential. Overtime includes evenings at PTA meetings, school pageants, soccer games, paper drives, and other activities you swore you'd never become involved in. Your job includes being social secretary, responsible for scheduling child's birthday party, gymnastic practices, music lessons, soccer practices, and current list of best friends.
>
> Wanted: Parents of Teenager. Must have extraordinary degree of pa-

tience. Knowledge of current fads and slang helpful. You will be treated as if you have lost some or all of your mental acuity, but don't panic! Ability to fade into woodwork at appropriate times a plus. Driver's license no longer necessary, since teen will inevitably have a car when you need it, or will be out of gas. (p. 3)

It is to matters and issues relevant to developing these directions in parenting research to which we next turn.

Mechanistic versus Contextualistic Views of Parenting Effects

One barometer sometimes used for evaluating the significance of a parenting construct to child development has been to demonstrate the generalizability of effects across different developmental periods. However, this particular approach for gathering validity data is based on a mechanistic assumption about the nature of human development; that is, it assumes that the phenomena under study (e.g., parenting, child adjustment) are inherently inactive, static, and passive. Any failure to demonstrate generalizability within this orientation, then, is considered to be a reflection of problems with (1) the theoretical assumptions underlying the construct, (2) translating theory into a valid operationalization and assessment of the variable, and/or (3) limitations accompanying statistical models (e.g., statistical power).

Influenced by contextualistic worldviews, many developmental psychologists eschew this static view of child development in favor of conceptualizing changes in the system and its components as basic or fundamental. Applied to parenting, this means that charting changes in parenting dimensions and their evolving, dynamic relations to the larger network of systemic (e.g., family, ecological) and child variables is an integral task of developmental psychopathologists. For example, based on a meta-analysis of the large literature pertinent to continuity and change in parenting, Holden and Miller (1999) have shown that multiple dimensions of child rearing evidence similarities, but also differences, across time (and also situations and children), and have argued that change and variability in child rearing must be recognized in theoretical models of parenting in order to advance understanding of the nature of parenting and its effects on children. They concluded:

> Acceptance of the assertion that child rearing is simultaneously enduring and different implies a fundamental change in the way that parents are thought of and studied. Thus, in addition to recognition of the enduring characteristics of parents, the question of paramount importance is under what conditions, in what ways, to what extent, and why does child rearing change or vary? (p. 26)

Because there are many developmental strategies for conceptualizing this dynamic unfolding of relations among context, parenting, and child adjustment over time, we selectively focus on the value of a subset of these approaches.

Stage-Salient Tasks

Despite the demonstrated utility of embedding parenting models in the context of a series of developmental tasks for some risk samples (e.g., Cicchetti, 1989; Cole & Putnam, 1992; Elicker, Englund, & Sroufe, 1991), models of parenting have yet to capitalize on the value of using the developmental task model as a framework for understanding the interplay between parenting and children's normal and abnormal development. By way of introduction, Table 7.1 illustrates the value of examining parenting in the context of changing developmental tasks from infancy through childhood (Elicker et al., 1992). Each developmental level is accompanied by key developmental challenges, which, if successfully achieved by the child, may increase the probability of maintaining or reclaiming a healthy developmental trajectory. Further reflecting the transactional features of developmental models, effective parenting patterns in this dynamic model are not only conceptualized as regulating children's success in resolving the stage-salient task but are also, in turn, regulated or shaped by children's developmental level of functioning.

Within this developmental model, qualities of the emotional relationship between parents and children, that is, responsivity, sensitivity, and emotional availability, are conceptualized as central parenting dimensions in infancy that serve to facilitate at least two primary developmental tasks: physiological regulation and the formation of attachment relationships (Jacobvitz, Morgan, Kretchmar, & Morgan, 1992). The transactional interplay of the system during this developmental period is commonly manifested in one of two ways. First, infants with difficult temperamental characteristics may contribute to their own risk by evoking more rejection and insensitivity from the parent. Second, parental insensitivity and unavailability may cause an infant who falls in the normal range of temperamental characteristics to become more irritable and troublesome, thereby setting the stage for further increases in parental insensitivity. By the end of this period, this pattern of parent–child interaction may place the child at considerable risk for developing an insecure attachment to the parent (Shaw & Bell, 1993).

The transition from infancy to toddlerhood is paralleled by a change from resolving tasks that involve the regulation of physiological arousal and the formation of secure attachment relations with the parent to a focus on goals of effectively exploring the world and developing a sense of mastery, autonomy, and individuation (Edwards, 1996; Jacobvitz, Morgan, Kretchmar, & Morgan, 1992). Thus, the salience of parental sensitivity, predictable and responsive care, and emotional availability necessary to promote child resolution of developmental tasks of infancy increasingly evolves into serving as a secure base and exhibiting firm support that promote toddler mastery of the social and physical world. In addition, the parent needs to preserve the toddler's felt security without compromising the monitoring and limit setting necessary to protect the toddler physically from the trials and tribulations of exploration and curiosity (Lieberman, 1992). Given children's limited understanding of the rationale underlying physical and social rules during and prior to the preschool period (Hoffman, 1970; Johnson & McGillicudy-Dilisi, 1983), balancing the use of reinforcement contingencies (e.g., negative physical control, verbal corrections) with some modest use of inductive discipline (i.e., reasoning) may be more effective in instilling early moral understanding of rules than inductive discipline alone (Zahn-Waxler, Radke-Yarrow, & King, 1979). Parental use of internal state language (e.g., communication of feeling states) in emotion-laden situations is thought further to promote children's emotion regulation (e.g., monitoring of feeling states, identification of the source of emotion) and a developing sense of right and wrong (e.g., early forms of internalization of values) (Cicchetti & Lynch, 1993).

Developmental histories of negotiating developmental tasks are also theorized to influence how children and parents approach tasks during this developmental period. For example, the earlier developmental task of forming an attachment relationship may actually moderate parental reactions to these new stressful challenges. For example, mothers having an insecure attachment relationship with their infants may be especially prone to appraise their children's behaviors as troublesome, which, in turn, may fuel greater negativity, hostility, and withdrawal (Shaw & Bell, 1993). Further contributing to the parent–child interactive disturbance, insecurely attached children are also at greater risk for becoming increasingly noncompliant (Londerville & Main, 1981; Stayton, Hogan, & Ainsworth, 1971).

As children reach preschool and childhood periods, developing open lines of reciprocal communication and displaying acceptance are thought to promote positive internal representations (e.g., self as worthy, people as generally trustworthy), self-regulation patterns, and social skills (e.g., cooperation, self-disclosure) that are building blocks for the development of harmonious peer relations, close friendships, and self-confidence (Collins, Harris, & Susman, 1995). Similarly, effective monitoring and enforcement of rules through use of particular disciplinary techniques (e.g., induction, reasoning) appear to facilitate children's compliance with rules and acceptance of family and societal values as their own, and, as such, promote impulse management and constructive peer relations even in the context of challenge and conflict (Johnson & McGillicudy-Dilisi, 1983). Thus, children experiencing parenting styles characterized by responsivity with insistence or demandingness (i.e., authoritative) have been shown to fare better psychologically than their counterparts who experience responsivity without demandingness (i.e., permissive), demandingness without responsivity (i.e., authoritarian), or neither responsivity nor demandingness (i.e., uninvolved) (for exceptions, see the earlier section on *ecological and cultural characteristics*).

Periods of early and middle adolescence are characterized by substantial developmental changes and challenges, including (1) coping with peer pressure (Hogue & Steinberg, 1995; Windle & Davies, 1999); (2) undergoing transitions from the relatively intimate, personal confines of elementary school to ever larger and often more impersonal secondary schools (Eccles et al., 1993; Simmons & Blyth, 1987); (3) successively renegotiating balances between autonomy and relatedness in the family (Collins, Gleason, & Sesma, 1997; Holmbeck, Paikoff, & Brooks-Gunn, 1995); (4) coping with cumulative, stressful life events (Smolak, Levine, & Gralen, 1993; Windle, 1992); and (5) the development of heterosexual friendships and romantic relationships (Connolly & Johnson, 1996; Davies & Windle, 1997; Neeman, Hubbard, & Masten, 1995). As individuals continue through middle and late adolescence, identity formation, exclusive romantic relationships, and occupational preparedness (e.g., planned academic trajectory) become increasingly salient developmental tasks (e.g., Baumrind, 1991; Eccles, Lord, & Buchanan, 1996; Schulenberg, Maggs, & Hurrelmann, 1997).

The process of resolving these developmental tasks continues to precipitate new challenges for parenting. As adolescents negotiate levels of autonomy, effective ways of caretaking may change. Baumrind (1991), for example, illustrates how complex the interplay between parent and adolescent can be even within the narrow confines of negotiating autonomy. According to her model, early adolescence is characterized by shedding the simple acceptance of influential adults as authority figures in favor of what Baumrind terms the "practicing" phase of differentiation. In an effort to underscore their emerging appraisals of autonomy and individuation, and to downplay any "immature," child-like signs of dependence, early adolescents unequivocally oppose rules made by parents and authority figures, especially conventional rules that maintain the status quo but serve little or no purpose in promoting social or individual good (Smetana, 1995). As children progress through midadolescence, they commonly experience the second phase of differentiation, termed the "rapprochement" phase. Recognizing that the threat of regressing to overdependence on parents is waning, midadolescents attempt to renegotiate a more sound balance between autonomy and relatedness to parents. According to this contemporary view, the developmental outcomes of adolescents during each of these phases are fostered by parents who ultimately develop and enforce rules of conduct. However, although power in decision making is decidedly assymetrical, parents respect the differences of opinion expressed by their children and, as part of this expression of respect, provide reasonable, sound explanations for the rule formulation and enforcement. Furthermore, as children progress through adolescence, a key task of parents involves granting increasing autonomy in the context of maintaining relatedness with their children. Granting autonomy without parental support and warmth is likely to increase adolescents' risk for following maladaptive developmental pathways (Fuligni & Eccles, 1993; Holmbeck, 1996; Steinberg, Elmen, & Mounts, 1989).

Working from a biopsychosocial model, Holmbeck (1996) has also underscored how new developmental tasks brought about, in part, by puberty may also affect parenting and adolescent development. Emotional distress resulting, in part, from hormonal changes of puberty may directly challenge the caregiving resources of parents (Buchanan, Eccles, & Becker, 1992), particularly in high-risk dyads characterized by preexisting parent–child relational disturbances, parental psychopathology, or family alcoholism (Holmbeck, Paikoff, & Brooks-Gunn, 1995). Illustrating a more complex, indirect pathway, empirical evidence indicates that physical and reproductive maturity also prompt parents to increase their expectations for mature behavior and their desire to monitor their adolescents' affiliations with heterosexual peer groups (Hill & Lynch, 1983). According to the gender intensification hypothesis, part of this process involves increased pressure, both by the self and parents, to conform to gender-stereotypical roles emphasizing agency among boys (e.g., independence, competition) and communion among girls (e.g., interpersonal concern). Thus, the maturational process is conceptualized as prompting changes in developmental challenges for both parents and adolescents that are moderated by the gender of the adolescent.

Given the considerable changes in physiological, psychosocial, and emotional functioning experienced by adolescents, the parenting task of striking a balance between exercising control (i.e., maturity demands, monitoring peer activities, and supporting adolescent autonomy) and expressing warmth and support is best conceptualized as a dynamic one (Collins, Henninghausen, Schmit, & Sroufe, 1997). Parental flexibility during this developmental period is critical, as concretely evidenced by continual renegotiation of the balance between control and autonomy-supportive parenting that is commensurate with adolescent development (Holmbeck, 1996). Inflexibility, in which parents continue to retain high levels of control without increasing their support of adolescent autonomy, is thought to hinder adolescents' ability to resolve developmental tasks, including the establishment of supportive peer relations, intimate romantic relationships, autonomy (i.e., behavioral, emotional, cognitive), and identity formation (Hauser, Powers, & Noam, 1991). Successive difficulties in achieving these developmental milestones place these individuals at risk for psychopathology by increasing the probability of their failing to resolve adult developmental tasks (e.g., stable occupational trajectory; involvement in intimate, long-term relationship; parenthood) (Fullinwider-Bush & Jacobvitz, 1993; Windle & Davies, 1999).

While casting development as a series of stage-salient tasks negotiated by parents and children underscores the considerable change and discontinuity of child development, a developmental framework is also useful in uncovering the continuity that underlies these dynamic changes. For example, whereas intrusive caregiving during infancy, parental overprotection during childhood, and parent–child role reversal during adulthood are considered distinct parenting dimensions from an adevelopmental perspective, a developmental psychopathology perspective suggests that these caregiving patterns reflect the same underlying family systems process of parent–child symbiotic boundary disturbances that are simply manifested in somewhat different ways across developmental periods (Jacobvitz, Morgan, Kretchmar, & Morgan, 1992). Thus, despite important differences in parenting, heterotypical continuity is evident in the thematic coherence of parent–child enmeshment and the accompanying constraint of children's autonomy and individuation over an extended part of the life span. Furthermore, within family systems theory, these different caregiving patterns serve the same function of over time of stabilizing a chaotic family system through the rigid emotional entanglement of parent and child (Sroufe, 1989; Sroufe, Jacobvitz, Mangelsdorf, DeAngelo, & Ward, 1985).

Sensitive Periods

Sensitive periods, which are integral to an understanding of stage-salient tasks, refer to the notion that many of the developmental changes in neurobiological, socioemotional, and cognitive processes may precipitate increases in sensitivity to parenting practices during certain developmental periods. It is useful to differentiate this term from "critical period" models that have sought to identify environmental events that have their maximal and often irreversible effects on some developmental system within a limited developmental period and have a negligible effect prior to or following this critical temporal window. Sensitive periods are also developmental periods during which the effects of an event, or series of events, may become particularly pronounced; however, it is also acknowledged that the sequelae of the events do retain some plasticity (i.e., potential for change) and that the event, or events, may still exert appreciable effects on individuals both prior to and following the sensitive period (Myers, 1984; Rutter, 1989b).

Specific developmental periods are accompanied by changes in social, emotional, cognitive, and physiological functioning that may increase or decrease children's risk for psychopathology. However, the changes occurring across all these domains make it difficult to pinpoint any one time period as being differentially sensitive to general parenting styles. For example, adolescents could be considered to be more vulnerable to parenting disturbances than children by virtue of (1) increases in sensitivity to family and parental distress (e.g., Buchanan, Maccoby, & Dornbusch, 1991; Cummings & Davies, 1994b), (2) having to simultaneously cope with peak occurrences of stressful life events (Windle, 1992), and (3) simultaneously attempting to negotiate very challenging developmental tasks (e.g., autonomy, establishment of intimate relations, identity formation). On the other hand, this vulnerability may be offset by adolescents' broader, more effective repertoire of coping strategies, greater independence from family relationships, and utilization of extrafamilial relationships (e.g., peers) as sources of support (Garmezy & Rutter, 1983; Sim & Vuchinich, 1996).

Perhaps as a result of the difficulties of disentangling cohort (e.g., date of birth), adaptational (e.g., length of time between stressor and adjustment), and maturational (e.g., age) effects in research designs, few researchers have attempted to examine whether age moderates the relationship between parenting and child outcomes. In an attempt to address this gap, Sim and Vuchinich (1996) tested the hypothesis that the greater psychological and social resources available to adolescents would dilute the effects of parental emotional disengagement relative to their younger counterparts. Contrary to their hypothesis, the findings indicated that the relationship between parental disengagement and child antisocial behavior was actually greater in magnitude for adolescents than children or young adults. Although this study was not without methodological limitations (e.g., different measures of parenting and child antisocial measures across the age groups appear to have different levels of face validity), the findings do support the notion that adolescence may be a sensitive period for the effects of parental emotional disengagement.

Different theoretical models of parental discipline have been posited to vary in their utility as a function of the child's developmental period. Hoffman (1970), for example, suggested that processes of reinforcement, punishment, and observational learning may be particularly powerful early on by instilling an awareness of simple rules and conventions. Yet the behavioral contingencies and modeling processes may fall short of explaining how different disciplinary strategies instill a deeper understanding of the reasons for the rules and, ultimately, the inculcation and acceptance of moral values or rules. Hoffman theorized that once children achieve some knowledge base of rules and conventions during the toddler and early preschool years, inductive discipline, in which parents stimulate children's own thinking about the reasons underlying the acceptability of the behavior, is likely to foster children's internalization of the reasons for rules. Relative to children's awareness of rules or the acceptability of certain behaviors, children's understanding of the rationale underlying rules may require more sophisticated cognitive and interpersonal understanding that may not emerge until the early or middle years of childhood.

Delineating age as a moderator is only a first step in understanding the operation of sensitive periods. As Rutter (1989) points out, age changes are not explanations for behavioral development; rather, they are only very rough markers for maturational and experiential processes. Since changes in different developmental systems may actually offset each other, age differences (or the lack thereof) in the effects of parenting may even be misleading. Thus, an important task for developmental psychopathologists is to begin to understand the underlying processes that mediate or account for the moderating effects of age in the link between parenting and child functioning.

Peak Periods for Risk Exposure

Differences in vulnerability and resilience to caregiving practices across developmental periods may also be the result of differences in exposure to caregiving practices. In interpreting some reports, for example, investigators have concluded that the incidence of child maltreatment tends to decline with age (Powers & Eckenrode, 1988). Belsky (1993) has suggested that young children may be at greater risk for experiencing maltreatment because caregivers are more likely to use physical force with them in disciplinary situations. At the same time, he notes that age differences in the incidence of maltreatment are far from resolved, with some studies even indicating that adolescents experience higher rates of maltreatment than children. Furthermore, whether the differences in the incidence of maltreatment across age periods reflect differences in exposure to a broad susceptability of parenting disturbances is questionable. For example, there is some evidence that parental adjustment problems are more common in middle childhood than in adolescence (Harrington, Rutter, & Fombonne, 1996).

Developmental Pathways and Trajectories

Risk and resilience models of parenting have commonly been tested within the confines of cross-sectional and static longitudinal research designs that only investigate each key construct at a single point in time (e.g., parenting patterns at time 1 and child functioning at time 2). These designs are very important and necessary first steps in establishing a reliable set of findings on basic relations between parent and child functioning before ultimately moving on to more costly and complex longitudinal designs. Yet in many areas of parenting research, the well-documented associations between various forms of parenting and child adjustment call for the move to a more complex developmental model of parenting. First, making more firm conclusions about the directionality of effects and transactional interplay between parenting and child adjustment is hindered by a reliance on cross-sectional designs even at the most basic interpretive level; that is, cross-sectional designs violate the principle stipulating that a variable can only be caused by values of a preceding variable. Second, both cross-sectional and static longitudinal designs fail to capture the dynamic nature of developmental psychopathology centering on (1) the continuity, variability, and transformation of parenting patterns over time and development, and (2) the interindividual differences in intraindividual change (i.e., diversity in the pathways or trajectories of adjustment experienced by children).

As another example, the association between children's conduct problems (e.g., aggressive, disruptive behavior), and parental control tactics (e.g., coercion), and low levels of affection are well-documented in both cross-sectional and static longitudinal designs (e.g., Hart, DeWolf, & Burts, 1993). Thus, on the one hand, developmental psychopathology research has made appreciable progress on the first goal of drawing firmer, though not definitive, conclusions about the directionality of the interplay between parenting and child adjustment. Yet slight modifications, such as the incorporation of child functioning measures at time 1, as well as time 2, may allow for much more powerful tests of parenting as predictors of change in functioning. Autoregressive models that statistically control for preexisting psychological functioning (i.e., time 1) allow for a more powerful test of whether parenting practices assessed at time 1 predict change in psychological functioning from time 1 to time 2. Use of this approach has yielded important results on the modest but consistent association between parenting styles and dimensions and changes in children's functioning (e.g., Herman, Dornbusch, Herron, & Herting, 1997; Pettit, Bates, & Dodge, 1993; Steinberg, Lamborn, Darling, Mounts, & Dornbusch, 1994; see also Davies, Dumenci, & Windle, 1999). Cross lagged models, which use repeated measures of parenting and child functioning at multiple occasions of measurement, are especially useful in modeling the dynamic, reciprocal nature of family processes by simultaneously specifying pathways running from (1) parenting to subsequent changes in child functioning and (2) child functioning to subsequent changes in parenting (Campbell, Pierce, Moore, Marakovitz, & Newby, 1996; Ge, Conger, Lorenz, Shanahan, & Elder, 1995; Stice & Barrera, 1995).

However, although cross-legged approaches do capture individual differences in change in parental and child functioning, they fail to map individual differences in the slope, starting points, and endpoints of children's developmental trajectories (Willett, Singer, & Martin, 1998). Thus, they cannot address a fundamental task in the developmental psychopathology of parenting: explicating the structure, and parenting origins and correlates of specificity, equifinality, and multifinality of children's developmental trajectories. Complementary methodological strategies and statistical models are thus needed to address change. For example, growth curve analyses have revealed that elevated negative maternal control (e.g., yelling, threatening) is associated with high, stable trajectories of disruptive behavior problems, whereas low levels of negative control predicte initial low disruptive behavior problems that continue to decline over a 3-year period. Therefore, over time, differences in exposure to negative maternal control have been associated with diverging trajectories of behavior problems (Spieker et al., 1999). McFayden-Ketchum, Bates, Dodge, and Pettit (1996) used regression analyses to identify eight different developmental trajectories of child disruptive problems that captured the initial level of problems and their subsequent slopes over four measurement occasions. Consistent with the previous findings, negative maternal control and lack of affection predicted among boys initially high levels of disruptive behavior that continued to increase over time. However, unlike the earlier results, gender was found to be a moderator. Although negative maternal control predicted initial levels of disruptive behavior problems in girls, it also predicted decreasing, rather than increasing, trajectories of disruptive behavior over time. Applied to coercion theory (Patterson, 1992), this suggests that the negative reinforcement value of escalating aversive behaviors in discipline situations and, hence, prompting mothers to withdraw their aversive threats and demands, may only operate for boys. Similar models have also been applied to understanding the parental and family precursors to different pathways of peer relations (see Pettit, Clawson, Dodge, & Bates, 1996).

Toward a Process Conceptualization of Developmental Outcomes

Another goal for a developmental psychopathology perspective is a richer characterization of relations between developmental pathways and children's developmental outcomes. Research programs traditionally have been designed to unravel the origins of different forms of adaptation and maladaptation in isolation from one another. For example, parenting researchers attempting to understand the social functioning of children have often focused on children's problems in one of the following domains: (1) behavioral problems or externalizing symptoms (e.g., interpersonal hostility, aggression, delinquency), (2) emotional disturbances or internalizing symptoms (e.g., depressive symptoms, loneliness, anxiety), and (3) peer competency, status, or relationship quality (e.g., peer victim, victimizer). However, there may be important similarities as well as differences in pathways to different types or forms of adjustment problems, and the examination of such comparisons may be highly informative with regard to the specific origins of childhood disturbances. Moreover, although identifying the socialization and intrapersonal mechanisms underlying each of these dimensions of functioning is useful in its own right, newly emerging person-based approaches to children's functioning provide a new way of looking at process by simultaneously capturing functioning across multiple response domains and thus more significant "chunks" of the child. Work by Schwartz and colleagues, for example, provides a convincing case for integrating multiple response domains into larger profiles of interpersonal functioning (Schwartz, Dodge, Pettit, & Bates, 1997). Simultaneously considering children's externalizing symptoms and peer functioning, these researchers classified children into four profiles of interpersonal functioning: (1) passive victims of bullying, (2) aggressive victims of bullying, (3) non-victimized aggressors, and (4) normative children. Guided by social information-processing frameworks (e.g., Crick & Dodge, 1996), they specifically hypothesized that aggressive victims of bullying emerged partly as a function of long histories as both witnesses and victims of family rejection and hostility. The underlying rationale was that being a victim and witness of rejection and hostility, rather than simply a witness, would lead to hostile attributional styles, explosive, dysregulating bouts of negativity, and hypervigilance to stressful situations that would leave children prone to both aggressive outbursts and victimization by peers. Consistent with the hypothesis, aggressive victims of peer bullying were at greater risk for witnessing and experiencing hostility and rejection in the family than the three other groups.

PARENTING IN THE CONTEXT OF THE NORMAL AND ABNORMAL: PARENTAL MALTREATMENT AS AN ILLUSTRATION

As a final theme in our coverage of parenting, we illustrate the importance of considering the mutually informative nature of abnormal and normal parenting in formulating developmental models of the effects of parenting on child development. As we have noted, considering the normal and abnormal together is considered by some to be the "essence" of developmental psychopathology (Sroufe, 1990). However, the common focus of parenting research is on normal parenting behaviors in community populations. This is a major limitation of parenting research with regard to understanding the range of adaptive and maladaptive developmental trajectories associated with various parenting practices. Developmental psychopathologists have argued that it is important to refrain from making assumptions about the generalizability or specificity of relations between normal and abnormal developmental contexts. Extended more specifically to parenting research, this means that the similarities and differences in the nature and adaptational value of developmental processes and trajectories across normal and abnormal caregiving contexts cannot be fully explicated without a more comprehensive focus on both healthy and at-risk samples (Cicchetti, 1996). The study of maltreatment provides an excellent example of the problems and challenges of studying samples characterized by abnormal parenting practices, and it is one of the relatively uncommon instances in which parenting practices clearly linked with abnormal child development have received extensive study. As we will see later in Chapter 9, the effects of parental depression on children are another example, but in this instance, multiple family problems, not just parenting, are clearly implicated in children's adjustment problems.

Challenges in Defining Maltreatment

Guarding against making premature conclusions about the applicability of normal processes to the study of abnormal development has been particularly challenging in exploring the effects of parental maltreatment. A primary problem for developmental psychopathologists lies in devising a strategy for exploring the boundaries between parenting in the normal, suboptimal, and abnormal ranges. The trials and tribulations of conceptualizing and defining psychological maltreatment in the 1991 special issue of *Development and Psychopathology* is an excellent illustration of this conundrum (see Barnett, Manly, & Cicchetti, 1991). Social policy, service, and treatment approaches have used deductive, sociological approaches to defining maltreatment by relying heavily on the consensus of society regarding the inappropriate nature of parenting practices (Giovannoni & Becerra, 1979). Conversely, working from an inductive, empirically driven approach, McGee and Wolfe (1991b) proposed that maltreatment should only be defined following the establishment of a predictive relationship between specific quantitative measures of caregiving behavior and children's maladaptive outcomes. Thus, psychological maltreatment would be defined as only those specific parental behaviors that predict negative child outcomes.

However, this approach by itself is of limited use to many developmental psychopathologists for several reasons. First, the narrow empirical focus is at odds with the eclectic, interdisciplinary goals of developmental psychopathology. Developmental psychopathologists replying to this article have thus underscored the importance of integrating the inductive approach with the deductive approach rather than replacing one with another (e.g., Barnett,

Manly, & Cicchetti, 1991; Thompson & Jacobs, 1991). For example, Barnett and colleagues (1991) recommended that empirical findings from developmental and clinical research be used as a way of refining definitions derived from societal standards.

Second, conceptualizing maltreatment as a specific set of parenting behaviors along a continuum may obscure the distinctions between suboptimal parenting and maltreatment. Finding a statistically significant relationship between parenting practices and children's maladjustment cannot in itself be used as an evaluative criterion for classifying acts as maltreatment. Moderate and large sample sizes, for example, can detect significant relationships that are of trivial magnitude from clinical and social policy perspectives. Classifying maltreatment on the basis of the magnitude of relations between a continuous score on a parenting dimension and child outcome is also problematic given our current state of knowledge and psychological tools. The specific difficulty lies in ascertaining the threshold at which parenting becomes problematic enough to warrant the label of maltreatment (Thompson & Jacobs, 1991)—a problem that cannot be fully resolved even with statistical models designed to chart curvilinear effects. Many developmental psychopathologists therefore believe that neither the nosological nor continuum approach to conceptualizing maltreatment is superior. Rather, conceptualizing maltreatment as part of a continuum and as a qualitative threshold requiring a distinct classification are complementary perspectives that usefully inform one another (Barnett, Manly, & Cicchetti, 1991).

Third, the implicit mechanistic assumptions underlying the empirical strategy of defining maltreatment are at odds with the organismic tenets of developmental psychopathology. Recommendations for defining maltreatment involve isolating the effects of a discrete set of parenting behaviors from each other and the larger ecological and developmental context. According to McGee and Wolfe (1991a), ascertaining maltreatment is best approached by examining the specific additive, independent, and interactive effects of specific parenting practices and child characteristics within multiple regression models (i.e., age, intrachild vulnerabilities and protective factors). Although these recommendations are useful in understanding the specific developmental and intrachild moderators of the association between parenting practices and child outcomes, the assumption that the parent–child functioning link is a product of parenting practices that cause child maladjustment is specious. Dynamic transactional models of maltreatment, for example, highlight the role the child plays in also changing caregiving quality over time, and the role that third variables (e.g., neighborhood violence, poor schools, interparental aggression) may play in creating or at least bolstering the coincidence of parenting disturbances and child maladjustment (e.g., Cicchetti & Lynch, 1993; Cicchetti & Toth, 1995). The full complexity of these models cannot be captured within simple regression equations that examine the additive, unique, and interactive effects of caregiving and intrachild variables.

Furthermore, although McGee and Wolfe (1991a, 1991b) recognize that the same parental act can have a different impact on children across different developmental periods, they fail to embrace fully the concept of holism. Thus, despite acknowledging that the same parental behavior may have different meanings at different levels, for example, "isolating a teenager from his peers may be damaging, but doing so to an infant may not be" (p. 10), at the structural level of analysis (i.e., regression models), they ultimately fail to recognize that different developmental levels may alter parts of the measurement model, that is, that the specific acts of parenting may "load onto" or be indicators of different parenting constructs across different developmental periods. Whereas preventing teenagers from interacting with peers may be considered a core index of a larger parental isolation factor, this same act probably plays little or no role in ascertaining the degree of parental isolation in infancy. Thus, the process of operationalizing and tracing the effects of any parenting behavior cannot be conducted in a developmental or ecological vacuum. Models of parenting at both the measurement and structural level (in this case, regression analyses) gain essential meaning from developmental context (Cicchetti & Toth, 1995).

Specifying the Process Dimensions of Maltreatment and Caregiving Quality

Early research programs on maltreatment were commonly geared toward understanding (1) the basic relationship between global measures of maltreatment (e.g., different forms of maltreatment combined into a single category) and child vulnerability and/or (2) the risk incurred to children who experienced a very narrow range of maltreatment experiences (e.g., physical abuse) without consideration of other forms of maltreatment (McGee & Wolfe, 1991a). The results of these studies have clearly shown that children experiencing a wide range of maltreatment experiences, from physical and sexual abuse to neglect and psychological maltreatment, are at risk for developing a number of psychological disturbances, including internalizing symptoms, externalizing problems, impairments in social skills, and disharmony in peer relations (e.g., Ammerman, Cassisi, Hersen, & Van Hasselt, 1986; Cicchetti & Toth, 1995; Egeland, Sroufe, & Erickson, 1983; Hoffman-Plotkin & Twentyman, 1984). As findings on the basic association between maltreatment and child psychopathology continue to accumulate, researchers have now increasingly turned to providing a more comprehensive, detailed portrayal of the context in which maltreatment occurs.

The developmental psychopathology model of maltreatment proposed by Cicchetti and colleagues is particularly valuable as a heuristic for process research and theory development (e.g., see Cicchetti & Lynch, 1993; Cicchetti & Toth, 1995). Within this framework, the degree of risk posed by maltreatment is contingent on several characteristics of the maltreating acts, including form (e.g., physical abuse, neglect, sexual abuse, psychological maltreatment), severity, frequency, duration, and relationship to perpetrator. As one step toward understanding pathways to risk and resilience, this more precise explication of maltreatment characteristics has proven to be useful and informative. Although definitive conclusions about the specificity of effects of different forms of maltreatment await the resolution of inconsistencies in operational definitions of maltreatment, sample characteristics (e.g., control samples), and recruiting procedures (McGee & Wolfe, 1991a), some researchers have reported differential profiles of functioning among children exposed to different maltreatment experiences. For example, illustrating potential specificity in developmental pathways, Egeland, Sroufe, and Erickson (1983) found that (1) neglected children were characterized as lowest in self-esteem, positive affect, and agency; (2) psychologically maltreated children (i.e., psychological unavailable) were characterized by heightened noncompliance and negative emotional tone in school and family contexts; and (3) physically abused children, although similar to psychologically maltreated children in noncompliance and negativity, also appeared to exhibit the greatest dependence on teachers in attempting to cope with the challenges of preschool (see also Manly, Cicchetti, & Barnett, 1994). In addition to serving as a caution against overinterpreting the specificity of outcomes of different maltreatment experiences, additional findings documenting that all maltreatment groups exhibit similar difficulties in impulse control and behavior regulation reflect the importance of understanding equifinality, or why children who appear to have very different family experiences may reach the same endpoint (see also Crittenden, Claussen, & Sugarman, 1994).

However, this greater precision yields only modest or moderate advances in predicting children's risk. Children experiencing the same forms of maltreatment often exhibit a diversity of outcomes. How can we better understand such multifinality in development? Part of the heterogeneity may be due to the operationalization and measurement of maltreatment. Although it is clear that nature conspires in ways that commonly lead children to be exposed to multiple, co-occurring forms of maltreatment, the common practices of (1) targeting a single form of maltreatment and (2) force-classifying children into single, exclusive maltreatment categories fail to capture this holistic organization of maltreatment experiences. Future researchers should consider the promise of employing person-based analyses that are designed to classify individuals into groups on the basis of their profile of experiences with multiple forms of maltreatment (e.g., cluster-analytic techniques) rather than their rank-ordering (or dichotomy of presence–absence) on a single, isolated form of maltreatment.

Even if the scope of the study encompasses a single form of maltreatment such as physical abuse (which is justifiable from the perspective of floating holism), more precise specification of children's developmental pathways hinges, in part, on greater empirical articulation of the various caregiving contexts experienced by children (Trickett, Aber, Carlson, & Cicchetti, 1991). As Diana Baumrind (1995) aptly notes, "The actual childrearing practices and attitudes of abusive parents are seldom if ever examined in depth and using a prospective design" (p. 55). Various parenting styles (e.g., uninvolved parenting in child neglect cases, combinations of uninvolved and authoritarian parenting in child abuse cases) and practices may very well map onto different forms of maltreatment in reliable ways and thus serve as interpersonal mediators in the risk incurred by children of maltreating caregivers. By the same token, since a one-to-one correspondence between maltreatment type and quality of child-rearing contexts is unlikely, it might also be hypothesized that variability in exposure to different parenting styles may moderate the link between maltreatment and child outcomes and, in the process, explain the multifinality of maltreatment. For example, even though many children from physically abusive homes may experience high levels of authoritarian and uninvolved parenting, they may be protected from deleterious effects of maltreatment if the larger child-rearing context is characterized by relatively high levels of authoritativeness.

Richer conceptualizations of maltreatment experiences as multidimensional constructs also raise the possibility that specific characteristics such as form, severity, chronicity, and type of perpetrator may interact in ways that cannot be captured in main effects models. One question pertains to whether the presence of one form of maltreatment may catalyze or synergistically exacerbate the deleterious effects of another form of maltreatment. In addressing this very issue, Wolfe and McGee (1994) found that a significant interaction between physical and psychological abuse reflected that boys were particularly vulnerable to adjustment problems if they reported experiencing high levels of the two forms of maltreatment. Likewise, interactions between severity and frequency of maltreatment are beginning to be identified in the literature (Manly, Cicchetti, & Barnett, 1994). However, rather than reflecting a synergistic effect, the findings suggest that severity of maltreating acts has a detrimental effect on children's development irrespective of the frequency. Frequency only appears to have an impact on children if it occurs in combination with maltreatment acts that are judged to be relatively low or moderate in severity. Thus, in accordance with the principle of equifinality, the interaction suggests that the same maladaptive outcome may be reached by many different experiences, including (1) infrequent severe acts of maltreatment, (2) frequent severe acts of maltreatment, and (3) frequent acts of maltreatment of low to moderate severity.

Weaving Maltreatment Back into the Ecological Web

Maltreatment researchers have long recognized that maltreatment does not occur in a biopsychosocial vacuum. For example, underlying the conventional standard of recruiting a comparison group that is similar to maltreatment groups along relevant demographic and social variables is the acknowledgment that maltreatment is often accompanied by a constellation of other risk factors. Although these designs have been particularly valuable in disaggregating the predictive power or "effects" of maltreatment from the larger web of sociodemographic variables, excessive reliance on this conventional practice may obscure the goal of understanding the larger pattern of organization and holistic experiences within which caregiving is embedded; that is, unpacking maltreatment experiences from the larger context is one strategy of developmental psychopathologists that must be complemented by another strategy, that of examining the interplay between maltreatment and various dimensions of the ecological climate. This latter approach does not treat ecological variables as nuisance variables to be controlled by methodological design or statistical procedure; rather, it regards them as playing a central conceptual role in understanding the diversity of developmental trajectories experienced by children (Okun, Parker, & Levendosky, 1994).

Thus, although links between child maltreatment and risk remain robust even after considering sociodemographic variables, Trickett, Aber, Carlson, and Cicchetti (1991) note that such methodological control techniques fail to capture the complex interplay among maltreatment experiences, socioeconomic status, and subculture. Their specific findings indicate that differences between abusive and nonabusive families on indices of family and child adjustment become progressively weaker or nonexistent at lower socioeconomic levels (see also Okun, Parker, & Levendosky, 1994). Whether this is due to the overriding effects of danger and poverty (Elmer, 1977), greater difficulty identifying and documenting relatively mild abuse cases in higher socioeconomic level homes, or another process, awaits further investigation; but the findings do highlight that the "effects" of physical abuse on the quality of family relationships and child psychopathology may differ vastly across different ecological contexts (Crittenden, Claussen, & Sugarman, 1994). New research programs also point to the value of examining how relations between abuse and family and child functioning may differ across ethnicity and subculture, although it is still too early to provide definitive answers as to the extent and nature of moderating effects (e.g., Crittenden et al., 1994).

Although charting the more specific pathways underlying the diversity of functioning among maltreated children remains an important and relatively neglected task, the emerging consideration of components in the larger transactional model strongly reflects the multiplicity of experiential trails children take in the journey of development. For example, Fergusson and Lynskey (1997) reported that part of the linkage between physical abuse and child psychopathology is the direct result of caustic effects of abuse. Even after considering a number of co-occurring risk factors, adults who reported experiencing greater physical maltreatment as children were at risk for alcohol problems and violence in roles as victims and victimizers. At the same time, it appears that concurrent exposure to family (e.g., family instability, interparental conflict, sexual abuse) and ecological (e.g., poverty) adversity partly accounted for the degree of adjustment difficulties that these physically abused children were experiencing. These findings provide at least some initial support for the contention that the chronicity and quality of caregiving disruptions underlying specific acts or forms of maltreatment may play a central role in explaining children's developmental difficulties (Wolfe & McGee, 1994).

Early models of maltreatment and child psychopathology have also implicitly regarded children's relatedness or positive affiliation with parents as fixed, static protective factors or "inherent" buffers across a wide range of contexts of maltreatment. In fact, we believe that the assumption that parent–child relationship quality as a protective buffer shielding children from the deleterious effects of maltreatment has become so deeply ingrained in the scientific community that it has been treated as an obvious fact. However, the principle of contextual relativism in developmental psychopatholog, which espouses that the adaptive and maladaptive value of any factor or process depends on the context within which it is embedded, warns against such premature assumptions. Toth and Cicchetti (1996), for instance, reported that secure or optimal patterns of relatedness to the mother moderated the relationship between maltreatment and child adjustment in a way that is contrary to conventional models of protective factors as static traits. Although secure or optimal patterns of relatedness have been demonstrated to predict greater psychological adjustment in the nonmaltreated sample, optimal patterns of mother–child relatedness were actually associated with poorer psychological adjustment. While replication using different methods is necessary before drawing firm conclusions, it appears that the same factor that promotes resilience and adjustment in a normative sample operates very differently in an abnormal sample. Consistent with this perspective, Toth and Cicchetti (1996) propose that optimal parent–child relatedness may prompt children to identify with and emulate their maltreating parents' aggressive dispositions.

Developmental Models of Maltreatment Experiences

In reviewing the application of developmental models to the study of child maltreatment, Trickett and McBride-Chang (1995) concluded that "little can be said about developmental effects largely because, as noted earlier, most of the studies were not designed to address developmental questions and no longitudinal study with a long-enough time frame has been conducted" (p. 327). Fortunately, the growing field of developmental psychopathology has made significant headway in remedying this oversight. We briefly highlight how some of the developmental themes championed by developmental psychopathologists have resulted in fruitful directions in understanding when parenting disturbances break the threshold of the "average expectable environment."

"Developmental" Unfolding of Events

The search for processes and conditions that more precisely specify the nature of the link between caregiving contexts and child adjustment in the research reviewed above is also evident in process research on maltreatment. The maltreatment literatures have been particularly interested, for example, in identifying the underlying social, emotional, and cognitive processes that may mediate the link between maltreatment and maladaptive child outcomes (for a comprehensive review, see Cicchetti & Toth, 1995).

Although initial studies in this area have been primarily cross-sectional, they are still developmental in nature because they provide a beginning foundation for understanding the unfolding events that ultimately manifest themselves in the form of child adaptation and maladaptation. For example, supporting the application of social information-processing theory to maltreating samples (Crick & Dodge, 1994), new evidence supports a pathway whereby parental physical abuse increases children's risk for conduct problems by compromising their social information processing of stressful peer situations (i.e., encoding in processing relevant social cues, generation of aggressive reactions) (Dodge, Pettit, Bates, & Valente, 1995). Interpreted theoretically, repeated victimization in abusive relationships with parents may alter children's representations of relationships in a way that makes them hypervigilant to signs of threat in other social contexts. This hypervigilant processing pattern, although adaptive in situations of actual family threat, may fuel children's hostile and aggressive reactions in peer interactions, thereby evoking negative reactions from peers that, in turn, further crystallize their aggressive dispositions.

A complementary direction for delineating the emotional and behavioral mechanisms mediating the effects of maltreatment is also beginning with some notable success. Examining school-age children, Shields, Cicchetti, and Ryan (1994) reported that the relationship between experiential histories with maltreatment and children's difficulty in peer relationships was accounted for, in part, by disruptions in their ability to regulate their behavior. Moving along the life span to adolescence, additional research has found support for a developmental pathway whereby maltreatment experiences predict greater destructive conflict in adolescent girls' romantic relationships, mainly by virtue of their caustic effects on girls' emotion regulation abilities (i.e., angry, hostile dispositions) (Wolfe, Wekerle, Reitzel-Jaffe, & Lefebvre, 1998).

Stage-Salient Frameworks

Comprehending the myriad possible developmental processes that maltreatment may set in motion within children is a very daunting task for researchers. As a guide for the process-oriented study of maltreatment, an increasingly common approach taken in developmental psychopathology is to anchor the study of mechanisms of maltreatment within a model of stage-salient tasks. Resolving developmental tasks poses significant challenges and require considerable resources from children even in optimal contexts. Moreover, the ways in which children negotiate these developmental challenges are thought to be contingent, in part, on the dynamic transaction between the caregiver and child. Thus, given that maltreatment represents a significant perturbation in the caregiving system, the integration of maltreatment in a developmental framework may elucidate the mechanisms underlying maltreatment and the

nature of developmental deviations from normality. Given our detailed overview of stage-salient tasks earlier in the chapter, we selectively illustrate the
utility of this approach (for a more comprehensive account of the interplay between maltreatment and children's negotiation of developmental tasks, see
Cicchetti, 1989; Cicchetti & Toth, 1995).

Forming a secure attachment relationship or enduring, trusting emotional
bond with the caregiver is a key developmental task in infancy that has been
the subject of considerable research by maltreatment researchers. Relative to
sociodemographically matched comparison children, maltreated children have
been shown to be at considerably higher risk for developing insecure attachment relationships (e.g., Carlson, Cicchetti, Barnett, & Braunwald, 1989;
Cicchetti & Toth, 1995; Crittenden, 1992). Further underscoring the value of
examining the entire continuum from abnormal to normal, the study of maltreated children has actually resulted in a more expanded view of the diversity
of different patterns of attachment relationships that may occur in contexts in
which caregiving is not within the bounds of the "average expectable environment." More specifically, whereas attachment research has generally identified three primary attachment patterns, the study of maltreated samples has
also revealed additional patterns of insecure attachment characterized by (1)
disorganization, paralyzing fear, and lack of a coherent strategy for regaining
emotional security; and (2) role reversal or parentification in which the child
assumes the role of the caretaker of the parent (Crittenden & Ainsworth,
1989; see Chapter 6, this volume).

As the attachment relationship emerges and is continually negotiated between parent and child, a new set of developmental tasks focusing on self-
development (Cole & Putnam, 1992), individuation (Macfie et al., 1999),
emotion regulation (Cummings, Hennessy, Rabideau, & Cicchetti, 1994;
Smetana et al., 1999), and social representational models (Toth, Cicchetti,
Macfie, & Emde, 1997) come to the fore during the toddler and preschool periods. Research indicates that maltreatment experiences do in fact predict difficulties in successfully resolving these developmental tasks over and above the
effects of community impoverishment. Consistent with this notion, the self
systems of maltreated toddlers and preschoolers are characterized by additional disruptions in the development of an autonomous self and the self in relational context, as evidenced by greater representations and enactments of
role reversal in parent–child relations (Crittenden & DiLalla, 1988; Macfie et al.,
1999), diminished use of internal-state words reflecting physiological and emotional need states (Beeghly & Cicchetti, 1994), exaggerated (perhaps in a defen-
sive way) self-appraisals of competence (Vondra, Barnett, & Cicchetti, 1989),
and negative representations of the self and caregiver (see Toth et al., 1997).

Maltreated children continue to exhibit difficulties in key developmental
tasks in middle childhood, including the development of peer relationships,
friendship formation, and school adjustment. Not only do maltreated children
evidence more frequent experiences with peer rejection and isolation (Dodge,
Pettit, & Bates, 1994b), and more disengaged, uncooperative play with peers
(Shields, Cicchetti, & Ryan, 1994), but their high rates of school disciplinary

referrals and suspensions, truancy, poor academic performance, and difficulties with authority figures clearly reflect substantial difficulties adjusting to school settings (e.g., Cicchetti, Toth, & Hennessy, 1989; Crittenden, Claussen, & Sugarman, 1994; Eckenrode, Laird, & Doris, 1993; Toth & Cicchetti, 1996).

Difficulties adjusting to school settings commonly persist or escalate as maltreated children progress through adolescence. Teachers, for example, report that maltreated adolescents continue to engage in high levels of aggression and harassment in school settings. As psychological characteristics of friends become increasingly prominent features of friendship formation and maintenance, maltreated adolescents report difficulties establishing close, trusting relationships with friends (Wolfe, Wekerle, Reitzel-Jaffe, & Lefebvre, 1998). Adolescents not only must continue to negotiate these earlier developmental tasks, but they must also increasingly cope with resolving emergent tasks such as the establishment of romantic relationships, autonomy, and plans toward becoming productive, self-sufficient members of society (e.g., identity formation, occupational plans). Although little is known about the development of maltreated adolescents (Crittenden, 1995), the available evidence does suggest that they have considerable difficulties with these developmental tasks. For example, maltreated adolescents report being more frequent victims and perpetrators of verbal and physical abuse in romantic relationships than nonmaltreated youth (Wekerle & Wolfe, 1998; Wolfe, Wekerle, Reitzel-Jaffe, & Lefebvre, 1998). Tentative cross-sectional evidence indicating that maltreated children display elevated aggressive–disruptive problems as early as infancy and toddlerhood through adolescence further suggests that maltreatment may be accompanied by a stable, life-course persistent pattern of antisocial conduct (Moffitt, 1993a) or an orientation toward "moving against the world" that ultimately deters adolescents from achieving tasks relevant to becoming productive members of society (Dodge, Pettit, Bates, & Valente, 1995; Erickson, Egeland, & Pianta, 1989; Wolfe & McGee, 1994). More firm conclusions about maltreated children's vulnerability for life-course-persistent antisocial behavior await longitudinal designs that track the level and slope of aggressive behavior across childhood and adolescence.

Developmental Pathways and Trajectories

Applying stage-salient frameworks to the study of maltreatment is useful not only in cataloging the manifestation of psychosocial difficulties across development, but also as a way of understanding how maltreatment and earlier histories of negotiating developmental tasks may lay the foundation for children's success in resolving subsequent developmental tasks and achieving adaptive developmental outcomes. This may occur through the operation of two primary developmental pathways.

In the first "cascading" pathway, maltreatment experiences may prompt an unfolding series of failures to resolve successfully central developmental tasks that, in turn, further compromise the probability of resolving future developmental tasks. Consistent with the tenets of developmental psychopathology, this model makes two assumptions: (1) The experience of maltreatment will be especially likely to jeopardize performance in stage-salient domains of functioning (e.g., attachment in infancy, representational models in toddlerhood), and (2) the skills and resources developed from successfully resolving earlier developmental tasks are conceptualized as important tools for adaptively coping with and resolving subsequent developmental challenges. In support of this model, Shields and colleagues (1994) reported that the persistent difficulties with earlier, stage-salient tasks into middle and late childhood (i.e., self-regulation in early childhood) mediated or accounted for the relationship between maltreatment and difficulties with current developmental tasks centering on the establishment of harmonious peer relationships. Although this study provides substantial support for a cascading developmental model, the move to longitudinal designs may afford an even more convincing demonstration of the developmentally ordered pathways from maltreatment to later functioning. Rogosch, Cicchetti, and Aber (1995) reported that the prospective relationship between maltreatment in early childhood and poor peer competence around middle childhood (e.g., peer isolation, low acceptance) is mediated by children's difficulties in resolving two early childhood tasks relevant to emotion and self-regulation (i.e., cognitive control functioning, negative affect understanding) around their transition into elementary school (for another example of a developmentally guided mediational model, see Wolfe, Wekerle, Reitzel-Jaffe, & Lefebvre, 1998).

In the second "potentiating" pathway, children's history of resolving developmental tasks may moderate the link between maltreatment and the subsequent resolution of critical tasks. Maltreatment may thus have particularly toxic effects on children's developmental competence when they have failed to resolve earlier stage-salient tasks. For example, Beeghly and Cicchetti (1994) hypothesized that maltreatment will have especially toxic consequences on toddlers' development of internal-state language when they have formed insecure attachments with their caregivers. The underlying theoretical premise is that disturbances in the development of representational models of emotional relationships are conceptualized as natural outgrowths of insecure attachments that serve to potentiate difficulties in developing internal-state language in the emotionally labile and restrictive climates of maltreating families. In support of the model, toddlers' internal-state language ability is particularly compromised when maltreatment is coupled with insecure parent–child attachment.

While systematic research on the developmental sequelae of maltreatment pathways is only beginning, even less is known about the interrelationship between these socialization pathways and children's developmental slopes and trajectories of adjustment. Without rigorous prospective designs that can capture dynamic change in maltreatment, context, and developmental outcomes (e.g., autoregressive and cross-lagged models), the developmental processes underlying the static associations will remain a mystery. For example, although Lynch and Cicchetti (1998a) reported that prior maltreatment and exposure to community violence predicted adjustment problems 1 year later, more rigorous prospective analyses revealed that only prior maltreatment predicted increases in maladjustment over the subsequent year (i.e., after statistically controlling for prior maladjustment). Furthermore, children's prior externalizing behavior (time 1) predicted increases in exposure to community violence over the subsequent year, after controlling for prior exposure to community violence. Thus, these findings run directly counter to social mold models that specify community violence as a key etiological factor in the development of psychopathology. Rather, consistent with transactional models of developmental psychopathology, the results suggest that children with behavior problems may play an active role in perpetuating or increasing their exposure to community violence by evoking aggressive reactions from others, electing to inhabit violent niches, or both.

Charting the relationship between maltreatment and developmental trajectories will require even more assessments of children's adjustment over time (i.e., three or more assessments). According to Dodge, Pettit, and Bates (1994a), the developmental trajectories of maltreatment may take at least three shapes (see Figure 7.4). First, in the transient developmental model, maltreatment is a significant stressor that has deleterious effects on children's adjustment in the short term, but with time, children's self-righting tendencies and active use of psychological and social resources offer protection, allowing them to reclaim a healthy developmental trajectory. Second, in the enduring developmental model, the experience of maltreatment alters children in a way that has immediate, enduring, and stable effects on their adjustment. Third, in a potentiating developmental model, maltreatment poses for children an immediate risk that becomes progressively worse over time, resulting in increasingly divergent developmental trajectories for maltreated and nonmaltreated children. Supporting the potentiating model, the findings from Dodge and colleagues study indicated that the prior maltreatment significantly predicts impairments in peer relations in early elementary school that continue to intensify throughout childhood. Although follow-up studies designed to identify underlying developmental processes are needed, the results are consistent with two central notions in developmental psychopathology. First, within a stage-salient framework, maltreatment may compromise the resolution of developmental tasks, which, in turn, further increases the probability of difficulties with subsequent critical tasks and, ultimately, susceptibility to psychopathology and impaired developmental competence. Second, illustrating the conceptualization of an active child, the negative internal working models, ineffective coping styles, and maladaptive behavioral dispositions (e.g., aggression) that may develop, in part, from maltreatment experiences may guide children actively to select out similarly aggressive peers and, at the same time, evoke rejection by normal peers. Affiliation with deviant peers in the broader context of peer rejection may serve further to intensify aggressive tendencies, intrapersonal distress (e.g., alienation, disengagement, depression), and a negative peer reputation (Dodge et al., 1994a).

Model 1. Transient developmental model of maltreatment

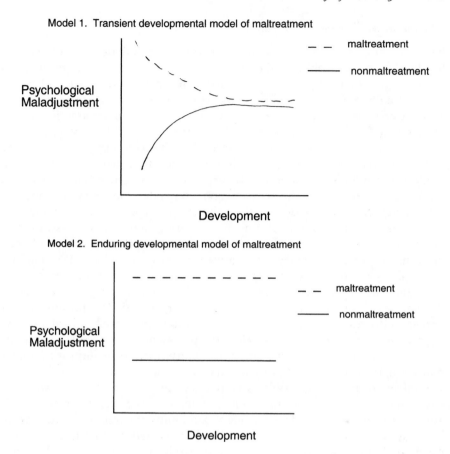

Model 2. Enduring developmental model of maltreatment

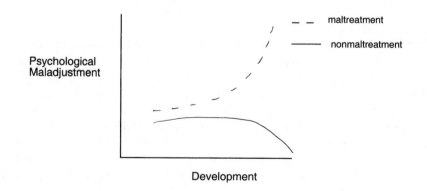

Model 3. Potentiating developmental model of maltreatment

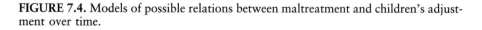

FIGURE 7.4. Models of possible relations between maltreatment and children's adjustment over time.

Intergenerational Transmission of Parenting

Earlier theories on the origins of maltreatment often took the form of main effect models in which childhood experiences of maltreatment were regarded as being the predominant, overpowering force that drove individuals to become maltreating parents (e.g., Steele, 1976). At the other extreme, other researchers have concluded that the intergenerational transmission of parenting disturbances is a "myth to be placed aside" (Kaufman & Zigler, 1989, p. 135). Which view is correct? Most developmental psychopathologists eschew either of these extreme views in favor of the conclusion that there appears to be a modest transmission of parenting disturbances across generations. However, the key to understanding this transmission from a developmental psychopathology perspective lies not only in ascertaining the magnitude of effect, but also in focusing on answers to questions that specify context and process. Central questions include the following: (1) For whom and under what conditions does the risk of experiencing maltreatment carry over and affect an individual's role as a parent? Alternatively, (2) can we identify the people and conditions that are most likely to break the cycle of maltreatment? (3) Why or through what specific channels does this intergenerational transmission of parenting distress operate? The first two questions are geared toward identifying the intrapersonal (e.g., personality, temperament, coping styles) and interpersonal (e.g., social support, family instability, marital quality) moderators that strengthen (i.e., potentiating factors) or weaken (i.e., protective factors) the linkage of parenting problems across generations. The final question focuses on the complementary task of identifying the processes that play a mediating role in maintaining developmental continuity of parenting disturbances. Thus, these are the directions and avenues indicated by the developmental psychopathology perspective for future research on understanding the intergenerational transmission of parenting practices associated with maltreatment.

CONCLUSION

A salient theme in our review of parenting from a developmental psychopathology perspective is the need for broader contextual models of parenting as an influence on child development. Moreover, it is evident that certain additional aspects of parental behavior in families (e.g., the quality of marital relations or the lack thereof), in particular, merit consideration as dimensions of parenting (i.e., significant parental influences on children within families). Thus, in addition to supporting broader, familywide models of influences on children, Chapters 8 and 9 are also relevant to future directions in the conceptualization of parenting as a factor in children's development in families.

Children and the Marital Subsystem

Models of family and child development have focused on parent–child relationships. While these relationships are primary influences on development, it is increasingly apparent that other family factors also affect children's adjustment in families (Belsky, 1984; see Figure II.1). Research over the past two decades provides substantial support for the proposition that interparental relations have considerable influence on children's development in families. Given their relevance for conceptualization of family influences on children, the issues raised by a developmental psychopathology approach to the study of families and children merits consideration at the outset.

The study of marital functioning and child development provides striking examples of the need for more complex models of relations between human development and contexts of development provided by the developmental psychopathology approach. For example, scores of studies, with the earliest published in the 1920s and 1930s (e.g., Towle, 1931; Watson, 1925), document relations between marital discord and child adjustment (Emery, 1982; Grych & Fincham, 1990). Dozens of studies have also documented that children are distressed by exposure to marital conflict. A summary of these studies is shown in Table 8.1, indicating that there is ample evidence based upon carefully controlled studies to document the idea that exposure to adults' anger and conflict is disturbing to children.

Research based on parents' reports of children's reactions to marital conflict in the home also documents these associations. The following example is based upon a mother's report of the reactions of a 20-month-old child.

"I was very upset about, well, I still had the flu virus and I wasn't feeling very well. And the house was a shambles, where the children had been running and

TABLE 8.1. Studies Showing Exposure to Marital Conflict Is Distressing for Children

Study	Sample	Comparison	Response
	Studies of behavioral emotional responding		
Cummings, Zahn-Waxler, and Radke-Yarrow (1981)	24 children between 10 and 20 months of age; behavior in the home reported over a period of 9 months	Naturally occurring anger > naturally occurring affection	Distress, no attention and response
Cummings, Iannotti, and Zahn-Waxler (1985)	90 2-year-olds	Adults' anger > adults' positive emotions	Distress
Cummings (1987)	85 5-year-olds	Adults' anger > adults' positive emotions	Negative emotions, positive emotions, preoccupation
El-Sheikh, Cummings, and Goetsch (1989)	34 4- to 5-year-olds	Adults' anger > adults' positive emotions	Freezing, facial distress, postural distress, verbal concern, anger, smiling, preoccupation
Klaczynski and Cummings (1989)	40 first- to third-grade boys	Adults' anger > adults' positive emotions	Facial distress, postural distress, freezing
	Studies of self-reported emotions		
Cummings, Vogel, Cummings, and El-Sheikh (1989)	121 4- to 9-year-olds	Hostile verbal and nonverbal anger all > friendly interactions	Negative emotional responses (anger, fear, sadness)
Ballard and Cummings (1990)	35 6- to 10-year-olds	Verbal, indirect nonverbal, destructive, and aggressive anger all > friendly interactions	Anger, distress
Cummings, Ballard, El-Sheikh, and Lake (1991)	98 5- and 19-year-olds	Unresolved anger partially resolved anger > friendly interactions	Anger, sadness, fear
Cummings, Ballard, and El-Sheikh (1992)	60 9- and 19-year-olds	Hostile verbal and nonverbal anger all > friendly interactions	Negative emotional responses (anger, fear, sadness)

Note. From Cummings and Zahn-Waxler (1992). Copyright 1992 by Springer-Verlag. Adapted by permission.

pulling out toys, and the dishes had not been done, and there were clothes on the floor (they played mommies). So the house was in bad shape. So I put Clara to bed and I made Tommy go to his room to rest. And then I ran down to the kitchen to put away some of the things that were out of the refrigerator in there, and things that would spoil. And Dick was in the kitchen and I yelled at him, 'I don't care if this house stays a mess forever, I am not picking up another damn thing.' And I screamed to the top of my lungs, I was mad and I was furious. . . . And in a squeaky voice . . . I heard Clara say, 'Mommy, shut up.' She said this about three times. The whole incident didn't last longer than 15 seconds." (Cummings, Zahn-Waxler, & Radke-Yarrow, 1981, p. 1276)

However, matters are far less clear-cut than simply that the occurrence of marital discord directly affects children's adjustment. As we will see, research on the effects of children's exposure to marital conflict aptly demonstrates the importance of multidimensional assessment of both interparental conflict and children's reactions to discord. For example, not all forms of marital conflict are distressing for children to observe as bystanders. Whereas conflicts that include physical aggression between the parents are highly disturbing to children, those that are fully resolved, or constructive, may not be distressing at all (Cummings, Ballard, El-Sheikh, & Lake, 1991; Jenkins & Smith, 1991). As a reflection of the relevance of holism to the assessment of children's reactions, research indicates that children's reactions are indicated by emotional, cognitive, social, and even physiological responding (El-Sheikh, Cummings, & Goetsch, 1989; Katz & Gottman, 1995a), but no one response dimension in isolation is necessarily a reliable index of the impact of marital conflict. Thus, some children do not show distress behaviorally when faced with marital conflict but report covert feelings of anger or distress. Other children even smile or laugh during conflicts, then later act out aggressively toward peers, suggesting that the exposure induced considerable negative emotional arousal (Cummings, 1987).

However, it has clearly been shown that one must look beyond direct relations between exposure to marital conflict and children's reactions to understand the effects of these events on children within families. This illustrates even further the value of a holistic perspective. In particular, parenting practices are affected by high marital conflict, with parents from conflictual marriages more likely to evidence lax or inconsistent discipline, hostility, emotional unavailability or unresponsivity toward children, or other parenting deficits (Erel & Burman, 1995). Moreover, the emotional relationship or attachment between parents and children may be undermined by high marital conflict, with children from conflictual homes more likely to develop insecure attachments (Davies & Cummings, 1994). Interestingly, a recent meta-analysis on relations between marital discord, parenting, and child adjustment suggested that good parent–child relations do *not* moderate the effects of high marital conflict on children; that is, a buffering hypothesis, despite its appeal (Emery, 1982), failed to find support in an important meta-analysis (Erel & Burman, 1995) of the substantial literature in this area.

There is also evidence for the importance of the active organism assumption; that is, characteristics of individual children are factors in outcomes resulting from marital discord. Thus, boys and girls may react quite differently to conflict (Cummings, Iannotti, & Zahn-Waxler, 1985), and these reactions may be mediated by quite different processes of responding to these events (e.g., threat, self-blame; Cummings, Davies, & Simpson, 1994; Grych, Seid, &

Fincham, 1992; Kerig, 1997). As another example of the relevance of individual child characteristics, children who show aggression as a personality characteristic are more prone to react to conflict exposure with emotional arousal (Klaczynski & Cummings, 1989) and aggressivity (Cummings et al., 1985) than children who are less aggressive.

Another fundamental assumption of developmental psychopathology, the principle of directionality, is illustrated by the repeated finding that children are sensitized by repeated exposure to high marital conflict. Thus, children repeatedly exposed to intense marital conflict are more emotionally (e.g., angry, distressed) and behaviorally (aggressive, prone to mediate in parental disputes) reactive to these events and report cognitive reactions indicative of greater threat and self-blame (Cummings, 1994). Heightened reactivity to conflict, in turn, has been related to increased risk for adjustment problems in children. Accordingly, there is evidence for a cumulative effect of exposure to marital conflict on children, which is hypothesized to set in motion more general processes that underlie the greater risk for adjustment problems in children from these home environments (i.e., a greater sense of emotional insecurity about family functioning; Davies & Cummings, 1994). Over time, it is presumed that these cumulative effects influence pathways and trajectories of development, including risk for psychopathology and specific forms of psychopathology.

There also is evidence that the broader family environment moderates the effects of marital conflict on children, further illustrating a holistic perspective on risk factors and children's adjustment. Notably, the risk for adjustment problems associated with marital conflict may vary as a function of parental adjustment, quality of interparental attachments, and family emotional climate, including emotional expressiveness. Socioeconomic and other family factors may also play a role, although these issues have only begun to be explored.

Finally, if we are to agree with Sroufe (1990) that considering the abnormal and normal together is the "essence" of developmental psychopathology, then the study of marital conflict is inherently a good fit; that is, marital conflict is, at the same time, normal and abnormal. It is normal in the sense that it is inevitable, taking place in virtually all marriages, and by no means necessarily dysfunctional or problematic. In fact, the avoidance of important marital and family issues may be far more problematic than their discussion (Gottman, 1994). Marital discussion of significant and real areas of disagreement, which qualifies it as a "conflict" event by most definitions (Shantz, 1987), can be beneficial, helpful, and even necessary, with good outcomes for both parents and children. On the other hand, some forms of conflict are caustic for marriages, poisonous for children, and a major source of emotional and adjustment problems for parents and children alike. Thus, it is important to study all forms of conflict in relation to each other, and to examine the outcomes of the many ways that families handle disagreements to determine the forms are ultimately constructive and "normal," and those that are destructive and "abnormal."

We provide a template from a developmental psychopathology perspective for the matters to be considered in much greater depth as the chapter unfolds. As an introduction, we present a topical overview of what is to come. To stress the importance of these issues for understanding children's normal and psychopathological development, we briefly examine general relations between marital functioning and child adjustment, with a focus on marital conflict, which has been most closely linked with children's adjustment problems. Highlighting the importance of studying the normal and abnormal together, we consider evidence suggesting that the effects of marital conflict vary as a function of the risk status of families and children; thus, risk status is a moderator of the effects of marital conflict on children (see Chapter 5).

Next, we introduce a developmental psychopathology framework for understanding children's development as a function of marital conflict and discuss a variety of pathways through which marital conflicts affect children, examining direct effects of marital conflict on children, including identification of the dimensions of marital conflict associated with risk and vulnerability, and protection and compensation. We then consider indirect effects, that is, effects due to the impact of marital conflict on parenting and family functioning, then examine important moderators of effects (e.g., parental psychopathology, children's gender). Consistent with a holistic emphasis on understanding patterns and processes at an overall level of analysis, we review theoretical models that serve to unify the study of mediating and moderating processes associated with marital conflict. This discussion focuses on the "emotional security hypothesis" as an example of a model that has received empirical support. Finally, we look at a relatively new area for research, that is, research concerning pathways of development associated with marital conflict, and briefly outline future directions. Consistent with the notion that the developmental psychopathology tradition and corresponding research on childhood disorders are only beginning to emerge, we see that the parameters defining *comprehensive* models of factors linking marital conflict to children's adjustment are only beginning to be articulated. Throughout, we note key principles and issues from the developmental psychopathology perspective as they relate to understanding the impact of marital conflict on children.

MARITAL CONFLICT AND THE DEVELOPMENT OF PSYCHOPATHOLOGY IN CHILDREN

Positive marital relations form a powerful foundation for healthy family functioning. The importance of the support and positive foundation for optimal parenting and family functioning that is provided by healthy, happy, intact marriages merits emphasis at the outset. Thus, marital satisfaction is linked with secure parent–child attachment and with positive father–child and mother–child relationships (Cummings & O'Reilly, 1997). Recent research suggests that secure interspousal relations compensate when marital partners have had insecure attachments to their own parents in childhood, and, as a consequence, foster the development of secure attachments with their own children (Colin, 1996). There are also numerous correlates of intact marital relations (e.g., more optimal parenting practices) that serve to foster the healthy socioemotional development of children.

On the other hand, conflict-ridden marital relations have been consistently linked with children's adjustment problems, which makes such behaviors immediately relevant to developmental psychopathology models for children's development in families. As we have noted, support for the association between marital conflict and child adjustment has been consistent over the years (Baruch & Wilcox, 1944; Gassner & Murray, 1969; Jouriles, Bourg, & Farris, 1991; Porter & O'Leary, 1980; Rutter, 1970) and is also reported cross-culturally (Lindahl & Malik, 1999) (extensive reviews are provided by Cummings & Davies, 1994a; Grych & Fincham, 1990). However, early research simply established relations between general marital adjustment and adjustment problems in children. The findings did not necessarily implicate marital conflict per se as the causal agent, or clarify the nature of the processes involved. Other aspects of dysfunctional marriages also might contribute to adjustment problems in children, for example, partners' unhappiness with each other or the absence of intimate communication between them (Jouriles, Bourg, & Farris, 1991). Recent work, however, identifies marital conflict as a particularly important aspect of marital functioning with regard to children's development. First, marital conflict has been shown to be typical of distressed marriages. Second, it has been found to be a better predictor of a wide range of children's problems than general marital distress. Finally, marital conflict is more closely associated with children's problems than other individual aspects of distressed marriages (Cummings & Davies, 1994a).

Thus, the notion that "problem" marriages increase the likelihood of "problem" children is thus certainly not new. However, recent work suggests that the way parents handle their differences or conflicts is related to children's risk for psychopathology. As a consequence, research is increasingly concerned with discriminating between constructive and destructive interparental conflict styles from the perspective of the children, on the assumption that understanding such a distinction holds a key to predicting positive and negative outcomes for children due to the quality of interparental relations (Davies & Cummings, 1998). Adult-oriented research on marital quality and trajectories of marital relations over time have shown the importance of differentiating between constructive and destructive marital conflict styles, both for the purposes of scientific explanation and as a foundation for more effective therapeutic interventions (Gottman, 1994; Notarius & Markman, 1993). Consequently, reflecting these emphases in the literature, this chapter carefully examines children's vulnerability or protection due to different ways in which parents handle their differences. Notably, consistent with the view that the normal and abnormal need to be studied together, recent work suggests that when marital conflict is resolved positively, children learn valuable lessons about handling their own inevitable conflicts that result in more adaptive social conflict resolution strategies with peers and others; that is, conflict can have a positive, as opposed to simply a non-negative, outcome (Beach, 1995; Davies, 1995). On the other hand, children's exposure to interparental hostility and violence is a significant source of adversity and contributes to their risk for psychopathology (Holden, Stein, Ritchie, Harris, & Jouriles, 1998). Oddly, despite the evidence on the association between interspousal violence and adjustment problems in children, this was not widely recognized until recently. Accordingly, Jaffe, Wolfe, and Wilson (1990) noted in *Children of Battered Women* that "it was not until the past decade that family discord and spousal violence reached center stage as possible predeterminants of developmental psychopathology" (p. 33).

Relations between marital conflict and children's adjustment problems, often reported in nonclinical samples, are even more robust predictors of childhood disorders in clinical samples, particularly when there is marital violence (Jouriles, Bourg, & Farris, 1991); that is, consistent with the notion that process relations are best illustrated by examining the normal and abnormal together, more powerful effects of marital conflict on children are observed in family environments that are also otherwise at-risk. While mild to moderate relations between marital conflict and child adjustment are found in studies of normal community samples, moderate to strong relations are reported when at-risk samples (e.g., violent marriages) are examined (Fincham & Osborne, 1993; Wolfe, Jaffe, Wilson, & Zak, 1985). Thus, marital conflict is reported as a highly significant factor in children's adjustment in families with parental divorce (Amato & Keith, 1991; Emery, 1988, 1994; Hetherington et al., 1992), parental psychopathology, especially depression (Downey & Coyne, 1990), alcoholism (El-Sheikh & Cummings, 1997; West & Prinz, 1987), and sexual and physical abuse (Browne & Finkelhor, 1986; Jouriles, Barling, & O'Leary, 1987). Thus, different pictures emerge with regard to the extent of relations between marital conflict and child adjustment as a function of the relative normality of family environments, implicating the broader family environment as significant to the effects associated with high marital conflict. Accordingly, the magnitude of relations between marital conflict and child adjustment is moderated by the overall adaptiveness and level of resources that characterize the family environment.

Consistent with the point that healthy interparental relations form a strong foundation for family functioning and child development, the absence of marital relations can present considerably greater problems. A number of factors may account for this, including a severe lack of socioemotional and financial supports for the custodial parent and children; fewer consistent, close adult–child attachment figures for children; reduced opportunities for parental warmth and supervision, greater stress on the remaining parent; and reduced safety and educational/societal resources associated with conditions of lower socioeconomic status (McLanahan & Sandefur, 1994). However, the absence of a marital partner should not be understood to mean that children in single-parent families are not exposed to interadult anger and conflict, or violence, for that matter, in their socioemotional environment. Other adult partners who do not become spouses, relatives, or other adults in the context of unstable family situations may each serve to continue or increase the level of conflict and violence in the child's environment. Moreover, conflict may continue, or worsen, with ex-spouses or ex-partners, despite the absence of current, or even past, formal and legal relations (Wallerstein & Blakslee, 1989).

While marital conflict has traditionally been associated with children's risk for aggressiveness, conduct disorder, and other "externalizing" problems, in fact, it has repeatedly been linked with a variety of other disturbances in children, including behavioral and emotional disturbances, social and interpersonal problems, and school problems (Cummings & Davies, 1994a). In fact, recent research relying on methodologies that are more sensitive to children's covert as well as overt processes of adjustment suggests that marital conflict may be more closely linked with internalizing problems of anxiety, sadness, and insecurity than with "acting-out" disorders per se. In other words, the impact of marital conflict is pervasive rather than specific to any particular disorder, suggesting, again, the importance of broadband or holistic assessments of the effects of these family processes.

On the other hand, it is important to bear in mind that many other factors in families affect children's development besides marital conflict. Furthermore, children are active contributors to their own development and may be quite resilient even in the face of considerable adversity, including extreme marital discord and violence. Relatedly, consistent with a developmental psychopathology perspective and advancing understanding of pathways of development, the children who do not develop disorders in highly adverse circumstances are just as interesting as those who do. Currently, the emphasis is on the study of the psychopathological outcomes that occur in these homes, but it is important also to pay attention to children who do not develop disorders.

A FRAMEWORK FOR A PROCESS-ORIENTED PERSPECTIVE OF THE IMPACT OF MARITAL CONFLICT ON CHILDREN'S ADJUSTMENT

As we saw in Chapter 2, a hallmark of the developmental psychopathology approach is a focus on the processes that account for relations between predictors and outcome variables. A framework that reflects the complexity of family processes and factors associated with the effects of marital conflict on children is presented in Figure 8.1, which makes a distinction between constructive and destructive marital relations. Marital relations are portrayed as having not only direct effects on children's psychological functioning but also indirect effects mediated by effects on parenting. Psychological functioning (i.e., emotional, social, behavioral, cognitive, physiological reactions) is hy-

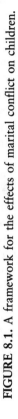

FIGURE 8.1. A framework for the effects of marital conflict on children.

259

pothesized as mediating children's adjustment, with marital conflict processes either increasing vulnerability or competence. Moderator variables are hypothesized to include family context (e.g., parental adjustment, family emotional climate, socioeconomic scale, and other family factors), and child characteristics (e.g., gender, personality, or temperament). With regard to specific mediating processes of psychological adjustment, children's sense of emotional security is represented as one significant class of psychological processes likely to be affected by marital conflict, either directly, due to exposure to marital conflict, or indirectly, due to the effects of marital conflict on parenting practices. In Figure 8.1, the relevance of pathways of development is signified by the notation "development over time."

The framework in Figure 8.1 thus places emphasis on studying specific contexts of exposure to marital conflict and its effects on the family and individual differences between children in their reactions to it, including their histories of exposure and the multidimensional nature of coping processes, which are central, as is the impact of marital conflict on changes in the family system's overall level of functioning. The intent is to capture a holistic perspective on marital relations, family functioning, and child development. Recent findings in the literature on marital relations and child development have served to underscore the need for a familywide perspective on influences on children's development in families, rather than a focus on any one subsystem (e.g., parent–child) (Emery, Fincham, & Cummings, 1992). Nonetheless, even this relatively complex model does not account for all possible pathways of effect. For example, marital conflict may also have effects on children's relationships with siblings, with implications for processes of adaptation and maladaptation over time. Thus, Stocker and Youngblade (1999) reported that marital conflict is associated with problematic sibling relationships, and that the link between marital conflict and sibling rivalry is mediated by children's self-blame for interparental conflicts.

The model thus provides a basis for conceptualizing multiple pathways of effect associated with marital conflict and incorporates other forms of child and family adversity. Consistent with a developmental psychopathology perspective, emphases are placed on dynamic processes of interaction between multiple intra- and extraorganismic factors, as contrasted with traditional, relatively static notions of associations between relatively global characterizations of marital discord and child outcomes. The study of process is assumed to require the examination of multiple domains and responses (e.g., cognitive, emotional, physiological) and also effects that emerge over time (i.e., "sleeper" effects). For example, with regard to "sleeper effects," a young child exposed to high marital conflict may act as a caretaker for the parents and appear to be functioning well. However, these undue burdens on the child may contribute to the development of problems that emerge much later in development, that is, "sleeper effects," as illustrated in the vignette in Chapter 2.

DIRECT EFFECTS OF EXPOSURE TO MARITAL CONFLICT:
DIMENSIONS OF MARITAL CONFLICT ASSOCIATED WITH
RISK VERSUS PROTECTION

The effects of exposure to marital conflict on children depend a great deal on precisely how marital conflict is expressed. Marital conflict is normal, even inevitable. Thus, the issue is not whether marital conflict occurs, but how it occurs. Moreover, it is clear that (a) children react to the perceived meaning of conflicts for themselves and their families, not the occurrence, or even the form of the conflict; (b) the meaning is personal and emotional, evident in children's cognitive appraisals, emotional reactions, and coping behaviors; and (c) historical as well as current experience with marital conflict influences reactions.

Moreover, current theory and research suggest that children's stress and coping reactions provide a valuable window into the meaning of marital conflict from their perspective and also reflect broader patterns of response that mediate development (Cummings & Cummings, 1988; Emery, 1989; Davies & Cummings, 1994, 1998; Grych & Fincham, 1990); that is, marital conflict induces powerful emotional, cognitive, and behavioral responses in bystanding children (Cummings & Davies, 1994a). Correlational studies have long indicated that children's stress and coping responses are related to their marital conflict history on the one hand, and their risk for adjustment problems on the other (e.g., Cummings & Davies, 1994a; Laumakis, Margolin, & John, 1998; Margolin, Christensen, & John, 1996). Empirical support for mediational models, albeit limited in the measurement of mediating processes, is now reported (e.g., Davies & Cummings, 1998; Harold & Conger, 1997; Harold, Fincham, Osborne, & Conger, 1997). Moreover, recent theory provides a rich conceptual foundation for mediational and moderational models (e.g., Cummings & Davies, 1996; Davies & Cummings, 1994; Emery, 1992; Grych & Fincham, 1990). Thus, there is evidence that children's stress and coping reactions reflect dynamic, process-level mediators of their adjustment over time.

Recent research is beginning to clarify the distinction between constructive and destructive marital conflict styles from the children's perspective. The former class of marital conflict styles might be considered protective or compensatory in terms of their effects on children and family functioning, whereas the latter can be regarded as increasing children's risk for adjustment problems. In the absence of long-term prospective studies and comprehensive, rigorous assessments of critical variables, any conclusions about distinctions between constructive and destructive conflict must be regarded as tentative. Nonetheless, certain tentative conclusions are suggested by current research.

Making distinctions between contexts of development that contribute to the emergence of children's problems versus those elements that foster more positive outcomes is consistent with the notion that contexts of development need to be carefully defined and, when relevant, desegregated into their constituent parts (e.g., Boyce et al., 1998). This issue is particularly pertinent to the case of marital conflict because of the quite different effects on children depending upon how marital conflict is expressed. Thus, some forms of conflict expression appear to increase children's risk for adjustment problems, whereas other forms may be benign and even teach children valuable lessons about how to handle their own conflict. A reason for focusing on this topic is that understanding the distinction between constructive and destructive marital conflict behaviors can provide a basis for intervention in marital and family problems and also serve as an informed basis for the prevention of the development of problems, as well as full-blown psychopathology, in children.

As we will see later in this volume, prevention is an important direction within the developmental psychopathology tradition. Consistent with the pathways model of development outlined in Chapter 4, research must delineate those specific risk factors for children that predict the later development of problems, before they become severe enough to merit clinical diagnoses. Such models also support clinical or preventive interventions that are instituted before children develop serious problems and are aimed at ameliorating children's problems before they become chronic and severe, and, therefore, more resistant to treatment. We first consider the forms of marital conflict that appear to be associated with increased risk for maladjustment in children.

Physical Aggression or Violence

There is considerable evidence that physical violence in marital disputes is highly distressing to children observing such behaviors and increases their risk for adjustment problems (Emery, 1989). In analogue studies, children report that they perceive conflicts involving aggression as more negative, and they describe more negative emotional reactions to them (e.g., Cummings, Pellegrini, Notarius, & Cummings, 1989). Of course, analogue research conducted in the laboratory, as is the case for all experimental studies, leaves questions about whether the results generalize to other contexts. However, this finding has also received support based upon parental reports of children's reactions in the home (Cummings, Zahn-Waxler, & Radke-Yarrow, 1981). The pattern of results indicates that physical violence is among the most disturbing forms of marital interaction for children, and the form most clearly linked with their adjustment problems. However, other forms of aggression are also disturbing to children and related to adjustment problems, as is interparental violence. Thus, Ballard and Cummings (1990) reported that children react as negatively to analogue presentations of parental aggression toward objects as to inter-partner aggression. In addition, Jouriles, McDonald, and Norwood (1996) found that other forms of marital aggression (e.g., insulting or swearing at the partner; throwing, smashing, or kicking something; threatening to hit or throw something at the partner) and marital violence were each correlated with children's adjustment problems in both a marital therapy and a women's shelter sample. Furthermore, other, assessed forms of marital aggression still related to children's adjustment problems even after controlling for the frequency of marital violence.

Also, some types of conflicts may contain messages that children find as disturbing as marital violence. Thus, Laumakis, Margolin, and John (1998) reported that conflicts involving threats to leave physical aggression elicited similar, high levels of negative reactions from children. Moreover, conflicts involving threats to leave and physical aggression elicited more negative emotional reactions and predictions of negative outcomes than conflicts with name-calling, negative voice, or conflicts with positive affect. These results support the notion that children react to the negative implications of marital conflict for marital and family relationships, and support also the consideration of multiple types and expressions of marital and family conflict and violence in models of the effects of extreme marital discord on children.

Nonverbal Conflict or the Silent Treatment

Nonverbal forms of conflict expression are not adequately assessed by any of the questionnaire instruments used to record rates of different forms of marital conflict in the home. However, children's reactions to analogue presentations of nonverbal conflict, or "the silent treatment," indicate that they are significantly distressed by these behaviors, and, in some studies, reactions are indistinguishable from reactions to overt verbal conflicts. A disadvantage of nonverbal conflict expressions is that they are unlikely to lead to resolution of the possibly significant marital issues that motivated the behavior. A failure to address marital problems over time is associated with problems both for marriages and for children in families (Cummings & Davies, 1994a).

Intense Conflicts and Conflicts about Child-Related Themes

It makes sense that more intense conflicts would be more disturbing than less intense conflicts. Presumably, more intense anger expressions reflect more negative feelings toward the spouse and are more often accompanied by highly negative conflict expressions (e.g., contempt; Gottman, 1994). However, an important caveat is that greater emotionality may sometimes simply reflect expressiveness and be a matter of personal style of communication rather than an index of disrespect or anger toward the spouse. In such instances, intensity would *not* be expected to increase children's distress given that they understood the intent of the communication. There is support (Grych & Fincham, 1993) for the view that more intense conflicts elicit more negative reactions than less intense conflicts, but effects may vary to some extent as a function of children's family history. For example, Nixon and Cummings (1999) found that children from homes experiencing greater stress and distress due to the presence of a disabled sibling had a lower threshold for intensity of responding emotionally and behaviorally to conflict than children from homes without a disabled sibling.

It makes sense intuitively that child-related themes of conflict would be more disturbing than other themes. Conflicts about child-related themes are linked with adjustment problems (Jouriles, Bourg, & Farris, 1991) and elicit more self-blame from children than conflicts about other issues (Grych & Fincham, 1993). However, themes of child-related conflict have been found either to elicit no differences in children's distress (Davies, Myers, & Cummings, 1996; Davies, Myers, Cummings, & Heindel, 1999) or even to reduce distress reactions, although a recent study was inconclusive on this point (Grych, 1998). Grych has speculated that these surprising results regarding distress reactions may reflect the possibility that children have a greater sense of personal control when conflicts are about them and, thus, less concern about whether something can be done to ameliorate the conflict. Thus, more important than whether themes involve the children may be whether the themes have relatively serious, negative implications for the family, regardless of the presence or absence of child content. Such a conceptualization is consistent with theoretical notions that children evaluate the meaning of conflict in determining how they will respond, rather than simply responding to the overt elements of conflict expression (e.g., emotional expressiveness, thematic content of the discussion). In fact, numerous studies have failed to support the hypothesis that children differentiate between the content of conflict scenarios in their responding when all other elements are made comparable (e.g., the relative seriousness vs. triviality of the issues for the marriage).

Withdrawal

In addition to overt conflict behavior, the withdrawal of parents from conflict may signal marital distress to children. The findings in this regard support the notion that children do not simply react to the expressiveness of conflict behavior. Katz and Gottman (1997a, 1997b) reported that husband withdrawal, indexed by observationally based codes of husband anger and stonewalling, predicts children's increased risk for adjustment problems. Notably, spousal withdrawal has been found consistently to predict future marital distress and is an even more significant predictor of future marital problems than overt marital conflict in some studies (Gottman, 1994). Pertinent to this point, Cox, Paley, and Payne (1997) found that marital withdrawal is more predictive of negative child outcomes than marital conflict. Again, the point is that these behaviors, while perhaps relatively subtle, can be reflective of significant marital distress, and it would appear from recent work that children, as well as spouses, are highly sensitive to the negative meaning of these communications.

In contrast to these forms of conflict expression, which appear to increase children's risk for problems, other ways of handling conflict have been found to have little negative effect and may possibly function as protective or compensatory events in the context of family functioning.

Mutually Respectful, Emotionally Modulated Conflicts

Only one study has examined the issue of mutually respectful conflict styles: Easterbrooks, Cummings, and Emde (1994) reported that toddlers evidenced little distress in reaction to conflictual discussions between parents in a sample that almost always expressed conflicts in mutually respectful, emotionally well-modulated tones. On the other hand, parental anger expression, which was relatively uncommon, was associated with negative emotional reactions by children even in this study.

Conflict Resolution

A long series of analogue studies has demonstrated that children's distress and other negative reactions are dramatically reduced when conflicts are resolved (Cummings & Davies, 1994a). In analogue studies, children are exposed to conflict on video- or audiotaped vignettes enacted by actors unknown to them. Frequently, children are asked to imagine that the actors are their parents and to respond as they would in the home to such conflict scenarios. The highly controlled presentation of stimuli in these analogue studies leaves little doubt that conflict resolution, rather than other factors, was responsible for the reduction in negative responding, which has significant theoretical implications regarding the importance of the meaning of conflicts, rather than simply their occurrence, for children's reactions (discussion to follow). Moreover, a recent field study based on a new questionnaire that assesses conflict resolution reported that marital conflict resolution is more consistently associated with child adjustment (i.e., reduced adjustment problems) than even negative elements of conflict (e.g., frequency, severity) (Kerig, 1996).

Furthermore, conflict resolution may sometimes ameliorate the negative impact of children's exposure to marital violence. Thus, Cummings, Simpson, and Wilson (1993) found ameliorative effects of conflict resolution on children's emotional responses to conflicts that were nonverbal, verbal, or that included physical aggression. However, again, it should be noted that children were responding to analogue presentations in this studies. Also, the actors' resolutions appeared genuine, and there was no history of prior conflict to compromise the apparent sincerity of the resolutions. As we will see later, children react to the meaning of conflicts for marital and family relations based on *both* their past histories of exposure to conflict, and the nature and form of current conflict stimuli. Although the question awaits empirical tests, children's responses to resolution may not be positive if chronic marital violence has occurred in the past within the family, even following supposed resolutions. On the other hand, conflict resolution may be relatively uncommon in high-conflict homes, so that such endings to conflicts might well carry *more*, rather than less, weight for such children. Consistent with this notion, Hennessy, Rabideau, Cicchetti, and Cummings (1994) found that physically abused children from high-conflict homes benefited more, rather than less, from conflict resolution than a comparison group.

However, a distinction should be made between reduced marital violence and constructive conflict. The model for disrespect, hostility, and negativity toward a loved one, indicated by violent behavior, mitigates against marital violence ever being constructive. Nonetheless, the meaning of marital violence for children may be modified by conflict resolutions/apologies; that is, the perception of immediate threat and danger to the self, marriage, and family may be reduced. The extent to which children's emotional security is increased is likely to depend upon the broader pattern of marital interactions. The severity and chronicity of violence is likely to be critical; that is, constructive messages may be more perceptible when marital aggression is relatively low in intensity (e.g., a single, low-intensity behavior) than when violence is intense, prolonged, and chronic. In summary, the relative impact of marital violence followed by resolution/apologies depends upon children's past and current appraisals and emotionality in response to marital conflict and violence; at the same time, children (marriages and families) are likely to benefit from any progress toward resolution and positive endings, even in the most negative family contexts.

Progress toward Resolution and Other Information about Resolution

Analogue studies also indicate that children benefit from any progress toward resolution; that is, distress reactions are reduced even when parents (actors) do not fully resolve conflicts. Furthermore, and somewhat surprisingly, children's distress reactions are much reduced even when adults have resolved conflicts behind closed doors, indicating resolution only by changed (to positive) affect after emerging from another room, entered in the midst of conflict. Children also benefit from hearing brief explanations that indicate conflicts have been resolved (Cummings, Simpson, & Wilson, 1993), or even that conflicts have *not* yet been resolved, but parents expect that they will be (Cummings & Wilson, 1999). Furthermore, children are sensitive to the emotional as well as thematic content of conflict resolution (Shifflet-Simpson & Cummings, 1996); that is, children are slightly more distressed by an angry apology than a friendly apology, but any form of apology elicits much less self-reported concern about the parents (actors) and personal distress than continued conflict.

However, examining children's reactions to specific elements of conflict can provide no more than an approximation of how the average child will react to family conflict, since children react to the meaning of conflict in the context of broader family functioning, including past histories of exposure to conflict and an understanding or interpretation of what parental communications mean. Consider the following:

> Eddie and Mike, both preschoolers, were playing together in the living room of Eddie's house. Suddenly, there was a crash from the kitchen as a door slammed, and the children could hear Eddie's parents arguing

loudly. The argument went on and on, with both parents storming about, making demonstrative statements, and slamming kitchen cabinet doors. Mike was scared, because his own parents never fought in such a manner, but looking over at Eddie, he could see that his friend was not concerned at all. Eddie got up and went into the kitchen. When his parents saw him, they stopped fighting and the daddy said, "Your mother makes ravioli the wrong way. My mother did it the right way." The mother said, "Well, it is so sweet that your daddy cares so much about the cooking." The Daddy said, "And your Mother is such a great cook." Next, they kissed a lot and made up.

Eddie knew that his parents were not really all that mad at each other; it was just that they were both very demonstrative, cared a lot about cooking, and enjoyed the fun and stimulation of a vigorous back-and-forth on a topic. On the other hand, Mike's parents, who also had a happy marriage, were reserved and undemonstrative in their interactions about everyday problems. If Mike's parents had ever fought in the same manner as Eddie's parents, the meaning for Mike would have been that his parents' relationship was in a terrible state. The point is, research suggests that children are very sensitive to the meaning of parental communications, even differentiating between relatively subtle nuances of emotional communication and how conflicts end. However, more than that, children appear to take into account past histories of interaction when evaluating how to respond to current events. Thus, in learning that children respond to specific elements of conflicts in certain ways, we are only beginning to understanding the impact of specific forms of marital communication on children. Consistent with the developmental psychopathology assumption of holism, it is necessary to understand the broader context and meaning of marital communication in order to understand its effects. Many of these questions ultimately await the conduct of appropriately data-intensive prospective longitudinal research; that is, they are open, empirical questions. However, as we have shown, considerable information suggests of what the answers may prove to be.

DEVELOPMENTAL PATHWAYS AND EXPERIENTIAL HISTORIES

Contextual factors associated with person–environment interactions are assumed to underlie process. Thus, as we have noted, the meaning and interpretation that children ascribe to marital conflict and violence in the broader context of the family may be at least as significant as the occurrence of particular interparental behaviors. Conceivably, children may evidence little negative outcome if parents are very expressive and emotional during conflicts but usually resolve their disagreements. On the other hand, children may have difficulty adjusting when parents rarely fight openly, but any occurrence of conflict seems to carry serious implications for the future intactness of the family. Certain nonviolent anger expressions may be as distressing to children as violent behaviors. For example, parental threats to leave the family have been shown in research to upset children as much as exposure to physical violence (Laumakis, Margolis, & John, 1998).

Consistent with the developmental psychopathology premise that one should study the abnormal in relation to the normal, research in this area also emphasizes understanding the development processes underlying both normal development and the development of adjustment problems (Cummings & Davies, 1994a; Emery & Kitzmann, 1995). It is assumed that a focus only on extremes is likely to provide a limited window into mediating processes. With regard to marital conflict, as we have seen, specific types and intensities of conflict elicit very different responses from children, so that a focus on one element of conflict (e.g., overt violence) may yield limited information about the effects of conflict and violence on children, and a potentially narrow, even misleading, perspective on key mediating processes and developmental sequelae. Thus, studies of both harmonious and adverse family contexts are mutually informative and essential to characterize the broader patterns of both expressions of conflict and marital relations and other family and extrafamilial relations, in order to understand the processes that mediate child development outcomes.

Furthermore, from the standpoint of understanding process, children who do not develop problems despite growing up in high-risk environments are just as interesting as those who do, but the focus has traditionally been on those children who develop psychopathology. What protective factors, or personal or environmental sources of resiliency, account for children's adaptive outcomes in very adverse family circumstances? Relatedly, some children from low-risk family environments do develop adjustment problems, and they are at least as interesting in terms of understanding mediating processes as those who develop competently. What stress factors, or personal or environmental sources of vulnerability, explain why some children have difficulty when most do not? Again, the study of the range of family environments around issues of marital conflict and violence is most likely to advance understanding. There has been limited development of these issues and questions to date.

Research on stress and adversity associated with marital conflict has neglected positive processes and events, but the developmental psychopathology perspective also calls attention to the significance of these events for understanding development in adverse family circumstances. The concepts of resiliency, compensatory, and protective factors, in particular, require an understanding of the role of positive processes in children's functioning when there is marital conflict or violence. For example, the *absence* of positive marital communications may be as significant as the presence of negative conflict behaviors. Beach (1995) reported that children's perceptions of *low* positive marital communications are a significant predictor of children's adjustment problems, independent of conflict behaviors. In conclusion, while significant progress has been made in desegregating marital conflict as a context for child development, it is undoubtedly the case that other dimensions that have not yet been articulated are important to children's functioning in families and related to the manner in which parents handle their disputes.

Exposure to Marital Hostility and Violence: Persistent, Not Short-Term, Effects

Acts of hostility and violence between the parents may be relatively rare and short-lived, even in discordant marriages. However, the effects of exposure to these events are *not* short-lived or limited to the time of exposure to these events. Children's fundamental notions of the quality and safety of marital and family relations may be profoundly influenced by their relatively infrequent exposure to marital conflict and violence. Thus, these events may have very significant effects on children's *general* patterns of emotional, cognitive, and behavioral functioning. Accordingly, histories of exposure to marital conflict and violence have been linked to patterns of emotional, behavioral, and cognitive coping with stress in other contexts, and these response patterns, in turn, have been linked to risk for adjustment problems (Cummings & Davies, 1994a). Appreciating the potentially wide-ranging impact of children's exposure to relatively infrequent acts of interparental conflict and violence is essential to conceptualizing the mediating processes that may be set in motion by their exposure to violence.

The Sensitization Hypothesis: Accounting for the Direct Effects of Exposure to Marital Conflict

A critical question for researchers concerned with the clinical implications of marital conflict for child development is whether there are cumulative effects of exposure to chronic marital conflict. How or why does exposure result in the development of adjustment problems over time? Following the assumptions of the developmental psychopathology perspective, we would expect to observe maladaptive behaviors in children's dynamic interactions with environmental contexts of marital conflict that would gradually lead, as a function of day-to-day responses to these experiences, to what would be classified as adjustment problems. What would these changes be? At a concrete level, what would be happening to the children? Consider the following examples:

> Lois and John came from families with very different relationships between the parents. Lois's parents fought all the time and were very angry with each other. John's parents discussed areas of disagreement periodically but were always mutually respectful and resolved most disagreements. One day, Lois's and John's fathers were both late picking them up from a first-grade school play. In both cases, the mothers were very worried. Both yelled at the fathers, even John's mom, because she was so up-

set. Lois got visibly anxious when her mother behaved that way and tried to make excuses for her father. John, on the other hand, simply went inside to play with his toys and did not even look up at his arguing and distressed parents.

This vignette illustrates a key finding of research on this question. One might expect at a glance that children would get used to marital conflict if it occurred all the time, and perhaps they do learn not to be as surprised by it as children who have little experience with such events. However, they do *not* get used to it. This is the consistent and repeated message of research. It is important to bear in mind that marital conflict is a stressor, even for children to observe as bystanders, and a threatening event in the context of the family. People do not get used to stressors, and repeated stressors, which have even more serious negative implications for the individuals involved as a function of their being repeated, become more, and not, less stressful. At a process level, the repetition of this stressor has effects evidenced by children becoming more dysregulated emotionally, behaviorally, and in their capacity to appropriately control their social behavior. For example, children from high-conflict homes are more aggressive than others following exposure to marital conflict (Cummings, Hennessy, Rabideau, & Cicchetti, 1994).

Thus, the process or mechanism by which exposure to chronic marital conflict leads to children's adjustment problems over time appears to have to do with its effects on children's regulatory capacities, experiences of stress and distress, and capacity for appropriate social behavior, particularly when threatened. Interestingly, some of the research we considered was reviewed in the section on principles. For example, work by Post and colleagues suggests that even biological systems for regulatory arousal in animals are altered by repeated exposure to stress (Post & Weiss, 1997; Post, Weiss, & Leverich, 1994). There is no doubt that marital hostility and violence, and other forms of marital communication that have negative implications for family intactness, continuity, or effective functioning, are significant stressors for children.

Thus, we know that children's conflict histories in the home predict their responses to conflicts; that is, histories of exposure to background anger, marital conflict, and interparental violence are predictors of children's greater emotional (e.g., distress), behavioral (e..g., aggression), social (e.g., mediation in parental disputes), and even physiological (e.g., heart rate, blood pressure, galvanic skin responses; El-Sheikh, Ballard, & Cummings, 1994) reactions, and their own reports of greater perceptions of threat and negativity about future marital interactions. These findings have been observed even in response to presentations of conflict that are the same across groups, so that children's reactions in relation to other groups must be attributed to their past histories rather than the current stimuli. The results suggest that conflict histories lower children's thresholds for responding negatively and increase their reactivity to conflict; hence, the phenomenon has come to be termed the "sensitization hypothesis." This result is reported in field studies of children's reactions to actual marital conflicts (Cummings, Zahn-Waxler, & Radke-Yarrow, 1981, 1984), laboratory simulations of conflict (Cummings, Iannotti, & Zahn-Waxler, 1985), and parental reports of marital conflict histories and children's reactions (e.g., Ballard, Cummings, & Larkin, 1993; Cummings, Pelligrini, Notarius, & Cummings, 1989; Cummings, Vogel, Cummings, & El-Sheikh, 1989; Gordis, Margolin, & John, 1997; Myers, 1997; O'Brien, Bahadur, Gee, Balto, & Erber, 1997; O'Brien, Margolin, John, & Krueger, 1991; Rogers & Holmbeck, 1997). Thus, Laumakis et al. (1998) reported that children from high-conflict homes evaluated conflicts more negatively than children from low-conflict homes, with boys exposed to high-conflict marriages more likely to report an intervention response, particularly in response to marital physical aggression. As another recent example, Grych (1998) reported that children exposed to higher levels of conflict between their parents perceived the conflicts as more threatening and verbalized more negative expectations about their own efforts to intervene in marital conflicts. Histories of marital violence have been associated particularly with sensitization to parental conflicts (e.g., Cummings, Pelligrini, et al., 1989), which makes sense given the likely emotional impact of violence between the parents on children. Furthermore, when conflict "histories" are artificially created in the laboratory, results are consistent with the predictions of the sensitization hypothesis (e.g., Cummings et al., 1985; Davies, Myers, Cummings, & Heindel, 1999; El-Sheikh & Cummings, 1995; El-Sheikh, Cummings, & Reiter, 1996).

These results have important theoretical implications for understanding the processes that mediate the impact of marital conflict on children's adjustment. They suggest that emotional, behavioral, and social dysregulation in the face of parental conflicts (actors or actual parents) at least partially mediates the direct effects of marital conflict and violence on children; that is, repeated exposure to destructive forms of marital conflict undermines children's capacities for regulating their emotional and behavioral functioning. The weight of the evidence suggests that the reduction in children's regulatory capacities is limited not only to situations of marital conflict but also may be related to a more general reaction tendency in response to distressing or stressful situations (e.g., Ballard, Cummings, & Larkin, 1993; see also Davies & Cummings, 1994). Moreover, repeated exposure to certain destructive forms of conflict is reflected in more negative representations of cognitions about the family. It can be readily seen how such an increased proneness to responses of emotional, behavioral, and cognitive negativity and dysregulation might contribute to children's development of problems over time.

Repeated episodes and instances of dysregulatory functioning in multiple social contexts and situations might result in successive changes in functioning that constitute a gradual emergence of developmental deviations. Cummings and colleagues (Cummings & Cummings, 1988; Cummings & Davies, 1994a) have argued that children's stress and coping reactions provide a powerful window into the meaning of marital conflict from their perspective and also reflect broader patterns of response processes that underlie development, thus holding out the possibility that these responses index dynamic, process-level mediators of adjustment over time. Interestingly, Davis, Hops, Alpert, and Sheeber (1998) recently reported impressive evidence based upon sequential analyses of observed family interactions that interparental conflict predicted children's aggressive behavior and was linked to increased adjustment problems. Their findings directly implicated interparental conflict in accounting for problems of aggression in children. The emotional security hypothesis, which we describe later as it relates to children's responses to marital conflict, provides a specific theoretical model for explaining how sensitization processes might result in developmental deviations over time.

Other findings support the framework in Figure 8.1. For example, there appear to be consistent individual differences in reactions to conflict organized around patterns of emotional responding (Cummings, 1987); these individual differences appear to be stable over time, with tests indicating stability for periods up to 5 years (Cummings, 1987; Cummings, Zahn-Wazler, & Radke-Yarrow, 1984). Moreover, broader patterns of family violence (e.g., child physical abuse) are associated with increased sensitization to parental conflicts (e.g., Cummings, Hennessy, Rabideau, & Cicchetti, 1994). These findings suggest that processes mediating responses to marital conflict are psychologically meaningful, since they tend to be stable over significant periods of time and relate to broader patterns of behavior and organizations of individual functioning, particularly surrounding emotional regulation. Thus, they may reflect important organizations of children's responses to threat and challenge, and also be related to general patterns of conflict and violence in the family.

MARITAL CONFLICT AND PARENTING: INDIRECT PATHWAYS OF EFFECT

Recent research documents the finding that exposure to marital conflict affects children *both* directly, due to exposure and indirectly, by changing parenting practices (e.g., Harold, Fincham, Osborne, & Conger, 1997; Margolin, Christensen, & John, 1996; O'Brien, Bahadur, Gee, Balto, & Erber, 1997). In fact, a rather substantial literature has emerged to support relations between marital conflict and negative changes in parenting (Erel & Burman, 1995). The relations are illustrated in Figure 8.1.

Demonstrating an indirect pathway, parenting problems have been shown to be mediators of the effects of marital conflict on children (Davies & Cummings, 1994). One possible explanation is provided by the spillover hypothesis, in which distress and hostility accompanying marital conflict are carried over into parenting practices, leading to changes in parental emotional availability (e.g., rejection, hostility, unresponsiveness) or control (e.g., lax monitoring, inconsistent or harsh discipline) (Jouriles & Farris, 1992; Mahoney, Boggio, & Jouriles, 1996; Margolin, Christensen, & John, 1996).

Traditional models of family and child development have focused on parent–child relationships and paid scant attention to broader family functioning, including marital (or interpartner) relations. For example, family violence and abuse are often considered primarily in terms of parents' physical abuse of children. However, marital relations, including conflict, are central to children's well-being. In fact, evidence that the quality of marital relations affects the quality of parent–child relations is quite strong (Erel & Burman, 1995). Thus, marital relations are a significant underlying influence on parenting and the quality of parent–child emotional relationships. These results underscore the importance of a holistic perspective on family functioning and child development, consistent with the precepts of a developmental psychopathology perspective (Emery & Kitzmann, 1995).

Marital Relations and Parenting Practices

Marital relations are predictive of the quality of parenting; that is, the consistency of parenting, the extent to which parenting is hostile or appropriate, the emotional availability of parents, and other parenting dimensions may be affected by the quality of marital relations. Emotional dimensions and qualities of parenting practices are particularly influenced by the quality of marital relations (Davies & Cummings, 1994), with support for causal relations between marital conflict and parenting (Jouriles & Farris, 1992).

For example, relationships marked by the presence of violence or a high frequency of overt conflict have been linked to inconsistent child rearing and disciplinary behavior (Holden & Miller, 1999; Holden & Ritchie, 1991; Stoneman, Brody, & Burke, 1989). Marital conflict has also been associated with increased parental negativity and intrusive control (Hetherington et al., 1992) and low levels of parental warmth and responsiveness (Holden & Ritchie, 1991). Parental rejection has been identified as a mediator of marital conflict for both externalizing and internalizing problems (Fauber, Forehand, Thomas, & Wierson, 1990). Specifically, parental behaviors such as withdrawal and hostility have contributed to the prediction of social withdrawal, depression, and anxiety in children (Denham, 1989; Hoffman-Plotkin & Twentyman, 1984; Pettit & Bates, 1989) and externalizing problems in children (Bousha & Twentyman, 1984). Marital conflict can thus be viewed as an important contributor to disruptions in the parenting process, which impacts a variety of indices of relevant parenting behavior and influence.

Marital Relations and the Attachments between Children and Parents

Marital relations are also predictive of the quality of the emotional bond or attachment that forms between parents and children, that is, the emotional security of the attachment between parents and children (Davies & Cummings, 1994). This fact is particularly important since, as we saw in Chapter 6, the quality of attachment relations predicts children's outcomes over time, including their risk for adjustment problems. Studies show that increases in marital conflict during the child's first 9 months or even prenatally (Cox & Owen, 1993), are linked to insecure attachment at 12 months of age. Another study found that exposure to high marital conflict at age 1 year predicted insecure attachment at age 3 (Howes & Markman, 1989). Moreover, children's relationships with their parents may also change because of the negative effects on their sense of trust or high regard for parents due to watching them behave in mean or hostile ways toward each other. Thus, the impact of marital conflict on parenting may be quite direct (Owen & Cox, 1997). In summary, the research seems to be quite clear that destructive conflict has a particularly negative impact on emotional relationships within the family.

The Co-Occurrence of Marital Conflict, Divorce, Adversity, and Abuse within the Family

Further highlighting the importance of a holistic perspective on how marital conflict affects children, marital conflict and violence, adversity, and abuse often occur together (e.g., Cummings & Davies, 1994a; Davies & Cummings, 1994; Emery, 1989; Grych & Fincham, 1990). Marital conflict is often a factor in children's adjustment because they reside in families that are characterized as disturbed for other reasons. For example, marital conflict is a significant factor in the effects of divorce on children. It may influence children's development long before the divorce occurs (Block, Block, & Gjerde, 1986), and children's postdivorce adjustment is often related to the extent and form of marital conflict (Amato & Keith, 1991). The effects of custody arrangements following divorce also vary significantly as a function of the type and level of marital conflict (Emery, 1994). There may be a recommendation against joint custody when there is chronic interparental violence, whereas joint custody might otherwise be recommended. As another example, marital conflict and parental depression are highly correlated in both men and women (Whisman, 2000). Recent analyses suggest that marital conflict is a more significant predictor of some forms of adjustment problems than parental depression per se (Cummings, 1995a; Cummings & Davies, 1994b, 1996; Downey & Coyne, 1990). Marital conflict and alcoholism are also interrelated. Interparental conflict and violence are among the most disturbing aspects of parental alcoholism from the children's point of view and may be a predictor of problems in children's adjustment (El-Sheikh & Cummings, 1997; West & Prinz, 1987).

In summary, multiple forms of adversity are associated with marital conflict. Minimally, models of family adversity, violence, abuse, and child development need to incorporate the effects of the marital (or interpartner) system on the functioning of the family. Including marital factors in the equation is likely to increase the prediction of child outcomes, and provide a more sophisticated view of the familial causes of child outcomes at a conceptual level.

Marital Conflict Co-Occurs with Dysfunction in Other Family Systems

As we have seen, a sole focus on the parent–child system offers a limited and oversimplified view of pathways of influence within the family. The behaviors of parents and children in the parent–child interaction are *each* influenced by the quality of the marital relationship, as well as by other family events and relationships outside of the parent–child system (Cummings & O'Reilly, 1997). Relations are frequently reported between marital conflict and violence, and problems in other family systems (Holden & Ritchie, 1991; Katz & Gottman, 1995a; Jouriles, Bourg, & Farris, 1991; Jouriles & Farris, 1992). Marital conflict is correlated with difficulties in parent–child discipline and child-rearing practices, patterns of coercive family interactions, and negative sibling relationships (Cummings & Davies, 1994a, 1995). Furthermore, marital conflict fosters the emotional and psychological unavailability and lack of responsiveness of parents, increasing the insecurity of parent–child emotional bonds and decreasing the quality of parent–child attachments (Davies & Cummings, 1994). Associations have also been reported between marital conflict and various forms of child abuse. Thus, interspousal aggression and child physical abuse have been linked (e.g., Jouriles, Barling, & O'Leary, 1987). Marital conflict has also been associated with child sexual abuse (e.g., Browne & Finkelhor, 1986). Thus, interrelations among marital conflict, the functioning of other family systems, and children's problems are indicated. Accordingly, Cummings and Davies (1994a) concluded: "Children's mental health problems do not develop out of parallel and independent disturbances within the family. Rather, disturbances in each family subsystem affect the other subsystems, and broad problems in family functioning are likely to be associated with negative child outcomes" (p. 106).

On the other hand, positive marital relations and conflict resolution styles may foster positive outcomes in other family systems and may be a protective factor and source of resilience. Thus, conflict resolution may ameliorate negative emotional reactions to marital conflict and violence, and may lead to positive outcomes (e.g., Cummings, Simpson, & Wilson, 1993).

The Cumulative Impact of Family Stress

Marital (or interpartner) conflict and violence may be central to negative emotional and behavioral processes in families. Marital discord is associated with children's emotional and behavioral dysregulation, attempts to control or regulate the dysfunctional interactions between the mother and father, and representations of the self and family members' relationships that are more negative and pessimistic about the future (Davies & Cummings, 1994). These negative processes bear similarities to those linked with the impact on children of dysfunction in other family systems, such as coercive parent–child relations or insecure parent–child attachment (e.g., Cummings & Davies, 1994a; Davies & Cummings, 1994). Problems in family functioning also interact with children's dispositions in influencing the likelihood that children will develop dysfunctional coping responses, processes, and styles (Davies & Cummings, 1994). Dysfunctional behavioral styles, in turn, are linked with the development of psychopathology.

Figure 8.1 also illustrates how multiple family systems may affect common processes in children. In this regard, it has been proposed, based on a survey of the literature, that "family adversity may affect children's development through its action on common processes and mechanisms. Consequently, . . . joint effects may occur, which could be additive, interactive, or multiplicative" (Cummings & Davies, 1994a, p. 108).

Several recent studies further advance our understanding of these issues. Lindahl (1998) found that dimensions of parental, marital, and family functioning each distinguished whether boys had no behavioral problems, attention-deficit/hyperactivity disorder (ADHD), oppositional deviant disorder, or both ADHD and oppositional defiant disorder (a comorbid group). With regard to marital functioning, oppositional defiant and comorbid groups were found to have experienced much greater marital distress and discord than the control group. In comparing the clinical groups, parenting, marital, and family problems were more elevated for the oppositional defiant and the comorbid groups in relation to the ADHD group. These results indicate that behavior problems may have quite different familial origins depending upon the nature of the disorder, again underscoring the relevance of conceptualizing pathways of development and etiology, including careful differentiations among predictors, mediating and moderating processes, and childhood outcomes.

Owen and Cox (1997) provided additional support for the finding that chronic marital conflict interferes with warm, sensitive, and involved parenting for both mothers and fathers. Chronic marital conflict predicts insecurity in father–infant attachment and is linked with a particularly disturbed dimension of attachment relations, that is, the degree of disorganization in both mother–infant and father–infant attachments (Carlson, 1998). Owen and Cox attributed the effects of marital conflict on attachment disorganization to children's exposure to frightened or frightening parents in the context of repeated interparental conflict situations. Their results thus supported both direct and indirect pathways by which marital conflict can disrupt parenting. Moreover, while most reports of the direct effects of marital conflict have focused on effects influencing children's emotional security about marital functioning, these results provide evidence for how marital conflict may also directly reduce children's emotional security about their own relations with their parents, as illustrated in Figure 8.2. Thus, children's confidence in the availability and sensitivity of their parents may be reduced by observing parents' mean and hostile behavior toward each other (i.e., direct effects) as well as spillover of parental hostility in terms of behavior toward the children (i.e., indirect effects).

Learning, negative reinforcement, and modeling may also be factors in the common impact of marital and parent–child systems on children; that is, children may learn behavioral and cognitive styles for coping with everyday events from both observing their parents in interparental situations and interacting with them. Thus, Beach (1995) recently reported that maternal attributional styles in analogue conflict situations with a "spouse" were significantly correlated with similar attributional styles in their children's responses to analogue conflict situations with a "peer." Interestingly, statistically significant relations were also found between maternal positive communications and reciprocity in analogue conflict situations with a "spouse" and children's similar behaviors with a "peer," suggesting that children may learn constructive lessons about handling conflict situations from positive parental models.

As another example, children who are *witnesses* of spousal abuse exhibit adjustment problems similar to those of children who are *victims* of parental violence (Jaffe, Wolfe, Wilson, & Zak, 1986; Jouriles et al., 1998). Similarly, exposure to one form of violence in the family may affect reactions to others (e.g., Hennessy, Rabideau, Cicchetti, & Cummings, 1994). With regard to the physical, emotional, and sexual abuse of children, Jaffe, Wolfe, and Wilson (1990) stated that "it is widely acknowledged that . . . different forms of maltreatment also give rise to many of the same developmental adjustment problems, suggesting that very similar psychological processes may be commonly responsible for the children's reactions to trauma" (p. 68).

In summary, there is accumulating evidence that (1) marital conflict is a significant source of adversity and risk for children's adjustment problems in families, and (2) marital conflict and other forms of adversity in the family are interrelated. Similarly, positive marital relations and marital satisfaction may support positive functioning in families, fostering children's adaptive develop-

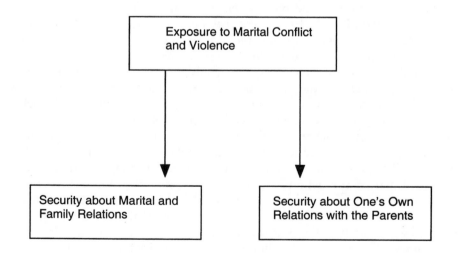

FIGURE 8.2. Marital conflict and direct effects on security of attachment.

ment (Cummings & O'Reilly, 1997). Thus, an emerging literature supports the notion that marital relations are central to an understanding of family processes and events, including the negative impact of extremely adverse family events such as violence or abuse. Marital relations serve as a foundation for emotional processes and their regulation within the family, and thus have a role in modulating, ameliorating, or exaggerating the risk associated with other family events. However, an important caveat is that our understanding of these processes and relationships is at an early stage, and the evidence is far more suggestive than conclusive, particularly since it is based largely on global assessments of family events and their interrelations, correlational analyses, and studies based on concurrent rather than longitudinal assessments of variables.

A MODEL FOR MEDIATING PROCESSES: AN EMOTIONAL SECURITY HYPOTHESIS

As we have noted, another important direction for a developmental psychopathology perspective is the articulation of theory to make sense of the complex empirical directions that are demanded by this approach to the study of the etiology of children's adjustment problems. While relations between marital conflict, violence, and children's adjustment problems are long established, until recently, there was little progress toward articulating theories about mediating processes. In the case of relations between marital conflict and child adjustment, two major theories have been proposed: (1) Davies and Cummings's (1994) emotional security hypothesis, and (2) Grych and Fincham's (1990) cognitive-contextual framework.

These two models, and other recent theoretical directions (Crockenberg & Forgays, 1996; Emery, 1989, 1992; Feldman & Downey, 1994; Wilson & Gottman, 1995), are generally complementary and emphasize similar points. For example, these models highlight children's reactions to and interpretations of marital conflict for themselves, the family, and the marriage, suggesting that it is more than just the occurrence of conflict that affects children. Moreover, the meaning of conflict is personal and emotional, and related to children's appraisals of the conflict as well as their emotional reactions to it (see, especially, Harold, Fincham, Osborne, & Conger, 1997). Furthermore, both models emphasize the significance of the particular context of marital conflict, past as well as present, in children's adaptation and maladaption; that is, both history of marital conflict and the specific characteristics of any current conflict behaviors are seen as having substantial influence on children's current functioning according to both the cognitive-contextual framework and the emotional security hypothesis. A difference between the theories is that Davies and Cummings emphasize the importance of emotion, whereas Grych and Fincham put more stress on the role of cognition.

We focus here on the emotional security hypothesis, but the other model also merits examination for further theoretical understanding of these processes. Davies and Cummings (1994) propose that, logically, children's reactions to conflict must be related to and understood within the context of other developmental and family processes, part of the whole of child and family development, and not a new process unrelated to reactions to other family events. Based on the data, which in the view of Davies and Cummings suggest the primacy and immediacy of emotionality in reactions to conflict, and a functionalist perspective positing that emotions serve appraisal and organizing functions (e.g., Campos, Campos, & Barrett, 1989), an emotional security hypothesis describes a key domain of processes mediating relations between marital conflict, violence, and children's adjustment. This hypothesis is described in further detail.

Theoretical Tenets

The emotional security hypothesis specifies a *particular* meaning against which children appraise the implications of marital and family conflict for themselves and their families, suggests how that meaning is personal, and indicates why children respond emotionally (Davies & Cummings, 1994). In important respects, this model builds upon and, in particular, complements the cognitive-contextual model proposed by Grych and Fincham (1990), which stresses how children's cognitive processing and coping behaviors are shaped by the characteristics of marital conflict and contextual factors such as past experience with conflict, gender, expectations, and mood. However, while cognition is acknowledged as being important to coping processes, the present model places greater emphasis on emotionality in the very emotion-laden domain of family conflict and, specifically, the significance of emotional security to children's reactions to marital conflict. Davies and Cummings's (1994, p. 387) key theoretical proposition follows:

> Children's concerns about emotional security play a role in their regulation of emotional arousal and organization and motivation to respond in the face of marital conflict. Over time these response processes have implications for children's long-term adjustment. Emotional security is seen as a product of past experience and a primary influence on future responding (to emotionally charged events).

Operationalization in Terms of Specific Component Regulatory Systems

When confronted with marital conflict, children seek emotional security. Thus, emotional security describes the goal of children's functioning in the face of marital conflict. However, various specific regulatory systems are subsumed under the rubric of emotional security as an operating process (Cummings & Davies, 1996). These specific components are separate, but also interdependent, in the service of emotional security. The definition of emotional security in terms of these specific systems also articulates specific measurement requirements and avenues toward the precise assessment of emotional security as a mediating process in the face of marital conflict. Each component is assumed to be a function of not only current stimuli but also past exposures to interparental relations. In recent research, specific, multi-method strategies toward the operationalization of these processes have been proposed (Cummings & Davies, 1996; Davies & Cummings, 1998).

Emotion Regulation

Consistent with conceptualizations of security in attachment theory, insecurity may be reflected in emotional reactivity characterized by heightened fear, distress, vigilance, and covert negativity. This component is not the equivalent of emotional security, but a subset or component of it. It consists of children's emotional reactivity and arousal, and their capacity to reduce, enhance, and/or maintain their emotionality in the face of conflict. It can be inferred from subjective reports of feelings, overt expression of emotion, and physiological arousal. Because children from high-conflict homes exhibit more distress, fear, aggression, and preoccupation in reaction to parental conflicts (Cummings & Davies, 1994), we suggest that emotion regulation strategies may play a mediating role between exposure to conflict and children's emotional reactivity to it.

Internal Representation of Family Relations

While rarely tested, representations of marital and family relations are expected to be influenced by marital hostility (Davies & Cummings, 1994). Representations most relevant to children's emotional security consist of their interpretation of the meaning and potential consequences of marital conflict for their own well-being. These representations are proffered to be relatively accurate depictions of family life (Bowlby, 1973); thus, it follows that children with histories of negative conflict should be prone to developing insecure representations of family relations. Children's internal representations reflect their appraisals of family events and their active processing of the meaning that events have for their own well-being. These appraisals are a reflection of their sense of emotional security and the implication of events for emotional security. As noted by Grych and Fincham (1990), these internal representations also include children's primary assessment of the self-relevance and threat of events, and their secondary appraisal of who is responsible, why these events are occurring, and whether they have adequate coping skills. Insecure representations, in turn, are hypothesized to increase children's risk for psychological disturbance. There is initial support for the hypothesis that negative representations of marital relations serve as a mediator of relations between high conflict and children's adjustment problems (Davies & Cummings, 1998).

Regulation of Exposure to Family Affect

Children may also attempt to regulate their emotional security by controlling their exposure to marital conflict. Emotional security serves a motivational function by guiding children to regulate their exposure to stressful parental emotion. The issues with regard to an assessment of emotional security include the repertoire of children's regulatory activities and behaviors (e.g., forms and styles of mediation behaviors), their threshold for onset, and their appropriateness in specific contexts. Insecurity in this domain may be manifested in the "overregulation" of exposure to parental affect, shown through overinvolvement. Children's behavior as mediators in parental conflict may reflect direct attempts to control parental emotions and thereby minimize negative sequelae for the family. Research has shown that children from high-conflict homes more often use intervention in an attempt to alleviate conflict (Cummings & Davies, 1994). Moreover, there are developmental differences in children's ability to avoid, confront, or effectively intervene in marital conflict and other family disputes.

Specific Theoretical Definition

Emotional security, as a construct, appears to have à shared, implicit meaning in the literature. However, the concept has rarely been subject to precise definition. To address this gap, an explicit definition of emotional security is proposed:

> Emotional security is a latent construct that can be inferred from the overall organization and meaning of children's emotions, behaviors, thoughts, and physiological responses, and serves as a set goal by which children regulate their own functioning in social contexts, thereby directing social, emotional, cognitive, and physiological reactions. (Cummings & Davies, 1996, p. 126)

Thus, while recent theory stresses that children react to conflict in terms of their assessment of its meaning for family functioning and their own well-being, the emotional security hypothesis proposes that a particular meaning is especially important, that is, the emotional security implications of conflicts. Building upon attachment theory (Sroufe & Waters, 1977a), emotional security is seen as a paramount factor in children's regulation of emotional arousal, organization of emotion, and motivation to respond in the face of marital conflict. Emotional security is conceptualized from a contextual perspective, emphasizing the interplay between socioemotional and biological processes. While emotional security is described as the set goal of regulatory functioning, as noted ealier, various specific regulatory systems are conceptualized as being subsumed within emotional security as an operating process, that is, emotional regulation, regulation of exposure to family affect, and internal representations of family relations. Thus, similar levels of emotional insecurity may be evidenced by different organizations of emotional and behavioral responding in different children. Therefore, one must consider children's responding in terms of higher-order organizations of responding across multiple domains of functioning in order to evaluate their emotional security. Consider the following example:

> LeeAnn is a 4-year-old whose parents fight constantly and rarely resolve their differences. Furthermore, the conflicts often escalate from a relatively conversational discussion of the issues to very hostile remarks exchanged between the parents. Sometimes LeeAnn's mother throws things at the father, and he sometimes pounds the table or wall with his fist. On several occasions, after particularly angry conflicts, the mother has taken LeeAnn and her sister, Kris, to their grandmother's for the night. At this point, whenever her parents even begin to discuss a problem, LeeAnn becomes visibly distressed, sometimes begins to cry, but generally stays away from her parents as much as possible. She now often tells her older sister that she doesn't think that Mommy and Daddy love each other anymore. Even though her parents are warm and responsive to LeeAnn in their own interactions with her, she much less often seeks their help in times of stress and sometimes feels uneasy around them even when they are being nice to her or each other. On the other hand, LeeAnn's 10-year-old sister, Kris, often gets involved in the conflicts when the parents fight, trying as best she can to mediate and umpire the discussion but sometimes also becoming overtly angry with one parent or the other. Kris has also become her mother's confidant, and having taken over many of the household responsibilities, is constantly working to make things go more smoothly within the family, even to the point that she has neglected her own friendships and schoolwork.

Thus, we can conclude that both LeeAnn and Kris experience heightened emotional insecurity in the family on a frequent, even daily, basis due to their parents' frequent and intense conflicts. The fact that a set goal of emotional security is not achieved for these girls in their day-to-day family living is evident in their heightened, day-to-day emotional arousal levels, their obvious negative representations of the well-being of the marriage and family, and various aspects of how they are clearly motivated to regulate exposure to the parents' conflicts. However, emotional insecurity has organized different patterns of responding in the two girls and has motivated different patterns of behavioral responding in direct reaction to the conflicts. Thus, LeeAnn is overtly emotionally dysregulated and has clearly developed more negative representations of the parent–child relationships, the marital relationship, and the family as a source of emotional security. However, LeeAnn does not become involved in the parents' conflicts. On the other hand, while Kris is also very emotionally dysregulated by the parents' problems, her sense of emotional insecurity has motivated very different patterns of behavioral responding, namely, constant efforts to take care of things around the house so that fights do not start or end as quickly and amicably as possible if they do start. She also tries as much as possible not to reveal her own emotional distress overtly to the parents when they fight, although she sometimes loses control of her own anger.

The emotional security perspective also has important implications for the distinction between constructive versus destructive conflict from the children's perspective. Contexts of marital conflict are evaluated by children in terms of their emotional security implications for the child and the family, and these appraisals in turn serve to motivate and regulate children's emotions, their exposure to marital conflict, and their internal representations of marital relations. In other words, children react not only to the *occurrence* of marital conflict but also to *whether* marital conflict has destructive versus constructive implications for personal and family functioning from their point of view. The example of Edie and Mike, described at the outset of the chapter, illustrates this point. Edie's parents often fought, but she knew from experience that these conflicts did not have negative implications for the family. Thus, due to her evaluation, that her set goal of emotional security was not altered by these events, her functioning did not change due to her parents' conflicts in terms of her own emotional regulation, representations of family, or efforts to regulate exposure to family. The comparison between traditional attachment theory, which has focused on emotional security as derived from parent–child relations, and the emotional security hypothesis of Davies and Cummings merits consideration. According to the emotional security hypothesis, it is limiting to view children's experiences and representations of emotional security *solely* in terms of the attachment relationship as assessed by the Strange Situation. Children's emotional security *also* originates from children's experiential histories with interparental emotional events and other interwoven family factors (e.g., parental adjustment, family emotional climate, child characteristics). Thus, the central hypothesis is that emotional security plays a mediational role in the impact of parent–child relationships (Sroufe & Waters, 1977a), marital relations (Davies & Cummings, 1994), and other family factors (e.g., Cummings & Davies, 1999) on children's adjustment. In particular, it is proposed that destructive marital conflict increases children's vulnerability to adjustment problems by reducing their emotional security. Children have sound reasons for being concerned about destructive marital conflict. Severe interparental conflict increases insecurity by signifying a loved one's unhappiness and possible emotional instability, and raising the possibility of divorce or family dissolution, with accompanying hardships. Children may also fear that parents will become less emotionally responsive to them or carry unresolved hostility from marital conflicts into parent–child interactions.

As we have noted, emotional security is theorized to be a control system within which interrelations among the three component processes (i.e., marital relations, parent–child relations, and exposure to marital conflict) operate with an overarching latent goal of emotional security. Figure 8.2 illustrates this model. Thus, emotional security is at the same time a set goal and a regulatory system that governs the expression of the specific component processes according to immediate and historical context, age, gender, and other intra- and extraorganismic influences. For example, insecurity resulting from marital discord may increase children's incentive to reduce their exposure to the threatening event by escaping or intervening in the conflict. By the same token, emotional security is regulated by these response processes. Extending the previous example, the escape or intervention that was originally motivated by felt insecurity subsequently serves as a means of restoring some sense of emotional security, at least in a temporary, superficial way. Notably, the emotional security hypothesis posits the preseveration of emotional security as a significant goal in itself (e.g., see Sroufe & Waters, 1977a), thereby shifting some of the emphasis away from an evolutionary and ethological account of the origins of security. This shift towards a functionalist perspective permits a broader, more inclusive, familywide model of the etiology of emotional security, also providing a theoretical foundation for testable hypotheses about the meditating role of emotional security derived from factors other than parent–child interaction.

Supporting Evidence

For a comprehensive test, a rigorous, multivariate, longitudinal design is required that can effectively test the Davies and Cummings model and distinguish cause-and-effect relations during children's development over time. While the marshaled data can only be suggestive until the model is tested formally in this way, a considerable body of evidence to support more extensive testing has accumulated. The following summarizes some of the suggestive as well as more cogent supporting evidence:

1. The notion of emotional security is consistent with more general family and child development models, specifically, the literature on parent–child attachment. This construct has a long history in psychiatric, psychoanalytic, and clinical traditions. The concept is that emotional security is more than a secure base, but is posited as an internal state. As Sroufe and Waters (1977a) proposed, emotional security is seen as an internal set point that serves as a basis and source of motivation for responding to the environment. The new element is an extension; that is, children's emotional security also derives from the marital relationship, in addition to the parent–child relationship.

2. This notion can explain why negative reactions to conflict are so dramatically ameliorated by conflict resolution, and why children are so sensitive to any evidence about possible resolution, even when resolutions may be much briefer than conflict episodes; that is, children are concerned about the meaning of conflicts for themselves and their families, not just the occurrence of conflict. Conflict resolution greatly changes the familial implications of

otherwise anxiety-arousing social situations. Specifically, conflict resolution changes the emotional security implications of conflict. Moreover, a similar point regarding the applicability of the emotional security construct can be made for the family climate more generally; that is, other forms of family conflict (e.g., parent–child conflict) also induce negative reactions in the children that are similarly ameliorated by conflict resolution.

3. The emotional reactivity construct can account for why children evidence sensitization, rather than habituation, when they have histories of exposure to high marital conflict in the home, especially violence. It makes sense that children from such homes would become more aroused, since these events are more threatening, realistically, for them; that is, when there is high marital conflict, there is more likelihood that conflicts will proliferate to include the children, that a parent will be injured, and that the occurrence of conflicts will have more negative short- and long-term implications for the child and family. Even though these children are more distressed, it makes sense for them to also be more likely to try to intervene in conflicts, given the implications (Emery, 1989). In other words, conflicts pose a greater threat to their sense of emotional security. Similarly, high rates of parent–child conflict, especially when conflicts involve physical aggression, induce heightened reactivity in children, that is, sensitization, and this sensitization may pertain to multiple forms of family conflict (e.g., other forms of conflict involving the parents; Cummings, Hennessy, Rabideau, & Cicchetti, 1994).

4. Emotional reactions predict behavioral responses, aggression, self-reported cognitions and feelings, and even heart rate responses (e.g., Cummings, 1987), whereas other levels of responding thus far have not, which suggests an organizing role of emotionality.

In an analogue test, inducing different emotional states systematically predicted differences in multiple types of reactions to interadult conflicts, supporting the basic proposition that emotionality, or the emotional set point, motivates responding (Davies & Cummings, 1995).

5. The most convincing support is a recent study indicating that multimethod assessments of emotional security mediated relations between qualitative aspects of marital conflict and qualitative differences in child outcomes (Davies & Cummings, 1998). In this concurrent test, support was found for a theoretical pathway, whereby negative marital conflict led to children's adjustment problems as mediated by reduced emotional security about marital relations. By contrast, greater emotional security mediated a pathway between constructive marital conflict properties (e.g., marital conflict resolution) and reduced adjustment problems (Davies, 1995). Of the components of emotional security, children's regulation of negative emotionality in reaction to marital conflict mediated pathways to both internalizing and externalizing (e.g., aggressiveness) disorders, and the children's representations of the quality of marital relations also mediated relations between marital conflict and children's internalizing problems (e.g., anxiety, depression).

Figure 8.3 provides an illustration of the pathways supported in this study for the emotional security processes mediating relations between marital conflict and child adjustment. Notably, consistent with the methodological assumptions of the developmental psychopathology approach outlined in Chapter 3 that constructs should be measured by multiple methods and assessments, each of the psychological variables portrayed in Figure 8.3 were measured by multiple assessments. Moreover, consistent with the statistical approaches for demonstrating process models outlined in Chapter 5, the analyses were based upon structural equation modeling.

These analyses are based on an assumption that subprocesses at this level of assessment provide the best characterization of the mediating processes. Sometimes higher-order patterns may better capture the processes mediating relations between family events and childhood disorders. Pattern-level analyses are consistent with a person-oriented approach to understanding individual differences in organizations of the dynamic processes underlying adjustment. Attachment research has demonstrated the virtues of analyses of patterns of functioning to predict children's development (Ainsworth, Blehar, Waters, & Wall, 1978; Greenberg, Cicchetti, & Cummings, 1990b). With regard to organizations or patterns of responding to interparental conflict, various attempts have been made to assess patterns of children's responding to marital conflict (e.g., Cummings, 1987; El-Sheikh, Cummings, & Goetsch,

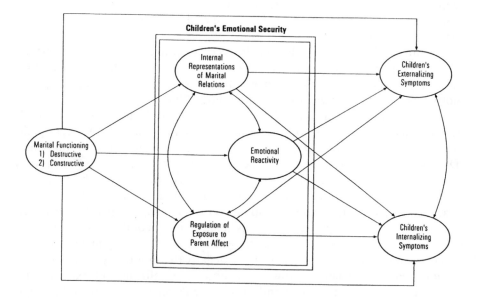

FIGURE 8.3. Marital conflict, mediating processes of emotional security, and child adjustment. From Davies and Cummings (1998). Copyright 1998 by University of Chicago Press. Adapted by permission.

1989). Recent research suggests that certain patterns of avoidance in the context of interparental conflict may possibly signify successful perseveration of emotional security in the interparental subsystem (O'Brien, Margolin, & John, 1995). Notably, however, subprocesses of emotional security are also conceptualized as subsuming multiple domains and dimensions of responding, consistent with an organizational perspective on children's adaptation.

The Distinction between Process and Outcome Variables

The emotional security hypothesis of Davies and Cummings was explicitly inspired by the principles and notions of the developmental psychopathology perspective, which is another reason for its emphasis here. A key issue from the developmental psychopathology perspective is the distinction between process and outcome variables. This notion merits consideration. Descriptive, symptom-based classification systems of child outcomes fail to acknowledge the complex nature of individuals' adaptations and transactions within their environments, leaving major gaps with regard to understanding the processes underlying the development of psychopathology (Cicchetti & Cohen, 1995a). Consequently, such static models of the development of psychopathology have inherent limitations with regard to the adequacy of explanatory models, and relatedly, the adequacy of models for diagnosis, prevention, and treatment (Jensen & Hoagwood, 1997; Richters, 1997). Thus, Sroufe (1997, p. 251) has stated that maladaptation is not something a person " 'has' . . . [but] the complex result of a myriad of risk and protective factors operating over time." Guided by these notions, process-oriented approaches (e.g., Cummings & Cummings, 1988), or more broadly, the discipline of developmental psychopathology (Cicchetti, Ackerman, & Izard, 1995), aim, as a primary goal, to identify specific processes and process relations-in-context that, over time, underlie what is broadly conceptualized as normal development, psychopathology, and symptomatology. A distinction is drawn between process variables (e.g., indices of emotional security assessed in the specific context of parental or marital relations) and outcome variables (e.g., scores on instruments designed to assess general adjustment beyond relational contexts) at the level of theory, specificity, and level of assessment. For example, illustrating this distinction, a significant body of research on relations between emotional security in close interpersonal relationships and adjustment problems classifies emotional insecurity at a different (i.e., process) level of analysis in relation to outcomes, reflecting that the constructs are distinct domains of functioning in models of developmental psychopathology (Greenberg, Cicchetti, & Cummings, 1990a). By extension, this theory reflects a corresponding "second generation" of research on children and marital problems that aims to move beyond simply documenting correlations between global notions of marital relations and child outcomes, toward understanding the more precise processes that account for or mediate the linkage, both at the level of family process (e.g., destructive and constructive dimensions of marital conflict) and child process (e.g., emotional security in different family subsystems).

Emotional Security across Different Family Subsystems

Consistent with the developmental psychopathology perspective on the importance of considering the context and organization of psychological functioning, the emotional security hypothesis acknowledges that the operation, interrelations, and meaning of concrete indicators of emotional security may be somewhat different across the different relational contexts of parent–child and interparental family subsystems. Different responses may have similar, or different, functional value in achieving a goal of emotional security within and across family subsystems. For example, although avoidance strategies are hallmarks of "avoidant" or "dismissing" attachment styles, the emotional security hypothesis posits that certain patterns of avoidance in the context of interparental conflict may possibly signify emotional security with regard to the interparental subsystem. Thus, children from low-conflict homes in which the parents have harmonious marriages may appear unconcerned about marital conflict, sometimes leaving the room in the middle of the argument. In such situations, when the parents' conflicts have been found by the child in the past to have little or no negative meaning for the family, the child is not motivated to respond or even stay in the room. Moreover, since the parents have been observed by the child to work things out well themselves, the child may assess that leaving the parents alone may foster even quicker resolution of marital issues.

While the emotional security hypothesis eschews claims that the exact behaviors have the same meaning or functional significance in achieving emotional security across family subsystems, comparability is expected in the operation of emotional security at other levels of analysis. First, the emotional security hypothesis suggests that emotional security is a goal of primary and comparable significance across the multiple family subsystems. Second, although the meaning and effectiveness of any discrete behavior are not necessarily equivalent across different relational contexts of the family subsystems, the emotional security hypothesis postulates that coherency in higher-order or organizational-level patterns of security may exist. Thus, emphasis is placed on individual differences or person-oriented levels of analyses and the meaning of patterns across multiple response systems, consistent with core concepts of attachment theory specifically, and the developmental psychopathology approach to the study of children's organizations of functioning during development more generally.

In closing, we wish to emphasize the caveat that this is a new theory and that much of the current support is suggestive, or supports only some propositions, rather than conclusive. In particular, a prospective, longitudinal test of the causal propositions of the model is needed. Moreover, there are undoubtedly other classes of processes and mechanisms that account for children's development in families as a function of marital conflict (see Figure 8.1). For example, children may learn how to handle conflicts from observing their parents' behavioral, cognitive, and emotional styles of resolving, or failing to resolve, interparental disputes (Beach, 1995). Cognitive styles of discussing and resolving disputes in the marriage may be especially influential in what children learn from their parents' behavior (Grych & Fincham, 1990). Thus, no claim is made that the emotional security hypothesis accounts for all important mediating processes in the effects of marital conflict on children. Instead, we would describe it as a midlevel, rather than grand, theory. However, consistent with the developmental psychopathology perspective, after decades of study in the absence of theory, it is important to get on with the business of proposing and improving upon theoretical models of the impact of marital conflict and violence on children.

CONTEXTUAL INFLUENCES IN THE FAMILY: MODERATING FACTORS

The size of the relationship between marital conflict and children's adjustment may also vary with other aspects of parental and family functioning. These factors are moderators of the relations between martial functioning and child adjustment. From the perspective of the developmental psychopathology approach, these might be regarded as contextual influences in the family. These elements are shown in Figure 8.1 as distal predictors of family functioning and child adjustment; that is, their influence occurs by affecting family processes that have a more proximal influence on children's dynamic processes of responding in the contexts of the family, leading over time to adaptive or maladaptive response dispositions in the context of the family and other social contexts. Current research supports a number of factors as potential moderators.

Parental Adjustment

Close relations between marital conflict and parental adjustment, particularly depression, make inclusion of parental adjustment essential to any comprehensive model of developmental pathways associated with marital conflict and family functioning. Parental depression and marital conflict are highly correlated, and causal relations between the two variables have been demonstrated (Whisman, 2000). Moreover, marital conflict accounts for important variance in the effects of parental depression on children, and parental depression, correspondingly, accounts for variance in the effects of marital conflict (see Chapter 9 for much more on these topics). Parental depression has been linked with children's emotional security, partly due to its association with marital conflict (Cummings, 1995b; Cummings & Davies, 1999).

However, little is known about the specific forms of marital conflict that are linked with parental depression, and how these particular forms of marital interaction affect children. Given the high interrelation between parental adjustment and marital conflict, joint study of these variables promises to be mutually informative. It is hypothesized that parental adjustment, particularly depression, will moderate developmental pathways. Furthermore, there has been almost no investigation of relations between *paternal* adjustment, marital conflict, and child adjustment (Cummings & O'Reilly, 1997). It is also important to assess parental adjustment more broadly than depression, in order to explore whether other parental adjustment problems may also moderate effects.

Parental Alcohol Problems

A primary mode through which parental alcohol problems affect children is the marital conflict and discord associated with parental alcohol abuse (West & Prinz, 1987). For example, some studies have reported that children are more distressed by parental conflicts than by alcohol-related behaviors (El-Sheikh & Cummings, 1997). Children of parents with alcohol problems may be especially sensitive to interparental conflicts. Thus, Ballard and Cummings (1990) found that children of parents with alcohol problems were more reactive emotionally to marital conflict than children of parents without alcohol problems. In addition, these children even suggested interventions for interparental behavior that was *not* conflictual in the course responding to a series of maritally conflictual and nonconflictual interactions presented on videotape. For example, children were shown a tape of two adults interacting in a friendly way and asked what they would do in the situation. Typically, children of parents without alcohol problems said "nothing," whereas parents of children with alcohol problems frequently described a response, typically some behavior or act designed to keep the parents in a good mood (e.g., get the parents refreshments, do housework chores). Notably, parental depression, parental alcohol problems, and marital conflict are interrelated (El-Sheikh & Cummings, 1997), so that parental depression and alcohol problems may jointly affect children's functioning by causing disruptions in family processes (West & Prinz, 1987).

Family Emotional Climate

Characteristics of the family emotional climate may also affect children by influencing marital conflict and parent–child relations. Especially important in this regard are *family emotional expressiveness* and *interparental emotional bonds* (i.e., trust, happiness, security). For example, marital anger expressions may reflect a family tendency to express more overtly both positive and negative emotions, a pattern that has been associated with social competence in children (Cassidy, Parke, Butkovsky, & Braungart, 1992). Thus, family emotional expressiveness may act as a protective factor in the context of high levels of family anger. The vignette about Eddie and Mike made this point. Eddie was not distressed about his parents' loud argument because he understood that such conflicts were usually resolved and had no broader negative implications for the family's functioning. Moreover, there was a high rate of positive affect expression between his parents as well. One possibility, from the perspective of the emotional security hypothesis, is that high rates of positive affect in the proximal context of anger and conflict may reduce children's emotional insecurity, thereby "freeing" them to understand better how people effectively manage and resolve disputes (Davies & Cummings, 1994). However, it was clear that Mike would have been quite distressed if his parents had behaved in such a manner, since, in the context of his family's patterns of expressiveness, such behavior would have indicated problems that could have serious and negative implications for future family stability and happiness. Similarly, the quality of emotional bonds between the parents has implications for how parental conflicts should be interpreted. When parents are securely attached to one another, they are likely to be more effective at parenting, and there is a greater likelihood that children will develop secure attachments to the parents. This relationship holds even if one of the parents has an insecure attachment history, which has otherwise been shown to be linked with insecure attachments between parents and children (Colin, 1996). Other research provides evidence that insecure attachment between adults and more marital conflict are associated, and that parents' histories in this regard are linked with children's functioning in conflict situations (Hall, 1997). Thus, the broader emotional climate in the family may be a significant moderator of the effects of marital conflict, and marital relations more generally, on children, and thus merits consideration in developmental tests of process-oriented models of childhood disorders.

Children's Characteristics

Children's individual *temperaments* may also affect their responses to marital conflict and other marital problems (Emery & Kitzmann, 1995). With regard to emotional security as a mediator of outcomes, temperament has sometimes been viewed as weakly related to emotional security. However, other research suggests a more important role in children's emotional security (Calkins & Fox, 1992; Vaughn et al., 1992) and its interactive effects with attachment on subsequent social development (Kochanska, 1995). Consequently, temperament is conceptualized as (1) a possible precursor of susceptibility to some dimensions of insecurity in the face of marital conflict and hostility (e.g., negative emotional reactivity), or (2) a possible buffer with regard to insecurity, with implications for subsequent social development.

Children's characteristics may also affect interparental functioning; that is, there is a bidirectional nature to family environments. This notion is consistent with the assumption of the developmental psychopathology approach that children actively influence their own adjustment and are not just passive recipients of experience. There is evidence that aggressive children respond with particular arousal to marital conflict or other forms of interadult conflicts that they witness as bystanders. One study reported that aggressive toddlers showed the greatest increase in aggression toward a same-age peer following exposure to conflict between adults (Cummings, Iannotti, & Zahn-Waxler, 1985). In a second study, children with behavior problems were more distressed than others by exposure to interadult conflict (Cummings, Vogel, Cummings, & El-Sheikh, 1989). A third study found that school-age boys classified by their teachers as aggressive were the most aroused by background anger (Klaczynski & Cummings, 1989).

Despite considerable research on the topic, a clear picture with regard to *gender differences* has not yet emerged. Early work focused on conduct problems, suggesting that boys experienced greater disturbances than girls (e.g., Emery & O'Leary, 1982), perhaps due to males' greater constitutional susceptibility to stress (e.g., Eme, 1979; Zaslow & Hayes, 1986). However, it now appears that girls may manifest distress in forms that are more difficult to detect, resulting in a serious underestimation of the effects of marital conflict. Due to socialization experiences and norms for gender-based aggression, girls may express distress in more socially acceptable ways by internalizing symptoms such as anxiety, worry, and distress (Crockenberg & Forgays, 1996; Lytton, 1991). Close scrutiny of preschoolers' responses in experimental analogues of marital conflict suggests that girls may even be more sensitive and emotionally reactive than boys to interadult conflict. The findings suggest that girls are more threatened by intense conflict, make discriminations between forms of conflict at earlier ages, and are more sensitive to whether conflicts are resolved and conflict histories between the parents are constructive versus destructive (Cummings, Pellegrini, Notarius, & Cummings, 1989; Davies, Myers, & Cummings, 1996; Davies, Myers, Cummings, & Heindel, 1999; El-Sheikh, 1994; El-Sheikh & Cummings, 1995; El-Sheikh, Cummings, & Reiter, 1996; Grych, 1998). Moreover, mediating processes appear to be different for boys and girls, with the appraised destructiveness of interparental conflict related to perceived threat in boys and self-blame related to perceived threat in girls (Cummings, Davies, & Simpson, 1994; Kerig, 1997). Thus, emotional security may be reflected in quite different psychological processes for boys and girls, with different implications for their development of competencies and vulnerabilities. On the other hand, complicating the picture, frequently, no differences are found when boys' and girls' reactions to marital conflict are *observed*. This is in contrast to the differences in reactions that seem to be more reliably found when children are interviewed about their covert emotional and cognitive reactions. For example, with regard to the former, Davis, Hops, Alpert, and Sheeber (1998) recently reported that both boys and girls evidence aggressive behavioral patterns in response to martial conflict. Thus, the differences in the immediate and observable responses of boys and girls to marital conflict may be relatively small; more important may be the role of their internal reactions that cannot be seen, especially their more subtle, and covert, appraisals and emotional responses, as mediators of differing trajectories of long-term development.

Parent Gender × Child Gender

Differentiating between children's responses to mothers' and fathers' marital conflict behaviors and parenting practices may further advance understanding of gender differences (Cummings & O'Reilly, 1997). Interparental conflict is uniquely related to children's perceptions of the father–child relationship, even after taking into account perceptions of mother–child relations (Osborne & Fincham, 1996). More specifically, fathers' positive qualities appear to be more likely to deteriorate than those of mothers in the face of marital stress and conflict (e.g., Amato & Booth, 1991; Howes & Markman, 1989; Jouriles & Farris, 1992). If so, it is possible that fathers' parenting practices play a more robust role than those of mothers in linkages between marital conflict and child adjustment. However, plausible hypotheses for this possible difference require further examination. For example, women may be better at compartmentalizing the spousal and parental roles, resulting in less carryover from marital relations to parenting for mothers (Belsky, Youngblade, Rovine, & Volling, 1991). Another hypothesis is that motherhood is a more fundamental role than is fatherhood (Belsky, Gilstrap, & Rovine, 1984).

Further complicating the issue, new evidence suggests that one must consider the match between the sex of the parents and children. Girls have been reported to exhibit more negative emotional responses than boys only in response to their fathers' behavior during marital disagreements (Crockenberg & Forgays, 1996). Fathers' parenting quality and relationships with their daughters are particularly prone to decline as marital discord increases (Belsky, Rovine, & Fish, 1989; Booth & Amato, 1994; Goldberg & Easterbrooks, 1984; McHale, 1994). On the other hand, interparental conflict has been shown to be a better predictor of negativity in mother–son relations than in mother–daughter and father–son relationships (Osborne & Fincham, 1996). Interestingly, Grych (1998) recently reported that father-to-mother and mother-to-father aggression were each independent predictors of children's adjustment. Another intriguing recent finding is that aggressive behavior directed by adolescents toward the mother in interparental conflict predicted adjustment problems for both boys and girls, but these responses were most significant predictors for boys when the mother had attacked the father, whereas they were most significant for girls when the father had initiated conflict with the mother (Davis et al., 1998).

Race

Race may relate to differences in family systems, sensitivity to contextual factors, and differential attributions about contextual factors. However, there are no published comparisons of black families and white families on marital conflict and its effects on children. The higher incidence of single parents (excluded in this study) and extended families in the black community may possibly affect the nature of marital conflict and its meaning for children. For the value of research in this area to have pertinence to all families, there is an urgent need for researchers to examine the effects of marital conflict on children in African American and other minority groups, as well as conflict with extended family members or live-in partners, given family structures in different ethnic niches.

Histories of Family Distress

We have seen that children's reactions to marital conflict are a function of their histories of exposure to conflict, with elevated responding associated with histories of greater past exposure. However, there is reason to believe that children's sensitization to marital conflict may reflect more general appraisals of family functioning as well. Thus, studies comparing physically abused and nonabused boys from low socioeconomic backgrounds have reported that abused boys are more likely to become aggressive following exposure, to intervene in marital conflicts, and to benefit in terms of reduced distress reactions by observing the resolution of conflict (Cummings, Hennessy, Rabideau, & Cicchetti, 1994; Hennessy, Rabideau, Cicchetti, & Cummings, 1994). Moreover, children from families that are distressed for reasons other than conflict or abuse histories also appear to be more reactive to exposure to marital conflict, and other forms of family conflict as well. Thus, Nixon and Cummings (1999) found that children with disabled siblings reported more anger, sadness, fear, personal responsibility, and dispositions toward intervening in marital and other forms of conflict involving family members (e.g., parent–child conflict, sibling–peer conflict) than children without disabled siblings. The literature suggests that families with disabled children experience more general distress than other families, including more marital conflict. Interestingly, Nixon and Cummings did *not* find significantly more marital distress in their sample, although maternal depression was elevated in relation to the control group. Other studies found that children *report* distress in response to a variety of types of family conflict other than marital conflict, although reactions are typically significantly greater to marital conflict (El-Sheikh & Cheskes, 1995; Hall & Cummings, 1997), and distress reactions in response to other forms of family conflict are reported less frequently (Grych, 1998).

   Behavior problems also may be more elevated in children from families with spousal violence than in families without spousal violence, whether or not the children directly observe the incidents of violence (Jouriles et al., 1998). This may be due to the fact that information about violence is just as upsetting to a child's sense of emotional security as actually observing the events. For example, with regard to positive information about conflict, children's distress is allayed just as much by hearing an explanation that the conflict was resolved as by actually observing the resolution (Cummings, Simpson, & Wilson, 1993). Thus, children's heightened reactivity to marital conflict may reflect an elevated sense of emotional insecurity based on a familywide analysis of current and past family functioning, and not necessarily a reaction to histories of marital conflict per se, although that is clearly the most commonly reported, and likely the most important, single family predictor of sensitization to marital conflict. On the other hand, children's distress in response to other stresses may be related to marital conflict. For example, El-Sheikh (1997) reported that in comparison to children from low-marital-conflict homes, children from high-marital-conflict homes were more distressed by *mother–child* disputes. These findings also suggest that there may be significant interactions between interparental and other conflict histories in the family in predicting children's adjustment over time (Grych, 1998).

STUDYING DEVELOPMENTAL PATHWAYS PROSPECTIVELY: A DIRECTION FOR FUTURE RESEARCH

As noted in Chapter 4, the study of developmental pathways is a critical element of the developmental psychopathology perspective. However, most studies, particularly studies that comprehensively test multiple dimensions of children's stress and coping with marital conflict, and that disaggregate the forms of expression of marital conflict, have been based on cross-sectional designs; that is, data-intensive assessments of multidimensional, multidomain, and multimethod assessments of the effects of marital conflicts on children have typically been based upon cross-sectional research, which has limited capacity to support causal inferences about the course of development over time. Marital conflict has been shown, prospectively, to predict children's adjustment problems (e.g., Block, Block, & Morrison, 1981), but such tests have been based upon limited model testing and assessments with regard to constructs concerning marital relations and children's adjustment (e.g., Harold, Fincham, Osborne, & Conger, 1997; Howes & Markman, 1989). These studies are even more limited in terms of assessing mediating processes and moderating factors that link marital conflict and child outcomes.

While there is not yet firm evidence on developmental pathways associated with marital conflict, some points can be made about age effects based on research to date. The evidence concerning how children are affected early in life by exposure to marital conflict is quite remarkable. Thus, observational studies based on children's reactions to marital conflict in the home indicate that *even 1-year-olds* react, often with vigorous emotional and behavioral responses as bystanders to their parents' conflicts, including overtly angry, even aggressive displays, crying, yelling, distressed vocalizations, and sadness or scared facial expressions (Cummings, Zahn-Waxler, & Radke-Yarrow, 1981). Even at this age, children sometimes try to intervene in their parents' conflicts. For example, in one case, a 1-year-old heard his parents arguing in the kitchen and then urgently cried, "Mommy, mommy!" Hearing her son's cries, the mother had to break off her argument with her husband and go to the living room to see how her son was. The child's response was to smile broadly! In another instance, a little 1-year-old girl kissed and wiped off her mommy's tears after her mother had a terrible fight with the father. It is remarkable how many parents are unaware of the sensitivity of even very young children to their conflicts.

While young children may not understand the content of the parents' arguments, they are highly sensitive to their conflicts and remain highly sensitive to unresolved and chronic fighting between the parents throughout childhood. As we have noted, some developmental psychopathologists posit that there are stage-salient tasks for children during development. In some instances, relatedly, there are stage-salient stressors. For example, separation from parents is a stage-salient task that reflects the significance of early attachment relations to infant's functioning, but separation from parents becomes dramatically less stressful for children as they get older. From this perspective, it is interesting to note that marital conflict does not appear to be a stage-salient stressor for children; that is, it is stressful for children throughout their development, and there is evidence that adults and the elderly report that marital conflict is stressful for them as well (Hall & Cummings, 1997).

Reactions do change with age. Thus, younger children are also less able to interpret the distinction between resolved and unresolved conflicts, and otherwise understand the implications and causes of conflicts (Davies, Myers, & Cummings, 1996; El-Sheikh & Cummings, 1995; Grych, 1998). They also react in a manner that suggests a greater sense of helplessness and are more prone to self-blame. On the other hand, older children are more likely actually to become involved in the conflicts and may more often become enmeshed in these situations. However, these differences are not at all readily interpretable in terms of making decisions about which age groups or developmental levels are more vulnerable to exposure to high levels of marital conflict. On the other hand, with regard to age effects, it is difficult to disentangle whether developmental level or children's different length of histories of exposure to marital conflict account for differences in patterns of responding. There are a variety of additional complicating factors, such as the possibility that parents fight differently in front of children of different ages, children at different ages are vulnerable to different problems, or furthermore, that there may be differences for boys and girls in the problems exhibited at different ages. There are certainly studies documenting disorders associated with marital conflict at all of the ages of childhood. Thus, the findings to date do not support conclusions that one age or another is more vulnerable to high levels of marital conflict in the family, although expressions of vulnerability may vary with age as well as other factors, such as gender.

CONCLUSION

The study of relations between marital conflict and child adjustment has been guided in recent years by models that are quite consistent with the principles of the developmental psychopathology approach to uncovering the processes that underlie children's development and risk for adjustment problems (Cummings & Cummings, 1988; Cummings & El-Sheikh, 1991; Davies & Cummings, 1994). Thus, the great progress in understanding that has taken place over the past 10–15 years is a tribute to the utility of this approach for making scientific progress on questions that are complex and quite difficult to study. As we have shown in the course of our discussion, multiple factors and pathways have been implicated as possibly important and as therefore meriting inclusion in future research designed to study these questions. Prospective, longitudinal research is required, and urgently needed, for testing causal pathways over time, including models of mediating and moderating processes. As we have seen, information about pathways of development constitutes a significant gap in our understanding of relations between marriages, children, and families. The potential significance for clinical science and practice of more sophisticated and complex studies for an adequate developmental psychopathology of families and children is notable given the clear links with childhood disorders. In addition, more complex models of mediating and moderating processes that examine development over time are needed, and these fit well with the principles outlined in the developmental psychopathology perspective. Thus, this area of research and theory should have obvious practice implications and, thus, should be a proving ground, in a sense, for the promise of this approach if we are to advance to a second generation of research on the study of childhood disorders.

For example, longitudinal research needs to examine changes in children and marital functioning over time. Thus, it will be especially important to investigate how stability and change in marital conflict forecast change in children's behavior problems, an issue heretofore never systematically studied. Children whose parents reduce marital conflict (or learn to manage it better) should show diminished difficulties. When conflict begins or is exacerbated, there is likely to be an escalation in children's emotional difficulties. The study of these questions has particularly important clinical implications, especially when studies provide insights into the critical processes underlying childhood outcomes. Research that aims to test the tenets of the emotional security hypothesis further is thus especially promising given the already developed theoretical and empirical foundation for the tenets of this model. Fortunately, several laboratories, including investigators with considerable experience in this area, are now undertaking such complex longitudinal studies. Armed with the extensive body of research that has accumulated in recent years about process relations between marital conflict, children's functioning, and child adjustment, investigators in the area of marital relations and children's development are poised to undertake research that comprehensively addresses the questions and issues at hand.

Finally, since the quality of interparental relations has such significant implications for children's development and is a function of the parents' behavior, marital relations might properly be conceptualized as another dimension of parenting. The view that marital relations (or the termination or lack of marital relations) are a dimension of parenting is consistent with a holistic perspective on parental behavior in families and the implications of parental behavior for child development. This perspective on marital relations as parenting is consistent with the developmental psychopathology perspective, which emphasizes a broader organizational view of the multiplicity of influences on children's development in families.

CHAPTER NINE

Applications of Developmental Psychopathology: Parental Depression, Families, and Children's Development

In this chapter, we consider yet another approach used by developmental psychopathologists in the study of children and families; that is, instead of being concerned with a specific family subsystem, this chapter examines multiple family processes that affect a specific group of children. Developmental psychopathology is often focused specifically on groups of children at risk for psychopathology.

We illustrate this fact of developmental psychopathology by examining a particular group of children at risk, that is, children of depressed parents. Over the past two decades, parental personality and adjustment have increasingly been regarded as a one of the determinants of a multiplicity of processes linked with family functioning and broader ecological contexts (Belsky, 1984; see Figure II.1). Specifically, we focus on children at risk for adjustment problems as a function of the constellation of familial variables associated with parental depression. Consider the following cases:

Joe's father had been diagnosed with major unipolar depression. Joe's paternal grandfather had also experienced episodes of depression. Nonetheless, Joe's parents were both attentive and responsive as parents, and Joe's father spent a great deal of time with him when he was growing up. Even during his bouts of depression, Joe's father remained attentive and emotionally warm toward Joe except when his symptomatology was particularly severe. Joe's mother was very supportive of her husband, and they had a secure attachment relationship with each other as married partners. Both parents were highly educated and hardworking, and the family enjoyed a middle- to upper-middle-class lifestyle. Relations between Joe and his two sisters, Kelly and Mona, were close and supportive. Joe did well in school and was popular, although he tended to be shy in large groups. He was admitted to an excellent university and studied medicine, becoming a pediatrician after many years of schooling. His eventual marriage was happy and both Joe and his wife were themselves attentive and responsive as parents. Joe experienced periods of anxiety and, on occasion, mild to moderate symptoms of depression, but he never sought therapy, and his symptoms were rarely more than subclinical.

Frank's mother was diagnosed with major depressive disorder, and her mother had been depressed before her. Frank's mother and father divorced when he was 10, after many years of intense marital conflict, which included sometimes dangerous episodes of reciprocal and mutual interparental aggression during the last years of the marriage. Until the time of the divorce, both parents had also been generally emotionally unresponsive toward the children, often inconsistent and negligent in parenting, and they constantly involved Frank and his sister, Edie Jo, in their marital conflicts, frequently blaming them for their marital problems. Frank and Edie Jo constantly fought and were never close to each other. Frank was highly aggressive and difficult in preschool, and over the years, his behavioral problems worsened. By adolescence, Frank was habitually delinquent, and he dropped out of high school. As an adult, Frank also was diagnosed with depressive disorder, just like his mother, and his interpersonal relationships were tumultuous and typically short-lived.

These cases illustrate some of the different pathways of development that may be evidenced by children with depressed parents. Note that both children came from families with histories of depression. However, despite depression in family members, family interactions in Joe's family were positive, supportive, and loving. On the other hand, members of Frank's family were conflictual and emotionally unsupportive toward each other. Not surprisingly, quite different outcomes were found for the children from these different family environments, despite the fact that both Frank and Joe could be characterized as children of depressed parents.

These examples make an important point: Children's psychological outcomes and the quality of family relations vary widely in families with parental depression or other problems known to increase children's risk for adjustment problems (e.g., alcoholism). Accordingly, children's risk for adjustment problems is probabilistic, not certain, and many children in even the most adverse family circumstances will develop normally, or may even become high functioning (Garmezy, 1985). These facts are not puzzling, but actually make good sense if one understands children's development from a dynamic, process-oriented perspective rather than as a function of the presence, or absence, of static marker variables (e.g., parental mental illness); that is, children's development stems from the complex, and multiple, processes of functioning that emerge from the transaction of intra- and extraorganismic factors over time in specific familial and extrafamilial contexts. In every circumstance, there may be protective factors that serve as sources of resiliency. Some of these protective factors may come from within the child. For example, the child may have an easy temperament, with a high capacity to adapt, or even profit, from adversity. On the other hand, some protective factors may be external to the child. For example, a girl's father, despite being alcoholic and depressed, may remain very loving and caring toward her. While she may experience the negative sequelae of the father's problems, she may also firmly understand that she is loved and may treasure and benefit from those experiences that are supportive and special.

However, the message is not simply that many different familial experiences may be subsumed within the fact that a parent is diagnosed with a disorder. Returning to the issues in Chapter 2, the most significant point, from a developmental psychopathology perspective, is that children's adjustment must be understood at a process-oriented level of analysis that reflects the multiple and complex social, emotional, cognitive, physiological, and other elements of the child's functioning in multiple specific contexts, and that are continuously being adapted to circumstances throughout the course of development over the days, weeks, months, and years of the child's life. Admittedly, this fact does not make matters easier, at least at first, for the clinical researcher or practitioner hoping to understand or treat children at risk for disorder, or children who have developed disorders. However, over the long term, this perspective is likely to result in models of development that account for much more of the variance in the scientific prediction of child outcomes, and that provide a much firmer foundation for insightful and effective interventions with children and families. These assumptions are at the heart of the second generation of research on childhood psychopathology.

In this chapter, we see that children of depressed parents are at greater risk for adjustment problems than children with nondepressed parents, and we review evidence that suggests the significant role of interpersonal relations in families in outcomes associated with depression in families. On the other hand, we again wish to emphasize: Many children of depressed parents do not develop psychopathology, and family relations, despite depression in a parent, can nonetheless be positive and supportive. As we see quite clearly in this chapter, consistent with the themes of the developmental psychopathology perspective, many different intra- (e.g., genetics) and extraorganismic (e.g., family relations) factors influence children's development.

Thus, in this chapter, we begin with a sample or group rather than a family subsystem. The focus on at-risk groups fosters a person-oriented perspective on developmental processes and pathways, which, as we have seen, provides an important perspective on the development of adjustment problems (Sroufe & Rutter, 1984). There are other advantages to a focus on at-risk groups as well, as we will see later. This is not to claim that the study of at-risk groups is the best method to advance a process-oriented perspective. The emphasis of the developmental psychopathology perspective is on fostering multiple methods and perspectives rather than valuing one approach to the exclusion of others. A more appropriate statement is that the study of the normal and the abnormal in relation to each other is the most effective way to advance a developmental psychopathology perspective, and the study of at-risk groups in relation to normal groups is a means of examining the abnormal in relation to the normal from a family environment (or other contextual) perspective.

We show that the literature on children of depressed parents indicates the importance of taking into account family influences, and, in fact, multiple family influences, when conceptualizing the development of children. In a sense, we are making good here on a promissory note that has appeared repeatedly in the volume to this point: We have frequently used children of depressed parents as examples, and we now proceed to elaborate. As we will see, these examples of children of depressed parents illustrate that (1) patterns of adaptation and maladaptation have multiple sources within the family and the individual, and (2) a narrow view focusing on only one familial, or individual, factor ultimately is likely to be misleading about the course of children's development in these families. Since considerable, accumulated evidence indicates that children of depressed parents are at risk due to dysfunctional marital relations as well as problematic parenting, a consideration of this sample is particularly appropriate to the presentation of a familywide perspective on risk processes that may lead to psychopathology in children. However, we also see that even in this instance of a much-researched risk group, we are only beginning to glimpse some of the critical processes that mediate children's development, and much progress remains to be made in order to reach a process-oriented understanding of children's development in these family environments.

THE IMPORTANCE OF THE STUDY OF AT-RISK SAMPLES FOR THE DEVELOPMENTAL PSYCHOPATHOLOGIST

Understanding the development of children at risk for adjustment problems is an important aspect of developmental psychopathology research; that is, for the developmental psychopathologist, the study of at-risk samples is an important topic in its own right. Because the study of such samples is a frequent focus of the developmental psychopathologist, this topic merits brief discussion and elaboration.

The study of at-risk samples is an area of special interest to the developmental psychopathologist because of not only the high incidence of maladaptation but also the occurrence of normal adjustment, with the corresponding diversity of pathways, and myriad influences on pathways, of development. More broadly, the multiple and essential processes underlying development are likely to be particularly illuminated in such samples, with a higher base rate of processes underlying the development of psychopathology. This fact makes understanding the development of children at risk especially likely to have a high payoff for clinical work: An understanding of the processes underlying developmental deviations is of inherent interest to the clinician. The relatively high incidence of developmental deviations (e.g., diagnoses of psychopathology) makes the study of these groups especially informative for those in clinical practice, including directions concerned with the articulation of preventive and intervention strategies. Moreover, since rates of clinically significant outcomes are elevated in such cases, clinically relevant pathways of development are more likely to be observed. In addition, a range of outcomes, from high social competence to extreme disorder, are more likely to be found in such samples, so that processes of risk and vulnerability, protection and competence, may each be much more evident here than in community samples. In unselected community samples, by contrast, there may be an overrepresentation of positive outcome and influence processes, so that negative outcomes, and the processes underlying negative outcomes, may occur too infrequently for meaningful analysis. There is a double-edged sword here: In terms of time and resources, the cost required for comprehensive analysis of processes of child and family functioning (e.g., detailed and multilevel analyses of familial interactions in the laboratory or home) is likely to be very high, so that the study of only relatively small samples may be practical. When only relatively small sample sizes can be studied, however, the incidence of maladaptive child and family processes with potential clinical significance may be very small indeed in an unselected community sample. This reality also argues for the focus on, or at least the inclusion of, at-risk groups in research on childhood psychopathology.

Advances in process-oriented understanding of pathways of development for at-risk groups also have implications for the conceptualization of strategies for clinical practice and intervention within the family, because these children and families are more likely to be referred for clinical assessment. In addition, perhaps even more important from a developmental psychopathology perspective, understanding pathways of development for at-risk groups lays the groundwork for the possibility of intervention before disturbances become full-blown and therefore, typically, much more difficult to ameliorate effectively (Kazdin, 1994f; Reid, 1993); that is, by being able to identify children at-risk for later adjustment problems, perhaps even years before their problems reach the level of diagnostic disturbance (e.g., major depression, conduct disorders), clinicians may be able to provide prevention programs that greatly reduce the likelihood of the later development of disturbances, based on an informed understanding of pathways and processes of development (e.g., Conduct Problems Research Group, 1992; Reid, 1993). Thus, a virtue of being able to begin to identify and track pathways of development that predict later disturbance before disorders become manifest is that interventions may be initiated when they are more cost-effective (i.e., briefer, less intensive) and more likely to succeed. With regard to the centrality of preventive directions to the developmental psychopathology movement, Cicchetti and Cohen (1995a, p. 13) have made the following points:

> Because the discipline of developmental psychopathology is concerned with the detection of developmental deviance before an actual disturbance crystallizes, as well as the course of disorders once exhibited (Sroufe, 1989), knowledge derived from research in this field possesses considerable relevance for application to the prevention and treatment of high-risk and psychopathological conditions. The value of applying a developmental psychopathology perspective to prevention and intervention efforts was captured by Sroufe and Rutter (1984), who have stated: "[B]y throughly understanding factors that pull subjects toward or away from increased risk at various age periods, one not only acquires a deeper understanding of development but one also gains valuable information for primary prevention" (p. 19). Additionally, once a disorder has become manifested, knowledge of the mechanisms that contributed to the maladaptive outcome can be applied to remediation.

That is, the study of at-risk, but not yet psychopathological, groups provides bases for identifying, and helping, individuals before problems become clinically significant, stable, resistant to change, and, consequently, much more difficult to treat successfully. There is considerable theoretical and empirical foundation for these assumptions (e.g., Coie, Terry, Lenox, Lochman, & Hyman, 1995; Kellam, Ling, Merisca, Brown, & Ialongo, 1998). These directions are a logical outgrowth of the articulation by the developmental psychopathologist of children's problems as developmental deviance rather than static, diagnostic entities, points that we covered in some detail in Chapters 2 and 3. Thus, the study of developmental pathways that may lead to later disturbance, and the corresponding search for preventive interventions to be initiated before problems develop or become entrenched, provides a promising direction for clinical researchers and for clinical practice, with the promise of better, cheaper, and more effective approaches to the amelioration of social and emotional problems.

The example of children of depressed parents also provides an instance of risk for psychopathology that often runs in families. This topic is of considerable interest for the student of families and children. The problem of the intergenerational transmission of risk has significant societal as well as clinical importance; that is, there is great cost to society when the problems of groups are chronic and continue from one generation to the next. How does one break these insidious cycles? Is society doomed to repeat continuously its past problems? How does society cope with the fact that individuals from high-risk environments may have higher birth rates, thus increasing the proportion of children in at-risk settings from one generation to the next? Unfortunately, these problems are not solvable simply with good intentions (a necessary but insufficient ingredient!). There is a need for knowledge to inform efforts to break the cycles of risk.

Evidence emerging from recent prospective, longitudinal studies is particularly cogent in demonstrating the role of familial factors in the intergenerational transmission of risk (Serbin & Stack, 1998). Thus, there is accumulating evidence for the intergenerational transmission of risk, and the role of family processes in the transmission of risk. In addition to parental depression, a number of other familial factors associated with children's risk for adjustment problems have been identified, including teenage pregnancy, which may be an intergenerational phenomenon (Hardy, Astone, Brooks-Gunn, Shapiro, & Miller, 1998), parental aggression and withdrawal (Serbin et al., 1998), and antisocial behavior in parents (Capaldi & Clark, 1998). Thus, while the focus of this chapter is on parental depression, we intend these data and this discussion to exemplify much wider issues of interest to the developmental psychopathologist. Thus, a variety of other familial factors have also been associated with children's risk for adjustment problems and the intergenerational transmission of risk; that is, in a variety of respects, parental depression illustrates a problem of broader interest to the developmental psychopathologist than the impact of this particular pattern of symptoms on families. We return to the practice implications of this research and address these matters at length in Part III of this volume.

RISK IS ASSOCIATED WITH MULTIPLE FAMILY PROCESSES IN CHILDREN OF DEPRESSED PARENTS

Parental depression presents particularly intriguing subject matter for the developmental psychopathologist concerned with familial influences on development. Familial influences reflect genetic inheritance; at the same time, complex patterns of social and emotional family processes also factor into children's risk for the development of psychopathology, which may or may not have some basis in genetics but are certainly to an important extent environmental at both distal and proximal levels of analysis. With regard to parental depression, it is important at the outset to appreciate that depression does not occur in isolation from other family processes related to children's risk for the development of adjustment problems, whether or not there is a genetic disposition toward depression. In fact, the opposite is certainly the case. The following example illustrates one possible scenario:

Mary was the child of a mother diagnosed with major depression. By adolescence, Mary had developed significant problems with anxiety and depression. However, numerous family circumstances complicated Mary's and her mother's problems. In therapy, it emerged that Mary's problems appeared to have multiple sources. Mary's mother and father fought a great deal, often over money and the father's job problems and stresses. In addition, Mary's mother attempted to self-medicate with alcohol, developing a serious drinking problem. Moreover, it appeared that it was in response to these conflicts, the alcohol abuse, and other stresses, that Mary's mother developed symptoms of depression. Accordingly, for the good of all family members, and because she loved her mother, Mary felt that she had to mediate the parents' disputes and alleviate her mother's sadness. Over time, these multiple family problems took a heavy toll on Mary's psychological well-being.

Thus, on the surface it would appear that Mary's problems were due to her mother's depression, and that it might well be the case that the risk was genetic in origin. However, closer examination suggests that many environmental aspects of family functioning, as well as her mother's depression, were pertinent. In particular, it is evident in this example that feeling she needed to care for her mother had a considerable psychological impact on Mary. In fact, it is worth noting that even such complex chains of family circumstances have been documented (Cummings & Davies, 1994b, 1999; El-Sheikh & Cummings, 1997; Nixon & Cummings, 1999).

The message of this vignette is that children's development is not influenced by individual family systems in isolation from the rest of the family environment. Instead, children's adjustment derives from a complex set of transactions between the individual and multiple family systems. Risk for disorder can have origins in multiple, different sources within the family, including genetic inheritance, and there may be cumulative risk associated with the combined effects of multiple family influences. Moreover, the risk may be cumulative rather than merely additive. Family systems are not independent, but mutually influential (Cummings & Davies, 1994a). The example of Mary and her mother provides an illustration of how multiple family factors may be related to children's risk for adjustment problems.

FAMILY INFLUENCES RELATED TO THE ADJUSTMENT OF CHILDREN OF DEPRESSED PARENTS

Returning to the main themes of this chapter, research also indicates notably heightened risk for adjustment problems among children of depressed parents. Moreover, with regard to family processes, compelling evidence concerning multiple possible modes of familial transmission of risk has accumulated for these children. Thus, this group serves as a pertinent example for making more general points about the development of children in high-risk families, illustrating how multiple familial factors can contribute to risk for children's adjustment problems. In particular, family researchers have often focused exclusively on parenting as a mediator of risk (Patterson, 1998), ignoring, or only very weakly assessing, the effects of other family systems, such as marital relations. Inadequate assessment of family variables makes it inevitable that those variables will emerge statistically as poor predictors, regardless of their actual status as formative influences on children's development (i.e., error variance due to weak assessment will submerge prediction, especially in competition with more rigorously measured constructs). Moreover, if an important family variable is not assessed, it will not even be a weak predictor! Adequate assessment of the effects of family systems beyond parenting requires considerable care in the design of research (Fincham, 1997). Researchers concerned with parental depression have made notable attempts to go beyond simply paying lip service to broader family systems both in assessment and in the design of prospective, longitudinal tests of causal models of the effects of different family systems on children's development. This fact alone makes this literature of special interest to the developmental psychopathologist concerned with multivariate models of family relations and child development.

Risk for Adjustment Problems

There is a considerable basis for viewing children of depressed parents as being at greater risk for adjustment problems than children without a depressed parent. Children of depressed parents have been found to be two to five times more likely to develop behavioral problems than children of normal parents (Beardslee, Bemporad, Keller, & Klerman, 1983), with even higher rates of disorder reported in some studies. A significant percentage of children of depressed parents develop depression, and over one-third of parents with a depressed child are depressed themselves (Puig-Antich et al., 1989). Children of depressed parents are at greater risk not only for depression and mood disorders but also for a variety of other forms of psychological and medical dysfunction (Weissman, Warner, Wickramaratne, Moreau, & Olfson, 1997). On the other hand, as many children of depressed parents do *not* develop psychopathology, the study of children of depressed parents is also of interest for the knowledge that can be gained about how children may cope effectively despite adversity. The mechanisms involved in intergenerational discontinuity (i.e., protective factors) are as interesting and important for developmental models as the mechanisms contributing to intergenerational continuity (Rutter, 1998). In summary, the multiplicity of pathways of risk and normalcy that are reported among children of depressed parents makes this a fascinating family context for the study of processes pertinent to a developmental psychopathology perspective.

A Framework of Familial Influences

Figure 9.1 provides an outline of the factors that we consider with regard to the effects of parental depression on children's adjustment. Consistent with this, we examine children's development as a function of genetic factors, extrafamilial influences, parental symptoms of depression, parenting, parent–child attachment, marital influences, and children's own characteristics.

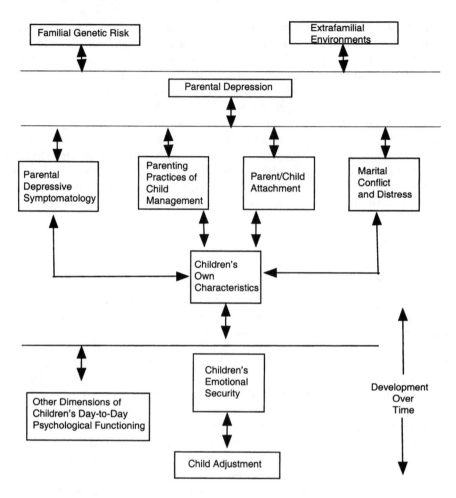

FIGURE 9.1. A framework for the effects of parental depression on children.

Genetic Inheritance as a Family Factor

While this chapter focuses on social and emotional aspects of family functioning that influence the risk for depression among children of depressed parents, it is important to recognize that another source of familial risk concerns the genetic inheritance of depression and/or susceptibility to psychopathology in children of depressed parents. A simple explanation for risk among children of depressed parents is that genes control certain biological processes that, in turn, lead to the development of depression. In line with this reasoning, neurophysiological investigations into the operation of various antidepressant medications have implicated the neurotransmitters norepinephrine and serotonin in the occurrence of depression (Garbutt et al., 1994). Various research directions indicate the significance of biological processes in the occurrence of depression, including animal investigations of the pharmacokinetics of antidepressant medications, studies of cerebrospinal fluid and plasma metabolites in depressed people (e.g., Goodwin & Jamison, 1990), and investigations of neurotransmitter receptors (e.g., McNeal & Cimbolic, 1986). Also, children may inherit temperamental characteristics or mood states–personality factors that increase risk for depression that may have biological bases (Cicchetti, Rogosch, & Toth, 1998).

However, the implication of biological processes in the onset and course of depressive episodes or symptomatology does not indicate genetics as a sole, or even the originating, cause. For example, with regard to the notion that biological factors may not be the original cause of depression even when they are implicated, it has been shown that environmental events and experiences can induce or influence change in biological systems; that is, the direction of effects may be from environmental experience to biological change, rather than the other way around. Thus, environmental stress can cause a neurophysiological sensitization that then enhances subsequent stress reactivity (Gold, Goodwin, & Chrousos, 1988; Post, Rubinow, & Ballenger, 1986). Moreover, even when genes play a role in influencing biological structures, the resulting biological manifestations require an eliciting environment in which to be expressed, and an environment of particular importance for children and adolescents is the family. Genetic factors are most likely to be important to risk for depression among children with parents and families having a significant history of depression (e.g., a history of depression in multiple family members and across multiple generations). However, even when the genetic diathesis for depression is significant, and depression is likely to emerge at some point in children's development, the family environment may be the penultimate link in the causal sequence that begins with genes and culminates in a major mood disorder. Hence, it is important to bear in mind that "family" studies of depression, directed at establishing genetic/biological causes, do not rule out the significance of other causes, both biological and environmental ones, in the family.

More specifically, traditional family studies that focus on genetics may underestimate the causal variance in psychopathology arising from social and emotional aspects of family environments in which one parent is depressed, particularly when the only familial source examined is family history of depression. In studies such as these, only instances of depression among children of depressed parents support familial transmission of depression. Depressed children of, say, overly punitive parents in the same studies would not support familial transmission of depression unless the punitive parents were also depressed. Family processes other than depression, no matter how profound their effects, would not be exposed by "familial" studies of this sort.

Evidence concerning the parental-depression-to-child-depression link says nothing about the effect of parental depression on other indicators of child adjustment; nor does it say anything about the effect of other forms of parental adjustment on child depression. In fact, parental depression is a broadband predictor of children's adjustment problems, including depression, but also a variety of other disorders, including conduct disorders and other externalizing problems (Downey & Coyne, 1990). Moreover, many individuals who develop depression do not have depressed parents. These various lines of evidence strongly indicate that biological models can only partially, and quite incompletely, explain the association between depression in parents and maladjustment in children.

Parental Depression and Marital Conflict

There are interrelations between multiple family processes associated with parental depression even when children's functioning is not specifically considered. For example, it is quite intentional that in Figure 9.1, a bidirectional arrow is drawn between marital conflict and parental depression. In our example at the outset of the chapter, we suggested that depression in Mary's mother was related, in part, to marital conflict. As we see later, there is considerable support for the particular proposition that parental depression and marital conflict are linked.

Research on relations between parental depression and marital conflict merits careful examination given the evidence we consider later: that marital conflict is an important predictor of children's adjustment problems in families with parental depression; that is, these data are also persuasive regarding the need for a familywide model of the effects of depression in families, and for the inadequacy of examining only one family subsystem in accounting for the effects of depression. In a sense, this particular line of research might be seen as less relevant than others to the goals of this chapter, because it focuses on spousal functioning when adults (who may also be parents) have depression. However, in another sense, it is a particularly pertinent line of research, since it makes the case quite clearly that parental depression has significant effects on family subsystems other than parenting. The notion that marital relations and other broader family contexts are affected by parental depression is central to the cogency of a familywide model describing children's adjustment in families with depression. For example, parental depression may explain variance in the relationship between marital conflict and child adjustment; at the same time, marital conflict may account for elements of the relationship between parental depression and child adjustment. It is also in the spirit of the developmental psychopathology approach to consider wider, rather than narrower, patterns of influence processes in the family.

Considerable evidence has accumulated to indicate that parental depression and marital conflict and distress are linked (Beach, Smith, & Fincham, 1994). While these relations have long been suggested by correlational studies (Cummings & Davies, 1994a), recent work supports causal relations between these variables, although the directions of effects go both ways (Whisman,

2000). The data also suggest that the provision of support by the non-depressed spouse is significant, although, as we will see, support and reassurance seeking by depressed individuals does not necessarily have the desirable long-term effect of ameliorating depression.

Marital Conflict

Depressed individuals are more negative, unsupportive, critical, and intrusive with their spouses, frequently experiencing high levels of marital conflict, including overt hostility, poor communication, avoidance and withdrawal, and sexual dissatisfaction (Beach, Smith, & Fincham, 1994; Downey, Feldman, Khuri, & Friedman, 1994). The significance of the relations between parental depression and marital conflict receives support in an emerging body of research. One study found that more than 50% of depressed persons in treatment reported significant marital disputes (Coyne, Schwoeri, & Downey, 1994). Another study reported that individuals who have conflictual marriages are 10 times more likely to experience depressive symptomatology than individuals who do not report marital conflict (O'Leary, Christian, & Mendell, 1994). Yet another study found that in conflictual marriages in which the husbands are depressed, the wives have an increased risk of suffering both mild and severe husband-to-wife violence (Pan, Neidig, & O'Leary, 1994). Finally, Beach and Nelson (1990) reported the correlation between marital adjustment and depression to be −.35 after 6 months of marriage and −.56 after 18 months of marriage.

Epidemiological data on relations between depression and marital conflict make similar points. Epidemiological data are relevant to the pervasiveness of a phenomenon, since concerns about sampling biases are minimized (e.g., studies based on clinical samples are subject to the concern that biased samples of individuals may seek treatment). In one such study, depression was found to be 25 times more likely among those who reported unhappy marriages than among those who said their marriages were happy. Even though men were half as likely as women to be depressed, this 25-times rate also held for men from unhappy versus happy marriages (Weissman, 1987). Less compelling evidence, but results nonetheless consistent with substantially higher rates of depression among both men and women in distressed marriages also have been reported in more recent epidemiological studies (Whisman, 2000).

Marital *improvements* have also been found to precede recovery from depression (Brown, Lemyre, & Bifulco, 1992). Conversely, in a study based on a clinic sample, 70% of both depressed and maritally discordant women believed their marital discord preceded their depression (O'Leary, Riso, & Beach, 1990). Using a prospective, longitudinal design, which is particularly relevant to questions about cause-and-effect relations, Beach and Nelson (1990) found that newlyweds who were discordant 6 months into the marriage experienced relatively elevated levels of depression 12 months later, even when levels of depression at 6 months were statistically controlled. Finally, demonstrating the relations between parental depression and marital conflict with another type of evidence, Beach and O'Leary (1992) showed that marital therapy was an effective treatment for depression even without medication, and was effective for both marital discord and depression. Evidence that marital therapy is effective for both depression and marital discord suggests that common processes underlie depression and marital disturbance at least for some individuals.

While causal arrows between depression and marital functioning appear to go both ways, there is evidence that direction of effect may be somewhat different for men and women. In a study that examined relations between marital discord and depressive symptoms in newly married couples, causal paths emerged from marital dissatisfaction to depression for wives, whereas for husbands, causal paths emerged from depression to marital dissatisfaction (Fincham, Beach, Harold, & Osborne, 1997). Thus, while these two factors were significantly correlated in both men and women, marital relations were more significant as a causal agent for depression in women, whereas depression was a significant contributor to marital dissatisfaction in men. In addition, recent tests of causal models based on prospective longitudinal designs, and using structural equation modeling approaches, support the notion that certain interpersonal and cognitive processes associated with marital distress lead to depression, and, conversely, processes associated with depression lead to marital distress (Beach, Fincham, & Katz, 1998).

Social Support

There is also research to indicate that the onset and course of depression may be a function of the availability of support, as well as the incidence of interpersonal stress (Beach, Sandeen, & O'Leary, 1990); that is, the positive, as well as the negative, side of marital relations is pertinent to the likelihood of depression in adults. For example, the availability of a secure attachment relationship with one's spouse is an indicator of the availability of support, whereas an insecure attachment reflects less reliable or satisfactory emotional support. In this regard, Hammen and colleagues (1995) showed that anxious or dependent attachments to other adults, negative interpersonal events, and their interaction, predicted depressive symptoms in late adolescent women. Relatedly, spousal "warmth," that is, reports of feeling understood by one's spouse and being able to depend upon, trust and open up to her or him, has been shown to predict recovery from depressive episodes (Jacobson, Fruzzetti, Dobson, Whisman, & Hops, 1993; McLeod, Kessler, & Landis, 1992), where warmth is indicated by self-reported feelings of being understood by one's spouse and being able to depend upon, trust, and open up to him or her. With regard to marital discord, Pasch and Bradbury (1998) reported that social support activities predicted positive marital outcomes 2 years later.

A particularly important domain of interspousal dynamics may be spousal attitudes and behavior toward the depression itself; that is, partner reactions to the disorder per se have substantial bearing on the course and magnitude of symptomatology. Hooley and her associates (Hooley, 1986; Hooley & Teasdale, 1989) have reported that high rates of hostile and critical statements made by spouses of depressed individuals predict relapses of depression even after treatment. Furthermore, the quality of one's interpersonal support system may range from helpful to unhelpful, and can shade into even being harmful of its own accord. While initial expressions of depressive symptomatology may elicit sympathy and encouragement, significant others may tire of the depressive symptoms and the maintenance behaviors they prompt, leading to avoidance, aversion, criticism, and rejection of the depressed person (Coyne, 1976). A vicious cycle can result when these interpersonal signals are detected by the depressed person, who then experiences even further reductions in self-esteem and increased neediness and persistence, exacerbating depressive symptomatology. Thus, the nondepressed spouse may grow impatient and weary of the depression, while the depressed spouse becomes further depressed by (often accurately) perceived signs of frustration, hostility, and overt criticality (Beach, Sandeen, & O'Leary, 1990).

Relatedly, depressed people explicitly solicit reassurance from others (Joiner, 1995; Joiner & Metalsky, 1995). However, partly because the feedback received is explicitly solicited, and partly because they disbelieve positive information because of their negative self-view, depressed individuals may discount any reassurance received and seek, on other occasions, negative feedback. The tiresome, chronic reassurance seeking and frustrating inconsistency of the kind of feedback sought may lead to eventual rejection by significant others. In addition, when depressed people with low self-esteem receive positive feedback from their partners, it may lead to a reduced sense of predictability and control. On the other hand, when depressed individuals with low self-esteem receive self-verifying feedback, this feedback increases depression (Katz & Beach, 1997). Therefore, the motivation to have others view the self in a way that is consistent with preexisting self-conceptions may further increase depression (Swann, 1983). The evidence thus suggests that not only interspousal attachment and support but also negative expressed emotion about depression are relevant to characterizing the effects of the reactions of spouses to depression in their partners.

Effect Sizes: Community and Clinical Samples

A recent series of meta-analyses by Whisman (2000) provides another take on the evidence regarding relations between parental depression and marital conflict. An impressive element of the Whisman meta-analyses is the exclusion of studies that introduce possibly important confounds or limitations on the interpretation of the results. One meta-analysis, based on 11 studies, indicated that lower marital quality was consistently linked with more depressive symptoms, with correlations of .44 for women and .36 for men. In this instance, studies were included only if they met various criteria for adequate methodology (e.g., standardized measures of the two key constructs; relatively large samples). The results for these meta-analyses were based on samples that, overall, included over 1,000 men and 1,000 women, respectively, and included a wide range of demographic characteristics. The findings on the association between depression severity and marital conflict met the statistical criteria for a medium effect size, which is a relatively robust outcome for research on psychological processes and variables. A similar analysis of four studies that focused on samples of clinically depressed individuals yielded results that met the criteria for *large* effect sizes, which are, as those of us immersed in the research enterprise well know, quite rarely reported in psychological research.

Marital Therapy in the Treatment of Depression

Another intriguing series of findings comes from treatment outcome research indicating that marital therapy may be effective for the treatment of depression. Beach, Fincham, and Katz (1998) recently reviewed evidence from research concerned with the efficacy of marital therapy as a treatment for depression. This line of therapy was inspired by the findings from research, just reviewed, which suggested that marital relations and adult depression might be causally linked. As noted by Beach and colleagues, a first series of studies showed that marital therapy had potential for the successful treatment of depression and could be adapted for that purpose. A subsequent series of studies has provided evidence that well-defined marital therapies can be an effective treatment for depression in comparison to a control group and even to other therapies for depression. The theoretical value of treatment outcome research of this sort is that it implicates the processes contributing to psychopathology when it shows that treatments oriented toward changing the targeted processes (i.e., marital distress) result in other therapeutic outcomes as well (i.e., alleviated depression). Hence, evidence that therapy for depression targeting marital function does indeed reduce depression provides another type of evidence indicating that marital problems contribute causally to the maintenance of depression.

In summary, research underscores the salience of marital relations in families with parental depression. It is important not to be too pat at this point in drawing conclusions. For example, many individuals have their first onset of depression before they marry. Thus, marital distress may cause a reoccurrence of depression, rather than being the initial or originating cause of depression. Moreover, individuals prone to depression may have a predisposition to select partners who will engender marital distress. Nonetheless, this work suggests the importance of considering familywide factors beyond the depressive symptomatology of the parents, and especially the marital relationship and marital conflict, in accounting for the effects of parental depression on children.

A Framework for Familial Influences on Children in Families with Parental Depression

We have argued that family environmental factors, including marital conflict and distress, affect the development of children in families with parental depression (Coyne, Schwoeri, & Downey, 1994; Downey & Coyne, 1990; Schwoeri & Sholevar, 1994). Figure 9.1 presented a framework illustrating a variety of familial factors related to children's adjustment in families with parental depression. We continue our discussion of these factors, focusing on family environmental influences, including exposure to parental characteristics of depressive symptomatology, various elements of marital distress and conflict, parenting practices, parent–child attachment, and children's own characteristics. As the framework illustrates, these influences are not conceptualized as "main effects" but are seen as interrelated rather than independent. Thus, as we saw in Chapter 8, there is persuasive evidence that marital conflict and parenting are interrelated (Erel & Burman, 1995).

A particularly important additional element to Figure 9.1 is the representation that these various family and child factors are seen as predicting children's outcomes as mediated by changes in their psychological functioning over time. This point is consistent with, and thus illustrates, some of the central points about the developmental psychopathology perspective made elsewhere in this volume. As we saw in Chapter 2, the developmental psychopathology perspective puts great emphasis on the study of the processes of adaptation and maladaptation that mediate child development outcomes; understanding the development of psychopathology is not simply a matter of assessing correlations between family factors and child adjustment problems.

Thus, from this perspective, the goal of research on children of depressed parents should be to determine the mediating processes that emerge from the transactions between intra- and extraorganismic factors in the various socioemotional contexts in which children develop over time. As we saw in Chapter 5, the study of moderating, as well as mediating, processes is also important, as these factors (e.g., age, gender) may importantly qualify the size or strength of relations between predictors and outcomes as mediated by processes of adaptation and maladaptation. In other words, development cannot be seen as simply a function of some interaction between various classes of influences on the child, but, consistent with the fundamental assumptions of active organism, holism, and directionality that we discussed in Chapter 1, must be seen in terms of the patterns of adaptation and maladaption that the child develops over time. However, it bears repeating that such matters run the risk of becoming overwhelmingly complex without the structure and organization provided by theory. Given the inherent complexity of family models for child development, there is a particular need for theory about mediating processes to guide research (even when postulating testable theoretical models puts one at risk of being wrong!), a matter to which we return at the end of this chapter.

This framework for relations between parental depression and child outcomes is consistent with, and in a sense an extension of, earlier family models for the effects of parental depression on children. Thus, Rutter and Quinton (1984) articulated several possible modes by which parental depression might influence children's functioning. These modes of influence included (1) parental depression exerting an adverse impact on child functioning through disturbances in parent–child relations; (2) parental depression leading to family disruption (e.g., foster care, breakup of the family), and these difficulties, in turn, leading to child psychopathology; and (3) marital discord, a correlate of depression, causing psychological problems.

This framework places special emphasis on parent–child relations and marital conflict as key pathways of influence on children, consistent with the bulk of the findings in this literature to date, but it also recognizes the role of the child in reciprocal family relationships. While the focus is on intact marital relationships, interparental relations are also a factor in children's risk in nonintact families, or after the breakup of families. Thus, when parental depression leads to family disruption (e.g., divorce and breakup of the family, foster care), children are also at increased risk for psychopathology (Hetherington, Stanley-Hagen, & Anderson, 1989; Rutter & Quinton, 1984). The role of parental depression in divorce, and effects associated with divorce, has received little attention, and even less attention is given to the role of depression in family functioning in single-parent families. However, given the relations between parental depression and marital problems, particularly when marital distress is severe, it may be that depression is a significant factor in the functioning of marriages, families, and children when there is a divorce. Also, relationship discord may be a significant factor in the risk for depression in single parents. These issues merit consideration in future research.

Characteristics of Parents with Depressive Symptomatology

Parental depression may impact children as a result of how the depression affects the behavior, cognitions, and/or emotions of the parent. In other words, one way in which children may be affected by parental depression is simply through their exposure to the depressed behavior of parents. With regard to models of causal processes within families with parental depression, this might be regarded as the most direct and unambiguous pathway through which parental characteristics associated with mental health disturbances of depression can exercise an influence on child development.

Depressed persons evidence distinctive patterns of emotional and behavioral expression (Beck, 1976). Their symptomatology may carry over into their behavior in the presence of their children. Particularly intriguing are studies that demonstrate the direct impact on children of the affective behavior associated with depressive symptomatology in the parents. For example, in face-to-face interactions, maternal displays of dysphoria and withdrawal have been shown to elicit responses of reduced activity, dysphoria, and social withdrawal in infants (Cohn & Campbell, 1992; Cohn, Campbell, Matias, & Hopkins, 1990). Prolonged exposure to such interactions has been linked with the development of depressive behavioral styles in contexts outside of mother–child interactions (Field, 1992). There are other characteristics of the socio-emotional behavior of depressed persons that may also affect children. For example, depressed people have characteristic speech patterns, including greater response latencies, hesitations and silences, poor eye contact, and negative self-disclosures (Gotlib, 1982; Gotlib & Asarnow, 1979). In remarkably short order (3–5 minutes in some studies), they can cause strangers with whom they interact to feel anxious, dysphoric, and hostile, and to behave in rejecting ways (Gotlib & Robinson, 1982; Strack & Coyne, 1983). However, relatively little is known about children's immediate reactions to more general behavior styles associated with parental depression in daily interactions, or about the lasting and long-term effects of such exposures. As we saw in Chapter 8, re-peated exposure to high marital conflict has been associated with children's lowered thresholds for high reactivity in such situations. Does exposure to pa-rental depressive behavior have similar sensitizing effects, except that the heightened reactivity is to the symptomatology associated with depression? For example, do children of depressed parents become particularly emotion-ally distressed and more likely to respond verbally, or in other ways, when ex-posed to silence, lack of explanation or resolution of issues, or withdrawal in interpersonal situations?

Moreover, depressive symptomatology is also characterized by high rates of irritability and aggression, which may become heightened during depressive episodes. As we discussed in Chapter 8, exposure to parental and interspousal expressions of anger induce distress, anger, and behavioral reactions of vari-ous sorts from children (e.g., aggression), even when the children are merely bystanders not involved in such expressions (Cummings, Zahn-Waxler, & Radke-Yarrow, 1981).

Differences in cognitive behaviors and expressions in depressed persons compared to nondepressed persons are also defining features of depression. Children may also be affected by exposure to the cognitive as well as emo-tional symptomatology of depression. The negative social-cognitive processes of depressed persons may shape and organize their responses to children's behavior, thereby affecting the children. Associations have been reported be-tween maternal depression, negative cognitions about the children, and par-enting impairments (Christensen, Phillips, Glasgow, & Johnson, 1983). An-other study reported evidence that negative attributions of child behavior mediated relations between maternal depressed mood and child psychological problems by fostering harsh parenting practices (Geller & Johnson, 1995). On the other hand, Whiffen and Gottlib (1989) reported that while depressed par-ents had more negative attributions about their children's behavior (e.g., saw them as more bothersome), independent observers also found that their chil-dren were more difficult on a variety of dimensions (e.g., more tense, less con-tent, deteriorating more quickly under stress), so that parental attributions may to some extent be an accurate reflection of children's functioning rather than a distortion due to depression. Finally, children's exposure to negative attributional strategies, that is, mixed expressions of personal responsibility and helplessness, may also have more subtle effects on their functioning (Garber, Braafladt, & Zeman, 1991b); that is, these types of communications may increase the children's sense of personal responsibility and guilt for their parents' depression.

The criteria used for research on depression in families and the distinction between depressive symptomatology and clinically significant syndrome of depression warrant close consideration when discussing the effects of depressive symptomatology on children's functioning. Depression is assessed in two ways in the literature: depressed symptomatology and diagnoses of depression. Coyne and Downey (1991) have persuasively argued that it is important to distinguish between studies that assess depressive symptomatology based on self-report instruments such as the Beck Depression Inventory (BDI; Beck, Rush, Shaw, & Emery, 1979) and those based on direct clinical interview instruments and formal diagnostic criteria, such as the Schedule for Affective Disorders and Schizophrenia (SADS; Endicott & Spitzer, 1978). People from community samples with high scores on self-report depression scales may not meet the diagnostic criteria for clinical depression, even though people with diagnosable depression typically score quite high on self-report instruments. On the other hand, both sets of criteria tap significant elements of depressive phenomena in families. These various issues bear on the likely effects of exposure to parental symptomatology on children's functioning; that is, the pattern of findings, and their interpretation, may vary depending upon the criteria for the assessment of depression.

Another issue is the relative sizes of effects due to exposure to the cognitive versus socioemotional symptomatology of depression. While it is premature to draw conclusions, evidence at this time suggests that socioemotional processes play a particularly important role in explaining the links between parental depression and child development. Thus, in a recent review, Cummings and Davies (1999) reported that on tasks related to cognitive functioning (e.g., teaching, linguistic communication), parental depression was often a weak or nonsignificant predictor of parental, child, and family functioning, whereas repeated, and sometimes strong, support was found for the role of emotionality, emotion regulation, and related socioemotional processes in relations between parental depression, child and family functioning, and children's adjustment. Furthermore, since children have no direct access to internal processes of parental cognitions, such constructs are more precisely seen as indirectly affecting children by affecting parental interaction in the family. Socioemotional processes have also been implicated in studies that identify the operation of cognitive processes. Thus, one recent study reported that depressed and well mothers could not be distinguished in their description of child behavior expressed in affectively neutral tones, but that depressed mothers were more negative when affectively hostile statements were considered (Goodman, Adamson, Riniti, & Cole, 1994).

Depression and Parenting Practices

Parental depression also has implications for parenting practices. On the one hand, in comparison to nondepressed parents, depressed parents are more inconsistent, lax, and ineffective in child management and discipline. On the other hand, when not yielding to the child's demands, they are more likely to engage in direct and forceful control strategies, and less likely to end disagreements in compromise (Fendrich, Warner, & Weissman, 1990; see reviews in Cummings & Davies, 1994a, 1999). Support has been found for a model whereby parental symptomatology compromised child management practices, leading to children's deviance (Conger, Patterson, & Ge, 1995). Using a path analysis, Forehand, Lautenschlager, Faust, and Graziano (1986) reported a pathway whereby parental depression led to the use of ineffective child management techniques, and these impairments in turn contributed to the development of child noncompliance. Another study found that negative mother–child relations were a partial mediator of the link between maternal depression and children's externalizing problems, and that this model was a better predictor of child outcomes than a reduced model that deleted consideration of mother–child interaction (Harnish, Dodge, Valente, & the Conduct Problems Group, 1995).

However, there is considerable variability in outcomes, with many depressed parents evidencing normative parenting practices. The degree of risk is also a function of the chronicity of parental depression (Campbell, Cohn, & Meyers, 1995; Fergusson & Lynskey, 1993), with risk increasing when the chronicity of depression is greater.

For example, Campbell, Cohn, and Meyers (1995) studied first-time mothers who met diagnostic criteria for clinically significant depression in the postpartum period and who were followed up through 6 months. Women whose depressions lasted through 6 months were less responsive and positive when observed interacting with their infants during feeding and play at 2, 4, and 6 months; their infants were also less positive during face-to-face interaction. Women with short-lived postpartum depressions that had remitted by 6 months did not differ from nondepressed new mothers in their interactions with their infants across this 6-month period. This suggests that more chronic depression, which often is also more severe, is more likely to be a risk factor for children than briefer episodes of depression. The timing of the depression may be important as well as associated risk factors such as spouse support and the quality of the marital relationship. It is also possible that the manifestations of the depression itself may vary with chronicity (see Campbell & Cohn, 1997); for example, intense feelings of sadness and despondency may be more likely to interfere with positive mother–infant ineraction than vegetative symptoms such as fatigue, sleep difficulties, and appetite change. More research is needed on how the particular manifestations of depression predict qualities of mother–infant interaction because it is also clear that not all depressed women have difficulties responding to their newborns and that some depressed women see their infants as a source of delight despite their depressed mood. Furthermore, given the heterogeneity of depression in terms of its measurement, course, and symptom expression, it is not surprising that its impact on the mother–child relationship and children's outcomes varies as well. It is important to ask what aspects of depression and associated risk factors may account for the problems shown by some children with depressed mothers.

The effects of chronicity on maternal responsiveness and infant functioning are evident whether the depression is clinically diagnosed, as in the Campbell, Cohn, and Meyers (1995) study, or assessed via self-reported sad mood that may or may not meet clinical diagnostic criteria for depressive disorder. Data from the NICHD Early Child Care Research Network (1999) indicate that maternal reports of chronic depressive symptoms over the first 36 months of life were associated with lower levels of maternal sensitivity observed at 6, 15, 24, and 36 months. Chronic maternal depressive symptoms predicted lower levels of children's language development, school readiness, and cooperation at 36 months as well as higher levels of mother-reported behavior problems. These outcomes were partially mediated, however, by maternal sensitivity suggesting that the quality of maternal responsiveness across infancy and toddlerhood partly accounted for the impact of mothers' sadness on children. Mothers whose depressions were in evidence over the course of the first three years of the child's life were also probably less likely to spend time in conversation with their infants and or engaging in activities that facilitate cognitive and social development. Moreover, they showed the lowest level of responsiveness at 24 months, relative to other mothers with more intermittent depression or no depression, suggesting that they were less able to adapt to the changing demands of parenting. The presence of other risk factors associated with depression also was relevant to disentangling these effects.

Thus, other variables may be involved in the interrelations between parental depression, parenting, and child adjustment, suggesting the need for models that include assessment of more than just these three factors. Thus, in some studies, factors associated with parental depression have been found to be a better predictor of family problems than diagnostic status per se. Hamilton, Jones, and Hammen (1993) found that chronic life stress, low levels of positive events, and single parenthood were each linked with problems in parent–child interactions, independent of diagnostic status, and were better predictors of parent–child affective disturbances than parental diagnostic status. This is not necessarily a comment on the effects of parental depression on parenting. The fact that one significant predictor pulls more variance than another in an individual study does not negate the significance of the latter in family functioning. Moreover, statistical relations between parental depression and parenting have been repeatedly demonstrated. However, this result does suggest a caveat: Model testing that focuses exclusively on parenting and does not include, or adequately represent, other family processes associated with, or set in motion by, parental depression may lead to an oversimplified picture of family relations underlying the effects of parental depression. In families with parental depression, the combination of risk factors may be particularly significant with regard to child outcomes. Thus, Rutter and Quinton (1984, p. 866) stated, "For the most part, parental mental disorder does not give rise to an increased risk for the children that is independent of the family's psychosocial circumstances as a whole. Rather it should be seen as one of several psychosocial risk factors that are more damaging in combination than in isolation."

Depression and Attachment

There has been interest, both historically (e.g., Freud) and in recent years, with regard to disturbances in parent–child attachment as contributing to the transmission of depression in families (see Cummings & Cicchetti, 1990, for an extended discussion). There are compelling bases for postulating that parental depression contributes to the development of insecure parent–child attachment, which, in turn, increases the child's risk for the development of affective disorders. Parental emotional unavailability and psychological insensitivity are associated with parental depression and are also among the strongest and most reliable predictors of insecure parent–child attachment (DeWolff & van IJzendoorn, 1997). Furthermore, the cognitive and emotional contents of internal working models of the self and others that characterize children with insecure attachments (Oppenheim, Emde, & Warren, 1997; Oppenheim, Nir, Warren, & Emde, 1997) bear remarkable similarities to the cognitive and emotional patterns characteristic of depression (Beck, 1976). The concept of loss figures prominently in both the attachment and depression literatures as a core construct in the functioning of disturbed individuals (Beck, 1976; Bowlby, 1980).

Parental depression has repeatedly been linked with insecure parent–child attachment. The first such report was by Radke-Yarrow, Cummings, Kuczynski, and Chapman (1985), and there have been repeated replications of this finding in the subsequent years (Cummings & Davies, 1994b, 1999). Recent studies support the notion that parental depression may be causally related to insecure attachment. Thus, Murray (1992) reported that diagnoses of maternal depression at 2 months postpartum increased children's risk for developing insecure attachments with the mother 16 months later. Another study found that maternal depression during infancy predicted insecure attachment 13 months later in infants and preschoolers, in particular, disorganized–disoriented attachments, which were three to four times more likely in children of depressed mothers than in children of well mothers (Teti, Gelfand, Messinger, & Isabella, 1995). Notably, a repeated finding in this literature is that disorganized–disoriented attachments and related assessments of very insecure attachment (e.g., the A/C pattern; Radke-Yarrow et al., 1985) are particularly prevalent among children of depressed parents, which emphasizes the potential for parental depression to be highly disruptive to attachment relationships. Cicchetti, Rogosch, and Toth (1998) recently reported that more behavioral difficulties and insecure attachment were found among children with depressed than nondepressed parents. Again, exemplifying the interrelations among family influences, contextual factors, including marital satisfaction and family conflict, significantly added to the prediction of behavior problems in children of depressed parents. However, as with other studies of family processes, although depression increases the probability of dysfunctional outcomes, a wide range of outcomes are found, including outcomes of good adjustment in children of depressed parents.

The point that secure attachments are often formed between depressed parents and children merits emphasis. As with other family processes, the prediction of psychopathology is probabilistic, not certain. The severity of depressive symptoms increases the likelihood of disturbances in attachment relationships. For example, Radke-Yarrow, Cummings, Kuczynski, and Chapman (1985) found that insecure attachment was positively associated with how long the mother had been ill in the child's lifetime, the severity of the mothers's illness (e.g., bipolar disorder vs. minor depression), and the extensiveness of her treatment history. Other studies also indicate that the degree of risk is a function of the severity of parental depression as well as the timing of the depression in the child's life (e.g., Campbell & Cohn, 1997; Campbell, Cohn, & Myers, 1995; Fergusson & Lynskey, 1993). When parental depression is mild, transient, or short-term, there may be little or no impact on the child. Thus, depression increases the probability of dysfunctional outcomes, but a wide range of outcomes occur; that is, many children of depressed parents develop adaptively and competently, and some develop into well- or even high-functioning individuals. As we stressed in our discussions of developmental pathways, children's development is a product of the influence of many factors, but it ultimately reflects dynamic and active adaptation or maladaption to events and circumstances over time, with children having considerable potential for resilience even in the face of significant adversity.

Depression and Marital Conflict

A traditional view is that children are affected by their parents' behavior solely as a result of parent–child interaction. Similarly, a common assumption is that maternal depression affects children to the extent that it affects maternal–child interaction and parenting. However, as we saw in Chapter 8, recent work makes clear the need for a broader systems view of family influences on children, and there is particular support for the effects of interparental relations on children.

As we discussed earlier in this chapter, there is impressive evidence indicating that marital conflict and parental depression are interrelated. Rutter and his colleagues have been particularly influential in advancing a family systems perspective a step further, that is, by calling attention to relations between maternal depression and marital discord, and to the possibly causal role of marital discord in child outcomes. Based on their findings, Rutter and Quinton (1984, p. 876) concluded that "while parental mental illness constituted an important indicator of psychiatric risk for children, the overall pattern of findings showed that in most cases the main risk did not stem from the illness itself. Rather, it derived from the associated psychosocial disturbance in the family." Furthermore, they found that parental mental illness was associated, in particular, with children's adjustment problems through its effects on heightening marital anger and hostility.

More recent work continues to support the notion that marital discord plays a key role in the effects of maternal depression on children and may even be a more proximal predictor of certain outcomes than maternal depression per se. Thus, based on an extensive review of the literature, Downey and Coyne (1990, p. 68) concluded that "marital discord is a viable alternative explanation for the general adjustment problems of children with a depressed parent." Prospective, longitudinal studies conducted on this issue are particularly influential in suggesting that marital conflict and distress may be a significant variable in the effects of parental depression on children in families. For example, Caplan and colleagues (1989) reported links between maternal depression and marital conflict in the early years of child rearing, with marital discord more closely related to behavior problems than parental depression. In another longitudinal study, Cox, Puckering, Pound, and Mills (1987) found that marital discord was associated with maternal depression 6 months later, and maternal depression was correlated with marital discord 6 months later, suggesting that their interrelations were reciprocal rather than unidirectional. They also found that marital discord was more closely related to disturbances in mother–child interactions than maternal depression per se.

Other studies have begun to provide evidence for various pathways of influence within the family, as suggested in Figure 9.1. For example, Davies and Windle (1997) reported that adolescent daughters of depressed mothers experienced more depressive symptoms, conduct problems, and academic difficulties than did adolescent sons of depressed mothers. Mediational tests showed that daughters' greater vulnerability to family discord mediated the impact of maternal depression on their social and emotional development. Of course, an interesting, but unexplored, question here and, for the most part, in the broader literature on parental depression and children, is the relation between paternal depression and child development. With regard to this point, evidence has also emerged to support distinguishing between mothers' and fathers' conflict behavior when there is parental depression. Miller, Cowan, Cowan, Hetherington, and Clingempeel (1993) reported that fathers' depression was associated with increased marital conflict but the pathway to children's externalizing problems was based on decreased child control. However, for depressed mothers, both increased marital conflict and decreased positive affect and warmth in parenting were associated with children's externalizing problems via separate pathways. In addition to demonstrating multiple pathways of influence in families with parental depression, these studies also indicate that parental and child gender may moderate the nature of relations between parental depression, family functioning, and child outcomes.

Gender is also a relatively unexplored domain in this literature. Other recent research provides more support for greater effects on girls than boys. For example, Fergusson, Horwood, and Lynskey (1995) reported that maternal depressive symptoms were strongly correlated with subsequent depressive symptoms in adolescent daughters but not adolescent sons. However, little is known about differences between mother's and father's behavior in front of children as a function of marital conflict and the possibility of cross-gender effects in families with parental depression. Thus, a particularly intriguing direction is to examine mothers' and fathers' conflict behaviors in the context of families with parental depression, and the direct effects on their children of exposure to each parent's conflict behaviors. Significant issues for research include differentiating styles of marital conflict that are characteristic of depressed fathers versus depressed mothers. The prevalence and impact of nonverbal anger communication, anger mixed with dysphoria, unresolved conflict issues, and lack of explanation in families with depressed parents merit investigation (Cummings, 1995a).

Furthermore, the familial correlates and the symptomatology of depression suggest that children with depressed parents may be differentially exposed to particular forms and dimensions of interparental conflict (Hops et al., 1987; Hops, Sherman, & Biglan, 1990). There is a need for further examination of the effects on children of marital interaction patterns associated with parental depression. Much of the work thus far has been based on relatively global assessments of marital conflict and distress based on questionnaire assessments. It is uncertain whether such assessments capture the most important dimensions of marital conflict associated with parental depression; that is, relatively little is known about the conflict styles of depressed persons in comparison to nondepressed persons, particularly in contexts of everyday problem solving. It may be that a lack of constructive problem solving is just as significant as the presence of negative conflict behaviors. An interesting question is whether lower rates of positive affect expression by depressed parents exacerbate the impact of high rates of negative emotionality in these families. For example, Kochanska, Kuczynski, Radke-Yarrow, and Welsh (1987) reported that depressed mothers have difficulty resolving conflicts. Instead of attempting to reach a compromise, depressed mothers use less effortful strategies (e.g., withdrawal) in an effort to end conflicts, thereby leaving the underlying issues unresolved. This strategy may only serve to fuel marital conflict. For example, some studies report that while depressed wives typically withdraw after conflicts begin, their husbands become increasingly hostile (e.g., Hops et al., 1987). Thus, children of depressed spouses may be particularly likely to be exposed to marital communications that are especially ambiguous, changeable, unreliable with regard to meaning, and negative, which may contribute to their sense of emotional insecurity (Cummings, 1995a).

As with other elements of our model of parental depression, families, and children, an important direction for future research from a developmental psychopathology perspective is to account for the processes that mediate the effects of parental depression on children; theoretical accounts for these processes are particularly needed. In this regard, it is interesting to note that there is evidence that both parent–child relations and interparental relations affect children's adjustment by influencing their sense of emotional security. This premise has found support regardless of parents' depression status. In addition, problems in both parent–child and marital relations have been found to be associated with parental depression, and these factors, in turn, have been associated with adjustment problems in children of depressed parents. Thus, a groundwork is laid for a familywide theory of the effects of parental depression on children, that is, the notion that parental depression affects children by reducing their emotional security in the family. We return to this promising theoretical direction later.

Children's Characteristics

As we noted earlier, inherited dispositions may also play a role in increased risk for adjustment problems in children of depressed parents. Intraorganismic factors have often been implicated. The monozygotic:dizygotic rate is approximately 46:20 for unipolar mood disorder, and the rate for bipolar mood disorder is approximately 72:14 (McGuffin, Katz, Watkins, & Rutherford, 1996). Neurophysiological investigations of mood disorders, including studies of children (Birmaher et al., 1997), specifically implicate the neurotransmitters norepinephrine and serotonin, and also neuroendocrine dysfunction (Goodwin & Jamison, 1990).

However, as we have noted, it is also clear that biological influences can no more than partially explain the association between depression in parents and maladjustment in children (Rende, Plomin, Reiss, & Hetherington, 1993) and are most appropriately conceptualized as interacting with environmental factors in influencing an individual's development (Cicchetti & Toth, 1998) and susceptibility to depression in adolescence or early adulthood. Moreover, aside from evidence implicating genetics and biological processes, relatively little is known about these effects.

Difficult temperament may moderate children's responses to depressive familial environments (Crockenberg, 1986; Sheeber & Johnson, 1992; Wachs & Gandour, 1983). As we noted in Chapter 5, moderators specify the strength and/or direction of a relation between an independent variable and an outcome. One study found that during the first days of life, children of depressed parents were more unresponsive and lethargic, and displayed poorer orienting skills than children of nondepressed parents (Abrams, Field, Scafidi, & Prodomidis, 1995). Other studies have found a pattern of right frontal asymmetry in depressed mothers and their infants that may be an indicator of biological vulnerability (Field, Fox, Pickens, & Nawrocki, 1995; Field, Pickens, Fox, Nawrocki, & Gonzalez, 1995).

Thus, there is modest evidence that children of depressed parents (1) have more difficult temperaments, at least as rated by their own mothers, and (2) are more unresponsive and lethargic in the first days of life. These findings may suggest that constitutional vulnerabilities factor into children's relational problems within the family, including their proneness for difficulties in emotional regulation. However, studies identifying specific processes at risk in children of depressed parents, especially with regard to how child characteristics may affect family functioning, are scarce and much more study of this issue is merited. It is not enough to document in behavioral genetic studies that there is evidence of genetic risk associated with depression in families. Much more is needed to move from a "first generation" to a "second generation" of research-based understanding of these matters; that is, given the emphasis on process-oriented explanations as opposed simply to the identification of correlations between family variables and child outcomes, this is a significant gap in knowledge about the contributions of individual dispositions to processes of adaptation and maladaptation.

Gender provides another perspective on child characteristics associated with risk for depression. In addition to the issues already mentioned, gender differences are complexly intertwined with developmental level in predicting the risk for depression. In particular, it appears that whereas boys exhibit greater susceptibility to depressive family environments in childhood (Kershner & Cohen, 1992), this trend reverses in adolescence (Davies & Windle, 1997; Thomas & Forehand, 1991). Many questions remain as to why this shift in gender-based vulnerability to depression occurs at this time, but studies of high-risk groups parallel findings from epidemiological studies of depression prevalence as a function of age and gender (e.g., Offord, Boyle, Fleming, Blum, & Rae Grant, 1989).

Environmental Factors Outside of the Family

With regard to broader ecological contexts of depression, there are also conceptual bases (e.g., Bronfenbrenner, 1979) for expecting that extrafamilial factors, such as schools and neighborhoods, and the beliefs and values of the culture influence depression and risk for depression (Cicchetti & Toth, 1998). For example, geographical location, ethnicity, and socioeconomic status may account for significant variance in the continuity of risk from parents to children (Rutter, 1998). While this area has been the subject of relatively little systematic investigation, there is some support for the effects of extrafamilial factors. For example, perceptions of academic competence and school performance have been related to risk for depression in children and adolescence (Cole, 1991; Cole, Martin, Powers, & Truglio, 1997; Eccles, Lord, & Roeser, 1996). Community supports and the availability of high-quality treatment services, which are related to socioeconomic status, may also be relevant to the onset and course of depression (Cicchetti & Toth, 1998). There is obviously a great need for further systematic research on the role of extrafamilial factors in the risk for adjustment problems in children of depressed parents.

TOWARD A PROCESS-ORIENTED PERSPECTIVE

As we have seen, an important goal from the developmental psychopathology perspective is to account for the processes that underlie development. At this point, we consider the application of some of the principles discussed in Chapters 1 through 5 to the explication of processes accounting for relations between parental depression and family functioning on the one hand, and child outcomes on the other. As in other areas concerned with influences on the development of psychopathology in children, much of the work in this literature is limited by the incomplete conceptualization of process.

Pathways of Development

Another element implicit in Figure 9.1 is that adaptation and maladaptation as functions of familial factors also occur because of transactions between intra- and extraorganismic variables over time. Thus, it is important to conceptualize the development of children of depressed parents in terms of developmental pathways rather than simply as categorical outcomes of psychopathology versus normalcy. With regard to the prediction of depression, it is an error here, as elsewhere when considering developmental pathways, to assume that pathways between early and later development are relatively simple and straightforward.

Relatedly, this review has been concerned primarily with establishing the effects of multiple familial influences on children in families with parental depression. However, it is important not to take this discussion as offering a "pat" or oversimplified picture of how family influences affect children; that is, it should be kept in mind that different specific elements of family functioning do not affect children as "main effects" (i.e., as influences that are separate and distinct from other familial factors and characteristics of the individual). Instead, the various familial influences are likely to interact in affecting children's development, and there may also be interactions between the individual child's characteristics and family influences over time. Unfortunately, relatively little research to date has been conducted at a level of analysis that can detect the likely complexity of interrelations between familial influences and their transactions over time in affecting children's development. Such research ultimately will require not only measurement of multiple family influences but also rigorous measurement of these variables (e.g., observational measurement in the laboratory of multiple family subsystems, substantial records of family functioning made in the home over long periods of time); that is, weak, superficial, or only global assessments are unlikely to do justice to the possible effects of family factors. Moreover, study of the transaction between multiple familial influences ideally requires a prospective, longitudinal research design. Relatively few such projects have been undertaken to date. Hence, our level of understanding is limited. The following discussion also functions to provide additional concepts meant to facilitate more sophisticated family models of the development of children of depressed parents.

In this section we consider approaches to understanding pathways of development in children of depressed parents and the pertinence of a variety of the principles of the developmental psychopathology approach to the study of developmental pathways and processes in children of depressed parents. Some principles that will clarify our understanding pathways of development in these children are outlined, and points are illustrated with the findings from research in this area. Consistent with the developmental psychopathology perspective, it is assumed that a complex interplay of affective, cognitive, socioemotional, and biological components is involved in developmental pathways (Cicchetti & Toth, 1998). However, as we have noted, while progress has been made toward delineating pathways of development, longitudinal studies are rare, and even less common are longitudinal studies typified by the rigorous, multimethod and multidimensional assessment of the mediating and moderating factors needed for a full account of developmental deviance and normalcy from the developmental psychopathology perspective.

One set of pathways of interest is those pertinent to the development of depression. While children of depressed parents are at risk for a broad array of disorders, depression is a matter of particular interest given the evidence of the intergenerational transmission of depression and concerns about how, when, why, and where children develop depression in these families. Moreover, understanding pathways to the development of depression in childhood is central to the more general topic of depression and families. Thus, the matter of pathways to development of depression is especially pertinent to the themes of this chapter.

Childhood Depression

Work from the Institute of Psychiatry in London conducted on childhood depression over the past several decades, which is summarized in Harrington, Rutter, and Fombonne (1996), illustrates some of these various issues and questions. While there is a risk of some redundancy, as we briefly considered the results of these studies earlier in this volume, we revisit this research again because of its particular (and nearly unique) pertinence to illustrating pathways associated with depression. These studies have demonstrated that depressive symptomatology is not uncommon in childhood; that is, epidemiological studies have shown that depressive symptomatology (e.g., often miserable, unhappy) was reported in about 1 in 10 children. In addition, depressive symptomatology was related to an increased incidence of psychiatric disorders and a wide range of other problems in children (e.g., conduct disorders), underscoring its significance. Moreover, depressed children were at greater risk for adult depression than nondepressed children. These studies support the notion that pathways of risk for adult depression may have origins in early childhood. On the other hand, looking backwards from adulthood to childhood, it is also evident that most adult depression is not preceded by a depressive syndrome per se in childhood (i.e., most depression has an adult onset), but it may be preceded by a wide range of other childhood problems. In addition, depressed children are at risk for a variety of disorders other than depression in adulthood. Thus, the research supports the notion that the pathways associated with depression in childhood and adulthood are complex, clearly illustrating the concepts of multifinality and specificity.

Multifinality

The fact that two different individuals appear to be following a similar pathway at a given point in time does not mean their end results will be the same. Any one risk or protective factor apparent during development may have a different influence (e.g., having a parent with depression) depending on the organizational system in which it operates, thereby resulting in different outcomes later in development. Thus, even if two individuals have similar characteristics or experiences at one point in time (e.g., similar family patterns associated with parental depression), the events that follow may result in different outcomes later.

The research from the Institute of Psychiatry in London illustrates this point by demonstrating that depressive symptomatology in childhood may have quite different outcomes later in development. For example, Harrington, Fudge, Rutter, Ackles, and Hill (1991) found that depressed children without conduct disorders did not differ from depressed children with conduct disorders in the extent of depressive symptomatology at the initial point of assessment. However, depressive children without conduct disorder had a higher rate of depression in adulthood than did depressive children with conduct disorder; in fact, the rate of adult depression in the latter group was similar to the rate of depression in a group with conduct disorder but not depression in childhood. On the other hand, those with both conduct disorder and depression in childhood had a higher rate of adult criminality than those with childhood depression only. These results suggest that the developmental pathways to adult depression may be quite different for different groups of children with early depressive syndromes. Moreover, consistent with the principle of holism, the findings indicate that there is an interdependency among the elements of psychological functioning in childhood and that one needs to consider the overall organization of functioning and not just a subset of risk factors (i.e., depressive symptomatology) in order to understand and make predictions about pathways of development.

Equifinality

Consistent with the principles of developmental psychopathology, adult depression, like its childhood counterpart, does not result from a single causal chain of events but appears to develop along several different pathways. For example, for some, adult depression may be most influenced by genetic risk, whereas for others, one or more traumatic historical experiences (e.g., marital conflict, divorce, severe parental depression) may be most important. The notion that multiple pathways may lead to the same manifest outcome supports the need for relatively complex, person- rather than variable-oriented levels of analyses.

Another finding based on the longitudinal studies conducted at the Institute of Psychiatry illustrates this point (Harrington et al., 1994). The two risk factors assessed in childhood, again, were depression and conduct disorder, but the concern this time was with the prediction of a different adult outcome, that is, suicide attempts. Depression in childhood was a significant predictor of adult suicide attempts even when other childhood factors were statistically controlled. However, conduct disorder was also a predictor of adult suicide attempts even when childhood depression was controlled; that is, it was an independent predictor of suicide attempts. Thus, both risk factors led to a higher probability of the same outcome.

Syndromes and Continua

Another assumption of the developmental psychopathology approach is that it is meaningful to study disorders both as diagnostic categories and as continua or dimensions of symptomatology. The pertinence of these notions to the study of depression is also illustrated by the research from the Institute of Psychiatry in London. Even in childhood, several different forms of depressive syndromes can be identified, with comorbidity with other disorders related (e.g., conduct disorder) to the long-term risk for adult depression. Depression without conduct disorder increased the prediction of adult depression, whereas depression with conduct disorder predicted a broader range of adjustment problems. Thus, depression at the symptom level is not the only factor that must be considered in predicting outcomes (Harrington, Rutter, & Fombonne, 1996); that is, the extent to which symptoms form particular clusters or groupings bears upon the extent to which pathways from childhood depression to adult depression show continuity.

Familial Rates of Depression

We reviewed evidence to indicate that adult depression runs in families. However, as we have noted, in recent years, it has become evident that depressive symptoms, and even syndromes of depression, may appear well before adulthood (Harrington, Rutter, & Fombonne, 1996). Thus, the question arises, is there evidence that the intrafamilial transmission of depression also holds for childhood depression? If not, this would suggest that the processes that account for childhood and adult depression may be quite different. In another study based on data collected at the Institute of Psychiatry in London, Harrington and colleagues (1993) reported that first-degree relatives of depressed children had a greater risk for depressive disorder than first-degree relatives of nondepressed children. In addition, female relatives of both depressed and nondepressed children had a higher incidence of depression than male relatives. These findings thus support the notion that the depressive patterns identified in childhood, like depression in adulthood, also have a basis in family relations. As with adult depression, girls had higher rates of depression than boys. Of course, these family data do not increase the extent to which the risk associated with family relations has a biological versus family environmental foundation, but it likely that both influences are important for not only childhood but also adult depression.

Another, related question is whether the age of depression onset is related to family rates of depression and other family factors. Interestingly, the analyses of data from the British studies did *not* support the notion that an earlier age of onset of depression was associated with a greater lifetime familial risk for depression. This finding is interesting because early onset is linked to greater lifetime risk for some other important classes of psychopathology (e.g., aggression; Loeber, 1984). However, in the British studies, earlier onset of depression (i.e., prepubertal onset) was associated with higher rates of family discord, including marital conflict, suggesting that family environmental factors may be particularly important in prepubertal as opposed to postpubertal and adult-onset depression (Harrington et al., 1997).

Unfortunately, these data are not conclusive on this point. For example, results partly depend on where the cutoff is set for early- versus late-onset depression. Thus, there is evidence that early onset in adulthood may *increase* the familial risk associated with depression when the cutoff for early versus late onset is set at a different point in development. Research on an American sample reported by Weissman and colleagues indicated greater lifetime rates of depression in first-degree relatives in cases of early-onset adult depression (i.e., before age 20) in comparison to late-onset (i.e., 20–29 years) depression. Moreover, higher rates of the comorbid transmission of depression and alcoholism, and depression and antisocial personality, were found in first-degree relatives of individuals with early-onset depression (Rende et al., 1997). These results suggest that early-onset adult depression may indeed signal greater familial risk not only for depression but also for other disorders that are often comorbid with depression. These data are intriguing given the findings for other forms of psychopathology that early onset signals increased risk, but the matter is far from resolved based on the current evidence. In particular, as we have seen, early onset in the child area is pre- versus postpuberty, and the data based on these criteria may complicate the picture; that is, early onset by these criteria does *not* increase the risk for adult depression.

In summary, this research supports several of the notions of pathways of development that we reviewed in detail at a conceptual level in Chapter 4. However, it must be said that the quality and rigor of the data in these groundbreaking studies were limited (e.g., medical charts and other hospital records made before current advances in the assessment of depression; very scant detail on family functioning). Thus, greater understanding of these matters must await future prospective, longitudinal studies of depression in families based on multimethod, multidomain assessments of familial functioning and children's adjustment.

Other Issues Concerning Pathways of Development

Other issues pertaining to pathways of development in children from families with parental depression that are not systematically examined in the British studies merit consideration.

Quantitative and Qualitative Differences in Familial Functioning

While children of depressed parents may be exposed to more maladaptive forms of family functioning, it does not necessarily follow that these forms of functioning are unique to depression. In fact, when maladaptive forms of family functioning are identified in research, these processes are frequently linked to children's adjustment problems, regardless of whether or not the parents have depression (e.g., Hamilton, Jones, & Hammen, 1993; Tarullo, DeMulder, Martinez, & Radke-Yarrow, 1994). While some processes are clearly much less common in families without depression (e.g., Type D or A/C patterns of attachment; Radke-Yarrow, Cummings, Kuczynski, & Chapman, 1985), it is not evident that there are unique processes in families with parental depression that do not also occur in families without parental depression. While qualitative differences between families with and without depression may be found with the initiation of more rigorous and data-intensive family studies, at this point, it seems more likely that similar processes will be predictive of adjustment problems in children whether or not parental depression is present in the families. Thus, more maladaptive forms of the various aspects of family functioning linked with childhood psychopathology are likely to be found more often in families with parental depression, but it is not likely that qualitatively different family processes will be identified; that is, some constellations of family processes are surely likely to be more typical in families with parental depression, and these processes may be relatively deviant compared to the norm, but it is unlikely that they will be unique to families with parental depression.

It may well be that risk processes that are perhaps typical of dysfunctional families in general and predictive of children's general adjustment problems may primarily account for the child behavior problems associated with parental depression. For example, Cicchetti, Rogosch, and Toth (1998) found that when family contextual risk and maternal depression were both factored into an equation to predict externalizing behavior problems in toddlers, family contextual risk proved significant, with maternal depression not contributing further to the prediction. This result is consistent with the idea that although risk processes may be more preponderant in children of depressed parents, they may operate like those same risk processes do in other problematic families without depression rather than constitute a qualitatively distinct class of family process variables.

These notions are consistent with the precept of developmental psychopathology that highlights the importance of considering the normal and abnormal together (Sroufe, 1990), an issue that we developed at length in Chapter 2; that is, maladaptation is assumed to be a function of developmental processes that occur over time and in interaction with the environment, in response to stress, risk factors, and different transition points requiring reorganization. Viewing disorder as a "developmental deviation" is quite different from seeing a disorder as something one "has" or that one "gets." The implication is that one cannot compartmentalize disorder as qualitatively distinct from normal development in the way that is implied by the traditional medical model. Similarly, abnormal family processes are not distinct entities, separate and different from normal family processes. Instead, abnormal family processes are defined in relation to normal family processes, and one can only understand one in relation to the other. The search for deviance in family functioning as an "entity" of well-defined proportions and completely separate from what one observes in normal families is likely to be a futile endeavor.

Disorder as a Succession of Deviations over Time

For children in families with parental depression (or growing up in any other high-risk environment), the development of disorder, if it occurs at all, is assumed to occur as a result of repeated transactions between the individual and the environment over time; not as an immediate occurrence. Accordingly, when children of depressed parents develop disorders, this does not happen "all of a sudden," but as the outcome of a long history of responses to the conditions of a dysfunctional family environment. This assumption puts a premium on the careful, microanalytic study of response processes in context, as they are assumed to underlie child outcomes.

Change Is Always Possible

It is assumed that for children of depressed parents, as for all children, development involves continual, dynamic transactions between the individual and context. Accordingly, trajectories of development are never fixed, and change is always possible. In other words, since the process of adaptation during development is constant over time, change from psychopathology to normality, or from normality to psychopathology, may occur at any point. Thus, it is important *not* to infer that childhood problems (e.g., insecure attachment; peer problems, poor school achievement) necessarily presage long-term psychopathology for children of depressed parents (Cummings & Cicchetti, 1990) or those with other sets of family risk factors.

Change Is Constrained by Prior Adaptation

Also consistent with the principles of developmental psychopathology (Cicchetti & Cohen, 1995a), past adaptations influence future possibilities for development. As we saw in earlier chapters, it is assumed that during development, early psychological structures become incorporated into later psychological structures. Thus, the possibility of change is typically constrained by past functioning, although, as recent dynamic systems models indicate, change may sometimes occur much more rapidly or precipitously than at other times. Thus, signs of early problems in children from at-risk samples, such as children of depressed parents, *are* a cause for concern.

Risk Is Probabilistic, Not Certain

An outcome of psychopathology in children, even in the presence of multiple, significant risk factors, is never certain. At the outset of this chapter, we illustrated this point with the examples of Joe and Frank. Both were children of depressed parents, but they had very different familial experiences with depression and, relatedly, very different adjustment outcomes. Even the exposure to multiple risk factors (e.g., factors associated with parental depression; see Figure 9.1) does no more than probabilistically increase the likelihood of the development of psychopathology. On the other hand, some individuals confronted with apparently low-risk conditions may develop serious adjustment problems. Thus, it is important not to equate risk for psychopathology, including membership in a high-risk group, with the necessary outcome of maladaptive development. Relatedly, the degree of risk is a direct function of the *severity* and *chronicity* of parental depression (Campbell, Cohn, & Meyers, 1995; Fergusson & Lynskey, 1993; Seifer, 1995). Thus, when parental depression is mild, transient, or short term, there may be little or no impact on the children (Campbell et al., 1995; Radke-Yarrow, Cummings, Kuczynski, & Chapman, 1985). On the other hand, problems may be more likely when the duration of parental depression in the child's lifetime is high (Radke-Yarrrow et al., 1985) or when the depression is associated with multiple risk factors (e.g., Fendrich, Warner, & Weissman, 1990).

Risk and Resilience

It is also important in conceptualizing a family model of the development of children of depressed parents to articulate the specific factors that increase risk in this group, and also those factors that reduce risk and ameliorate outcomes. Children of depressed parents often cope effectively. In Chapter 5, we provided an extensive conceptual treatment of definitions and stressed the importance of considering buffers and resilience factors in considering children's development. Moreover, many families with depressed parents function in healthy ways in areas of marriage, child management, and the provision of love in rearing children (e.g., Cox, Puckering, Pound, & Mills, 1987). In addition, depression does not necessarily lead to an erosion or deterioration of social resources, either within the family or in terms of the social network outside of the family (Moos, Cronkite, & Moss, 1998). To some extent, positive aspects of the family variables outlined in Figure 9.1 (e.g., secure attachment) might be expected to buffer or protect children from the effects of exposure to parental depression. However, this assumption must be tested. Clinicians and researchers should not neglect the possible existence of buffers and resilience factors in even the most depressogenic family environments.

In addition, the effects of specific family processes may also depend upon the broader family context. For example, different relations between variables may be obtained when broader family environments are benign and well functioning versus deviant. Thus, in one study, it was found that negative maternal attitudes predicted child psychopathology in depressive family environments but not in nondepressive environments (Goodman, Adamson, Riniti, & Cole, 1994). Another study found that a good father–child relationship was a protective factor against the effects of high (but not low) levels of maternal depressive symptoms on children's adjustment problems (Tannenbaum & Forehand, 1994). Cicchetti, Rogosch, and Toth (1998) reported that contextual risk factors mediated relations between maternal depression and child behavior problems. Contextual risk was indicated by parenting hassles, low social support, stress, low marital satisfaction, and family conflict. In yet another study, Moos, Cronkite, and Moos (1998) found that family and extrafamilial resources were related to changes in depression over time. Specifically, family and extrafamilial social resources contributed to a decline in parental depression. More family independence predicted less depression 1 year later, whereas more family arguments were associated with more depression at the later time point. Thus, increases in independence, family organization, and family cohesion predicted declines in depression over time, whereas elevations in family arguments predicted increased levels of depression. With regard to extrafamilial variables, increases over time in the number of helpful friends, work support, and confidant support were associated with declines in depression.

Relatedly, it should not be assumed that depression in families has only negative implications for child development. There may be positive developmental outcomes, or special strengths, that are found in children from such backgrounds. For example, such individuals may learn to be especially attuned to others' feelings and sensitivities, which in some contexts may be especially adaptive and valuable. Outcomes associated with maternal depression are not necessarily pathological, and it is important not to assume that differences between children of depressed parents and of normal parents are always indices of risk for psychopathology.

In summary, these concepts and notions specify a variety of parameters that merit consideration in moving models of risk for psychopathology in children of depressed parents beyond correlational models to second-generation models that conceptualize development in terms of dynamic processes of interaction between the individual and the environment over time. In the next section, we consider another issue pertinent to the advancement of a developmental psychopathology perspective on the risk for psychopathology in children of depressed parents, that is, the significance of theory.

A THEORY ABOUT MEDIATING PROCESSES: THE EMOTIONAL SECURITY HYPOTHESIS

Finally, we consider a specific theoretical model delineating the processes that current theory and research suggest may underlie relations between parental depression, family functioning, and child development. As we have seen, there are multiple factors associated with the risk for adjustment problems in children of depressed parents. The complexity of these processes, and the often-complex patterns of findings generated by studies in this area, calls attention to the need for theory to organize and make conceptual sense of the data.

The emotional security hypothesis described here reflects an attempt to organize the complex multifamilial findings that have emerged regarding the processes mediating relations between parental depression and children's adjustment. At the outset, we want to make it clear that we do not consider the emotional security hypothesis a grand risk theory for children of depressed parents that fully accounts for childhood psychopathology or normalcy in these children. On the contrary, the emotional security hypothesis is proffered as a model for an important, but not exhaustive, subset of the processes mediating relations between parental depression and child adjustment (Cummings & Davies, 1996; Davies & Cummings, 1994).

On the other hand, we do not expect that any other grand theory will emerge either. Rather, we expect that a number of midlevel models or theories will probably be necessary to account for the multiplicity of processes operating in these family environments. Nonetheless, we hope a small set of (eventual) theories with some connections or interrelations between them will provide a more adequate scientific account and a more useful template for clinical prevention and intervention efforts than the current welter of complex empirical results.

As we have seen in this chapter, an important lacuna of research to date is that both parent–child and marital relations are significantly affected by parental depression, and both have been implicated in the development of psychopathology among children of depressed parents. Moreover, as we saw in Chapter 8, the emotional security hypothesis provides a model for how both parent–child and marital conflict affect children's adjustment. Thus, at the outset, there are bases for expecting that emotional security may account for important variance in the effects of both parent–child relations (Colin, 1996) and marital conflict and distress (Davies & Cummings, 1998) on children's adjustment in families with parental depression. Accordingly, the emotional security hypothesis has promise as an organizing construct for the effects of parental depression on child adjustment as affected by family processes (Cummings, 1995a).

There is a particularly urgent need for theory in the case of research guided by the developmental psychopathology perspective given the fact that this approach fosters multidomain, multimethod, and multidisciplinary studies of child development; that is, the complexity of results and findings that inevitably emerge from such sophisticated and diverse approaches to a phenomenon has the inherent potential to be overwhelming to researchers and clinicians alike. For the developmental psychopathologist, therefore, theory must always be a paramount and ultimate goal and concern while pursuing at the same time the highest standards of empirical research.

Searching for Common, Familywide Processes: Emotional Security and Family Functioning

As we have seen, children of depressed parents grow up in family environments that are more frequently typified by parental inconsistency, emotional unavailability, and marital conflict. The parenting and parent–child dimensions linked with parental depression increase the risk that insecure parent–child attachment will develop (see Chapters 6 and 7). In fact, as we have seen, children of depressed parents are more likely to have emotionally insecure, and even very insecure (Type A/C or D) attachments to their parents, which have been linked with their greater risk for adjustment problems (Colin, 1996). Moreover, children of depressed parents are also exposed to higher incidences of marital conflict, which has also been linked empirically with greater risk for adjustment problems. In addition, marital conflict has been linked both theoretically and empirically with emotional insecurity due to the negative quality of marital relations (Davies & Cummings, 1994, 1998). These threads of evidence thus point to the notion that emotional insecurity may be a mediator of these children's risk for adjustment problems, and as a risk factor, may have multiple sources within the family.

Put another way, one might ask how and why depressive family contexts shape children's developmental trajectories in such a way that developmental deviations are made more likely. The idea that increases in emotional insecurity due to dysfunctions in multiple family systems alter children's functioning so that maladaptive response processes are made more prevalent has appeal (Cummings, 1995a). Disturbances in attachment have long been implicated theoretically and empirically in the development, maintenance, and intergenerational transmission of depression in families (Cummings & Cicchetti,

1990). Given the higher incidence of marital conflict in homes with parental depression, the higher rates of insecure attachments, and the familial patterns of dysfunctional emotional communication and psychological unavailability, it seems logical that emotional security concerns would be elevated for children of depressed parents.

Similarities to Other Relations Systems Perspectives

This theory is a specific articulation of a relational systems approach, with similarities to other models for the development of children of depressed parents in its concern with family subsystems as developmental contexts and the importance of goals of interpersonal relations (e.g., emotional security) to the development of individuals. For example, Lee and Gotlib (1991) advanced notions as to why different forms of family disturbance predict common child outcomes, hypothesizing that different family stressors may affect child development through common emotional processes in the family system; that is, they suggested that because many different forms of family disturbance (e.g., marital discord, divorce, parental depression) are associated with similar child outcomes, then perhaps there is a common pathway through which they exert their effects. Similar to the tenets of an emotional security hypothesis (Cummings & Davies, 1996), there was a need for a family systems perspective that considered the comorbidity of family stressors. The most promising mediators identified were those involving emotional processes of "parental availability" and "children's sense of security or confidence in their parents."

Lyons-Ruth (1995) has also argued for theoretical frameworks that center on relational systems within depressive family contexts. Relational systems models maintain that an individual's well-being and functioning should be considered within an interpersonal context. Thus, patterns of behavior, including maladaptive patterns, are conceptualized as components and mechanisms that regulate interpersonal relations. Assuming fundamental importance for understanding the development of psychopathology is the specification of critical contexts of interpersonal relations, the goals within these contexts, and the success in achieving these goals. Lyons-Ruth contended that relational contexts that are particularly promising include (1) attachment relationships, (2) coercive parent–child interactions, and (3) hostile marital relations. The goals of interpersonal relations were seen as including (1) security in attachment relationships, (2) global self-worth, and (3) the extent of control in interpersonal relations. Lyons-Ruth also argued for the importance to children's development of implicit representational systems underlying relational and psychological disturbances.

General Propositions of the Emotional Security Hypothesis

It should be noted that we are extending a general theoretical model of emotional security for children's adjustment in families (Cummings & Davies,

1996; Davies & Cummings, 1994) to the specific instance of parental depression (Cummings, 1995a; Cummings & Davies, 1999). According to our extension of this model, parental depression and child outcomes are linked through a complex interplay among child-management impairments, child exposure to symptomatology, marital discord, and child characteristics such as temperament and developmental level. Among various direct and indirect connections, this diverse collection of phenomena and processes converges to threaten the child's emotional security, which then becomes an important locus for deleterious effects. Intermediary effects of threatened emotional security are evident in child responses to immediate family events and stresses. Ultimately, however, the cumulative effects of chronic threat to emotional security will be seen, probabilistically, in diagnosable childhood conditions.

The centrality (but not exclusivity) of emotional regulation to the emotional security approach is not unique. In fact, emotional regulation and emotional security are central constructs in other accounts of normal development and the development of psychopathology (Cole, Michel, & Teti, 1994). The idea that emotions serve regulatory functions is also not unique (Thompson, 1994; Thompson & Calkins, 1996). It is the hypothesized network of relations in which emotional security is embedded that marks its unique contribution to the parental depression literature, namely, that emotional security is central to the regulation of action (see also Emery, 1992). In fact, it is a constructive organizing process, not an epiphenomenal by-product of experience that needs to be controlled and modulated owing to any presumed disorganizing nature. Emotional security is the goal-state of a homeostatic apparatus encompassing not only emotions but also behavior, thoughts, and physiological responses. Hence, it extends beyond conscious thoughts and feelings and subsumes both present and past situational influences. Though broad in scope and necessarily explicated in abstract terms for theoretical purposes, various propositions of the emotional security model are readily tested with standard instruments and laboratory procedures (Davies & Cummings, 1998).

As we saw in Chapter 8, emotional security is specifically proffered to be reflected in three interdependent processes: emotional reactivity, representations of family relations, and regulation of exposure to family affect (Davies & Cummings, 1994). Assessing these component processes as distinct elements allows one not only to test the emotional security hypothesis but also to test the significance of the subprocesses as mediators of adjustment, without regard to assumptions of the higher-order organization posited by the emotional security hypothesis.

However, in theory, emotional security is conceptualized as a control system within which interrelations among these three component processes and the latent goal of emotional security are inextricable and bidirectional. Thus, emotional security is a goal that governs or regulates the expression of the concrete component processes. For example, insecurity resulting from marital discord due to parental depression may increase children's incentives to regulate their exposure to threatening parental events by escaping or intervening in the conflict. By the same token, emotional security is also a goal that is regulated by the component processes. Extending the previous example, the mediation in parental disputes that was originally motivated by felt insecurity subsequently serves as a means of restoring some sense of emotional security, at least in a temporary, superficial way. Thus, positing that emotional security is reflected in several specific, interdependent component processes advances the testability and specificity of the model, both in the general case and in the specific example of children of depressed parents.

CONCLUSION

The study of children at risk for adjustment problems is a central theme in the developmental psychopathology tradition because of the potential payoff for theoretical understanding of the range of pathways and processes that may contribute to child development, and the potential applicability of the lacunae of this research to clinical practice. This chapter calls attention to the significance of multiple family systems and processes in the impact of parental depression on children. Research and theory that support links between parental depression, family functioning, and child adjustment are discussed. While there are major gaps in specifying interrelations between different family systems in predicting outcomes for children of depressed parents, the case for the importance of multiple individual and family factors in children's risk for adjustment problems is already a strong one. Consistent with a developmental psychopathology perspective, next steps include a movement *toward* (1) articulating the specific processes linking these factors, and (2) adequately conceptualizing developmental pathways in children of depressed parents. While these directions *toward* a "second generation" of research meant to account for developmental deviance and normal development in children of depressed parents are in a relatively early stage, we outlined various guidelines for future research on a developmental psychopathology of depression in families. Finally, we advanced arguments for a testable theoretical model describing how the greater parenting dysfunction and marital conflict, in particular, in families with parental depression may initiate dynamic processes of emotional insecurity in children of depressed parents that mediate their greater risk for adjustment problems. A theoretical account such as this one, firmly based on research, is essential to the ultimate clinical applicability of research findings, as well as further scientific understanding of the processes accounting for developmental outcomes in children from high-risk family environments.

PART III

Clinical Implications

A Developmental Psychopathology Perspective on the Diagnosis, Classification, and Conceptualization of Children's Problems

So far, we have explained how the developmental psychopathology perspective structures our understanding of the complex determinants of children's adjustment and maladjustment. We have focused on the family as an important context that either supports or undermines healthy development. From this perspective, individual differences in child characteristics; in dyadic relationships within the family (e.g., attachment security and emotional security); in parental warmth, involvement, and limit setting; and in family functioning more generally (e.g., parental depression, marital adjustment) converge to predict which children will be well adjusted and better able to cope with developmental challenges and transitions, and which children will have difficulties dealing with new situations and experiences. The clinician working with disturbed children and families will consider these issues in conceptualizing the likely factors that may contribute to or maintain children's behavioral and emotional problems. Surprisingly, however, these issues are only included indirectly and unsystematically when the clinician assigns a formal diagnosis or classifies the child's problem using the usual nomenclature of child psychopathology.

Almost all clinicians use some system to classify children's problems, because it provides a shorthand way of communicating with other professionals, and most mental health facilities require that a diagnosis be assigned. Moreover, insurance companies will not reimburse in the absence of a diagnosis.

The current classification systems, however, focus almost exclusively on the child's behavior, with less emphasis on context and developmental level. Classification systems usually rely either on ratings of children's behaviors along dimensions such as aggression or social withdrawal, or they organize these behaviors into distinct categories of disorder or maladjustment, the most widely used system being the American Psychiatric Association's (APA) *Diagnostic and Statistical Manual of Mental Disorders* (DSM; APA, 1994). On the one hand, the description of children's behavior, whether along dimensions or as categories, can inform developmental psychopathology researchers about the range of problem behavior and levels of severity at one point in time, and over the course of development. On the other hand, however, classification systems run the risk of focusing too much attention on the overt manifestations of children's unhappiness and distress, thereby overlooking salient aspects of the child's environment. This can become a problem, because we know that maladaptive behavior such as aggression or severe social withdrawal have many different roots in development and follow many different developmental pathways depending upon a myriad of factors in the child, family, and wider social context in which the child is being raised. Thus, the question becomes which best captures the child's problem: We can describe 4-year-old Johnny as one standard deviation above the mean on aggression; we can diagnose him as *having* oppositional defiant disorder; or we can focus on the fact that his parents are constantly fighting and often use severe physical punishment with him as well. These different characterizations of Johnny's difficulties have implications for the conceptualization of his problems and, thus, for case management. It is these issues that we address in more detail in this chapter as we consider the diagnosis, classification, and clinical formulation of children's problems.

Because research in child psychopathology and clinical practice with children and families are both influenced by the systems used to assess and classify problem behavior, this is deemed an important topic to discuss. At one level, different diagnostic formulations may lead to different treatment recommendations, and the interpretation of research findings will be influenced by the classification of problem behavior as well. Thus, for example, despite symptom overlap and co-occurrence, different treatment recommendations may be made when a child is seen as anxious as opposed to depressed. At another level, children's problems may be conceptualized as reflecting a discrete psychiatric disorder or diagnostic entity, or be seen along a continuum of adjustment and maladjustment. This, too, will have implications for the interpretation of data at both a research and clinical level. The disorder concept implies relatively fixed assumptions about likely etiology and developmental course. In contrast, consistent with a developmental psychopathology perspective, when children's problems are seen as part of a continuum, a different set of assumptions about etiology and developmental course may apply (e.g., multidetermined and not necessarily likely to persist). Issues of assessment also are intertwined with the classification of children's problems. Placing children into categories of disorders and/or describing their behavior along dimensions of symptom clusters obviously means that children's behavior needs to be measured in some way.

Thus, in this chapter, currently accepted approaches to classification are discussed, and their strengths and weaknesses highlighted, along with some consideration of several assessment methods. Similar issues are raised in our examination of classification and assessment methods, because both focus almost exclusively on describing child behavior, with much less systematic consideration of family processes, family context, or the child's wider social environment (child care or school, peer group). Obviously, then, current methods of assessment and classification are in many ways more narrow and less theoretically driven than the perspective outlined in this book. At the same time, it must be remembered that, historically, the assessment of children's problems focused more explicitly on children's intrapsychic experiences and interpretations of events, with an emphasis on projective tests of limited reliability and validity (Gittelman-Klein, 1986). Although these traditional approaches did attend to family dynamics, the conceptualization tended to be deterministic, unidirectional (parent → child), and limited in considering the wider social environment. The more empirically based assessments that are common today are certainly a step forward, because they are well standardized and validated, but they run the risk of being insufficiently sensitive to the child's emotional security, relationship quality, and adaptation to family functioning.

In line with the themes of this book, current diagnostic systems and assessment methods are considered from a developmental psychopathology framework, which places a much larger emphasis on family processes and family/social context in understanding and predicting the onset, maintenance, and developmental course of children's problems. It is argued that children's problems cannot be understood in the absence of a consideration of the child's developmental stage, family context (marital, parental adjustment) and parenting behavior, extrafamilial social influences (school, peer group), and the child's history of adaptation and maladaptation to challenges and developmental transitions. In addition, problem definition is partly influenced by developmental and cultural expectations. Therefore, what is considered a problem in one community might be considered acceptable behavior in another and vice versa. Behaviors that concern families with unlimited resources might be overlooked by families struggling to meet basic needs, for example, moodiness or worry in a school-age child. Fears and worries may also vary as a function of cultural context and neighborhood. Moreover, there is evidence indicating that adult perceptions of psychopathology vary widely as a function of culture, both within a country and between countries (Lambert & Weisz, 1992; Mash & Wolfe, 1999; Weisz, Chayaisit, Weiss, Eastman, & Jackson, 1995). Despite this, the current diagnostic systems tend not to include cultural, ecological, or developmental considerations in definitions of disorder.

In order to illustrate these and other issues, case examples are discussed from a transactional, ecological perspective of the child in context, with a consideration of family processes, likely developmental pathways, and the balance of risk and protective factors. This is meant to illustrate the implications of the themes articulated throughout this book for the assessment, classification, and conceptualization of children's problem behavior.

Classification of children's problems is complicated further by the fact that most of the problem behaviors or symptoms that define childhood disorders may reflect normal variations in typical behaviors (e.g., noncompliance in toddlers, difficulty in sharing among preschoolers), problem behaviors that may be more serious but do not persist and never come to clinical attention (aggression between peers in preschool), or a constellation of problems that interfere with children's functioning and may lead to clinical referral (e.g., a combination of noncompliance, aggression toward siblings and/or peers, defiance, and tantrums). Thus, it is necessary to have some form of common metric or system to gauge the nature, severity, and clinical significance of problem behavior. If a researcher is interested in studying the developmental course of oppositional behavior, for example, it is important to know whether one is talking about age-appropriate oppositionality in a preschooler, a more serious problem that may be a sign of maladjustment, or a constellation of oppositional behavior and related symptoms that may reflect a diagnosable disorder (i.e., oppositional defiant disorder). The clinician working with family members concerned about their young child's defiance and tantrum behavior will need to assess the severity, nature, and context of the presenting problems before appropriate advice can be given to the parents. Likewise, depressed mood in children may reflect sadness that is part of normal, everyday variations in mood, sad mood that is a transitory reaction to a stressful event such as the loss of a pet, sad mood that is a correlate of other problems, or a prolonged sad mood that is part of a particular syndrome of depression or dysthymia. Obviously, these differences in the nature and severity of depressed mood have important implications for the assessment and diagnosis of a problem, for treatment, and for the interpretation of research findings. Therefore, in order to provide a common language about behaviors considered symptomatic of disorder, child psychopathologists have developed ways of assessing, conceptualizing, and organizing information about symptoms and clusters of symptoms. As is obvious, these methods of classification have relevance to both child psychopathology research and to practice with children referred to mental health clinics. However, as already pointed out, these methods tend to emphasize child behavior at the expense of considering the child in context, and the child's adaptation to adverse (or supportive) family circumstances.

CLINICAL AND EMPIRICAL APPROACHES TO ASSESSMENT, DIAGNOSIS, AND CLASSIFICATION

There are two widely used approaches to the classification of children's behavior problems: the diagnostic or clinical approach represented by the diagnostic nomenclature of the DSM (APA, 1980, 1987, 1994), and the empirical approach exemplified by the work of Achenbach (1991a, 1995). There are similarities and differences between the clinical and empirical approaches to classification, although most child psychopathology research relies on both when defining groups of children for study, and both are used widely in clinical practice. Thus, structured diagnostic interviews based on DSM criteria such as the Child Assessment Schedule (e.g., Hodges, Cools, & McKnew, 1989; Hodges, Saunders, Kashani, Hamlett, & Thompson, 1990), the Diagnostic Interview Schedule for Children (e.g., Shaffer, Fisher, Piacentini, Schwab-Stone, & Wicks, 1993), and empirically derived symptom rating scales, such as the Child Behavior Checklist (CBCL; Achenbach, 1991a), are used routinely to describe the nature and severity of children's problems. The information obtained from these interviews and questionnaires is basically descriptive, focusing on the child's current behavior. Two questions are addressed: What cluster of symptoms or problem behaviors best describes the child? Are they sufficiently severe to be considered clinically significant? Thus, the first step in the assessment and classification of children's problems, whether for research or clinical purposes, is defining what behaviors constitute symptoms, determining how they cluster together and how they differ from normal or typical behavior, and delineating how a particular cluster of problems differs from other clusters with different manifestations. Although at the level of clinical description the clinical and empirical approaches have similar goals, their methods and scientific underpinnings differ.

The Clinical Approach to Diagnosis

This approach to diagnosis is best represented by the DSM, and emphasis here is on the most recent version, the DSM-IV (APA, 1994). Childhood disorders were barely recognized systematically until the publication of the DSM-III (APA, 1980). The DSM has gone through two additional revisions since 1980. The DSM was derived initially from clinical experience and the consensus of practicing clinicians about what symptoms tend to go together. In more recent iterations of the DSM, descriptions of disorders have been backed up with confirmatory research on children referred to clinical settings, and with data from epidemiological studies of representative population-based samples (see, e.g., Lahey et al., 1994; Lahey, Loeber, Quay, Frick, & Grimm, 1992). Although the DSM-IV states explicitly that it is atheoretical and descriptive, making no assumptions about the causes of disorders (APA, 1994), at the same time, it is most vigorously espoused by those with a biological orientation, who adopt a medical model approach to psychopathology (see Jensen & Hoagwood, 1997, for a more detailed discussion of this issue). Moreover, the medical model is based on the assumption that one can define clusters of symptoms that go together to form syndromes. In turn, it is assumed that syndromes are categorical entities and, as such, they are relatively distinct from one another, with each syndrome having its own set of causes and correlates, a predictable developmental course and outcome, and response to particular, syndrome-specific treatments (Cantwell, 1996b; Caron & Rutter, 1991; Jensen & Hoagwood, 1997; Sonuga-Barke, 1998). Another implicit assumption of the diagnostic nomenclature is that the problem or disease entity is *within* the child rather than a function of inadequate environmental supports for the development of age-appropriate emotion regulation, communication and social skills, and so forth (e.g., Sroufe, 1997). Obviously, this view is quite different from the one espoused in this volume.

The most common childhood disorders discussed in the DSM-IV include the *disruptive behavior disorders (oppositional defiant disorder, conduct disorder), attention-deficit/hyperactivity disorder, separation anxiety disorder, attachment disorders, and the pervasive developmental disorders, including autism.* (Because the pervasive developmental disorders are more severe and likely to be totally biologically based, they are beyond the scope of this book.) Depression and anxiety disorders, other than separation anxiety, are defined by the same criteria used to describe adult depression and anxiety disorders. The reliance on adult criteria has obvious drawbacks because it does not place children's symptoms into a clear developmental or social context. Fear of strange people, for example, is normative, even adaptive, in some contexts and at some stages of development. Sad mood in young children is notoriously unstable (Lefkowitz & Burton, 1978) and needs to be considered in terms of the child's age and how well his or her emotional needs are being met. Whereas adults have some control over their environments, at least in most circumstances, children, especially young children, have only limited opportunities to seek out sensitive caregivers or to avoid family conflict or adversity. Thus, special consideration needs to be given to family context in assessing and diagnosing problems in young children, and this is missing entirely from the adult criteria.

For each DSM diagnosis, a series of specific criteria have been derived that must be met for the child to receive a diagnosis. These criteria always include a specified list of symptoms, a certain number of which must be present. A diagnosis is made on the assumption that the presenting symptoms are interfering with, or impairing, daily functioning on age-appropriate tasks and in age-related contexts (family, classroom, peer group). For some disorders, age of onset and duration criteria are also specified. However, developmental guidelines are extremely vague and provide the clinician with no real benchmarks for defining problem behaviors at different ages. To be considered a symptom, a behavior must occur more often than is typical in children of the same age. However, many of the symptoms that define disorders vary widely as a function of development (e.g., activity level, attention span, separation distress, noncompliance), and what is normal at one age may be abnormal at another (Campbell, 1990, 1998). Thus, the absence of developmental guidelines in the DSM-IV criteria remains a serious problem.

Because we consider the relevance of specific diagnoses to the conceptualization of cases, it is important to provide a brief overview of some of the criteria for the main disorders of childhood, summarized in Tables 10.1 and 10.2. One of the most common disorders of childhood is *attention-deficit/hyperactivity disorder* (ADHD), which is divided into three subtypes in the DSM-IV: inattentive, hyperactive–impulsive, and combined. To receive a diagnosis of *ADHD, inattentive subtype*, the child must have six of the nine symptoms that make up the inattention cluster. The inattention symptoms include difficulty sustaining attention, does not seem to listen, difficulty organizing tasks, and easily distracted by extraneous stimuli. To meet criteria for *ADHD, hyperactive–impulsive subtype*, the child must demonstrate six symptoms from the nine indicators of hyperactive–impulsive behavior, such as fidgets, leaves seat inappropriately, often "on the go," and blurts out answers. Children meeting criteria for both subtypes are considered to have *ADHD, combined subtype*. By definition, children with the combined subtype also have more severe problems, because they have more numerous and varied symptoms. In addition, for any ADHD diagnosis, symptoms must be present before age 7 and persist for at least 6 months. This is because these behaviors rarely appear "out of the blue," and when they do, they may be short-lived reactions to stressful life events such as family separation, the birth of a sibling, or family illness. (See Campbell, 2000, for a more in-depth discussion of attention deficit disorder from a developmental perspective.) Finally, impairment must be present in two or more settings (e.g., at home and school) in order to rule out situation-specific anxiety or agitation that may look like ADHD. Studies suggest that younger children are more likely to present with the hyperactive–impulsive subtype, whereas children are rarely diagnosed with the inattentive subtype prior to school entry, when the expectation that they pay attention and concentrate on school-related tasks becomes more salient (Applegate et al., 1997).

The diagnosis of *oppositional defiant disorder* depends upon the child showing four symptoms that reflect negative, hostile, and defiant behavior for 6 months. The symptoms that define the disorder include losing temper, argumentative, defiant, annoying, blames others for own mistakes, touchy, angry and resentful, and spiteful or vindictive. Negative affect is one core component of this disorder. However, many young children go through a prolonged period of noncompliance and difficult behavior, and the differentiation between clinically significant oppositional disorder and hard-to-manage but age-appropriate defiance is often difficult (Campbell, 1990). Moreover, defiant and uncooperative behavior is a common concern of parents, a common reaction to normative life events in young children, such as the birth of a sibling, and a common outcome variable in studies of young children's adjustment to normal developmental challenges and transitions (Campbell, Pierce, March, Ewing, & Szumowski, 1994; Crockenberg & Litman, 1990; Kuczynski, Radke-Yarrow, Kochanska, & Girnius-Brown, 1987; NICHD Early Child Care Research Network, 1998). Thus, it is important to understand both the normal and abnormal manifestations of defiant behavior in young children, as well as the fact that some types of noncompliance are adaptive (e.g.,

TABLE 10.1. Common Childhood Disorders in the DSM-IV

<u>Attention-deficit and disruptive behavior disorders</u>

<u>Attention-deficit/hyperactivity disorder</u>

Symptoms	Six or more symptoms (out of nine) of inattention (e.g., often has difficulty sustaining attention, often does not seem to listen) or six or more (out of nine) symptoms of hyperactivity–impulsivity (e.g., often fidgets, often blurts out answers) to a degree that is maladaptive and inconsistent with developmental level
Duration	At least 6 months
Onset age	Some symptoms causing impairment evident before age 7 years
Subtypes	ADHD, predominantly inattentive type: Six inattention symptoms, but fewer than six hyperactivity–impulsivity symptoms
	ADHD, predominantly hyperactive–impulsive type: Six hyperactivity symptoms, but fewer than six inattention symptoms
	ADHD, combined type: Meets criteria for both subtypes

<u>Oppositional defiant disorder</u>

Symptoms	Four out of eight negative, defiant, hostile, and argumentative behaviors that occur more frequently than is typically observed in children of the same age
Duration	At least 6 months
Onset age	Before age 18
Subtypes	None

<u>Conduct disorder</u>

Symptoms	Repetitive and persistent pattern of aggressive or antisocial behavior; violation of age-appropriate norms; three behaviors reflecting aggression to people and animals (seven specific symptoms, such as initiates physical fights, cruel to animals); destruction of property (two specific symptoms—fire setting, destructive); deceitfulness or theft (three symptoms); serious rule violations (three specific symptoms)
Duration	Behavioral pattern over the past 12 months
Onset age	May occur as early as age 5–6, but usually occurs later
Subtypes	Childhood onset (at least 1 criterion met prior to age 10)
	Adolescent onset (no signs prior to age 10)

<u>Internalizing disorders</u>

<u>Separation anxiety disorder</u>

Symptoms	Developmentally inappropriate and excessive anxiety about separation from home or from primary attachment figure, as evidenced by three of eight symptoms (e.g., excessive distress when separation is anticipated, excessive worry about harm befalling attachment figure, repeated complaints of physical symptoms)
Duration	At least 4 weeks
Onset age	Before age 18 (early onset if before age 6)
Subtypes	None

TABLE 10.2. Representative Internalizing Diagnoses Using Adult Criteria Regardless of Child Age

Major depression

Symptoms	Five of nine symptoms (depressed mood or loss of interest must be present; other symptoms include significant weight loss or gain, hypersomnia or insomnia, fatigue or loss of energy)
Duration	Symptoms must be present for the same 2-week period
Onset age	None; in children, sad mood can be replaced by irritable mood

Dysthymia

Symptoms	Chronic depressed mood (may be irritable mood in children), accompanied by at least two additional symptoms: poor appetite, sleep problems, low energy, low self-esteem, poor concentration, hopelessness
Duration	2 years; in children, 1 year
Onset age	Early onset is considered before age 21

Generalized anxiety disorder

Symptoms	Excessive anxiety and worry about a number of events and activities (e.g., school performance) that are difficult to control. The anxiety is associated with at least three of six symptoms, such as restlessness, easily fatigued, or irritability
Duration	6 months
Onset age	None

Crockenberg & Litman, 1990). Not surprisingly, this diagnosis has had its critics (Campbell, 1990) as well as its defenders (Lahey, Loeber, Quay, Frick, & Grimm, 1992).

In general, it is assumed that oppositional disorder is often a developmental precursor of more serious antisocial behavior (APA, 1994), as reflected in a diagnosis of *conduct disorder,* in which the child engages in more serious and persistent aggression toward people, destruction of property, deceitfulness, and major rule violations. Age of onset defines the two subtypes of conduct disorder (child-onset and adolescent-onset), which are hypothesized to follow different developmental pathways and to have different prognoses (Moffitt, 1993a; Patterson & Yoerger, 1997). Adolescent-onset conduct problems are seen as more likely to be age-related and transient, whereas early-onset conduct problems are more likely to reflect serious and persistent psychopathology that may begin as serious oppositional disorder in childhood and then continue into adulthood.

Of the anxiety disorders, only *separation anxiety disorder* has criteria based explicitly on child behavior, but even here, the developmental guidelines are vague and distinctions between normal variations in separation distress in young children and a pathological condition are far from clear. This weakness in the criteria is especially serious, since signs of separation distress may occur in young children as a normal reaction to stressful life events such as the hospitalization of a parent, family breakup, or entry into child care.

As already noted, childhood depression and most anxiety disorders are defined by adult criteria, regardless of age. This is a serious drawback, because almost no developmental guidelines are provided, although it seems obvious that children of different ages will manifest sadness and distress in different ways. To meet criteria for major *depression*, children must show a cluster of five out of eight symptoms for a 2-week period. Among these symptoms are depressed or irritable mood, or loss of interest in usual activities for most of the day, almost every day. Eating and sleeping problems, cognitive deficits (difficulty concentrating, excessive guilt, feelings of worthlessness, suicidal ideation) are also defining criteria. A more chronic, but less severe form of depression, *dysthymia*, is also diagnosed in children. Similarly, diagnoses of anxiety disorders (*generalized anxiety disorder, social phobia, panic disorder*) rely on adult criteria and are relatively rare in children. The criteria for depression, dysthymia, and generalized anxiety disorder are summarized in Table 10.2.

DSM diagnoses are usually made on the basis of interviews. In many research studies, structured and semistructured diagnostic interviews are used. These vary in how structured they are and how much they rely on clinical judgment to determine the presence or absence of a symptom, as well as whether the child meets criteria for a particular diagnosis. Many of these structured interviews have child and parent versions (e.g., Hodges, Saunders, Kashani, Hamlett, & Thompson, 1990; Shaffer, Fisher, Piacentini, Schwab-Stone, & Wicks, 1993), and combine information from both informants in making diagnostic decisions. The development of structured interviews has provided researchers with a useful tool for standardizing diagnostic decisions across laboratories and studies, and making diagnoses more reliable. At the same time, there has been some loss of coverage and clinical richness, a trade-off determined by the desire to achieve agreement among clinicians (Jensen & Hoagwood, 1997). In clinical work, the degree to which diagnostic decisions are made on the basis of standard interviews or less structured, individually developed interviews varies widely.

In general, the DSM approach is categorical (the child does or does not meet criteria for the diagnosis), descriptive, derived from clinical consensus, atheoretical, and lacking in developmental guidelines. On the other hand, the specificity of symptoms and other criteria (age of onset, duration, cross-situationality) makes it relatively likely that children who receive a diagnosis actually have significant behavior problems that interfere with their functioning in the family, school, and peer group. Clinically, by stipulating that a child must meet criteria for a DSM-IV diagnosis if the practitioner is to receive third-party payments, many insurance companies make political and economic considerations primary motivators for assigning a diagnosis. However, some children who are below threshold for a diagnosis may have serious problems that require treatment (Angold, Costello, Farmer, Burns, & Erklani, 1999), raising important issues about how well the diagnostic categories assess clinically significant problems. From a research perspective, too, it is now considered mandatory for investigators to use a common set of assessment methods, diagnostic criteria, and diagnostic labels that assure some comparability across samples and thereby facilitate the interpretation of research findings.

However, most important from the perspective of the clinician, knowing a child's diagnosis does not necessarily tell us much about the child or what to do about his or her problem. It is a shorthand label that is useful, at some level, as a brief communication among mental health professionals, educators, and researchers, but there are drawbacks as well, including reification of the label, potential stigmatization and misuse, and only limited prescriptive information for intervention. In addition, the proliferation of diagnostic categories means that diagnostic decisions are difficult to make reliably (i.e., different clinicians may not agree on which diagnosis or diagnoses are appropriate), and some researchers have questioned the validity of particular diagnostic categories, including oppositional defiant disorder, attention deficit disorder, and prepubertal depression (e.g., Angold & Costello, 1993, 1996). This means that despite the underlying assumption that each specific diagnosis is associated with a particular etiology or set of etiologies, a set of clinical correlates, a particular developmental course and likely outcome, and a predictable response to particular treatment regimens, the research on childhood disorders is not consistent with this degree of specificity. This lack of specificity is one major reason why the validity of several disorders remains debatable.

Furthermore, the diagnostic decision is based almost entirely on the child's behavior vis-à-vis the specific behavioral and impairment criteria that define the diagnosis. The implication of this entirely descriptive approach to diagnosis is that the problem is seen as being within the child. It is defined by the child's behavior in response to age-appropriate challenges and expectations, rather than as a transaction between the child and his or her environment. Although we have focused almost exclusively on the family as the context for the development of psychopathology in children, the DSM takes family factors into account only tangentially, and their inclusion is neither systematic nor central. Thus, the clinician may code the degree of psychosocial stress, but there is little concern with the family climate, the attachment relationship, emotional security, the quality of parenting and support for the child's development, or other issues that have defined our discussion so far. Although these factors will be part of any good clinician's case formulation, they will not necessarily influence the diagnosis.

Another major problem with the DSM is the tendency for most children referred to child mental health clinics to receive more than one or, often, multiple diagnoses, which is referred to as *comorbidity*. Because the DSM is a categorical system in which the child either meets or does not meet the criteria for a given diagnosis; because there are multiple categories, some of which overlap; and because children referred to mental health clinics often have a wide variety of problems, it is not surprising that multiple diagnoses are the rule rather than the exception. From a clinical perspective, it may be difficult to decide which set of problems to address first or to consider the most serious. From a research perspective, comorbidity may result in misleading interpretations of findings. For example, oppositional disorder and attention deficit disorder often co-occur, but failure to distinguish between children with one of these disorders and those with both has led to misinterpretations in studies of both family history (e.g., old Cantwell, Stewart studies) and developmental course and prognosis. It is now accepted that children with both ADHD and oppositional or aggressive behavior are more likely to live in dysfunctional families with high rates of psychopathology (e.g., Barkley, Anastopoulos, Guevremont, & Fletcher, 1992; Lahey et al., 1988) and to have a poorer outcome in adolescence (Barkley, Fischer, Edelbrock, & Smallish, 1990, 1991) and adulthood (Mannuzza, Klein, Bessler, Malloy, & LaPadula, 1993; Weiss & Hechtman, 1993). Moreover, the fact that comorbidity is so widespread, both in epidemiological studies of nonreferred children (e.g., Offord, Boyle, Fleming, Blum, & Rae Grant, 1989) and in clinical samples (e.g., Biederman, Newcorn, & Sprich, 1991; Hinshaw, 1987; Hinshaw, Lahey, & Hart, 1993), raises serious questions about the distinctness of the disorders defined in the DSM (Caron & Rutter, 1991; Nottelman & Jensen, 1995).

Finally, given the developmental perspective espoused in this book, the fact the DSM provides so little in the way of developmental guidelines and, in some instances, uses identical criteria for 8- and 80-year-olds, is troubling. This problem has been rectified somewhat by the American Academy of Pediatrics (AAP), which has published a revised version of the diagnostic nomenclature for children, with clearer developmental guidelines and criteria for severity (*Diagnostic and Statistical Manual for Primary Care* [DSM-PC]; AAP, 1996). This manual is meant for clinicians working in primary care facilities (rather than mental health clinics) and identifies three levels of severity (normal variation, problem behavior, clinical disorder). Thus, the DSM-PC takes into account the fact that many children may show problem behaviors as part of a normal developmental transition that may require short-term management but does not warrant a diagnosis of a major mental disorder.

The problems just outlined have led to many recent articles criticizing of the DSM (Caron & Rutter, 1991; Jensen & Hoagwood, 1997; Sonuga-Barke, 1998; Sroufe, 1997; Wakefield, 1997). Criticisms include the lack of specificity; the reliance on the medical model to conceptualize mental disorders, with an implicit assumption of biological cause; the atheoretical nature of the system; the tendency to be overinclusive but also to miss subthreshold cases; the failure to consider developmental issues; the difficulties encountered in making diagnoses reliably; and the fact that validity of some of the categories has not yet been established. The issue of comorbidity has also raised questions about the meaningfulness of the system. Because children, especially clinically referred children, almost always receive more than one diagnosis, it has been suggested that disorders either may not be distinct or they have not been defined appropriately (Caron & Rutter, 1991). The irony of this dilemma is captured by Sroufe (1997), who noted that "one might think that the discovery that children's problems often cut across the working categories would have led to a questioning of the entire system, not to a new medical term" (p. 257).

In summary, both child psychopathology researchers and clinicians working with children and families rely on the DSM-IV diagnostic system in describing children's problems. Although this is a step forward in that the criteria for each diagnosis are specified, there are major drawbacks that may in fact complicate both research interpretation and clinical decisions. In particular, the atheoretical and adevelopmental nature of the system is problematic, its underlying assumptions are untested, and the overlap among disorders and their questionable validity remain serious challenges.

The Empirical Approach to Classification of Children's Problems

The empirical approach to the classification of childhood disorders is likewise atheoretical and descriptive, but it is derived from research studies of children's problems rather than clinical consensus. In this approach, parents, teachers, or the children themselves rate the degree of severity of set lists of potentially problematic behaviors. Factor analyses of large numbers of such reports, usually from parents (e.g., Achenbach, 1995; Achenbach, Howell, Quay, & Conners, 1991), result in clusters of behavior that typically go together in large numbers of children recruited from both clinical and nonclinical sources. This approach has been used after the fact to validate some of the clusters of behavior used to define childhood disorders in the DSM (e.g., Lahey et al., 1992, 1994, 1998).

The Child Behavior Checklist (CBCL) epitomizes the empirical approach to the assessment and classification of children's problems. Four versions now exist: the parent CBCL for 2- to 3-year-olds (Achenbach, Edelbrock, & Howell, 1987); the parent CBCL for 4- to 18-year-olds (Achenbach, 1991a); and the Teacher Report Form (TRF; Achenbach, 1992) and the Youth Self-Report form for 11- to 18-year-olds (YSR; Achenbach, 1991b). Factor analyses of ratings on thousands of children across ages, cultures, and reporters (Achenbach, 1995) have consistently isolated two broad factors called *internalizing and externalizing*. These, in turn, are reflected in more narrow factors, such as anxious–depressed attachment style, somatic complaints, and social withdrawal, that make up the internalizing score. Aggressive and delinquent scales make up the externalizing score. Other narrowband factors (social problems, attention problems) lie midway between externalizing and internalizing factors. It should be obvious from this discussion that internalizing problems primarily reflect feelings of negative affect and worry turned inward, whereas externalizing problems are more explosive, annoying to others, and directed outward to the environment and other people. Children are rated on this scale and receive scores on each dimension of behavior; thus, this is considered a dimensional rather than a categorical approach to describing disordered behavior. Scales with representative items are summarized in Table 10.3.

TABLE 10.3. Child Behavior Checklist Scales and Representative Items

Internalizing

Anxious–depressed (lonely, feels unloved, worries)
Somatic complaints (dizzy, tired, headaches)
Social withdrawal (would rather be alone, shy, secretive)

Mixed internalizing–externalizing

Social problems (acts young, teased, not liked)
Attention problems (cannot concentrate, cannot sit still)

Externalizing

Aggression (mean, argues, fights)
Delinquency (no guilt when he or she misbehaves, lies, steals)

Years of research with the CBCL have led to the empirical derivation of age and gender norms for problem behavior and the definition of behavioral clusters that are evident across settings, reporters, and age groups (Achenbach, 1995). This means that the definition of problem behavior is less arbitrary than is the case with the DSM, since only children with CBCL scores above the 90th percentile (i.e., the top 10%) are considered at risk, and only children with scores at or above the 98th percentile (i.e., the top 2%, according to population norms) are considered to have clinically significant problems. Cutoff scores can be used, then, to make this dimensional system categorical for comparison with the DSM or for extreme group comparison studies. Indeed, research has indicated that children with highly elevated scores on the CBCL broad- and narrowband dimensions differ from low-scoring children on a wide range of other behaviors, family correlates, and the developmental course of problems (e.g., Campbell, Pierce, March, Ewing, & Szumowski, 1994; Campbell, Pierce, Moore, Marakovitz, & Newby, 1996; Coie, Terry, Lenox, Lochman, & Hyman, 1995; Greenberg, Leguna, Coie, & Pinderhughes, 1999; Shaw, Owens, Vondra, Keenan, & Winslow, 1996).

It is also important to note that there is some general correspondence between DSM-IV diagnostic categories and CBCL factor scores (e.g., anxiety/depression and anxiety disorders and depression, attention problems and ADHD, aggressive and oppositional defiant disorder, delinquent and conduct disorder). At the same time, some disorders considered distinct in the DSM system seem to merge together in the empirical studies (anxiety and depression), whereas other factors denote symptom clusters that seem clinically important but are not represented in the DSM (e.g., somatic complaints, social withdrawal). Additionally, in a dimensional system, the issue of comorbidity becomes moot. Children have profiles of high and low scores rather than specific sets of categorical diagnoses. The checklist items, however, do not map exactly onto the diagnostic criteria. This has led to the development of several more specific child instruments geared to assessment of anxiety and fearfulness (e.g., LaGreca & Stone, 1993; March, Parker, Sullivan, Stallings, & Conners, 1997; Ollendick, 1983a), depression (e.g., Kovacs, 1991), ADHD (e.g., Pelham et al., 1992), and oppositional behavior (Eyberg, Boggs, & Algina, 1995), as well as other problems such as suicidality (Reynolds & Mazza, 1994) and delinquency (Elliot, Huizinga, & Ageton, 1985). In addition, other broad assessments of children's behavior problems are in use (e.g., Reynolds & Kampaus, 1992). In general, like the CBCL, all these more or less empirically derived, standardized, checklists provide scores on dimensions of specific constellations of problematic behaviors. Discussion of these assessment instruments is beyond the scope of this chapter.

The empirical approach to the assessment and classification of children's problems is not based on assumptions about the behavioral clusters that emerge; the goal is purely descriptive at a dimensional level, and derived cutoff scores are based solely on normative data. In addition, the derivation of age and gender norms makes the empirical approach more sensitive to variations in problem behavior as a function of developmental and sex differences. At the same time, however, very large age spans are grouped together, making age norms less sensitive to variations than seems optimal. Moreover, the brief descriptions of behavior and the provision of only a 3-point scale may also obscure age differences in problem behaviors, especially in the 4–11 age range, where one would expect to find some variation (e.g., in anxiety–depression, aggression, and delinquency) as a function of age. On balance, however, the development of empirically derived dimensions of problem behavior with corresponding assessment measures provides a useful tool for both researchers and clinicians interested in the description and severity of children's behavior problems and their developmental course. These scales are also useful for gauging the change in symptom severity as a function of intervention.

In summary, both the empirical and clinical approaches to classification of childhood disorders systematize the description of children's behavioral symptoms and allow for some inferences about severity. Whereas the DSM approach is categorical and provides explicit criteria, but no age guidelines, the empirical approach is dimensional, based on symptom ratings, and provides norms by age and gender. These questionnaire measures can serve as useful tools for developmental psychopathology research because they allow researchers to describe their samples in more detail, thereby permitting more comparability across studies in the assessment of the nature and severity of adjustment problems, or when defining more clear-cut psychopathology. At the same time, as this discussion points out, the diagnostic categories in and of themselves remain problematic because of their limited specificity, lack of developmental guidelines, and focus on the child's behavior independent of context.

Comorbidity, or the tendency of referred children with one disorder to obtain more than one diagnosis, remains one of the main problems with the

DSM-IV categories. Research on the etiology, correlates, course, and outcome of disorders depends upon a clear definition of the disorder in question. If the boundaries between disorders are either fluid (in the sense of overlapping symptoms, as in depression and ADHD, where concentration difficulties and agitation figure prominently) or if the disorders themselves overlap (as in the case of the high rates of comorbidity between ADHD and oppositional disorder), it is difficult to know what to conclude about *specific* disorders as opposed to the comorbid condition or psychopathology more generally. Another possibility is that specificity beyond the broad constructs of internalizing and externalizing problems is counterproductive.

What are some of the implications of a developmental psychopathology perspective for these problems of assessment and diagnosis? On the one hand, more complex diagnostic categories may need to be developed, in which the child's behavior is considered in context. For example, a child with oppositional problems in the absence of other risk factors may well have a different disorder from the child whose problems occur in the context of multiple family and other risk factors, even though, on the surface, the behaviors look similar. Similarly, severe anxiety and fearfulness occurring in the context of family violence, a divorce accompanied by high levels of blame and retribution, a dangerous neighborhood, or other severe stresses may have very different roots than the anxiety and fearfulness that appear in the absence of these stressful events and negative experiences, although both children may present with similar symptoms (e.g., sleep problems, fear of being alone, somatic complaints, school refusal). Although the DSM-IV does include reference to stressors (Axis IV—psychosocial stressors), the assessment of social context is neither systematic, comprehensive, nor factored into the actual diagnosis. The DSM-PC does a better job of describing the nature of psychosocial stresses that affect children, but because the diagnoses are derived from the DSM, this manual only highlights the problem. It does not deal with it directly.

The developmental psychopathology approach also underscores the importance of considering children's problems as a function of age and gender. It is well known that both age and gender are associated with the prevalence of problem behaviors and their persistence over time. For example, boys show more externalizing problems across development; girls show more internalizing ones, especially in early adolescence and beyond (e.g., Bird, 1996; Verhulst & Koot, 1994). Furthermore, early-onset and pervasive conduct problems in boys are more likely to persist than conduct problems that have their onset in adolescence (Moffitt, 1993a). Clearer guidelines for assessment and diagnosis by age and gender are sorely needed.

In addition, more comprehensive assessment of children and families needs to be incorporated routinely into clinical work. Thus, whereas child behavior and cognitive functioning are often assessed systematically, and it is not uncommon to obtain teacher reports of children's problems (e.g., Achenbach, 1992), family context is often measured informally with unstructured interviews. Well-standardized assessments of marital functioning, parental adjustment and psychopathology, parenting, stressful life events, family process, family social support, and peer and sibling relationships need to be incorporated into standard assessment protocols not only in the laboratory but also in the clinic. Research protocols, including observational measures of family interaction and parenting behavior, need to move to the clinic as well, if the child's social and emotional context and family process measures are to be obtained systematically. Several case examples illustrate some of these themes.

CLINICAL IMPLICATIONS OF DIAGNOSIS

Hypothetical case examples are presented to illustrate some of the difficulties inherent in making a diagnosis and how a developmental psychopathology approach might enrich the typical-medical-model approach to children's disorders. If one assumes that children's problems arise from a complex mix of biological vulnerabilities and contextual factors in the family, peer group, and wider social environment, then one cannot also believe that the problem is a "disease entity" residing in the child. These viewpoints seem incompatible. Instead, in assessing the child's problems, one would need to focus not only on the presenting complaints, or even on the child's behavior across contexts, but also on the developmental course of the problem behaviors, and the social and emotional environment in which they emerged. This includes an assessment of the risk factors in the child's environment that might influence the onset of problems or their developmental course, and the balance of protective factors that might counteract or help the child overcome adversity (Masten, Best, & Garmezy, 1990; Masten & Coatsworth, 1998; Werner, 1993). Moreover, by assuming that even symptomatic behavior may reflect adaptation (Sroufe, 1997), one may get a different perspective on the meaning of a constellation of symptoms leading to referral.

The conceptualization of problem behavior, both for clinical and research purposes, is enriched by applying some of the theoretical issues discussed earlier in this book. For example, models of psychopathology in children partly consider the relative balance of risk and protective factors. Considering both proximal (e.g., the quality of parenting, the nature of the parent–child relationship, family discord) and distal (e.g., aspects of mother's job situation, the availability of social support from extended family, quality and availability of child care) aspects of the child's environment may suggest why the child is having difficulties adapting in general or coping with a specific developmental challenge, or, conversely, why the child's difficulties are not more severe despite high levels of adversity. Historical factors will be relevant as well (e.g., birth complications, the parents' own upbringing). A related issue is the relative role of early experience in shaping children's adjustment and adaptation, and the role of current challenges and supports. Case examples also illustrate the principles of *multifinality* and *equifinality* that were discussed earlier. It should be noted that these cases are hypothetical and prototypical to preserve confidentiality.

The Case of Billy

Billy, a 5½-year-old boy, was referred to a child psychologist because of difficult behavior at home and school. His mother, Mrs. M, complained that he was uncooperative, argumentative, and often threw temper tantrums when he did not get his way. She also complained that he could never sit still and was very disorganized and aggressive during play, often hitting and pushing other children, especially his younger brother, Jason, age 2½. Billy's kindergarten teacher felt that he might require special school services because of his poor language skills, his disruptive and aggressive behavior in the classroom, and his difficulties paying attention and completing worksheets.

Based on the behavior described so far, it would be appropriate to consider diagnoses of oppositional defiant disorder and attention deficit disorder, combined type, although one would need to get additional information about specific symptoms and their duration before these diagnoses could be considered definite. In addition, given Billy's early language and academic difficulties, it would be important to conduct a thorough cognitive assessment to rule out developmental delay, learning problems, or specific cognitive deficits. Because both Billy's mother and teacher are concerned about his behavior, his problems are likely to be relatively serious and pervasive, and to be impairing his functioning in the family, at school, and in the peer group. Billy's problems are not isolated to one setting or apparent only according to the report of just one adult. Moreover, the variety of Billy's problem behaviors suggests that he and his mother require some type of intervention. At the same time, some of Billy's troublesome behavior may reflect age-related, usual behaviors occasioned by the transition to kindergarten, typical squabbles between peers and siblings, inappropriate child management, and other challenges to adaptation.

Regardless of whether Billy meets criteria for oppositional disorder, attention deficit disorder, or both, his constellation of problem behaviors is characteristic of young boys showing externalizing symptoms. In addition, whether they are assessed with dimensional measures or categorical diagnoses, the behaviors characterizing oppositional behavior and attention deficit disorder often co-occur, especially in young children (Barkley, 1998; Campbell et al., 1991; Stormshak, Bierman, & the Conduct Problems Research Group, 1998). The psychologist who assessed Billy's problems was expected to derive at least one specific diagnosis. She, therefore, asked additional questions about relevant behaviors during a structured interview, based on the DSM-IV criteria, administered to Billy's mother. She asked both Mrs. M and Billy's teacher to complete the appropriate versions of the CBCL. Although there was only modest agreement on specific symptoms, Billy obtained elevated scores on the aggression and attention problem scales of the CBCL and TRF, as well as high scores on social problems. According to the structured interview, Billy met criteria for only four inattention and two hyperactivity symptoms, not enough to meet diagnostic criteria for an ADHD diagnosis, despite that fact that he met the age-of-onset criterion and his problems were apparent across settings. It was also less certain whether the problem behaviors all clustered together for 6 months. However, Billy did meet the diagnostic criteria for oppositional defiant disorder, since he had more than four symptoms and his mother had been worried about them for more than 6 months, although she had not sought help until Billy's kindergarten teacher confirmed her concerns.

Despite meeting criteria for one of these disorders, specific treatment recommendations will be determined by the family context, more than by the diagnosis per se. Based just on the behavioral descriptors defining the disorder and the subthreshold symptoms of ADHD, the clinician would not have clear directions for intervention. The relevant symptoms may be clear, but what to do about them is less certain. In order to get a more complete picture of the nature, course, and correlates of Billy's problems, the clinician needs to integrate information about Billy's current family situation and early development with relevant family history information.

Thus, the clinician also obtained a detailed family history that indicated Billy lives with his mother and younger brother; his father, an alcoholic, left the home shortly after his brother's birth, and his whereabouts are unknown. He does not pay child support. Billy's mother has a full-time job in a local department store, and she has managed to keep the family together. Because she has to work some evenings and weekends, she relies on her parents for help with child care and household tasks. Billy's mother has a good relationship with her parents, so this has not been a problem for her, and she is glad that her boys have her father as a male role model. This brief family history highlights several risk and protective factors that may play an important role in formulating hypotheses about the reasons for Billy's problems. They also suggest directions for treatment.

On the risk factor side, alcoholism and abandonment of the family suggest that Billy's father has serious problems himself. Moreover, Mr. M's drinking problems raise concern about whether Mrs. M was abused by her husband during her pregnancy, whether Billy was ever the target of abuse, or whether Mrs. M was ever abused in Billy's presence. Because of all the stresses on Mrs. M, the clinician also would be concerned about her mental health during her pregnancy, over the course of Billy's early development, and currently. In addition, it would be logical to ask whether she was depressed, used alcohol, or relied on medication. For example, if Mrs. M used alcohol or drugs, or was abused by her husband during her pregnancy, this might suggest that some of Billy's attentional, behavior, and academic problems reflect biological vulnerabilities. In addition, it is well known that both antisocial behavior and learning problems run in families, so it is possible that Billy's problems also reflect a genetic predisposition to behavioral problems and school difficulties, associated with his father's possible antisocial personality disorder.

Moreover, his parents' poor marriage and the sequence of events leading to his father's departure almost certainly exposed Billy to family discord, if not outright violence. Even if Billy did not witness violence, his mother would not have been able to shield him totally from family conflict or her own distress. There is also the possibility that her distress and upset interfered with her ability to provide highly involved and sensitive parenting during Billy's infancy and toddlerhood. Furthermore, Billy had to cope with the loss of his father and the birth of a brother at the same time, putting enormous stress on the resources of a 2-year-old. Even though Billy's father might have been explosive and inconsistent, his departure may still have triggered upset and fears of abandonment. Thus, piecing together Billy's developmental and family history suggests a number of risk factors that may have contributed to the early development of problems (risk and protective factors in this case are summarized in Table 10.4).

At the same time that there are multiple risk factors associated with Billy's early development, there are also protective factors, including his mother's resilience and ability to pull herself together, maintain a full-time job, and support the family; and the support that both Billy and his mother receive from his maternal grandparents. This indicates that Mrs. M has many internal strengths and adequate family support, as well as help with child care. The support provided by Billy's grandparents may be interpreted as having both direct and indirect effects on him. The direct effects are indicated by Billy's positive experiences when he spends time with his grandparents, because they provide him with warmth, stimulation, limit setting, and predictability in his daily routine. The indirect effects are mediated through the impact of their support on Mrs. M, who, because she has reliable and high-quality child care, can attend to her job and have some energy left to spend time with her children when she is not working.

During the initial interview, the clinician also obtained detailed information about the current family situation and Billy's developmental history. Systematic assessment of life events, depression, and social support indicated that Mrs. M was not currently depressed, she had adequate levels of social support from family and friends, and that although she had experienced numerous stressful events in the past and felt dejected and overwhelmed at these times, her current mood and social situation were much improved.

Additional developmental history indicated that Billy was born without complications and developed normally; he was an easygoing baby with a sunny disposition, but he became a bit more difficult to handle when he began to walk. Once mobile, Billy began to get into things that were prohibited, and he seemed very curious and determined, as well as less willing than he had been as an infant, to be redirected or distracted. However, Mrs. M did not become concerned about him until he was 18 months old and he had a difficult time adjusting to child care. At that time, Mrs. M decided to increase her work hours to full-time in order to supplement the family income. She also felt that Billy would benefit from exposure to other children. Although her marriage had been rocky from the start, with her husband sometimes going on drinking binges and becoming abusive, he had never been abusive toward Billy. Mr. and Mrs. M first separated when Billy was 18 months old, when Mr. M's drinking binges and fights over Mrs. M's work schedule became in-

TABLE 10.4. Risk and Protective Factors in the Representative Case of Billy

Risk factors	Protective factors
Child characteristics	
Early-onset problems	Healthy, full-term, easy baby
Across settings (home, school)	Responsive to positive caregiving
Across disorders (oppositional defiant disorder, ADHD)	
Difficulty adjusting to change	
Delayed language development	
Parenting	
Some inconsistency and lack of follow through	Basically supportive, positive, and involved
Use of threats	Willing to seek help
Family history and family context	
Alcoholic father	Maternal psychological adjustment and resources
Possible paternal antisocial personality disorder	Job stability and income
Single mother, no child support	Involvement of maternal grandparents
Early exposure to family conflict and spousal abuse	Paternal departure
Maternal mental and physical health during pregnancy	Availability of treatment
Frequent separations and reunions with Dad in early childhood	Maternal motivation and follow through
Timing of birth of brother	
School	
	Teacher involvement
	Support for Billy's learning
	Help with peer problems
Diagnosis	
Oppositional defiant disorder	
Subthreshold ADHD	
Prognosis	
Problems could remit, recur, or become more serious	

tense. This and subsequent separations were followed by periods in which Mr. M was contrite and begged for forgiveness, only to repeat the pattern. These frequent separations and reunions with his dad, paired with his mother's longer work hours, seemed to precipitate problems with Billy, who became very hard to manage. He often threw temper tantrums and became uncooperative and defiant as well as clingy and upset whenever his mother left him alone with a babysitter or in the family day care center; Billy also was reluctant to sleep alone, and he often awoke at night crying. It was at this point that Mrs. M's parents took over the child care, and Billy, who adored his grandparents, calmed down considerably. Billy's parents reunited briefly when he was about 28 months old, and at that time, Mrs. M became pregnant again, but the marital problems resumed despite some brief attempts at marital counseling; shortly after the birth of Mrs. M's second child, Jason, Mr. M left the household for good. Mrs. M was actually relieved after his final departure, and although she was stressed by the demands of caring for a young baby and a preschooler, her mood improved; she resolved to work hard to keep her family together and to give her boys a normal childhood. Mrs. M's parents, as well as other members of her social network, were invaluable supports for Mrs. M and her children at this difficult time.

Although Billy became more manageable after his father left the household and his grandparents became more involved in his upbringing, he still had to adjust to his younger brother, who was becoming more competition for Billy as he began to walk and talk, and was also able to grab Billy's toys. Billy also resented sharing his brother with his mother and his grandparents, especially since his brother was now at the stage where others found him cute and appealing. This seemed to exacerbate some of the tantrums and clinginess that Mrs. M had witnessed earlier and suggests that Billy was the type of child who has particular difficulties coping with normal developmental transitions. Some of the typical behaviors of preschoolers appeared to become exaggerated and to interfere with relationships and developmental achievements; in Billy's case, expectations that be become more independent and learn to accept and share attention with his younger brother became both overwhelming to him and the focus of conflict with his mother.

When he was 4, Mrs. M enrolled Billy in a small preschool in his local community center five mornings per week to give his grandparents a break and to give him some more structured time in a peer group. The preschool teacher was very warm and supportive, but also provided structure, and Billy flourished in this environment. He adapted easily, followed the routines, and played cooperatively with other children. Because of Billy's good adjustment to preschool, Mrs. M was not overly worried about his adaptation to kindergarten.

At the time of Billy's assessment, he had been in kindergarten for 3 months. Although his teacher was very experienced and warm with the children, she had quite a large class and could not give Billy the amount of personal attention that he had received in preschool. This may have contributed to his poor adaptation.

In addition to understanding more about the classroom setting, the clinician was especially interested in Billy's mother's approach to child-rearing and child management strategies. This was assessed with interview and questionnaire measures, as well as an observation in the clinic, in which Mrs. M was asked to teach Billy how to complete a difficult puzzle, ask him to follow a series of directions, and deal with his behavior while she completed questionnaires and had nothing else to do. Observations confirmed maternal reports; Mrs. M and Billy got off to a good start, but as the demands on Billy became more intense and he became less controlled, Mrs. M became less able to handle him and became more impatient, ineffective, and prone to threaten but not follow through.

This was consistent with her interview account. Although Mrs. M did not like to use physical punishment, she found herself more and more frustrated with Billy, and sometimes after a difficult day, when she came home exhausted, his tantrums and argumentativeness, as well as his high activity level, led her to banish Billy to his room after giving him a good smack on his bottom. Often, this sequence of events occurred after a buildup of tension, anger, threats, and yelling. Sometimes, Mrs. M would feel guilty and relent; other times, she would leave Billy in his room for up to 30 minutes, where he inevitably got into even more trouble, for example, by dumping out the contents of his toy box or pasting his socks together with glue.

The clinician saw that Mrs. M would clearly benefit from a child management group, where she would get some help in setting consistent limits and some support from other parents with similar problems. Mrs. M was doing what many stressed and upset parents do when they cannot manage their young child's behavior, and the child is upping the ante as well. She was using negative and authoritarian control, limiting her positive involvement, escalating to more negative control attempts in concert with her son's coercive and noncompliant behavior, and being inconsistent. Numerous studies have associated this type of parenting with maternal stress and children's problem behavior (e.g., Campbell, Pierce, March, Ewing, & Szumowski, 1996; Harnish, Dodge, Valente, and the Conduct Problems Prevention Research Group, 1995; McLoyd, 1998; Patterson, DeBaryshe, & Ramsey, 1989; Shaw, Owens, Vondra, Keenan, & Winslow, 1996). After talking with Mrs. M, it was also clear that although she was coping with many responsibilities, she was not depressed and was motivated to work to help Billy, and to cooperate with the school as well.

Billy's teacher, aware that Mrs. M was struggling to raise two boys on her own while maintaining a full-time job, was willing to work with the psychologist to provide more structure and positive attention for Billy. In addition, a teacher aide worked individually with Billy for 45 minutes each day to help him with his schoolwork. Billy's teacher also was concerned about the fact that he was getting into frequent battles with other children; as a consequence, he was often not chosen as a partner in group activities and some children avoided him. The psychologist suggested structuring some group activities and making sure that Billy was often paired with the more mature children who were not only less likely to tolerate aggression, but also were less likely to fight themselves. Her proactive response to these adjustment difficulties, paired with Mrs. M's more appropriate response to limit setting, more positive involvement with her son, and increased consistency, led to a marked decrease in problems, although Billy continued to have difficulties with transitions.

The family context and the resources available made it possible to work with this family. The diagnosis provided some systematic statement about the presenting complaints and suggested some very broad directions that treatment might take. However, whether the diagnosis had been oppositional disorder, attention deficit disorder, or both, treatment would have been likely to include parent management and school consultation. Because the history indicated that Billy had particular difficulties with transitions and seemed to require predictability, structure, and positive attention, the clinician was optimistic about Billy's response to more focused and short-term intervention, even though many children with the very same diagnosis, oppositional disorder, go on to have more long-term and serious problems that require much more intensive intervention.

This discussion highlights the relative balance of risk and protective factors, the various strands that came together to lead to Billy's adjustment problems, and how building on the family strengths allowed for some resolution of the difficulties. First, Billy seemed particularly sensitive to transition and change, but at the same time, he was responsive to warmth, structure, and attention from caring adults. In many ways, his symptoms at various developmental transition points, such as entry into child care, the birth of his brother, and the departure of his father, reflected typical reactions to both normative and atypical life events. Furthermore, his reactions became somewhat exaggerated, possibly partly because of the anxiety and emotional insecurity that arose from his awareness of family conflict. Thus, his mother's anxiety and upset may have led him to feel insecure and worried, but in children this young, worry may be expressed outwardly as noncompliance. In addition, his father's unpredictable behavior and frequent angry departures from the home left him feeling vulnerable and insecure, fearing abandonment despite his good relationship with his mother. In this context, his clingy behavior and upset at separation from his mother were hardly surprising. Moreover, the timing of these events in Billy's development, just as he was beginning to establish a sense of self, made him especially likely to experience problems, and this was exacerbated by the fact that Billy's father left and his new brother arrived at the same time. Billy's history reflects marked variations in adjustment that seem to be influenced by the intensity of demands on him and the availability of alternative sources of support and nurturance, making him more likely to benefit from intervention. On the other hand, further exposure to family stress and coercive interchanges with his mother, continued school difficulties, and problems in the peer group might place Billy on a pathway toward more serious problems later. For example, if additional problems occur in the family or things go poorly at school, Billy would be more likely to be vulnerable than other children with a different developmental and family history, especially given his father's serious personality problems. Thus, his ultimate outcome is difficult to predict.

The Case of Peter

Peter is 10 years old and in fifth grade. He was referred to the school psychologist in February because his teacher was concerned about his behavior in the classroom and academic achievement. In school, he often seemed to be daydreaming and not paying attention; he seemed unmotivated and completed his school work carelessly, although he had started the school year as a good student. Peter also argued with the other children and often stayed by himself, although at times, he joined in with the others at recess; when he did join in, he sometimes engaged in fights and tended to bully and threaten others. In general, Peter seemed angry and sullen, with a "chip on his shoulder." Since January, Peter had missed about 8 days of school, and he was falling even further behind in his work.

It is evident that although Peter is 5 years older than Billy, the first case discussed in this chapter, his presenting complaints of inattention, uncooperative behavior, aggression with peers, and poor schoolwork sound very similar. In this case, however, based just on the presenting information, the clinician might consider whether Peter was showing attention deficit disorder (attention problems, careless schoolwork), conduct disorder (aggression and bullying, possible truancy), learning problems (academic problems), depression (irritability, change in behavior), or separation anxiety or school refusal (missing school). Because Peter had started the school year as a good student, however, and he was already in fifth grade, it is probably safe to rule out learning disorders and attention deficit disorder. Learning problems should be apparent much earlier, and attention deficit disorder requires that the symptoms be present before age 7. Additional assessment confirmed these hypotheses of the clinician, since Peter had been an A student until recently and had never had attentional or related problems. However, a CBCL completed by his mother indicated that Peter's scores were moderately elevated on the depression and anxiety scale, the somatic complaints scale, and the aggression scale, confirming both internalizing and externalizing symptoms.

Further assessment revealed that Peter lives with his parents and a younger sister and brother in a middle-class suburb of a small city. His father and mother are both professionals, and the family is close. Recently, Peter's grandfather had been very ill and his mother was spending a lot of time in the hospital with him. Peter's parents were both very concerned when they received a call from the teacher to inform them that she wanted to refer Peter to the school psychologist; they immediately agreed to come in for an appointment at the school.

The family history did not reveal much in the way of significant historical information. The family was a well-functioning one, and Peter's development had been uneventful. He had always gotten on well with other children and been quite serious and responsible, maybe even somewhat anxious. His recent symptoms reflected a major change in functioning and clearly coincided with several stressful events in the family: the illness of Peter's grandfather; his father's job change, which also entailed more absences due to travel; and the move of his best friend to another city. The psychologist also inquired about Peter's frequent absences from school and found out that he was not a truant, but he complained of frequent headaches and stomach aches, and had actually had a bout with the flu. Taken together, it appeared that Peter's problems reflected anxiety and depression about loss. Although he did not technically meet diagnostic criteria for major depressive disorder, his irritability, social withdrawal, and somatic complaints indicated that he would benefit from brief intervention. The psychologist thought that given Peter's high intelligence and self-awareness, some individual treatment geared to modifying his mood and negative cognitions would be helpful. In addition, brief family intervention seemed important to help Peter better communicate his concerns to his parents to allow them to help and support him through an upsetting time. This case example, which illustrates a child going through a difficult period related to life events over which he has no control, may be exacerbated by personality characteristics and the onset of pubertal change. Although he does not meet diagnostic criteria for a major disorder, Peter is an excellent candidate for psychosocial intervention. However, the outcome of even these apparently benign problems is difficult to predict. Peter's early signs of depression and somatic complaints in the face of loss may set the stage for the onset of a major depressive disorder in adolescence, possibly of a recurrent nature; or these problems may be short-lived reactions to converging stressful circumstances. Only continued follow-up will determine Peter's later adjustment in adolescence and early adulthood, when major depression is most likely to emerge.

The Case of Sandy

Sandy came to clinical attention at age 12, when she appeared at the emergency room of her local hospital after a failed suicide attempt. Sandy had swallowed five of her mother's painkillers and was brought to the hospital after fainting several times. Sandy's mother was concerned about her daughter but very vague and uninformative when asked about the family situation. The disheveled and unhealthy appearance of both mother and daughter raised concerns in the emergency room physician, who recommended Sandy's hospitalization for observation on the psychiatric unit.

Sandy was admitted to the unit, and after recovering from the effects of the medication, she was eager to talk to the unit social worker. The history was complicated and suggested that Sandy's suicide gesture was really a cry for help and an attempt to escape from an impossible home situation. Sandy, the oldest of three children, lived with her mother, two younger siblings, and her mother's current boyfriend in a rural area. The boyfriend, Jack, had been in the household for the past 6 months, one of a string of men who had moved into the home over the 10 years since Sandy's father had been killed in an accident. Jack was also not the first of these men to abuse alcohol and drugs, or to become violent and sexually assaultive with Sandy's mother. Unfortunately for Sandy, now that she was a teenager, she, too, was more frequently the target of the verbal abuse, and she was realistically fearful of also becoming the target of the physical and sexual abuse that often followed drinking binges. Sandy did what she could to protect herself and her younger siblings, but unable to cope with an untenable situation, she had become increasingly desperate, depressed, anxious, and angry. Her mother, often inebriated herself, was little help. Although she herself was not abusive toward the children, she had a history of neglect and was currently being neglectful by exposing her children to danger. Because Sandy's mother was not very involved with her children, Sandy often took responsibility for getting her younger siblings ready for school while her mother slept off the prior night's binge drinking. Sandy's mother had been hospitalized several times for depression, and she noted that the only times she felt fine were when she was high on drugs or alcohol.

In the interview with the social worker, Sandy described a chaotic home life in a small house, with little privacy or a place to hide from the continuing verbal and physical battles between her mother and boyfriend. The house was dirty and ramshackle, meals were irregular, and there was constant noise and confusion. The situation had worsened since Jack had moved in. For the preceding year, there had been no live-in boyfriend, and Sandy's mother had been somewhat more available and involved, especially after the county child protective services came on the scene and threatened to remove the children because of inadequate care.

Sandy's mother did odd jobs from time to time, for example, cleaning other people's houses or babysitting, but she had dropped out of high school at age 16, when she became pregnant with Sandy. Jack had a steady job in construction and he put food on the table, but he also contributed to the substantial tension and disorder in the household. Most recently, he had slapped and punched Sandy's mother, giving her a big bruise on her cheek. On that night, Sandy ran away to a friend's house and stayed overnight, but she returned the next day, concerned about her younger siblings. On her return, she was threatened with a beating, but her mother was glad to have her back to take care of the children.

Sandy's schoolteacher was contacted and indicated that Sandy was polite, quiet, and withdrawn in school, and she tended to be picked on by others because of her disheveled appearance and hand-me-down clothes. Sandy was in the seventh grade in her local middle school. Her schoolwork was average, but she tried hard not to be noticed by either the teacher or most of her peers. Because the teacher had a large class and a number of unruly students, Sandy received little individual attention at school, and the school guidance counselor was not really aware of her because she was not a troublemaker in school.

Sandy's mother visited her in the hospital the next day and met with the social worker. The mother reported that Sandy had been born before she was ready to have children, and she had left Sandy at her own mother's from time to time because she could not stand to listen to her cry. A review of the child protective service records also indicated that Sandy had been sent by a family court judge to live with her maternal grandparents when she was a toddler, after her father died and her mother was charged with neglect. When the grandparents became infirm themselves and could not handle an active preschooler, Sandy was returned to her mother's custody and was monitored by child protective services. By then, Sandy's mother seemed to have a better living situation and to be more in control of herself; she was receiving some mental health counseling at the local community health center for her depression and working part-time at a local fast-food restaurant; she professed an interest in returning to school. Unfortunately, soon after Sandy's return, she became pregnant again and moved in with her boyfriend at that time, the father of Sandy's sister.

Sandy was born full-term without major complications, although it was never clear how much her mother used alcohol or drugs during the pregnancy. Sandy was a colicky baby and seemed to need a good deal of care early on, leading her mother to turn off and "just let her cry" because Sandy was "trying to get to me." Thus, from the beginning, Sandy and her mother had a troubled relationship, reflecting the typical problems of a teenage mother with limited emotional or material resources, or the ability to understand the needs of young infants.

By the time she reached clinical attention at age 12, Sandy had not experienced much in the way of a stable, nurturing home life, and it was amazing that she had not received any mental health services until then. Clearly, she was the type of child who had learned not to be demanding in order to avoid conflict; thus, she tended to fall through the cracks of the various service delivery systems (school, child welfare, mental health).

The child psychiatrist who interviewed Sandy was struck by her maturity and common sense, as well as her neediness, worry, and intense sadness and anger. On a structured diagnostic interview, Sandy met criteria for dysthymia and generalized anxiety disorder. In a case conference that included school personnel, child protective services, and professionals from the local mental health clinic, as well as hospital personnel, it was recommended that Sandy and her younger siblings be removed from the home, at least temporarily, and that she be placed in a special foster home for teenagers with problems (Chamberlain, 1996). The clinical team was concerned not only about the abuse that Sandy and her siblings might experience, but also about Sandy's long-term prognosis. Sandy was at risk to drop out of school and become pregnant herself, and the almost total lack of family support or resources for Sandy and her siblings meant that they were all at risk for serious adjustment problems in adolescence and adulthood.

However, consideration of this case underscores the problems of conceptualizing childhood disorders as reflecting problems within the child, especially when the child grows up under such adverse conditions. In Sandy's case, one would not ask why she was depressed and anxious at age 12, but how she had managed to function as well as she had all these years. Many young girls growing up in environments such as this have serious problems with delinquency, oppositional behavior, school failure, alcohol and drug abuse, and early pregnancy. Clearly, in this case, the diagnosis is almost irrelevant to the treatment recommendations, although the diagnosis allows for access to certain funds for adolescents requiring treatment as part of a combined intervention/prevention program.

DEVELOPMENTAL PSYCHOPATHOLOGY CONSTRUCTS REVISITED

The formulations of these three cases illustrate several of the constructs discussed earlier in this book. For example, both equifinality and multifinality are represented. Although both boys started out with somewhat overlapping symptom pictures and presenting complaints, they appear to have followed different routes to the development of problems. This is apparent from their different developmental histories, and the different family contexts and events surrounding the emergence of their problems, illustrating equifinality at the time of referral; that is, two boys with somewhat similar symptom patterns followed different developmental pathways to a similar point at initial referral (the equifinality). They also illustrate multifinality, because the end points, as of this writing, look quite different.

Furthermore, in all three cases, complex transactions among child characteristics and developmental level, parental behavior, and the wider family environment were implicated in the onset and course of problems. In addition, the convergence of and balance among risk and protective factors, in developmental context, helped us to understand the developmental course of problems and to see where intervention might be most effective. Focus on the protective factors in the family and wider environment, as well as the children's strengths, permitted some resolution of problems in the short term in the cases of Billy and Peter. In Sandy's case, it may be that by providing her with a more protective and nurturing environment, one can help her overcome her early negative experiences, at least to some degree, especially given her own inner strength and ability to function despite the adversity she had experienced.

These cases also illustrated issues of continuity and discontinuity. Continuity is evident in Billy's recurrent difficulties with major developmental transitions and his responsiveness to adult intervention and nurturance. Continuity is also evident in Sandy's tendency to become withdrawn and depressed, and to turn her problems inward. The suicidal gesture is consistent with this clinical picture, as were diagnoses of dysthymia and generalized anxiety disorder. Discontinuity is evident in the abrupt decline in functioning that Peter showed in the face of loss, which would not have been predicted from his prior level of functioning and adaptation. Finally, all these cases illustrated that the symptom picture is usually complex and often does not conform to the specifics of the diagnostic categories, that internalizing and externalizing problems are often evident simultaneously, and that problems in children are difficult to construe as residing in the child rather than in the family system and/or in the transactions between child and environment.

FUTURE DIRECTIONS

These problems with the diagnostic system have been the subject of debate for some time (e.g., Campbell, 1990; Garber, 1984; Jensen & Hoagwood, 1997). It will be incumbent on developmental psychopathology researchers to suggest ways to bridge the gaps between the clinical descriptive and more process-oriented and developmentally informed approaches to understanding and classifying children's problems. The DSM-PC of the AAP is a start in that different levels of severity, different developmental manifestations of specific problems, and different contextual stressors and supports are delineated. Zero to Three/National Center for Clinical Infant Programs (1994) has also attempted to describe young children's (0–3 years) problems in a developmentally informed way, although serious problems with overpathologizing and misconstruing some early problems have not been resolved. Finally, definitions of disorder, as well as assessment tools, need to take cultural issues into account.

This discussion suggests several directions for research. First, at a very basic level, we require descriptive studies that test the efficacy of the developmental psychopathology formulation and document the correlates, contexts, and manifestations of particular constellations of problem behavior in children of different ages more broadly and systematically than has been done in past epidemiological studies (e.g., Fergusson & Horwood, 1996; Lahey et al., 1996; Moffitt, Caspi, Dickson, Silva, & Stanton, 1996). Epidemiological studies have tended not to examine family processes adequately or to thoroughly consider the different developmental manifestations of apparently persistent problems. Although epidemiological studies suggest both similarities and differences in rates of particular disorders across cultures and ethnic groups (e.g., Bird, 1996; Verhulst & Koot, 1992), in general, cultural differences in the definitions of disorder, and in expectations for behavior, have not been examined in great detail, with the notable exception of the work of Weisz, Chayaisit, Weiss, Eastman, and Jackson (1995). Clearly, this is an area of increasing importance. Both definitions of disorder and assessment procedures need to be culturally sensitive, incorporating an awareness of different community norms and contexts, as well as adult expectations, for child behavior.

In addition, we need more longitudinal research on the life history of large samples of children identified early as showing particular problems that map onto the diagnostic categories at some level (e.g., noncompliance and argumentativeness, hyperactivity and poor impulse control, separation anxiety, extreme aggression). These children, then, must be followed over time, with in-depth assessments of the child, the family, and the wider social context (e.g., Campbell, Pierce, March, Ewing, & Szumowski, 1994; Conduct Problems Prevention Research Group, 1992; Greenberg, Leguna, Coie, & Pinderhughes, 1999; Shaw, Owens, Vondra, Keenan, & Winslow, 1996). This will allow for more process-oriented analyses as well as a better understanding of the factors associated with good and poor outcomes in children with early problems.

Another avenue for research involves decision making about treatment. How do clinicians make decisions about what and how to treat? How much does the actual DSM-IV diagnosis contribute to these decisions, and how much does the more comprehensive clinical case formulation underscore areas in need of intervention (e.g., academic skills, social skills) and possibly ways to intervene? Clearly, knowledge of the child's broader family and social context (including the peer group and the culture) will influence treatment decisions, and these may be largely independent of diagnosis. Another issue, forecast by Garber's (1984) article, involves broadening the diagnostic system to include aspects of the child's relationships family and environment into the categories. Zero to Three/National Center for Clinical Infant Programs (1994) has attempted to do this with diagnoses in young children ages 0 to 3, on the assumption that mood and regulatory disorders in infants and toddlers are almost always relationship-based. Although there are many problems with these diagnostic formulations, the attempt to consider the impact of parent–child and other relationships on children's adjustment is an important development.

We can also ask whether aspects of the classification of early problems prove valid as predictors of outcome, and the degree to which knowing something about the family and wider social context, including community and neighborhood factors, adds to the prediction of outcome (e.g., Campbell, Pierce, Moore, Marakovitz, & Newby, 1996; Shaw, Owens, Vondra, Keenan, & Winslow, 1996). Similarly, process-oriented and etiological formulations of children's problems can only be tested with prevention and intervention trials, making these a central tool of developmental psychopathology. It is to these issues that we turn in Chapter 11.

CONCLUSION

In this chapter, we have addressed issues in the diagnosis and classification of children's problems and noted some of the strengths and weaknesses of both the clinical and empirical approaches to categorizing childhood disorders. Whereas the assessment tools derived from these approaches to taxonomy have their usefulness as descriptive measures of the severity and nature of children's problem behaviors, they actually provide little in the way of actual help in case formulation or in understanding the likely developmental origins of the problems, their probable developmental course, or what to do about them. Three case examples were provided to illustrate the complexities and drawbacks of the diagnostic system, as well as to demonstrate how a developmental psychopathology approach informs the conceptualization of cases.

A Developmental Psychopathology Perspective on Prevention and Treatment

So far we have discussed the processes that may account for why some children show problematic behavior at some point in development, problems that may or may not reach clinical attention. We have also seen how an understanding of the cognitive, socioemotional, biological, and family/social processes underlying both adaptive and maladaptive development should either have implications for preventing problems from emerging at all or, at least, should make it possible to intervene at critical points in development to prevent problems from becoming more serious and debilitating once they are in evidence. Thus, from a developmental psychopathology perspective, it should be possible to change a child's developmental trajectory by changing something in the child and/or the child's environment, or both, thereby redirecting the child from a negative pathway to a positive or at least a benign one.

At the same time, it should also be clear that the developmental course of problems is difficult to predict because some children may overcome adversity without formal intervention. For example, some children may improve because their difficulties reflect a time-limited developmental stage (e.g., the transition to school) or because a change in life circumstances (e.g., a move to a neighborhood with better schools, the departure of an abusive father from the household) allows them to regroup and facilitates their development along a more positive pathway characterized by more adaptive functioning. Still other children's problems may remit in the absence of intervention or even apparent environmental change for reasons that are poorly understood. Developmental psychopathology principles have many implications for prevention and treatment, as well as for trying to understand why some children may improve without intervention despite adversity.

Thus, in this chapter, we discuss several issues in the prevention and treatment of children's problems, with a focus on the developmental psychopathology framework that we have addressed so far. We begin with a discussion of the distinctions between prevention and treatment and then consider the principles that underlie successful prevention programs. Using a theoretical model about the development of aggression as an example, we examine programs geared to the prevention of aggression, conduct problems, and their sequelae, with a focus on two ongoing programs that are especially promising. This discussion also illustrates how prevention trials can test theoretical models that derive from the developmental psychopathology approach. We also discuss the current state of research on the treatment of childhood disorders, contrasting the underlying assumptions inherent in most treatment research with those informing prevention trials. We examine one model of treatment for attention deficit hyperactivity disorder that, while relatively comprehensive, derives from different assumptions than do somewhat similar prevention trials. Finally, we attempt to bridge the theoretical divide between prevention and treatment. In so doing, we examine the practice implications of some of this material by returning to the case examples discussed in Chapter 10.

SOME INTRODUCTORY COMMENTS ON PREVENTION AND TREATMENT

There is a large body of research and theory on both prevention and treatment, and to some degree they complement and inform each other. At the same time, much of the work on prevention has grown out of a developmental psychopathology tradition (e.g., Allen, Philliber, Herrling, & Kuperminc, 1997; Conduct Problem Prevention Research Group, 1992; Dumas, Prinz, Smith, & Laughlin, 1999), because the complex theoretical framework and extant research suggest that we can identify particular groups of children and families who are at risk to develop problems, and then intervene in children's lives before problems become serious, debilitating, diagnosable, and resistant to treatment (Coie et al., 1993; Kazdin, 1993).

For example, it is well established that single, teenage mothers are at high risk themselves and are also more likely to place their infants at risk because they are more likely than older mothers to be neglectful, to provide inadequate parenting, and even sometimes to be abusive, often out of ignorance rather than malicious intent. Prevention programs geared to this population have shown promise, thereby stopping a negative cycle of parenting failures that gives rise to cognitive, emotional, and social problems in their offspring (e.g., Olds, Henderson, Chamberlin, & Tatelbaum, 1986).

Similarly, a wealth of data implicates childrearing and family stress in the onset of aggressive behavior in young children (e.g., Campbell, 1990, 1997; Greenberg, Speltz, & DeKlyen, 1993; Patterson, DeBaryshe, & Ramsey, 1989; Reid, 1993; Shaw, Owens, Vondra, Keenan, & Winslow, 1996). These children and their families are appropriate targets for a range of prevention efforts meant to change children's developmental trajectories by changing their behavior and cognitions directly, as well as by modifying the contexts (family, school, peer group) that support their development (Conduct Problems Prevention Research Group, 1992). Thus, these and numerous other prevention programs derive from a developmental psychopathology perspective on the complex determinants of children's problems, and on an understanding of developmental pathways, as well as factors associated with continuity and discontinuity in developmental trajectories.

Moreover, the large body of research identifying risk factors associated with problem onset, as well as the protective factors associated with healthy development, despite risk (Masten & Coatsworth, 1998; Werner, 1993) has been important in the design of prevention programs. Furthermore, prevention programs more often target infants, toddlers, preschoolers, and children making the transition to school, on the assumption that problems identified early may be more easily modified (Ramey & Ramey, 1998).

In contrast, most treatment research derives predominantly from a disease model of psychopathology (e.g., Arnold et al., 1997; Pelham, Wheeler, & Chronis, 1998). This means that treatment research is focused more explicitly on alleviating symptoms of a particular disorder, and although context and developmental course are considered to some degree (e.g., in the assessment of change), they play a relatively minor role in the selection of therapeutic techniques or in the underlying theoretical assumptions about the causes of disorder. For example, disease models may focus on underlying biological predispositions; other models of psychopathology emphasize learning histories, and these theories tend to be adevelopmental and limited in scope (Mash & Wolfe, 1999). Additionally, in contrast to prevention programs, treatment programs are most often geared to school-age children and adolescents who are much more likely to be referred for clinical services or to come to clinical attention through the school system.

What Distinguishes Prevention from Treatment?

Prevention and Early Intervention

It is necessary, first, to try to distinguish between prevention (including early intervention, primary prevention) and treatment. The term "treatment" usually implies that there is a problem or disease entity in need of intervention. In contrast, prevention programs are aimed at stopping problems before they develop, or before they escalate into a diagnosable disorder (Coie et al., 1993; Kazdin, 1993). Prevention programs can be universal, that is, delivered to a whole population of children or even an entire community. The addition of fluoride to the water in many communities is an example of a universal prevention aimed at preventing tooth decay. Antismoking and antidrug announcements on television and on billboards are also examples of community-wide attempts at prevention. Many school systems now include programs geared to the prevention of drug and alcohol abuse, teen pregnancy, and violence in their overall curriculum, targeting universal prevention for an entire school population in a particular community (e.g., Aber, Jones, Brown, Chaudry, & Samples, 1998; Allen, Philliber, Herrling, & Kuperminc, 1997; Coley & Chase-Lansdale, 1998). Thus, universal prevention programs aimed at encouraging better physical and mental health are widespread in our society.

More targeted or indicated prevention programs identify children and families at risk. For example, Olds and colleagues (Olds, Henderson, Camberlin, & Tatelbaum, 1986; Olds, Henderson, Kitzman, & Cole, 1995) initiated a home visiting program for poor, single, teenage mothers, whose children are known to be at risk because of unskilled parenting. Infants of single, teen mothers are also more likely to be victims of child abuse and neglect. Other parent education and well child care programs also select specific populations of high-risk families with young children (e.g., the Infant Health and Development Program; Ramey et al., 1992) in order to prevent problems related to poor nutrition and limited medical care, harsh and/or neglectful parenting, and inadequate cognitive and social stimulation.

The best-known prevention or early intervention program, Head Start, selects preschool children at risk because of poverty and associated risk factors, with the goal of enhancing cognitive and social skills prior to kindergarten entry, thereby facilitating the transition to school and preventing later school failure. Although most preschool early intervention programs that emerged in the 1960s as part of the War on Poverty were focused primarily on improving cognitive and language development, and school readiness, more recently, there has been renewed interest in the effects of preschool interventions on social development and more general adaptation as well (Ramey & Ramey, 1998). Evaluation of the first generation of Head Start and other early intervention programs suggested that cognitive gains were usually not maintained once the program ended, but that children in the more structured and comprehensive programs, especially those with parent involvement, still fared better than control children. For example, children in the intervention groups were less likely to be in special classes or to repeat a grade, suggesting improvement in classroom behavior and social skills (Lazar & Darlington, 1982; Zigler & Valentine, 1979). These early programs and the results of follow-up studies have led to the development of increasingly more complex and multifaceted preventive interventions based on an ecological model of development. These include two-generation programs that target both children and their parents, providing services that both help to support parents in their own lives and help them to help their children (St. Pierre & Layzer, 1998). We return to a discussion of specific programs shortly.

When is a program truly a prevention program, and when is it really early intervention? The line between these is blurred and many programs are both. Head Start, for example, provides intervention prior to school entry on the assumption that children living in poverty are universally at risk for poor school achievement, and that interventions meant to enhance cognitive, social, and academic skills will have both short-term effects on these skills and also prevent problems later, for example, school failure and its sequelae. Research, as already noted, confirms that well-structured early childhood programs enhance young children's cognitive and social skills in the short term (early intervention). These effects are also lasting to some degree, leading to a decrease in the rates of grade retention, as well as school dropout and delinquent behavior, thereby preventing problems later (Zigler, Taussig, & Black, 1992). Prevention programs are widespread and likely to become more so with the increase in social problems affecting children and families (Hetherington, Bridges, & Insabella, 1998; McLoyd, 1998). However, the relative cost–benefit analysis of universal versus targeted programs remains controversial. In addition, comprehensive programs for children truly at risk may be more useful than small-scale programs geared to everyone. This, of course, is also a question for research.

Research Issues in Child Treatment

As already noted, the term "treatment" implies a disease or disorder that needs to be modified or, better yet, cured. Thus, treatment is reserved for children with a diagnosed disorder. The literature on child treatment is voluminous, including a range of psychosocial and biological treatments with vastly different theoretical rationales and degrees of structure. For example, psychodynamic psychotherapy or play therapy tends to be relatively unstructured and to formulate somewhat vague goals of intrapsychic change. In contrast, parent training and behavior modification programs tend to be highly structured, with explicit goals that revolve around changing the environmental contingencies for the child's behavior. Psychoactive medication is widely used, with the aim of modifying biological processes hypothesized to underlie symptom expression, such as the balance among neurotransmitters or activity in certain brain areas. Although it is well documented that certain medications are extremely effective for certain disorders (e.g., methylphenidate and other stimulant medications for ADHD), the mechanisms by which they work are poorly understood (Hinshaw, 1994). Treatments may be directed at the individual child, the parents and child, or the entire family (e.g., Mash & Barkley, 1998), and may vary widely in goals and degree of structure. Moreover, children are treated as outpatients or inpatients, depending on the severity of disturbance and other factors (e.g., family motivation and severity of dysfunction, insurance coverage). Treatment may be provided in the therapist's office, in the school setting, at home, or in the natural environment. Actually, Kazdin (1995) has identified over 200 different treatment approaches to children's problems; these vary in many ways, including the degree of structure (didactic and focused vs. more psychodynamic vs. nondirective), who participates (child, parents, family), and the locus of treatment (therapist's office, classroom, community).

Despite the large literature on the treatment of childhood disorders, there is surprisingly little in the way of controlled outcome research that evaluates the effectiveness of various treatments for particular disorders (Lonigan & Elbert, 1998). Moreover, most treatment research has compared a treatment group to either a placebo treatment (e.g., attention from a therapist) or to an untreated group (e.g., waiting-list controls). These studies demonstrate that the treated group usually improves relative to the group without treatment (e.g., see Weisz & Weiss, 1993), although gains often are not maintained at 6-month or 1-year follow-up. In addition, because studies have rarely compared treatments varying along well-defined parameters with each other, we have little understanding of the active ingredients in treatment that facilitate behavioral change. Finally, most treatment research has been conducted in laboratory settings, and treatments that appear to be effective in this highly controlled setting, with carefully selected patients, are often less effective in the real world of the clinic (Ollendick & King, 1998; Weisz, Donenberg, Han, & Weiss, 1995; Weisz & Hawley, 1998; Weisz & Weiss, 1993). This is partly because children selected for such studies often come from middle-class, two-parent families and do not have multiple, co-occurring disorders.

The Society of Clinical Psychology (Division 12) and the Section on Clinical Child Psychology (Division 12, Section 1, now Division 53) of the American Psychological Association have been involved in identifying model treatments that appear comprehensive (Roberts, 1996), and that have withstood empirical scrutiny (Lonigan & Elbert, 1998). In general, more structured, focused, and educational treatments aimed at parents and/or the children themselves have proven most efficacious for school-age children (Brestan & Eyberg, 1998; Kazdin, 1997; Ollendick & King, 1998; Weisz & Hawley, 1998); parent training and relationship enhancement programs have worked best with preschoolers and younger, school-age children (Eyberg, Boggs, & Algina, 1995; Webster-Stratton, 1984, 1985). Although family interventions beyond parent training make theoretical sense, they have received less research attention than one might expect (e.g., Pinsof & Wynne, 1995). Nonetheless, comprehensive multidomain interventions targeting marital and other family systems, in addition to the parent–child system, offer the prospect of more effective prevention and intervention programs. Moreover, program efficacy is likely to be enhanced by comprehensive interventions in multiple settings (e.g., family, school, community) (see Cowan, Powell, & Cowan, 1998, for an excellent treatment of a family systems perspective on parenting interventions). Clearly, such directions are consistent with the systemic, contextual model of family functioning and child development implicit in the developmental psychopathology perspective. Medication has also proven useful for some problems (e.g., attention deficit disorder), although its use remains controversial (Safer, Zito, & Fine, 1996). In some ways, the use of medication may seem anathema to those with a developmental psychopathology perspective, although it may be possible to reconcile these apparently discrepant viewpoints under certain circumstances. Another issue is what type of treatment works best for each specific disorder (assuming disorders are really specific, an issue raised in the preceding chapter). Although a thorough review of the therapy literature is beyond the scope of this book, several of these issues are discussed in more detail later in this chapter.

It is also important to keep in mind the many apparent barriers to obtaining treatment. When children, such as the ones described in Chapter 10, are referred for clinical assessment and diagnosis, the logical result should be some form of treatment meant to help the child and family understand and deal with the problem. However, epidemiological studies suggest that only about 20% of children with potentially serious problems ever have any contact with the mental health profession (e.g., Offord, Boyle, Fleming, Blum, & Rae Grant, 1989). Thus, many children in need of help never receive it.

Many factors are likely to account for the limited access to and use of mental health services, including spiraling costs, program cutbacks, and lack of awareness on the part of adults responsible for children's well-being. Often, parents and teachers do not recognize that problems exist, or they may not know where to go for help. Even in the school system, the front line for the identification and management of many child problems, resources are inadequate to cope with the demand. Furthermore, interventions, especially for the more complex and severe problems, are often not effective, or when some change is in evidence at the conclusion of treatment, the short-term gains are not maintained over time (Hinshaw, 1994; Kazdin, 1993). The resistance of some problems to standard interventions favored by the clinical child psychologist, child psychiatrist, or social worker has contributed to a growing interest in prevention (Coie et al., 1993). Thus, we now turn to a more thorough discussion of prevention.

PREVENTION AND THE DEVELOPMENTAL PSYCHOPATHOLOGY PERSPECTIVE

Prevention and early intervention programs, by definition, must focus on some developmental issue or process if the course of development in some domain is to be modified. The assumption underlying targeted prevention and early intervention programs is that because of an array of risk factors in the child and/or the environment, children at risk are more likely than children without such risk factors to develop cognitive, social, emotional, and/or behavioral problems that may become stable or even worsen with development. It is also assumed that the earlier a child can be deflected from a maladaptive pathway to a more adaptive one, the greater the likelihood of a good outcome and the lower the overall risk for impaired functioning, problematic adjustment, or full-blown disorder. This perspective is rooted in the view that early experience sets the stage for later functioning (Hebb, 1949; Hunt, 1961), although it is recognized that later experiences play an important role as well.

From a developmental psychopathology perspective, prevention makes more sense than therapeutic intervention. This is because risk factors in the child, family, and/or wider environment may be identified early and may logically be implicated in a number of processes that place the young child on a problematic pathway toward maladjustment and psychopathology. Moreover, interrelated risk factors and their effects may escalate over time, making intervention more difficult as a function of the development of more serious problems. For example, maternal depression, inconsistent and rejecting care, and disorganized attachment, which have been shown to co-occur (see Chapter 9), may set the toddler on a pathway toward impaired cognitive and socioemotional development that are reflected in poor language expression, lack of mastery, and aggressive/explosive encounters with peers in child care. This risk for relatively serious impairments in early functioning across domains will be higher in a child who is already at risk because of biological vulnerabilities. This may lead to cascading problems as the young child is rejected by other children, thereby limiting experiences that facilitate the development of sharing, sociodramatic play with peers, better control of aggression, and so forth. Furthermore, the transaction between the child's escalating negative and problematic behavior and the mother's own problems may lead to a worsening of their relationship, which is further exacerbated by interparental conflict, eventually leading to the father's departure from the household. Possibly, by intervening early to deal with the mother's depression and the quality of the mother–child relationship, the quality of the attachment relationship, as well as other aspects of parent–child relations and the child's social and cognitive development can be modified, redirecting the child from a trajectory characterized by accumulating problems to a pathway that is possibly more benign, if not problem-free (Cicchetti & Toth, 1998). Numerous similar examples could be generated that theoretically link multiple early risk factors to problematic developmental pathways.

Earlier research on prevention has demonstrated the strengths and weaknesses of limited programs with highly specific foci, and has led to the development of more comprehensive programs based on transactional and ecological models that derive from the developmental psychopathology perspective (Cowan, Powell, & Cowan, 1998). However, that was not always the case. As noted by Dumas, Prinz, Smith, and Laughlin (1999), earlier prevention programs often focused on a single social context such as the preschool and/or on a single participant, such as the child. Moreover, the relatively brief interventions employed were not necessarily culturally or developmentally sensitive. Over the last few years, prevention trials have become more theory- and model-driven, more comprehensive and integrated, and have focused not only on reducing risk but also on building competence (Coie et al., 1993; Dumas et al., 1999; Masten & Coatsworth, 1998; Vitaro, Brendgen, Pagani, Tremblay,

& McDuff, 1999). Furthermore, as we already illustrated, it is generally believed that early prevention programs are more likely to be effective because they modify precursors of more serious problems before they become entrenched, habitual ways of functioning (e.g., Ramey & Ramey, 1998; Reid, 1993). In addition, programs that focus on the child in context, that is, two-generation programs that provide services both to high-risk children and their families, theoretically should be more effective (St. Pierre & Layzer, 1998).

What, How, When, and Who?

As should be evident from the discussion so far, prevention programs differ greatly in the scope and severity of the behaviors or problems they target (e.g., child abuse and neglect, social and cognitive delays, aggression, conduct disorder, depression, school dropout, drug use, teen pregnancy, suicide). Thus, programs vary widely in what they aim to prevent, that is, the goals of the prevention program. Not only do they differ on the specific behaviors or endpoints that define the ultimate goal of the program, but they differ also in terms of the underlying processes posited to account for change, or how change is thought to occur, as well as the actual components of the interventions themselves. Thus, some programs aim to reduce risk (e.g., poor parenting) on the assumption that if salient risk factors are removed, development will proceed along a more satisfactory course; other programs focus on enhancing protective factors, in order to counteract risk, for example, by providing support for involved parenting, in the context of poverty or a dangerous neighborhood; some programs are geared to modifying specific developmental processes (e.g., social cognitions such as hostile attributional biases; Dodge, Pettit, & Bates, 1994a) that are hypothesized to mediate outcomes (e.g., decrease aggression); still other programs attempt to build in skills, such as more competent social interactions—turn taking, sharing, negotiating, and perspective taking (Coie et al., 1993; Conduct Problems Prevention Research Group, 1992; Dumas, Prinz, Smith, & Laughlin, 1999; Masten & Coatsworth, 1998)—that facilitate positive interactions with peers and adults. Furthermore, a multitude of programs may be instituted with these goals in mind, including parent training, school-based tutoring and social skills training, parent support, and relationship building. In all cases, the ultimate goal, however, is to change the presumed developmental trajectory of children thought to be at risk for problems. The more comprehensive and multifaceted programs focus on all three pathways to change: risk reduction, modification of underlying developmental process, and the development of competence (e.g., Conduct Problems Prevention Research Group, 1992; Dumas et al., 1999), and they tend to use multiple means to reach these goals targeting children and their families.

In addition, the focus of the prevention program will partly determine when in development a program should begin. For example, programs geared toward preventing child abuse in the offspring of high-risk mothers may be initiated prenatally or shortly after the baby's birth (e.g., Olds et al., 1986).

Programs geared toward the prevention of cognitive delays often begin in infancy or toddlerhood, or at preschool entry at the latest (Ramey & Ramey, 1998). Programs meant to prevent aggression may begin in preschool, although more often, they begin during the transition to school (Reid, 1993). Drug or alcohol abuse or teen pregnancy prevention programs usually do not begin until middle childhood or early adolescence (Allen, Philliber, Herrling, & Kuperminc, 1997; Coley & Chase-Lansdale, 1998). In many ways, this seems logical. It would probably be a waste of resources to begin aggression or drug prevention programs in infancy, even if one's theory implicated certain aspects of the family environment as important in the eventual onset of the problem. However, it can also be argued that the reduction of overall risk in infancy may ultimately reduce aggression and drug use in adolescence, for example, by improving parenting and providing social support. Still, this is a tall order, and in the absence of continued family support, it is unlikely that early gains will be maintained.

In addition, the developmental timing of a prevention program will be determined partly by the scope of the program and whether it is universal or targeted to specific children at risk. This is because risk often cannot be determined until the child is a certain age, or because the program might not be meaningful until children have reached a certain level of cognitive and social development. For example, many programs target aggressive behavior and its sequelae. However, beginning aggression prevention programs in toddlerhood is probably misguided, because some degree of peer conflict is normative and even necessary for normal development (Shantz, 1987). Moreover, it would be difficult to determine which rough toddlers are really at risk for more serious aggression later; this may be partly because the perspective taking needed to understand negotiating and sharing is just beginning to develop (Campbell, 1990). Although an argument might be made for some universal interventions aimed at early aggression, targeted programs should probably be started somewhat later. By age 4 or 5, children who are highly aggressive are indeed at risk for persistent and more severe problems (Campbell, Pierce, Moore, Marakovitz, & Newby, 1996; Pierce, Ewing, & Campbell, 1999). They also stand out from their peers by age 4 or 5, and, because of cognitive development, may be in a better position to profit from structured guidance in peer interactions, although there are no data clearly supporting this position. Similarly, drug abuse or pregnancy prevention programs would not be very meaningful in kindergarten, but by middle childhood, they are both understandable and relevant to some children confronted with opportunities and conflicts about whether to go along with pressure from peers to engage in high-risk behaviors.

Prevention programs also vary in terms of who is targeted for services: specially selected children, all the children in a particular classroom or school system, parents, families, communities. Are these participants selected because they are at risk or because everyone theoretically may benefit (or not be harmed by) the program? If they are defined as "at risk," then on what basis is this designation made? And are there negative sequelae from defining someone as "at risk"? These complicated questions are pondered by prevention advocates.

Principles of Prevention

Because of the extensive body of research on early intervention, the area of prevention has a firm research base to guide program development and structure. Ramey and Ramey (1992, 1998) reviewed the well-designed outcome studies examining early intervention for infants, toddlers, and preschoolers at biological and psychosocial risk. Based on their extensive review of extant studies, they proposed six principles that should guide the formulation of new programs, if the goal is to obtain results that last beyond the life of the program:

1. Interventions that begin early and last longer are more likely to be effective.
2. More intensive programs (i.e., the amount of contact or involvement) are more likely to be effective, especially for those who attend regularly and follow through with program requirements (it should be noted that this means multiple contacts per week over 2 or 3 years).
3. Children need to receive direct interventions, if social and cognitive skills are to be enhanced. (It is sobering to realize that even long-term programs involving home visits were not effective if only the mothers were the recipients of the intervention.)
4. The most effective programs are those that are also the most comprehensive and multifaceted, and include social, cognitive, and health components for both the child and family, and also help the family to cope with other more basic needs (e.g., housing, negotiating social service delivery systems, job training). These are referred to as two-generation programs.
5. Regardless of how well-designed the program is, there will be individual differences as to who benefits, and not everyone improves or even stays with the program.
6. The initial positive effects of programs diminish in the absence of environmental supports meant to maintain gains in child and family functioning.

These six principles delineated by Ramey and Ramey (1998) provide important benchmarks for evaluating the few extant programs that deal with children's incipient psychopathology.

Early intervention work emerged primarily from early education and pediatrics, and focused on infants and young children at risk because of compromised prenatal and neonatal conditions, poverty, and parenting problems. In contrast, the primary prevention movement, spawned mostly by those in the mental health field who became concerned with the difficulties encountered treating disorders, has been influential in informing developmental psychopathology research. In addition, early advocates of primary prevention (Albee, 1983; Cowen, 1977) were motivated by strong ethical and social concerns, including an interest in avoiding the stigmatization of psychiatric diagnosis and treatment. Moreover, the increased body of evidence linking psychiatric disorders to a wide variety of risk factors, already discussed in earlier chapters, has strengthened the desire of some psychopathology researchers to utilize current knowledge in an attempt to modify problems before they emerge as a full-blown syndromes or disorders. The overlap with and convergence between primary and early intervention thus seems obvious; and likewise, their relevance to a developmental psychopathology perspective should be clear.

Based on a strong developmental psychopathology perspective, then, Coie and colleagues (1993) have argued for a science of prevention that is grounded in developmental theory and permits testing of developmental models of causal processes; that is, successful prevention trials should function as tests of specific hypotheses about the developmental and social processes that underlie the emergence of problem behavior in particular social and family contexts, and at particular points in development. Thus, these authors note that to be successful, prevention programs must recognize the dynamic nature of development and the fact that different developmental processes are salient at different points in time.

Therefore, static models linking specific risk factors at one age to a specific negative outcome at a later age will not suffice. Rather, multiple, co-occurring risk factors that are associated generally with psychopathology must be considered while simultaneously recognizing that the importance of specific risk factors will change with development. For example, parenting is more salient in early childhood, whereas the nature of the neighborhood or peer group becomes more central by adolescence (e.g., Dishion, Patterson, Stoolmiller, & Skinner, 1991), even though particular aspects of parenting remain important (e.g., warmth and involvement in infancy; proactive limit setting in toddlerhood; monitoring and supervision in middle childhood and adolescence). In addition, protective factors must be considered in developmental context, if meaningful preventions are to be devised. This raises issues of multifinality and equifinality (Cicchetti & Rogosch, 1996), and underscores the pivotal role of risk and protective factors in attempting to delineate the different developmental pathways that children follow to both normal and disturbed outcomes. Coie and colleagues (1993) also emphasize the need to recognize that only models describing "complex transactions between individuals and their environments, between systems of influence, and across periods of time" (p. 1017) will be adequate to account for the multiple causal factors in the onset and course of children's maladjustment. This is consistent with the theoretical perspective outlined in Chapter 2. This ambitious research agenda linking developmental psychopathology theory to carefully designed preventive interventions holds promise for helping us untangle causal processes that have so far eluded psychopathology researchers. Finally, Coie and colleagues caution against focusing only on diagnosable disorders as indicators of program success, but instead stress the importance of examining intervening or mediating processes that may be markers of, or explain, change. They also note the importance of more global markers of functioning that may be more predictive of outcome than specific symptom constellations or diagnoses. This perspective on prevention is highly consonant with the views espoused in this volume. Thus, it is not surprising that Coie has been a leader in developing a theory-driven model of prevention.

Theoretical Models and Prevention: The Example of Aggression and Conduct Disorder

It is probably safe to assert that no social problem has attracted more attention than aggression and its correlates and sequelae: oppositional disorder, conduct disorder, delinquency, and antisocial behavior (Coie & Dodge, 1998). Violence prevention programs have sprung up in many school systems (e.g., Aber, Jones, Brown, Chaudry, & Samples, 1998), and violence prevention has become a topic of sometimes emotional social policy and congressional debate. It is well recognized that the United States is a violent society, in comparison to many others, and this is clearly reflected in statistics: murders; violent crimes; family violence, including child and spousal abuse; gun ownership; and propensities for violence in the mass media. In the aftermath of the school shootings in Littleton, Colorado, the focus on this long-standing problem has become even more intense. Dramatic crimes such as this are often not predictable and may or may not be preventable. However, the voluminous research on aggression and antisocial behavior suggests that it may be possible to prevent some incidents of more typical types of physical aggression (fighting, bullying, reactive aggression), argumentative and explosive behavior, and other forms of antisocial behavior (theft, vandalism, truancy, drug use).

There is widespread consensus in developmental psychopathology that the array of risk factors discussed throughout this book is associated with the emergence of early aggressive and oppositional behavior that ultimately may become oppositional disorder, conduct disorder, and/or delinquency (Coie & Dodge, 1998; Conduct Problems Prevention Research Group, 1992; Dumas, Prinz, Smith, & Laughlin, 1999; Kazdin, 1995; Patterson, DeBaryshe, & Ramsey, 1989; Parke & Slaby, 1983; Reid, 1993): child factors (difficult temperament, poor self-regulation, poor cognitive and language skills); parenting factors (poor parent–child relationship reflected in low warmth and involvement and punitive, harsh discipline; limited stimulation and support for mastery; child abuse/neglect); family factors (single parent, parental mental illness, marital discord, substance abuse, low education, poverty, minority status); and community factors (dangerous neighborhood, low social support; poor community resources, such as inadequate child care, poor schools, limited recreational centers and structured activities). Moreover, numerous exiting theoretical models suggest problems that are evident early, for example, in toddlerhood or by preschool age (Campbell, 1990; Campbell, Pierce, Moore, Marakovitz, & Newby, 1996; Reid, 1993; Shaw, Owens, Vondra, Keenan, & Winslow, 1996), prepare the stage for a cascading set of difficulties that spill over from the early family environment (tantrums, noncompliance, sibling strife, poor parenting) to encompass the child's interactions with teachers and peers in child care and elementary school (aggression, uncooperative behavior). Ultimately, this pattern of behavior is reflected in peer rejection, unstable friendships with other aggressive children, and poor academic achievement (Dishion, Andrews, & Crosby, 1995; Patterson et al., 1989; Patterson & Yoerger, 1997; Vitaro, Tremblay, Kerr, Pagani, & Bukowski, 1997).

Thus, there have been numerous calls for comprehensive prevention programs designed to deal with this intransigent problem based on our knowledge of important risk and protective factors, the developmental course of aggression and antisocial behavior, and what we know about effective intervention. These programs attempt to modify the developmental pathways that at-risk children may follow by minimizing particular risk factors in children and their environment and by building in competencies in children and protective factors in their environment (e.g., Conduct Problems Prevention Research Group, 1992; Dumas, Prinz, Smith, & Laughlin, 1999). This includes some or all of the following: strengthening family support for children's academic achievement and appropriate social behavior; helping families cope with adversity that may undermine parenting; modifying children's social behavior and social cognition to maximize prosocial behavior with peers and limit aggressive, disruptive, and provocative behavior that alienates peers; and making the school experience a positive one by facilitating family and school communication, building academic and study skills, and working with teachers to help them better handle disruptive children.

Testing Models for the Prevention of Aggression and Conduct Problems

The model outlined in Figure 11.1 summarizes these programs and builds on the model presented in Chapter 3 (Figure 3.1). In so doing, it incorporates features of several models of the development of aggression, including those of Coie and Dodge (1998; Conduct Problems Prevention Research Group, 1992), Dumas, Prinz, Smith, and Laughlin (1999), Huesmann, Eron, Lefkowitz, and Walder (1984), Patterson (Patterson, DeBaryshe, & Ramsey, 1989; Patterson & Yoerger, 1997), Parke and Slaby (1983), and Reid (1993). This model suggests a number of places where intervention might be effective prior to or at school entry, or even later. Figures 11.1 and 11.2 also illustrate the pervasiveness of the influences on children's aggression, thereby highlighting the reasons why short-term, limited preventions are rarely effective. This serves as the backdrop for a more in-depth discussion of several prevention programs that have emerged from a developmental psychopathology perspec-

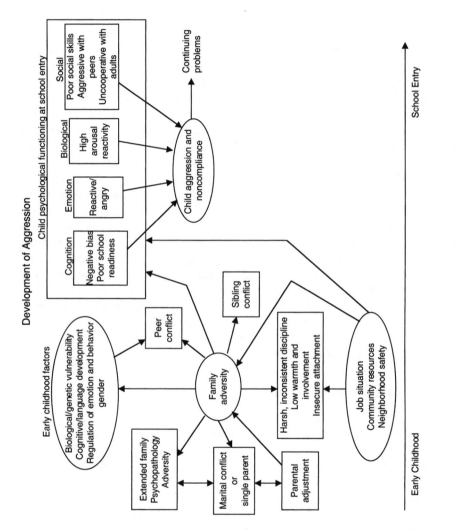

FIGURE 11.1. Model for the development of aggression from a developmental psychopathology perspective.

tive and share similar goals despite their differing underlying assumptions and definitions of risk.

A number of programs have been developed to decrease aggression in young children, with the ultimate goal of preventing conduct problems in adolescence. In general, programs that begin to reduce early conduct problems focus on both proximal goals, such as increased social cooperation, and distal goals, such as lower rates of delinquent behavior and school dropout. Proximal goals may be thought of as mediators of outcome in that they may change the child's developmental trajectory, leading a once aggressive child to become more cooperative and likable, for example, with possible longer-term consequences for peer relations (e.g., Vitaro, Tremblay, Kerr, Pagani, & Bukowski, 1997). Thus, many of these programs (e.g., Kellam, Ling, Mersica, Brown, & Ialongo, 1998; Kellam, Rebok, Ialongo, & Mayer, 1994; Vitaro, Brendgen, Pagani, Tremblay, & McDuff, 1999) have focused on relatively specific aspects of functioning, with the goal of testing particular models and, thereby, identifying possible mechanisms of change.

For example, Kellam and colleagues (1998) combined a universal and a targeted intervention directed at inner-city, mostly African American first graders, screened as aggressive at the end of kindergarten. The classroomwide intervention was meant to provide structure and feedback for good behavior at the group level, thereby changing the ecology of the entire classroom. For the intervention, called the Good Behavior Game, classrooms were divided into teams that then competed for rewards based on each team's ability to follow rules and behave prosocially. This preventive intervention was meant to test the assumption that group support from peers, paired with teacher support, would facilitate behavior change, and that structured rewards for positive, cooperative behavior, and consequences for disruptive and aggressive behavior would be adequate to socialize aggressive children to behave prosocially. A tutoring component was also included, with the aim of improving academic achievement. By including all children in a competitive bid for rewards, Kellam and colleagues hoped to change the social climate of the entire classroom, thereby modifying the social support that disruptive children often receive from peers, while simultaneously reducing the overall levels of classroom aggression.

Some data support the efficacy of this approach but highlight the importance of gender and context as moderators of outcome. Thus, Kellam, Ling, Mersica, Brown, and Ialongo (1998) found that the Good Behavior Game, implemented during first and second grade, was effective in reducing teacher-rated aggression in sixth grade, but only for highly aggressive boys in classrooms with higher overall levels of aggression. The aggression level of girls was not influenced by the intervention or the level of earlier classroom aggression. Highly aggressive boys in classrooms with only moderate levels of aggression were likewise less effected by the intervention than aggressive boys in aggressive classrooms. Rather, when first-grade classrooms had higher overall levels of aggression, the structure provided by the intervention changed the

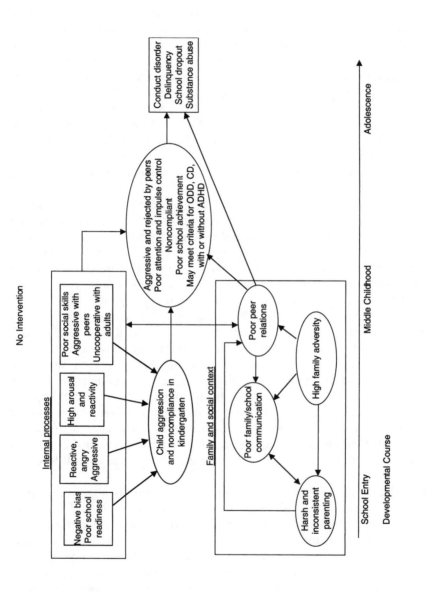

FIGURE 11.2. Internal and external processes that can be targeted for preventive intervention for the development of aggression.

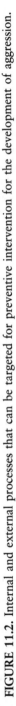

social climate of the classroom, and aggressive boys no longer reinforced and promoted aggression in each other. The program had less impact on boys who were aggressive in a less aggressive classroom, because the climate and ecology of the setting were likely to be less important in the emergence of aggression in these boys. These data may suggest something about the etiology and developmental course of aggression in young boys. Aggression may be more socially driven in some children than others, and these may be the boys who respond more readily to environmental structure. In contrast, children showing less change in response to the intervention may be the boys that Moffitt (1993a) has called "life-course-persistent," for whom family factors, especially child rearing and parental adjustment, may be more salient than social facilitation in encouraging aggression.

Tremblay and colleagues also tested a similar model of peer influence, where, rather than at the group level, the focus was social support for aggression at the dyadic level of the target child's best friend. These investigators instituted a more comprehensive program for aggressive and hyperactive boys, meant to reduce later conduct problems and delinquency in a moderately low income sample in Montreal (Vitaro, Brendgen, Pagani, Tremblay, & McDuff, 1999; Vitaro & Tremblay, 1994). It is noteworthy that only 13% of the boys were living in families on welfare, and 67% were living with both parents. This is in contrast to similar studies in the United States, where much larger proportions of children are living in poverty and in single-parent households (McLoyd, 1998). This underscores social and cultural differences that also influence definitions of risk status and reflect important variations in social context that may affect the likely efficacy of the program.

French-speaking boys in selected neighborhoods were screened in kindergarten using teacher ratings. Those above the 70th percentile were randomly assigned to prevention or control status. The prevention program, which was instituted when boys were in second and third grade, included basic parent training in behavior management, school-based social skills training focused on increasing prosocial behavior, and cognitive problem solving focused on improving anger control and negotiation strategies. Children were seen in small groups that mixed disruptive boys with more popular and socially appropriate peers. It was reasoned that prosocial boys would model more appropriate behavior, might become friends with the disruptive boys, and would remove any stigma from participation. In addition, it was argued, if disruptive boys can modify their social behavior with peers, their friendship patterns will change. Given the hypothesized influence of the peer group on children's social behavior and tendency to engage in delinquent behavior, modifying friendship patterns may be one mechanism of change; that is, if problem children socialize primarily with other problem children (Cairns, Cairns, & Neckerman, 1989; Patterson, DeBaryshe, & Ramsey, 1989), they will be more likely to get into trouble in early adolescence. This is partly because aggressive boys tend to engage in more coercive behavior with their friends and to model deviant behavior, while also providing less support to each other for prosocial behavior (Dishion, Andrews, & Crosby, 1995). Shifting friendship networks so that aggressive boys have more prosocial friends may help them to reject a pattern of escalating aggressive and antisocial behavior.

When boys were followed up at ages 10, 11, and 12, there were modest effects of the intervention program on teacher-rated aggression and self-reported delinquency. Boys in the treated group had best friends who were rated as less disruptive by peers; they were also slightly less likely to meet DSM-III-R diagnostic criteria for conduct disorder at age 13 (Vitaro, Brendgen, Pagani, Tremblay, & McDuff, 1999), suggesting modest effects of the prevention program. In a more detailed examination of potential models of change, Vitaro and colleagues asked whether these intervention effects were best accounted for by a decrease in disruptive behavior (direct child effects), by the influence of friends' behavior (indirect social facilitation model), or by an interaction between peer modeling and child behavior. The outcome of interest was the diagnosis of conduct disorder at age 13. Results were most consistent with the interactive model, in that boys who were low to moderate in disruptiveness at the end of the intervention were less affected by their best friends' level of aggression than were boys with higher levels. In this instance, highly aggressive boys postintervention were much more likely to meet criteria for conduct disorder if their best friends were also highly aggressive. Conversely, aggressive boys with nonaggressive best friends were less likely to meet criteria for conduct disorder, suggesting that prosocial peers may serve a protective function in some situations. These results highlight the difficulties of demonstrating dramatic effects even of relatively intense programs, as well as the complexity inherent in trying to disentangle mediators and moderators of change.

Other, larger-scale interventions target whole school systems in large communities (e.g., Aber , Jones, Brown, Chaudry, & Samples, 1998) or across the country (e.g., Allen, Philliber, Herrling, & Kuperminc, 1997), with the aim of modifying aspects of functioning that place school-age children and adolescents at risk for aggression per se, or for self-defeating behaviors such as teen pregnancy and school suspension associated with conduct problems and delinquency. Short-term results from several outcome studies examining the impact of these more universal and less intense programs suggest modest results, but only for certain subgroups of children. For example, Aber and colleagues (1998) evaluated the impact of a violence prevention program in the New York City public schools that focused on conflict resolution and was aimed at modifying children's hostile attributions and aggressive fantasies, and improving their interpersonal negotiation skills. The program did show modest effects in decreasing the rate of increase in hostile attributions in these middle-school students, but only among children in classrooms where violence was not accepted as normative. This seems similar to the findings of Kellam, Ling, Mersica, Brown, and Ialongo (1998), who also found that their preventive intervention was more effective for children in less violent classrooms, where peers did not encourage aggressive behavior in classmates.

Allen and colleagues (1997) focused on building general skills, such as more competent decision making around life transitions and choices, better interaction skills, and better control of one's own emotions in order to enhance school functioning and decrease teen pregnancy in high school students. This widely used national program, Teen Outreach, included volunteer work and classroom components. Allen and colleagues argue that the focus on the general developmental tasks of adolescence and on building competence, rather than on modifying specific problem behaviors or building specific skills, should affect a range of related, albeit diverse, problems of adolescence. Although this program does not focus on aggression per se, it clearly addresses problems that are often sequelae of aggressive or antisocial behavior. At the end of a 1-year period, adolescents in the treatment group had lower rates of teen pregnancy, school failure, and school suspensions than the control group, suggesting that this relatively simple program may have promise in the short term. However, the data do not indicate whether these youngsters are also less aggressive or conduct disordered, or whether results from the intervention will be maintained.

The prevention programs discussed so far illustrate how both targeted and universal programs can derive from a developmental psychopathology perspective, focus on an underlying developmental process or processes thought to be important in the onset or maintenance of problem behavior, and, at the same time, test theories of development. In addition, these programs illustrate the importance of context, especially the peer context, in determining which children are likely to fare better with the intervention. Although all these programs have been effective to some degree and have suggested that the issues that guided program development are important, they may not be intense or long term enough really to prevent conduct problems in children seriously at risk because of early-onset aggression. This argument is supported by the findings of both Kellam and colleagues (1998) and Aber and colleagues (1998), who found that level of classroom aggression mattered. In addition, with the exception of the Vitaro and colleagues (1999) program, these interventions focused solely on the child in the school context. For certain levels of early-emerging aggression, multifaceted programs that include interventions aimed at the child, family, peer group, and school may be necessary to effect longer-term change in a range of behaviors and contexts that support aggressive and other problem behaviors. Two such comprehensive programs are currently ongoing: the FAST Track program (Conduct Problems Prevention Research Group, 1992) and the Early Alliance Program (Dumas, Prinz, Smith, & Laughlin, 1999).

COMPREHENSIVE PREVENTION PROGRAMS FOR AGGRESSION AND CONDUCT PROBLEMS

The FAST Track Program

The FAST Track (Families and Schools Together) program (see Conduct Problems Prevention Research Group, 1992), a multisite prevention trial, illustrates many of the issues raised in this chapter, especially how a developmental psychopathology perspective and a theory-driven approach can inform the development of a large-scale, multifaceted prevention program, and how prevention trials can be used to test causal models of the development of psychopathology. Although the ultimate goal of FAST Track is to prevent conduct disorder, a problem usually not diagnosed before middle childhood or early adolescence (American Psychiatric Association, 1994; Hinshaw, Lahey, & Hart, 1993; Kazdin, 1995), the intervention begins at school entry and focuses on developmental processes that reseachers hope will be interrupted before they escalate into more serious and chronic patterns of negative and antisocial behavior. Thus, the long-term goal is the prevention of conduct disorder and associated problems, including school dropout, drug and alcohol use/abuse, and delinquency. However, early intervention aimed at more proximal mediating processes may be more effective than waiting until a diagnosable disorder is evident, or until more severe and chronic symptoms occur, especially given the intransigence of these symptoms to conventional psychological treatments (Kazdin, 1995). Returning to two crucial questions about prevention programs: The "what" of FAST Track is conduct problems, and the "when" is at school entry. FAST Track includes both universal components targeting all the first-grade classrooms in a school system and indicated components, targeting a group identified as "high risk." Given the nature of the problem to be prevented and the extensive literature on the emergence of conduct disorder (e.g., Coie & Dodge, 1998; Hinshaw et al., 1993; Kazdin, 1995; Patterson, DeBaryshe, & Ramsey, 1989; Reid, 1993), the program begins relatively early. This is because it is well established that highly aggressive young children at school entry are at high risk to continue to have problems with aggression, oppositional behavior, and poor school achievement, as depicted in Figures 11.1 and 11.2.

In order to select the high-risk group, a complex screening process was necessary. First, kindergarten teachers provided information on all the children in their classrooms at the end of the school year. Parents of the children who scored in the top 40% on a teacher screening measure of aggression and noncompliance were then contacted and asked about their child's behavior at home. The top 10% of aggressive, noncompliant children across both home and school settings were selected as target children. Then, schools containing these children were randomly assigned to intervention and control status. Thus, the "who" of FAST Track includes all first graders in participating schools for the universal components and all highly aggressive first graders in the participating schools for the more focused and intensive intervention components.

To answer the "how" question, a number of issues need to be considered. First, the integrated and comprehensive components of the intervention include parent training, case management, social skills training, academic tutoring, and a classroom intervention. Each of these components includes multiple subcomponents meant to facilitate generalization across settings (e.g., from home to peer group, from home to classroom, from peer group to home) and across relationships (i.e., with parents, teachers, siblings, and peers). Thus, parent training includes parent management training meant both to increase positive and consistent limit setting and decrease negative, inconsistent, and punitive behavior (e.g., Forehand & McMahon, 1981; Patterson, 1982). At the same time, parents are taught some of the same social skills that the children learn in the classroom setting (universal intervention) and in small peer groups (targeted intervention), including anger management and social problem solving around conflict resolution. The overall goal is building positive parent–child relations by modifying the behaviors and social cognitions of both parents and children, and by building in social and academic competence. Thus, the focus is on mediating processes hypothesized to link early aggressive and disruptive behavior to later conduct problems (Conduct Problems Prevention Research Group, 1999), some of which is illustrated in Figure 11.3, where the dotted lines reflect internal processes and environmental supports that are targeted for change. Conversely, Figure 11.2 demonstrates one possible pathway for a child with early onset problems that are not addressed with a comprehensive, multifaceted intervention.

Because academic problems often appear to exacerbate feelings of incompetence and fuel peer rejection (e.g., Patterson, DeBaryshe, & Ramsey, 1989), and because children living in high-risk, dysfunctional families are often ill-prepared for the demands of first grade (Dumas, Prinz, Smith, & Laughlin, 1999), intervention children also receive intensive tutoring, especially in reading skills. To help the parents learn to work with the school and to model more effective ways of helping their children with academic work, they are included in the tutoring sessions as observers and participants.

As already discussed, the importance of peer problems in the development of aggressive behavior and conduct problems has been the subject of extensive research indicating that peer rejection and the association with deviant peers are both important factors in exacerbating aggressive behavior evident in early childhood (Coie & Dodge, 1998). Thus, FAST Track includes multiple aspects of peer social skills training meant to facilitate both dyadic interactions with friends and appropriate social behavior in the larger peer group, such as effective group entry, self-control, prosocial behavior, and negotiation in the face of conflict. These skills are learned and practiced in different settings: dyadic, group-, and classroomwide. Teachers also are taught to use standard classroom management procedures such as clear directives, positive feedback, and time-out for misbehavior. Finally, case managers help parents deal with a range of other stressors that may interfere with family functioning. Thus, the components of the program are structured, comprehensive, and long term, with some components lasting from the beginning of first grade through the end of second grade.

The second aspect of the "how" question addresses processes of change. As illustrated in Figure 11.3, numerous internal and external processes are targeted by the intervention. In terms of internal processes within the child, interventions focus on building in cognitive and social skills, including improve-

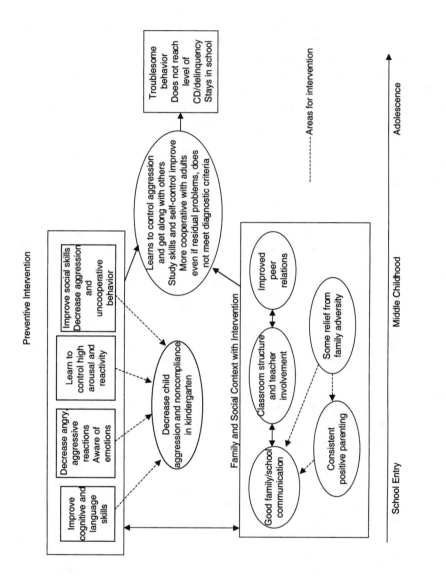

FIGURE 11.3. Preventive interventions for internal and external processes implicated in the development of aggression.

ment in academic functions such as reading and word attack skills, and teaching better study/homework habits. Peer relations and social skills are partly modified by changing children's ways of thinking about peers' internal states, social problems, and peer relations and friendships, as well as self-reflecting about the impact of their own behavior on others. For example, social-cognitive exercises are geared to help children develop more positive and adaptive ways of thinking about peers' intentions and internal states, especially recognizing their emotions. Thus, social perspective taking and empathy are involved. In addition, portions of the program build in specific social skills or behaviors meant to go along with the social cognitions. The link between thought and action is often not direct. Even though children may think differently about peers' intentions, they may not know how to behave or, even if they "know" how they should behave, they may not act accordingly when under stress. Thus, the social skills component of the program tries to give children alternative ways of behaving that are more appropriate and less confrontational. The anger management component is meant to teach children strategies for slowing down and not responding reactively without thinking. For example, when someone says something that upsets a child, he or she can talk to them about it and negotiate a solution to the problem or react with anger and get into a fight with them. At the same time, then, children should be learning to control negative emotions and reactive aggression, and to modulate some of their impulses and prepotent angry responses.

Interventions include both the child's family and wider social environment, based on the extensive research linking disrupted family environments, harsh and inconsistent parenting, lack of parental involvement, and limited family support for academic accomplishments to children's aggression and behavior problems (e.g., Campbell, Pierce, Moore, Marakovitz, & Newby, 1996; Dodge, Pettit, & Bates, 1994b; Gardner, 1987, 1989; Parke & Slaby, 1983; Patterson, DeBaryshe, & Ramsey, 1989; Pettit, Bates, & Dodge, 1997). Thus, the case managers are meant to help with family problems that might divert parental attention and energy from more adaptive involvement in parenting (Campbell et al., 1996; Harnish et al., 1995; McLoyd, 1998). At the same time, parents are engaged in skills building, both in terms of how better to help their child adapt to the demands of first grade and provide more consistent, positive, and structured limits, which should encourage more positive and involved parenting, and foster a better parent–child relationship.

At the level of the peer group, both targeted and universal interventions should lead to increases in social skills and awareness of peers' inner states, and the structured interactions in dyadic and group contexts should foster more positive interactions in the classroom generally, as well as with the specific children originally designated as aggressive. At the level of the classroom, teachers should learn more structured and systematic ways of coping with difficult children, while setting a tone in the entire classroom that promotes cooperation and awareness of classroom rules. Thus, this extremely comprehensive yet focused and directed preventive intervention should theoretically lead to decreases in problem behavior in multiple domains. Following the Patterson and colleagues model (1989), these youngsters should do better academically, should be accepted into better-functioning peer groups, and should not need to pair up with other antisocial children for recognition or kicks.

Outcome data on FAST Track through the end of first grade (Conduct Problems Prevention Research Group, 1999) indicate modest improvements in treated children's functioning across domains of outcomes that include parent and teacher ratings of social competence, observed parent–child interaction, observed child behavior at school, self-reported parenting behavior, peer ratings, and academic achievement. For example, treated children showed modest improvements in emotion recognition, social problem solving, and positive interactions with peers relative to high-risk children in the untreated group. Independent observers also rated parent–child interaction as more positive and less punitive; children's school behavior was also rated as more cooperative. In addition, treated children showed greater gains in reading and language skills at the end of first grade than did untreated children. Thus, several of the putative mediators of outcome (social cognition, social skills, academic achievement, and parent–child interaction) showed significant, albeit modest, changes at the end of first grade. Despite this, there were no differences between groups in actual ratings of externalizing symptoms according to either parent or teacher reports, and about 65% of the children in both groups received elevated scores on the CBCL/TRF externalizing scale. Thus, it remains to be seen whether continued intervention will affect developmental processes sufficiently to lead to greater reductions in symptoms at later follow-ups. In addition, mediators and moderators of treatment effectiveness still remain to be examined, as well as the role of treatment compliance in predicting outcome within the intervention group.

The Early Alliance Program

More recently, Dumas, Prinz, and colleagues (1999) have instituted a comprehensive prevention program for high-risk, predominantly African American children. The Early Alliance Program is based on a developmental model similar to FAST Track and also involves multiple components, with the goal of modifying conduct problems, school dropout, and substance abuse in adolescence. Like FAST Track, children are screened for this program prior to first grade; children who are aggressive and noncompliant at home and school are selected for the multifaceted indicated intervention, while whole classrooms receive a more complex, universal intervention than was the case with FAST Track. The main difference between these two programs appears to be the greater emphasis in the Early Alliance Program on building in structure and systematic positive feedback in classrooms, and working with teachers to create a positive classroom climate that rewards children for success. In addition, Dumas and colleagues have articulated a systematic theoretical model that emphasizes increased competence in communication skills and literacy, and both direct and indirect pathways to change. This program includes a very detailed behavioral management program implemented during first and second grade for all pupils in target children's classrooms, a structured, peer-interaction component meant to teach social skills and communication, an intense reading mentoring component, and family intervention in the home that focuses on parenting and social support. Thus, this program builds on some of the more promising features of other programs (Conduct Problems Prevention Research Group, 1992; Kellam, Rebok, Ialongo, & Mayer, 1994; Vitaro, Tremblay, Gagnon, & Pelletier, 1994), while focusing more specifically on classroom management and positive communication. Whereas the long-term goals include decreased rates of conduct disorder, substance abuse, and school dropout, the assumption is made that these will be achieved via the short-term goals of increasing social and emotional competence and school achievement, and decreasing aggressive and disruptive behavior. Like the other prevention programs discussed in this chapter, it is hypothesized that by modifying social-cognitive processes and social and academic behaviors in the child with adequate social and emotional supports across contexts (home, school, peer group), the developmental course of early-emerging aggressive and disruptive behavior will be altered.

Principles of Prevention Revisited

Both the FAST Track program and the Early Alliance Program are consistent with many of the principles of prevention and early intervention outlined by Ramey and Ramey (1998) and discussed earlier in the chapter. For example, both begin relatively early and last at least through first and second grade, extending beyond the crucial developmental transition to school; both are intensive, comprehensive, and multifaceted, including family, social, and cognitive components; both involve direct intervention with the child across contexts and also incorporate features meant to increase parental awareness of and involvement with the child's school. Furthermore, in line with the proposals of Coie and colleagues (1993), both programs derive from complex transactional and ecological models of developmental psychopathology, are theory- and model-driven, and permit tests of basic causal processes. Thus, on the one hand, these prevention programs provide strong tests of several developmental psychopathology models linking multiple risk factors to the development of aggressive behavior and conduct problems in children. If they are not successful, they will call many of our hypotheses into question. If they are successful, we will still not know exactly what led to change. Because so many aspects of the child and the child's environment are the focus of components of the interventions, it will be difficult to isolate the mechanisms of change, although it may be possible to identify some intervening or mediating processes (e.g., altered attributions about the intentions of others, better literacy skills, a more positive parent–child relationship, better self-esteem) that may account for change in some domains of functioning. As already noted, data on the effectiveness of FAST Track are just beginning to emerge, whereas the Early Alliance Program is just starting. Both studies will be theoretically and practically important to the science of developmental psychopathology, because they will provide crucial links from theory and model building to practice and social policy.

Concluding Comments on Prevention

Although the prevention programs discussed in this chapter have focused on aggression and conduct problems, they have also addressed more general features of the child's environment, such as family stress and positive parenting, implicated in the development of both internalizing and externalizing problems (e.g., Greenberg, Leguna, Coie, & Pinderhughes, 1999). They have also tried to enhance children's cognitive and social skills, emphasizing academic achievement (e.g., literacy) and social cooperation in the peer group. The families selected for program participation have been targeted based on their general high-risk status or because their children have screened positive for early-onset aggression and related problems.

Other program directions may be indicated for other groups. For couples with children, maritally focused psychoeducational programs that stress communication skills and understanding family processes may have advantages over parenting-focused programs. Thus, Cowan, Cowan, and Heming (1999) reported that maritally focused programs for two-parent, intact families improved both marital quality and parenting, but parenting-focused programs did not benefit marital quality. Further analyses assessing the direction of effects over time indicated that shifts in marital conflict in the maritally focused intervention group led to later shifts in parenting quality, whereas shifts in parenting for those in parenting-focused group were not followed by later improvements in terms of marital conflict (Cowan & Cowan, 1999). Thus, while beneficial effects on children's adaptation (internalizing and externalizing problems; academic achievement) over time (kindergarten to age 10) were found for both couple intervention conditions, the effects of the maritally focused condition on family functioning were more pervasive than those for the parenting-focused condition. Given that both marital conflict and parenting have been found to have direct effects on children's adjustment (see Chapters 6–8, this volume), these findings suggest the promise of maritally focused interventions as another direction for prevention or intervention programs for couples with children.

There has been little research on preventing of depression or anxiety in children, or on helping children cope with transitions such as divorce or remarriage (Emery, 1999). This is partly because it is easier to identify children at risk for aggression than for internalizing problems, and because aggression continues to be of such concern to educators, parents, and mental health professionals. However, a more systematic focus on depression is certainly needed given its prevalence in adolescence and early adulthood (e.g., Lewinsohn, Hops, Roberts, Seely, & Andrews, 1993), as well as the well-documented impact of more serious and chronic depression on parenting behavior (e.g., NICHD Early Child Care Research Network, 1999).

Some suggestive evidence implicates parental depression in the onset of depression in children. Based on this premise, one program meant to prevent depression in a small sample of children with depressed parents (Beardslee et al., 1997) indicates that this is a fruitful area for systematic research provided that multiple risk factors for depression can be identified (see Cicchetti & Toth, 1998). In general, it is likely that programs geared to the prevention of depression will either need to start early and identify offspring of mothers with chronic depression (Campbell, Cohn, & Meyers, 1995; NICHD Early Child Care Research Network, 1999), focusing on parental involvement and the mother–child relationship, or identify somewhat older children who show prolonged sadness in the context of family adversity and a family history of problems. In school-age children and adolescents, a focus on peer support and social competence might be one way to offset the development of the low self-esteem and feelings of worthlessness that are among the hallmarks of depression in adolescence. However, it is also likely given the co-occurrence of internalizing and externalizing problems that many of the programs meant to prevent conduct problems in adolescence, by virtue of their focus on enhancing social and academic skills, building competence, and improving parent–child relationships, will also decrease the occurrence of depressed mood in adolescents. This, too, remains to be seen.

Stressful life events and family transitions are also a likely focus of prevention efforts. It should be obvious from the discussion so far, and the data presented in Chapter 8, that marital conflict, separation, and divorce are extremely distressing to children. Therefore, it is not surprising that several programs, both parent- and child-focused, have attempted to prevent problems from developing in the aftermath of family separation and divorce. This is clearly a fruitful area for prevention because it is well-documented that children from divorcing families often have adjustment difficulties, and because the targets of prevention are quite clear. As Emery (1999) points out, children and parents must cope with feelings of loss, sadness, and anger, as well as learn to renegotiate family roles and relationships. Suggestive evidence, reviewed by Emery, indicates that didactic support groups for school-age children and adolescents adjusting to parental divorce can help youngsters communicate with family members, more realistically assess their own role in the process, and decrease anxiety and depression. There is surprisingly little research in this area, however, despite the fact that family dissolution is an obvious risk factor for children's adjustment, one that partly reflects decreases in parental support in the aftermath of divorce (Hetherington, 1989). Thus, it seems important to examine prevention programs geared to the family system as well.

TREATMENT OF CHILDHOOD DISORDERS

Limitations of Treatment Research

The discussion of prevention programs has linked components of intervention to underlying processes thought to set children on a developmental pathway toward poor adaptation, and possibly toward the emergence of more severe and chronic problems that interfere with functioning at multiple levels. In contrast, as already noted, treatment research has tended to be more narrowly focused and less comprehensive, despite the fact that children targeted for treatment have been identified by the mental health system or a related system (child welfare, special education) as needing help, thereby suggesting that their problems may be more severe and chronic than the problems of children targeted for prevention trials. In general, the child treatment literature is more fragmented and piecemeal, less theory-driven, less developmentally informed, and focused more specifically on alleviating symptoms of disorder than on testing theories of the development of psychopathology. Ironically, many of the components of prevention programs (e.g., social skills training, parent management training) were first developed as treatment packages for children with diagnosed disorders. This reflects the long history of treatment research derived from either a strict behavioral or a social learning theory perspective, where the emphasis is on modifying contingencies in the child's environment that appear to maintain maladaptive behavior (e.g., Patterson, 1982; Patterson & Yoerger, 1997). Research on social skills training and cognitive-behavioral treatments for children has been influenced partly by developmental research on peer relations and the potential impact of peer rejection on children (e.g., Lochman, 1992; Lochman & Curry, 1986), and partly by analogy from, and downward extensions of, effective treatments for adult disorders (e.g., Lewinsohn, Clarke, Hops, & Andrews, 1990). In general, the treatments that have been the subject of controlled research are highly focused, didactic, and short term, with an emphasis on symptom remission.

In addition, several features distinguish treatment research from prevention studies and make them less systematic. First, whereas the "who" and the "when" of prevention are usually tightly controlled by the researcher, in treatment research, the "who" and the "when" are more arbitrary. This is because participants ideally have been clinically referred, but who gets referred to what facility? This is rarely systematic and may be based on a number of unmeasured factors such as parental tolerance for troublesome and/or troubled behavior, parental resources (e.g., insurance coverage), or whether another adult in the child's environment initiates or mandates referral (e.g., schoolteacher, social worker in child welfare agency). The nature and severity of children's problems also may vary with both the source of referral and the type of facility (e.g., school psychologist, hospital specialty clinic, child welfare agency). In addition, children in treatment usually receive a diagnosis or multiple diagnoses, but treatment may be geared generally to family distress or to one aspect of the problem rather than to the complexity of issues that often surround referral. Furthermore, the problem may be long-standing but only come to clinical attention after a crisis.

Before addressing several important issues in child treatment research, it is crucial to point out that the worlds of the clinic and the laboratory rarely intersect (Weisz, Weiss, & Donenberg, 1992). Thus, as noted at the beginning of this chapter, the clinical science divisions of the American Psychological Association have emphasized the importance of empirically supported treatments for specific disorders, something that has become even more crucial with the emergence of managed care that mandates time-limited therapies of proven effectiveness. However, treatment research is often conducted on volunteers or participants screened in psychology department clinics or school settings rather than on clinically referred cases in clinical settings that cater to more severely impaired clients. As a result, treatments that appear promising for motivated parents and children may prove less so when offered to more dysfunctional families seeking treatment at community mental health centers, a point emphasized by Weisz and colleagues (1992). Moreover, the treatments offered in community mental health centers are more likely to be unsystematic and eclectic, with only limited follow-up or assessment of effectiveness and, hence, little evidence to support their use (Kazdin, 1995; Weisz & Hawley, 1998).

Empirically Supported Treatments

The emphases on empirically supported psychosocial interventions for children have led to the delineation of criteria to determine whether a treatment is well-enough established to be considered efficacious. These include the availability of data from at least two well-designed studies (e.g., including random assignment, adequate power, blind and independent assessment of change) by different investigatory teams that show the treatment to be more effective than an alternative treatment, or equivalent to an already-established treatment. Furthermore, the sample characteristics (e.g., age, gender, diagnosis) need to be clearly specified (Lonigan, Elbert, & Johnson, 1998). Moreover, there is a move toward manualizing treatments so that controlled studies can compare specific aspects of treatment. The fact that these basic aspects of research design must be specified underscores the state of treatment outcome research. Thus, despite the hundreds, if not thousands, of studies that have examined the effectiveness of various treatments for particular problems, there are surprisingly few that meet even these minimal criteria for empirical support. This is because most treatment outcome studies have used very small samples; they often do not compare the tested treatment with an alternative or even placebo treatment, but with a waiting-list control (no treatment); children often vary widely in age; comorbid diagnoses are often not considered; the range of co-occurring family problems and adversity is often not described or considered; and there are often problems demonstrating the generalization of treatment effects across settings and their maintenance over time once treatment is terminated (Brestan & Eyberg, 1998; Hinshaw, 1994; Kazdin, 1993, 1995, 1997a; Ollendick & King, 1998; Weisz & Hawley, 1998).

These limitations notwithstanding, there is evidence to support the use of particular treatment components for particular problems. For example, a substantial body of research supports the use of parent training for families of children with oppositional, conduct, or attention deficit disorder (e.g., Barkley, 1987; Brestan & Eyberg, 1998; Forehand & McMahon, 1981; Patterson, 1982; Pelham, Wheeler, & Chronis, 1998). Other studies suggest the effectiveness of various problem-solving and social skills training packages for children with oppositional and conduct problems (e.g., Brestan & Eyberg, 1998; Kazdin, Siegel, & Bass, 1990; Lochman & Curry, 1986), although their effectiveness in children with attention deficit disorder is less clear (Hinshaw, 1994; Pelham et al., 1998). Direct behavioral management in the classroom also appears to be effective for children with externalizing problems (Pelham et al., 1998). Thus, for children with problems of undercontrol, these very structured programs have proven effective in the short term, when the outcome measure is closely tied to symptom remission. For children with depressed mood or anxiety disorders, cognitive-behavioral and behavioral approaches appear to be promising (Kaslow & Thompson, 1998; Ollendick & King, 1998). However, these studies have been conducted on especially small samples, often not with clinically referred children. In addition, follow-up has often been short term. Moreover, children presenting to psychology clinics with internalizing problems in the absence of comorbid externalizing symptoms are often from higher-functioning families and/or have parents who are more aware of their moods, feelings, and concerns.

Thus, although studies suggest that particular approaches may indeed be beneficial for particular problems, it must be remembered that the studies considered in support of particular therapeutic approaches have usually examined a short-term and time-limited intervention geared to symptom remission. It is not likely that these individual treatment components by themselves are adequate to overcome serious, chronic problems in the context of family adversity. Thus, they neither normalize behavior nor generalize across contexts or time.

Toward More Conceptual Models of Child Treatment

The need for more theoretically driven, conceptual, and developmentally informed models for treatment development and research has been addressed most forcefully by Kazdin (1993, 1995, 1997a) who has called for treatment research that tests basic conceptual models about underlying processes and then establishes links between the hypothesized underlying process and the outcome. He also underscores the importance of considering the child's family and social context in designing treatments for complex problems. It is also noteworthy that almost no research has examined treatment effectiveness in a developmental context. Thus, it seems logical that certain treatments should work better for children of particular ages. Although there is some suggestive evidence that parent training programs are more effective for younger than older children (e.g., Brestan & Eyberg, 1998), studies have not examined treatment efficacy specifically as a function of children's age. Kazdin notes that most studies in support of these various treatment packages have been analogue studies with short-term follow-up. Moreover, even when they suggest that symptomatic improvement occurs after treatment, the hypothesized, underlying mechanisms (e.g., cognitive processes) do not always change, making it difficult to determine why the treatment might have worked. Because of the complexities of aggressive, oppositional, antisocial, and impulsive behavior, it is not surprising that short-term, small-scale treatments aimed at one or another symptom in one context (e.g., home or school) do not lead to major changes in behavior and adaptation that generalize across contexts and are maintained over time. This might be predicted from a developmental psychopathology perspective, where the complexity of interacting processes over time are the core of most developmental models. It is also a logical conclusion that can be drawn from the principles of prevention research and the description of comprehensive prevention programs discussed earlier in this chapter.

From a similar perspective, then, Kazdin (1993, 1997a) suggests that treatment researchers need to expand research questions to include aspects of the family and social context, to examine multiple outcomes, and to look for moderating effects, since it is well known that not all children and families respond in a uniform way to treatment. Child age, gender, and comorbid diagnoses seem to be logical candidates for moderating variables. In the family context, severity of family adversity, single- or two-parent status, and parental adjustment seem relevant, among a host of other variables to consider. Consistent with this, Kazdin notes that not all children and families are amenable to treatment. This is similar to Ramey and Ramey's (1998) admonition that not all families will respond to prevention trials.

Like Ramey and Ramey, Kazdin also argues for broad-based, more comprehensive and long-term interventions, taking into account the chronicity and pervasiveness of many clinical problems. Similar to the approach taken by the Conduct Problems Prevention Research Group (1992) and by Dumas, Prinz, Smith, and Laughlin (1999), Kazdin argues for testing a "high strength" intervention model in which large "doses" of theoretically meaningful treatment components are provided to carefully defined groups to determine whether a comprehensive treatment leads to improvement. If it does, then more systematic research can be undertaken to determine what components of the comprehensive treatment package contribute to the clinical impact of the treatment, and how much of them are necessary to lead to long-term gains in functioning.

Derived from an ecological and transactional perspective, several promising treatment strategies for adolescents with serious chronic conduct problems underscore the importance of a more broadly based and theoretically informed approach to the treatment of these pervasive and often intransigent problems (Chamberlain & Reid, 1998; Henggeler, Melton, & Smith, 1992; Henggeler, Schoenwald, & Pickrel, 1995). For example, multisystemic treatment (MST; Henggeler et al., 1992, 1995) fits in well with the principles of developmental psychopathology articulated in this book. MST focuses on adolescents with conduct disorder and delinquent adolescents, and considers their problems as reflecting dysfunctional relationships within the family, the school, the peer group, and the wider social network, including institutions that often work with troubled adolescents. Using an intensive, crisis-intervention approach with clearly articulated and concrete goals, and working across relationships and social systems, this treatment has proven quite effective when compared to treatment in the community. For example, Henggeler and colleagues report lower recidivism rates and better family and peer relationships at the end of treatment and after longer-term follow-up.

Another important issue raised by Kazdin is how one defines treatment effectiveness. Short-term symptomatic improvement is well established. But does the treatment lead to longer-term gains across domains of functioning? Does it improve family functioning or just the child's behavior? Among the various indicators of outcome, one may look at decreases in negative behavior or sequelae such as declines in symptoms, the absence of a diagnosis, or decreased use of various services (pediatric, mental health, juvenile justice, remedial education); alternatively, a more stringent test of therapeutic effectiveness involves monitoring increases in positive outcomes, such as improvement in social skills, competence, and feelings of well-being; improved parent–child interaction; decreased family stress; and the normalization of behavior. These outcomes, often assessed in prevention trials, are considered less often in treatment outcome studies.

Like research on prevention, some treatment research has examined several treatment components simultaneously. For example, Kazdin and colleagues (Kazdin, Mazurick, & Siegel, 1994; Kazdin, Siegel, & Bass, 1990) compared social problem solving, parent training, and combined treatments for children with conduct problems. Results suggested that the combined treatments were more effective than either component alone but depended on the outcome measure and who was reporting on the child's functioning. Teachers reported improvement across all three treatment conditions, whereas parents reported more improvement in the combined condition. In the ADHD area, several studies have examined the single and combined effects of parent training and classroom management, or parent training and cognitive behavioral interventions. Although symptomatic improvement is often evident from these treatments, they are rarely as effective as the standard treatment for ADHD—methylphenidate (see Pelham, Wheeler, & Chronis, 1998)—and they rarely last when treatment ends (Hinshaw, 1994; Pelham et al., 1998). Moreover, as Pelham and colleagues point out, even when these treatments lead to some improvement in home and classroom, they rarely lead to improvements in peer relations, an important facet of the difficulties experienced by children with ADHD. Thus, psychosocial treatments (and, to a large extent, medication) have not proved to provide long-term effects across contexts and domains of functioning. Thus, although numerous studies have demonstrated that stimulant medication results in marked symptomatic improvement in children with ADHD (Barkley, 1998), and many studies have examined psychosocial treatments in children with ADHD (Pelham et al., 1998), until recently, there had not been any large-scale, comprehensive treatment studies comparing them. Instead, most psychosocial treatments had been evaluated piecemeal in relatively small studies, although there was suggestive evidence that multicomponent psychosocial treatments might prove as effective as medication. Moreover, as noted in Chapter 10, the overlap between ADHD and conduct problems is substantial, increasing the urgency of identifying effective treatments for children with ADHD early enough to prevent the escalation of ADHD and oppositional/aggressive behavior to more chronic antisocial behavior and delinquency (Barkley, 1998; Moffitt, 1990; Weiss & Hechtman, 1993). With these various issues in mind, the National Institute of Mental Health recently sponsored a multisite, multimodal treatment study of children with ADHD.

The Collaborative Multimodal ADHD Treatment Study (MTA)

In view of what we have discussed so far, it is evident that a large-scale, comprehensive treatment study of the size and scope of the FAST Track is warranted. Until recently, there have not been any major multicomponent studies of child treatment involving state-of-the-art treatments put together into a package and presented over a long enough period to determine whether effects generalize and are maintained over time. Moreover, in line with Kazdin's call for larger questions beyond just "does the treatment work?", this ongoing study examines not only the effectiveness of a comprehensive psychosocial treatment package but also the combination of psychosocial treatment and medication, medication alone, and routine referral for treatment in the community (the typical or control treatment) (see Arnold et al., 1997). This study is the largest clinical treatment trial ever undertaken by the National Institute of Mental Health, in which 576 children, ages 7 to 9, with a primary diagnosis of ADHD, combined type, 96 at each of six sites, were randomly assigned to one of the four treatment conditions. Children with co-occurring diagnoses of oppositional defiant disorder, conduct disorder, depression, or anxiety were included given the marked overlap among disorders, especially ADHD and oppositional defiant disorder (Hinshaw, 1994). The three treated groups received 14 months of treatment and were followed for 2 years after study entry, that is, for 10 months after the termination of treatment. The goals of the study were twofold: to examine the relative effectiveness of an intensive psychosocial treatment package with and without medication, as well as medication alone; and to determine whether these three, intensive "state-of-the art" treatments were really any better than the routine treatment children and families receive in the community, for example, from their pediatrician or at school. This study was partly spurred by the controversies over medication usage and the possibility that intensive psychosocial intervention might be as effective as medication. Moreover, the study allowed the investigators to explore whether medication and psychosocial treatments interact to provide even greater benefits than either alone, or whether they interfere with each other.

Selection of the components of the psychosocial treatment was based on several criteria, including evidence supporting their short-term efficacy, as discussed earlier; the treatment had to be available in manualized form, so that it could be implemented consistently across sites; and it had to be intense, and not only capable of being integrated with other components but also able to stand alone. Thus, the psychosocial treatment package included standard parent training (Barkley, 1987; Forehand & McMahon, 1981), including both group and individual sessions over a 14-month period. It also involved biweekly teacher consultation in classroom behavior management. Children attended an 8-week intensive summer treatment program (Pelham & Hoza, 1996) that included cognitive-behavioral and behavioral treatments aimed at fostering academic, social, and sports skills. Once the summer treatment program ended, a teacher aide worked with the classroom teacher and the child to help bridge summer program and classroom, thereby facilitating generalization of skills across settings and helping the teacher to implement a structured classroom intervention, so that gains were not lost. Assessments of outcome compared these four treatment conditions on a range of measures of child functioning at home, school, and in the peer group, according to parental, teacher, and observer reports and child performance on standard measures of cognitive functioning (MTA Cooperative Group, 1999a; Wells et al., in press).

Results indicated that children in all four treatment groups improved relative to their initial levels of functioning across six domains of outcome: symptoms of ADHD, symptoms of oppositional defiant disorder, internalizing symptoms, social skills, parent–child relations, and academic achievement. However, in general, children in the medication management and combined treatment conditions showed the greatest improvement relative to those receiving psychosocial treatment alone or community treatment, especially on symptoms of ADHD. Further analyses indicated that children in the combined treatment condition showed greater improvement relative to those receiving only behavioral or community treatment on measures of oppositional symptoms, parent-reported internalizing symptoms, teacher-rated social skills, and reading achievement. Parents also reported using less power-assertive disciplinary techniques. Moreover, these gains were obtained despite the fact that children in the combined treatment group were managed on somewhat lower doses of medication.

In further analyses of this data set (MTA Cooperative Group, 1999b), several moderators of treatment efficacy were examined. Neither child gender (20% of the MTA participants were girls), co-occurring disruptive behavior problems, or prior experience with stimulant medication moderated outcomes. However, children with co-occurring anxiety who received the behavioral treatment package showed higher rates of improvement in ADHD and internalizing symptoms than children with ADHD without comorbid anxiety; moreover, for these children, the behavioral treatment was just as effective as medication management or combined treatment, at least for these outcomes. Finally, treatment compliance was moderately high and did not appear to mediate treatment effects.

Like the FAST Track, this multicomponent treatment underscores the need for longer-term interventions, but questions still remain about whether omnibus treatments are all that effective. The results suggest that the addition of an intensive behavioral treatment to medication management did have some beneficial effects, especially for self-regulatory and social problems that went beyond the ADHD symptoms themselves. At the same time, the magnitude of the differences was not large, raising questions about relative costs and benefits. Carefully monitored medication, including regular, face-to-face meetings with the child psychiatrist, proved quite effective in modifying behavior across domains of functioning. At the same time, even the more comprehensive treatment in the MTA study did not focus on factors beyond the management of child symptoms and related behavioral problems. The family context was not considered. Furthermore, although the researchers examined mediators and moderators of treatment effects, because this study derives strictly from a child psychopathology perspective rather than from a developmental psychopathology perspective, there is less emphasis on process and more emphasis on symptomatic improvement as a function of treatment modality. We cannot determine whether changes in parenting behavior or family context occurred as a result of treatment, or what processes explain the changes that occurred in children's behavior. This will require additional analyses of this data set as well as further research.

Family Therapy

Given our focus on family processes and contexts, it is important to comment on family therapy as a treatment modality. Family therapy per se was not included in the discussion of "empirically supported treatments," because family therapy covers a gamut of different treatments as already noted. Therefore, some of the parent training and other intervention efforts (e.g., multisystemic therapy) already discussed come under the rubric of family therapy, broadly construed to mean therapy with more than one family member present (e.g., Hazelrigg, Cooper, & Borduin, 1987). For example, family therapy has been defined as "any psychotherapy that directly involves family members in addition to an index patient and/or explicitly attends to the interaction among family members" (Pinsof & Wynne, 1995, p. 586). Using this broad definition, then, parent training for children with conduct disorder or ADHD, as well as psychoeducational approaches to working with families of children with ADHD (e.g., Barkley, 1998), or families coping with stressors such as marital separation and divorce would be considered family therapy. In addition, family therapy cuts across theoretical orientations, with most outcome research conducted on the more structured variants of family therapy, including behavioral and systemic approaches as opposed to more humanistic and psychodynamic family therapies that have not been evaluated systematically (Shadish et al., 1993). Another difficulty in assessing the specific impact of family therapy for childhood disorders is the fact that family-focused interventions tend to be included as components in larger treatment packages and are rarely evaluated alone. Indeed, recent reviews of the family therapy literature focus primarily on parent management training when discussing childhood disorders (e.g., Hazelrigg et al., 1987; Pinsof & Wynne, 1995) and explicitly state that it is difficult to evaluate systemic family therapy as it applies to childhood disorders. In general, it also appears that traditional structural or systems-oriented approaches to family therapy (e.g., Haley, 1976; Minuchin, 1974) are often applied to general family distress, with less attention paid to the specific diagnosis of individual family members, consistent with a systems view of family relationships and symptom expression (i.e., the symptom reflects the family distress or maladaptive interaction pattern rather than a disorder per se). Thus, the family therapy and the child psychopathology literature have remained fairly distinct except insofar as the focus has been on more didactic or structured behavioral interventions.

Despite these caveats, three recent reviews of the family therapy literature are consistent in suggesting that family therapy is useful for alleviating family distress in a range of situations, whether parents or children are the identified patients, and that, in many instances, family therapy may be more beneficial than individual therapy (Hazelrigg, Cooper, & Borduin, 1987; Pinsof & Wynne, 1995; Shadish et al., 1993). Moreover, there is consensus that despite the gaps in the literature, well-designed outcome studies support the use of more structured, pragmatic, and focused family interventions that attempt to modify patterns of interaction within the family system (Hazelrigg et al., 1987; Shadish et al., 1993). This fits in well with our transactional and ecological view of development and arguments made throughout this book that children must be considered within their family and wider social context. Indeed, the multifaceted prevention and treatment programs discussed earlier all include extensive work within the family system, while the FAST Track, the Early Parenting Alliance Program, and MST all include interventions beyond the family system (i.e., in the school, peer group, and community).

Concluding Comments on Treatment

Taken together, then, the voluminous research literature on child treatment tends to be less theory driven and developmentally oriented than is the case with research on prevention. Despite this, these two overlapping areas inform each other, so that programs with proven effectiveness in clinical work in the short term, such as parent training and social skills training, have been incorporated into prevention trials. At the same time, some of the principles that guide prevention trials appear to be equally important for treatment outcome studies and are reflected in the multisite MTA study. Overall, however, as Kazdin (1993) notes, research on child treatment has not been sufficiently concerned with developmental timing, process, or context. In addition, empirically supported treatments derive almost exclusively from learning theory and tend not to take family processes or emotion expression into account. Although family therapy and other forms of parent involvement (beyond parent training) are almost always included in clinical work with children and families, by and large, these specific components of treatment have not been systematically evaluated in treatment outcome studies. This is also a major drawback of much of the extant research. However, there is suggestive evidence from small-scale studies that ignoring family issues may impede the effectiveness of parent training, or may be associated with premature dropout from treatment (Dadds, Schwartz, & Sanders, 1987; Webster-Stratton, 1985). For example, Dadds and colleagues (1987) found that when marital issues were ignored in maritally distressed families, parent training was less effective, and Webster-Stratton (1985) found that in two-parent families, father involvement was associated with better treatment adherence. Finally, the work by Henggeler, Melton, and Smith (1992) on multisystemic family therapy suggests that viewing the adolescent with conduct disorder from a family and social systems perspective, and providing intensive, focused, and pragmatic crisis intervention, is effective in reducing recidivism in hard-to-treat populations.

Matching Clinical Problems to Clinical Practice: Case Studies Revisited

Before concluding this chapter, it seems worthwhile to revisit the cases discussed in Chapter 10 and to consider which children are candidates for prevention trials, as well as what types of empirically supported treatments would seem appropriate given the children's problems and the family context. Billy first came to clinical attention at the age of 5, shortly after beginning kindergarten. The presenting complaints of aggressive and noncompliant behavior evident across home and school settings would clearly make him a candidate for either the FAST Track or the Early Alliance Program in which the combined emphases on parenting, peer relations, academic and social competence, and classroom behavior would seem to be important areas for intervention. However, it is clear from the developmental history that Billy's problems were evident much earlier, during toddlerhood and the early preschool years, and that his problems tended to wax and wane with ongoing family problems. This suggests that a prevention or early intervention program for abused wives and their offspring might have helped Mrs. M cope with her marital and other difficulties, and possibly supported an earlier decision to separate from her alcoholic and abusive husband.

The description of Billy's problems illustrates a number of the issues outlined in Figure 11.1; that is, his problems appear to emerge in the context of ongoing marital problems, possible genetic liability, inconsistent parenting, and other indicators of family dysfunction and adversity. By school entry, these problems are expressed in extended peer and sibling conflict and aggression, poor self-regulation, noncompliance at home and school, and poor academic achievement. Thus, in the absence of either early intervention prior to school entry or enrollment in a prevention or treatment program, Billy would be at high risk for continuing problems despite the strengths in the family system.

In this case example, Billy was more fortunate than many boys with similar problems at age 5. He had an insightful and concerned teacher, and a motivated mother with adequate social support. Thus, Billy received clinical intervention early from a well-trained psychologist who made good treatment decisions. In terms of the empirically supported treatments discussed earlier, Billy's problems make him a logical candidate for classroom management and school consultation, social skills training, and academic tutoring. His mother is clearly a candidate for structured parent management training, although she may also require some emotional support to help her cope with the many demands on her as a single, working mother with two young children.

Although 10-year-old Peter was referred to a psychologist because of a mix of internalizing (social withdrawal, negative mood) and externalizing (aggression) problems, as well as inattention and a decline in academic functioning, the developmental history indicated that these problems had emerged only recently in the context of serious family stress and loss. In the absence of earlier or more clearly defined problems, Peter would not be a candidate for an indicated prevention program (e.g., to prevent aggression or depression), because he would be unlikely to be identified as "at risk." Furthermore, his problems appeared to be a reaction to several acute crises rather than chronic family adversity. Thus, he would be most likely to respond to short-term, structured cognitive-behavioral therapy, which has been demonstrated to be useful in small-scale studies of depressed children (Kaslow & Thompson, 1998), possibly with parental involvement as well. In this type of treatment, the therapist might help Peter control negative thoughts, cope actively with his feelings of sadness and despair around his losses (e.g., by arranging to write to or visit his friend, by having him think about the positive times he had had with his grandfather, by having him accompany his mother to the hospital), help him to develop other interests or find new positive activities in which to engage, and work on conflict resolution skills.

Twelve-year-old Sandy represents the failure of many social service systems to protect young children from family chaos and child neglect. Clearly, her problems, while seriously meriting intervention, might very well have been preventable if she had had a normal childhood with adequate parenting. It is possible that a very early prevention program for high-risk teenage mothers and infants (e.g., Olds, Henderson, Kitzman, & Cole, 1995; Ramey & Ramey, 1998) would have placed Sandy's mother on a better developmental pathway, thereby avoiding some of the intergenerational transmission of depression, substance use, and bad choices in partners that often appear to plague young women growing up in homes such as Sandy's. Sandy has few options in the current mental health or child welfare system, and the decision to place Sandy in a special treatment foster home for adolescents, assuming it is well monitored and can provide her with the structure and nurture that she needs, is probably among the better opportunities for her to move beyond her troubled childhood. In addition, she would clearly be a candidate for supportive therapy and structured interventions meant to foster feelings of competence, well-being, and informed decision making around life transitions (e.g., Allen, Philliber, Herrling, & Kuperminc, 1997).

This case also illustrates quite starkly the many gaps in service delivery systems that have followed Sandy from birth through early adolescence. Clearly, empirically supported treatments such as parent training or social skills training would be of little benefit in this complicated case of a child growing up in such a multiproblem family with such limited emotional and material resources. What is most striking about Sandy is her remarkable resilience, reflected in her concern for her siblings and her adequate school achievement. This suggests that even at this stage, given removal from her untenable family situation, along with appropriate emotional support, therapy for her anxiety and depression, and the provision of educational and other opportunities, Sandy may be able to overcome many of her problems (Masten & Coatsworth, 1998). Prediction in her case is difficult. Despite her grim history, she shows evidence of strengths that may belie both her family history of dysfunction and her personal experience of neglectful, rejecting, and unstable caregiving. In a sense, cases like Sandy's underscore the importance of a developmental psychopathology perspective, because they indicate that history and genes are not necessarily destiny, reflecting the principles of multifinality and discontinuity over time and across generations.

CONCLUSION

In this chapter we have considered how a developmental psychopathology approach informs research on the prevention and treatment of children's problems. We have reviewed several issues in prevention research and contrasted the differing goals and perspective of these two approaches to intervention. We have also described model prevention and treatment programs that are large-scale, comprehensive, and relatively long-term.

In the course of this chapter, we have emphasized the importance of intervention trials as both needed service delivery and sophisticated tests of theoretical formulations of the processes underlying maladjustment and disorder. Indeed, systematic evaluations of intervention trials, whether targeted to groups of children at risk to develop problems or to children referred to clinical facilities because of particular difficulties, are among the only ways we have to test theoretical models of causal processes. Because we cannot randomly assign children to receive poor parenting, to live in dysfunctional families, or to seek out deviant peers, and because risk factors tend to co-occur (Greenberg, Leguna, Coie, & Pinderhughes, 1999) and cluster together (Belsky, Woodworth, & Crnic, 1996a, 1996b; Campbell, Shaw, & Gilliom, in press), we must rely on experiments of nature to test theoretical models (Cicchetti, 1990b). Thus, the need to fall back on correlational research designs has stymied the investigator interested in unlocking causal mechanisms.

Theoretically driven research on both prevention and treatment, while time-consuming and difficult to conduct, is really one of the only ways we have to test models that may identify etiological factors and causal pathways leading from early developmental risk to later maladjustment and diagnosable disorder. The recognition that this research must be done on a large scale with well-defined, but still diverse and large samples, underscores the need for multisite studies such as the FAST Track and the MTA study. Only large-scale multidisciplinary studies that utilize the expertise of many investigators and obtain participants from wide geographic areas will give researchers adequate power to test complicated hypotheses and models about process, as well as about mediators and moderators of intervention effects. Such studies will permit the in-depth study of particular subgroups of children at especially high risk (e.g., comorbid oppositional defiant disorder, boys with early-onset ADHD problems), allow the consideration of context (e.g., inner-city neighborhood vs. rural town), and have large-enough groups of girls to permit a more complete assessment of sex differences in underlying processes and intervention effects than has been the case so far. It is noteworthy that the focus on ADHD and aggression means that we know much more about the problems experienced and pathways followed by boys than by girls, although there is a growing interest in behavior problems in girls across the age spectrum (e.g., Keenan & Shaw, 1996; Wangby, Bergman, & Magnusson, 1999; Zahn-Waxler, 1993).

Treatment studies of children with diagnosed disorders need to move from the university psychology clinic to the community mental health setting, where a larger number of impaired clients coping with more adversity and distress are likely to seek help (Weisz, Donenberg, Han, & Weiss, 1995). More community based treatments are also needed (e.g., Henggeler, Melton, & Smith, 1992) that take into account the wider social ecology of the child and family in distress. Finally, there needs to be better integration and collaboration across systems (e.g., mental health, educational, child protection, juvenile justice) to plan service delivery strategies for children and families in need of these services, to establish realistic goals for intervention, and to evaluate the effectiveness of integrated and comprehensive treatment packages. It seems obvious that short-term and small-scale interventions are generally not effective for children and families with more serious and chronic problems. From a developmental psychopathology perspective of highlighting the multiple influences on children over time, this is hardly surprising.

Epilogue

*T*he developmental psychopathology approach to the study and treatment of childhood psychopathology is quite different, one might say, radically different, from the traditional disease model of childhood disorders. As we have shown in these pages, there is a different epistemology about childhood problems, with substantial implications for (1) the theory of the origins, development, and nature of clinical disorders; (2) promising research directions that may help us to unravel some of the causal connections that underlie both disorder and normal development, and (3) new approaches to clinical work that offer the promise of both (a) more veridical and useful approaches to classification of problem behaviors, and (b) more effective interventions that can reach larger groups of people either at risk for or suffering from maladaptive patterns of functioning. After having immersed ourselves in this dynamic literature for the past several years, we have come to appreciate the idealism and dedication to advancing the human condition that obviously characterize so many of those who are grappling with these complex and daunting issues.

The prospects for future advances in our understanding of, and ability to ameliorate, psychopathology are promising and exciting. At the same time, the avenues outlined for future work are challenging. As befits the complexity of the subject matter, that is, the human psyche, the models required must be both rich in the characterization of influences and dynamic in their conceptualization of the processes underlying psychological functioning. Thus, there is a need for creativity and for researchers who are willing to go beyond traditional ways of thinking in order to approach these problems. Such a stance is never easy in the real world of either academia or clinical practice. Furthermore, since this approach and related disciplines are continuing to pioneer new directions in the study and treatment of disorders, the goal of this volume has been to articulate the state of the art of developmental psychopathology in addressing these challenges rather than to describe a finished product. Thus, we have raised more questions than we answered, something that may be frustrating to those new to the area. However, we hope we also inspired some researchers who are new to the area to embark on more study and research to address newly emerging questions in the field.

FUTURE TOPICS AND DIRECTIONS

Moreover, in endeavoring to convey the essential foundations of this approach, our aim has been not to treat all of its possible applications to specific disorders or to consider all elements of family functioning. Thus, for our purposes, it would have been redundant from a conceptual perspective, as well as prohibitive in terms of the number of pages required, to include additional chapters that addressed the application of a developmental psychopathology approach to the study of a broader range of disorders. In this volume, we have paid particular attention to depression. While efforts have been made to include coverage of a variety of problems in various places, we recognize that more space could have been devoted to other disorders, including conduct disorders, schizophrenia, autism, and learning disabilities, to give but a few of the possibilities. We encourage others to provide this more extensive treatment of these other disorders from a developmental psychopathology perspective in the future.

Similarly, some selection has been unavoidable in our choice of topics with regard to the family as a context for child development. In this volume, we have paid particular attention to the parent–child and marital subsystems. While efforts have been made to provide some coverage of other family subsystems and other influences on the family in various places, we recognize that much more attention could be paid to many other topics, including the influence of the sibling subsystem on children's development, the nature and course of genotype–environment interactions during development, and the importance of examining the family as embedded in larger ecological contexts, including schools, neighborhoods, and communities. Given the focus on children, we are also aware of the importance of the peer group, something that we have dealt with only in passing. Once again, we encourage others to provide a fuller treatment of these issues in the future.

Many important directions for future research can be readily identified, and these are implicit in the ambitious and broad canvas for future work outlined by this approach. A few examples illustrate the possibilities. It is one thing to advocate the study of development as a dynamic process, but it is yet another to measure adequately psychological functioning at this level of analysis and to integrate such microscopic levels of analysis into more macroscopic models that also convey the "big picture" with regard to children's patterns of adaptation and maladaptation over time in context. Similarly, it is one thing to advocate a multimethod approach to the study of children's functioning over time, but it is yet another to make good sense of the results of patterns of information that may diverge as well as converge on the picture provided about the children. For example, in Chapter 3, we discussed the problems created by the differing reports that are sometimes found when multiple informants (e.g., father, mother, teacher) give information about the child's functioning. Such problems are likely to be compounded when information about a child is obtained across multiple modalities (e.g., cognitive, emotional, biological, or physiological) as well as multiple informants, using multiple methods. As a final example of this sort, it is one thing to advocate that context and developmental history be incorporated into diagnostic systems, but it is yet another to develop a nosology or heuristic that can accomplish the integration of these different types of information pertinent to the appraisal of the individual's level of adjustment. This is not to say that we have not made substantial progress toward the goal of solving each of these problems (and many others). Indeed, at some level, even the articulation of the problem is progress in itself. At the same time, however, there remains much work to be done if the developmental psychopathology approach is to fulfill its promise as a new perspective on childhood disorder.

The developmental psychopathology approach also has important implications for public policy. Given the focus of this volume on the themes of theory, research, and clinical practice, we have not endeavored to address this matter directly, but it does merit comment in closing.

SOCIAL POLICY IMPLICATIONS

The developmental psychopathology approach also has obvious implications for social policy. At the first level of analysis, this includes an emphasis on the many possible prevention programs for children at risk. As stated in Chapter 11, a variety of prevention programs have now been demonstrated for infants and young children, ranging from home visiting programs for high-risk mothers to more comprehensive programs for toddlers and preschoolers at risk, such as Head Start and Early Head Start, that have promise. There is also evidence that the more intensive and comprehensive the program and the earlier it starts, the more likely it is to lead to concrete and measurable gains that last beyond the life of the program itself (Ramey & Ramey, 1998). Furthermore, programs that meld direct service provision to stressed parents, provide parent training, and work intensively with children have been shown to be most effective.

However, it is not clear that policy priorities and fiscal appropriations reflect these realities. Although President Clinton proposed a $1 billion increase in funding for Head Start (State of the Union Address, January 27, 2000) and there is even some consensus about the importance of universally available programs for young children living in poverty and other risk conditions, so far, funds have not been adequate to accommodate all children in need (e.g., Zigler & Gilman, 1996). For example, in the state of Pennsylvania, only half of all eligible children attended Head Start in 1999. Clearly, we have the tools needed to provide high-quality programs to children at risk, but this will require a commitment on the part of governments at all levels to make this a funding priority in the 21st century.

Programs such as the FAST Track also have promise and, indeed, many of its elements have relevance to high-risk families with both younger and older children. Other prevention programs that deal with internalizing problems such as depression, or that help children cope with stressful life transitions, also have been shown to be effective. The schools are the logical place to begin to intervene in the lives of some children at risk (Zigler & Gilman, 1996), as is evident from much of the work already discussed in this volume. However, programs tend to vary from one school system to another, and often the assessment of effectiveness is limited.

At the level of mental illness, the Surgeon General's report indicated that only a small proportion of people with disorders actually receive help. Access to mental health services for children are both better and worse. On the one hand, some insurance companies will not support treatments for chronic conditions such as ADHD, despite the obvious benefits of treatment (MTA Cooperative Group, 1999a). On the other hand, because most children are in school, those with problems are more likely to be identified as in need of services than is the case with adults. The best front-line system for identifying and working with children who have both diagnosable disorders and lower-level problems is clearly the school system. Mental health and school personnel need to work more closely together to identify children in trouble in the early grades and to put into place comprehensive programs that involve the family and the wider community. Such programs are beginning to appear, but regulations and turf battles hinder progress.

The developmental psychopathology approach also suggests that the 50-minute hour is obsolete. Psychologists and other mental health professionals need to work with children and families in their homes, schools, and communities (e.g., Conduct Problems Prevention Research Group, 1992; Henggeler, Melton, & Smith, 1992), rather than in therapists' offices. Moreover, comprehensive reviews of the child treatment literature indicate the importance of more didactic and structured programs, although most mental health clinics still provide eclectic and unsystematic treatments that may not be particularly effective (Weisz & Weiss, 1993).

Throughout this volume, we have identified a myriad of factors that place children and families at risk, including poverty, substance abuse, parental mental illness, poor nutrition and prenatal care, harsh and negative parenting, and family conflict. Some of these problems require societywide commitments, whereas others are specific to the individual. We have the knowledge about how to intervene in many of these problems, but it is not clear whether, as a society, such programs are enough of a priority. One message of the developmental psychopathology approach is that many children, despite formidable risk, overcome adversity. This is a positive and optimistic view of children's resilience, but it requires money—money that is much better spent on prevention and early treatment than on incarceration of serious adult offenders or on prolonged treatment of the seriously mentally ill adult.

In closing, the developmental psychopathology framework has broad implications for the conceptualization, investigation, and management of clinical disorders of childhood. In this volume, we have presented the fundamental elements of this approach, with particular concern for the relations between child psychopathology and family process. The intent of this work is to add to research and practice that will enhance the well-being of children and families in the 21st century.

References

Aber, J. L., Jones, S. M., Brown, J. L., Chaudry, N., & Samples, F. (1998). Resolving conflict creatively: Evaluating the developmental effects of a school-based violence prevention program in neighborhood and classroom context. *Development and Psychopathology, 10*, 187–214.

Abrams, S. M., Field, T., Scafidi, F., & Prodomidis, M. (1995). Newborns of depressed mothers. *Infant Mental Health Journal, 16*, 233–239.

Achenbach, T. M. (1988). Integrating assessment and taxonomy. In M. Rutter, A. H. Tuma, & I. S. Lann (Eds.), *Assessment and diagnosis in child psychopathology* (pp. 300–343). New York: Guilford Press.

Achenbach, T. M. (1990). What is "developmental" about developmental psychopathology? In J. Rolf, A. Masten, D. Cicchetti, K. Nuechterlein, & S. Weintraub (Eds.), *Risk and protective factors in the development of psychopathology* (pp. 29–48). New York: Cambridge University Press.

Achenbach, T. M. (1991a). *Manual for the Youth Self-Report and 1991 Profile.* Burlington, VT: University of Vermont, Department of Psychiatry.

Achenbach, T. M. (1991b). *Manual for the Child Behavior Checklist: 4–18 and 1991 Profile.* Burlington, VT: University of Vermont, Department of Psychiatry.

Achenbach, T. M. (1992). *Manual for the Teacher Report Form and Profile.* Burlington, VT: University of Vermont, Department of Psychiatry.

Achenbach, T. M. (1995). Developmental issues in assessment, taxonomy, and diagnosis of child and adolescent psychopathology. In D. Cicchetti & D. J. Cohen (Eds.), *Developmental psychopathology: Vol. 1. Theory and methods* (pp. 57–80). New York: Wiley.

Achenbach, T. M. (1997). What is normal? What is abnormal? Developmental perspectives on behavioral and emotional problems. In S. S. Luthar, J. A. Burack, D. Cicchetti, & J. R. Weisz (Eds.), *Developmental psychopathology: Perspectives on adjustment, risk, and disorder* (pp. 93–114). New York: Cambridge University Press.

Achenbach, T. M., Edelbrock, C., & Howell, C. T. (1987). Empirically based assessment of the behavioral/emotional problems of 2- and 3-year-old children. *Journal of Abnormal Child Psychology, 15*, 629–650.

Achenbach, T. M., Howell, C. T., Quay, C. T., & Conners, C. K. (1991). National survey of problems and competencies among four- to sixteen-year-olds: Parents' reports from normative and clinical samples. *Monographs of the Society for Research in Child Development, 56* (Serial No. 225).

Ackerman, B. P., Izard, C. E., Schoff, K., Youngstrom, E. A., & Kogos, J. (1999). Contextual risk, caregiver emotionality, and the problem behaviors of six- and seven-year-old children from economically disadvantaged families. *Child Development, 70,* 1415–1427.

Ackerman, B. P., Kogos, J., Youngstrom, E., Schoff, K., & Izard, C. E. (1999). Family instability and the problem behaviors of children from economically disadvantaged families. *Developmental Psychology, 35,* 258–268.

Ainsworth, M. D. S. (1962). The effects of maternal deprivation: A review of findings and controversy in the context of research strategy. In *Deprivation of maternal care: A reassessment of its effect* (Public Health Paper No. 14). Geneva: World Health Organization.

Ainsworth, M. D. S. (1967). *Infancy in Uganda: Infant care and the growth of love.* Baltimore: Johns Hopkins University Press.

Ainsworth, M. D. S. (1969). Object relations, dependency, and attachment: A theoretical review of the infant–mother attachment relationship. *Child Development, 40,* 969–1025.

Ainsworth, M. D. S., Blehar, M. C., Waters, E., & Wall, S. (1978). *Patterns of attachment: A psychological study of the Strange Situation.* Hillsdale, NJ: Erlbaum.

Albee, G. W. (1983). Psychopathology, prevention, and the just society. *Journal of Primary Prevention, 4,* 5–40.

Alessandri, S. M. (1992). Mother–child interactional correlates of maltreated and nonmaltreated children's play behavior. *Development and Psychopathology, 4,* 257–270.

Allen, J. P., Hauser, S. T., Eickholt, C., Bell, K. L., & O'Connor, T. G. (1994). Autonomy and relatedness in family interactions as predictors of expressions of negative adolescent affect. *Journal of Research on Adolescence, 4,* 535–552.

Allen, J. P., Philliber, S., Herrling, S., & Kuperminc, G. P. (1997). Preventing teen pregnancy and adolescent academic failure: Experimental evaluation of a developmentally based approach. *Child Development, 64,* 729–742.

Amato, P. R., & Booth, A. (1991). Consequences of parental divorce and marital unhappiness for adult well-being. *Social Forces, 69,* 895–914.

Amato, P. R., & Keith, B. (1991). Consequences of parental divorce for children's well-being: A meta-analysis. *Psychological Bulletin, 110,* 26–46.

American Academy of Pediatrics. (1996). *The classification of child and adolescent mental diagnoses in primary care.* Elk Grove, IL: Author.

American Psychiatric Association. (1980). *Diagnostic and statistical manual of mental disorders* (3rd ed.) Washington, DC: Author.

American Psychiatric Association. (1987). *Diagnostic and statistical manual of mental disorders* (3rd ed., Rev.). Washington, DC: Author.

American Psychiatric Association. (1994). *Diagnostic and statistical manual of mental disorders* (4th ed.). Washington, DC: Author.

Ammerman, R. T., Cassisi, J. E., Hersen, M., & Van Hasslet, V. B. (1986). Consequences of physical abuse and neglect in children. *Clinical Psychology Review, 6,* 291–310.

Anderson, K. E., Lytton, H., & Romney, D. M. (1986). Mothers' interactions with normal and conduct disordered boys: Who affects whom? *Developmental Psychology, 22,* 604–609.

Andrews, J. A., Hops, H., & Duncan, S. C. (1997). Adolescent modeling of parent substance use: The moderating effect of the relationship with the parent. *Journal of Family Psychology, 11,* 259–270.

Angold, A., & Costello, E. J. (1993). Depressive comorbidity in children and adolescents: Empirical, theoretical, and methodological issues. *American Journal of Psychiatry, 150,* 1779–1791.

Angold, A., & Costello, E. J. (1996). Toward establishing an empirical basis for the diagnosis of oppositional defiant disorder. *Journal of the American Academy of Child and Adolescent Psychiatry, 35,* 1205–1212.

Angold, A., Costello, E. J., Farmer, E. M. Z., Burns, B. J., & Erklani, A. (1999). Impaired but undiagnosed. *Journal of the American Academy of Child and Adolescent Psychiatry, 38,* 129–137.

Angold, A., & Rutter, M. (1992). Effects of age and pubertal status on depression in a large clinical sample. *Development and Psychopathology, 4,* 5–28.

Applegate, B., Lahey, B. B., Hart, E. L., Biederman, J., Hynd, G. W., Barkley, R. A., Ollendick, T., Frick, P. J., Greenhill, L., McBurnett, K., Newcorn, J., Kerdyk, L., Garfinkel, L., Waldman, I., & Shaffer, D. (1997). Validity of the age-of-onset criterion for ADHD: A report from the DSM-IV field trials. *Journal of the American Academy of Child and Adolescent Psychiatry, 36,* 1211–1221.

Arnold, L. E., Abikoff, H. B., Cantwell, D. P., Conners, C. K., Elliott, G., Greenhill, L. L., Hechtman, L., Hinshaw, S. P., Hoza, B., Jensen, P. S., Kraemer, H. C., March, J. S., Newcorn, J. H., Pelham, W. E., Richters, J. E., Schiller, E., Severe, J. B., Swanson, J. S., Vereen, D., & Wells, K. C. (1997). National Institute of Mental Health Collaborative Multimodal Treatment Study of children with ADHD (MTA): Design challenges and choices. *Archives of General Psychiatry, 54,* 865–870.

Bachman, J. G., Johnston, L. D., O'Malley, P. M., & Schulenberg, J. (1996). Transitions in drug use during late adolescence and young adulthood. In J. A. Graber, J. Brooks-Gunn, & A. C. Petersen (Eds.), *Transitions through adolescence: Interpersonal domains and context* (pp. 111–140). Mahwah, NJ: Erlbaum.

Bakeman, R., & Brown, J. V. (1980). Early interaction: Consequences of social and mental development at three years. *Child Development, 51,* 437–447.

Baldwin, A. L., Baldwin, C., & Cole, R. E. (1990). Stress-resistant families and stress-resistant children. In J. Rolf, A. S. Masten, D. Cicchetti, K. H. Nuechterlein, & S. Weintraub (Eds.), *Risk and protective factors in the development of psychopathology* (pp. 257–280). New York: Cambridge University Press.

Baldwin, A. L., Baldwin, C. P., Kasser, T., Zax, M., Sameroff, A., & Seifer, R. (1993). Contextual risk and resiliency during late adolescence. *Development and Psychopathology, 5,* 741–761.

Ballard, M., & Cummings, E. M. (1990). Response to adults' angry behavior in children of alcoholic and non-alcoholic parents. *Journal of Genetic Psychology, 151,* 195–210.

Ballard, M. E., Cummings, E. M., & Larkin, K. (1993). Emotional and cardiovascular responses to adults' angry behavior and challenging tasks in children of hypertensive and normotensive parents. *Child Development, 64,* 500–515.

Baltes, P. B., Reese, H. W., & Lipsitt, L. P. (1980). Life-span developmental psychology. *Annual Review of Psychology, 31,* 65–110.

Baltes, P. B., Reese, H. W., & Nesselroade, J. R. (1988). *Life-span developmental psychology: Introduction to research methods.* Hillsdale, NJ: Erlbaum.

Baltes, P. B., Staudinger, U. M., & Lindenberger, U. (1999). Lifespan psychology: Theory and application to intellectual functioning. *Annual Review of Psychology, 50,* 471–507.

Barber, B. K. (1992). Family, personality, and adolescent problem behaviors. *Journal of Marriage and the Family, 54,* 69–79.

Barber, B. K. (1996). Parental psychological control: Revisiting a neglected construct. *Child Development, 67,* 3296–3319.

Barber, B. K. (1997). Introduction: Adolescent socialization in context: The role of connection, regulation, and autonomy in the family. *Journal of Adolescent Research, 12,* 5–11.

Barber, B. K., Olsen, J. E., & Shagle, S. C. (1994). Associations between parental psychological and behavioral control and youth internalized and externalized behaviors. *Child Development, 65,* 1120–1136.

Barkley, R. A. (1987). *Defiant children: A clinician's manual for parent training.* New York: Guilford Press.

Barkley, R. A. (1998). *Attention-deficit/hyperactivity disorder: A handbook for diagnosis and treatment* (2nd ed.). New York: Guilford Press..

Barkley, R. A., Anastopoulos, A. D., Guevremont, D. G., & Fletcher, K. E. (1992). Adolescents with attention deficit hyperactivity disorder: Mother–adolescent interactions, family beliefs and conflicts, and maternal psychopathology. *Journal of Abnormal Child Psychology, 20,* 752–761.

Barkley, R. A., Fischer, M., Edelbrock, C. S., & Smallish, L. (1990). Adolescent outcome of hyperactive children diagnosed by research criteria: I. An 8 year prospective follow-up study. *Journal of the American Academy of Child and Adolescent Psychiatry, 29,* 546–557.

Barkley, R. A., Fischer, M., Edelbrock, C. S., & Smallish, L. (1991). Adolescent outcome of hyperactive children diagnosed by research criteria: III. Mother–child interaction, family conflict, and maternal psychopathology. *Journal of Child Psychology and Psychiatry, 32,* 233–256.

Barkley, R. A., Karlsson, J., Pollard, S., & Murphy, J. V. (1985). Developmental changes in mother–child interactions of hyperactive boys: Effects of two dose levels of Ritalin. *Journal of Child Psychology and Psychiatry, 26,* 705–715.

Barnett, D., Kidwell, S. L., & Leung, K. H. (1998). Parenting and preschooler attachment among low-income urban African American families. *Child Development, 69,* 1657–1671.

Barnett, D., Manly, J. T., & Cicchetti, D. (1991). Continuing toward an operational definition of psychological maltreatment. *Development and Psychopathology, 3,* 19–29.

Baron, R. M., & Kenny, D. A. (1986). The moderator–mediator variable distinction in social psychological research: Conceptual, strategic, and statistical considerations. *Journal of Personality and Social Psychology, 51,* 1173–1182.

Barrera, M., Li, S. A., & Chassin, L. (1995). Effects of parental alcoholism and life stress on Hispanic and non-Hispanic Caucasian adolescents: A prospective study. *American Journal of Community Psychology, 23,* 479–507.

Baruch, D. W., & Wilcox, J. A. (1944). A study of sex differences in preschool children's adjustment coexistent with interparental tensions. *Journal of Genetic Psychology, 64,* 281–303.

Bates, J. E., Pettit, G. S., Dodge, K. A., & Ridge, B. (1998). Interaction of temperamental resistance to control and restrictive parenting in the development of externalizing behavior. *Developmental Psychology, 34,* 982–995.

Baumrind, D. (1967). Child care practices anteceding three patterns of preschool behavior. *Genetic Psychology Monographs, 75*, 43–88.

Baumrind, D. (1971). Current patterns of parental authority. *Developmental Psychology Monograph, 4*(1, pt. 2), 101–103.

Baumrind, D. (1972). An exploratory study of socialization effects on black children: Some black–white comparisons. *Child Development, 43*, 261–267.

Baumrind, D. (1991). The influence of parenting style on adolescent competence and substance use. *Journal of Early Adolescence, 11*, 56–95.

Baumrind, D. (1995). *Child maltreatment and optimal caregiving in social contexts.* New York: Garland.

Baumrind, D. (1997). Necessary distinctions. *Psychological Inquiry, 8*, 176–182.

Beach, B. (1995). *The relation between marital conflict and child adjustment: An examination of parental and child repertoires.* Unpublished doctoral dissertation, West Virginia University, Morgantown.

Beach, S. R. H., Fincham, F. D., & Katz, J. (1998). Marital therapy in the treatment of depression: Toward a third generation of therapy and research. *Clinical Psychology Review, 18*, 635–661.

Beach, S. R. H., & Nelson, G. M. (1990). Pursuing research on major psychopathology from a contextual perspective: The example of depression and marital discord. In G. H. Brody & I. E. Siogel (Eds.), *Methods of family research: Biographies of research projects: Vol. 2. Clinical populations* (pp. 227–259). Hillsdale, NJ: Erlbaum.

Beach, S. R. H., & O'Leary, K. D. (1992). Treating depression in the context of marital discord: Outcome and predictors of response for marital therapy vs. cognitive therapy. *Behavior Therapy, 23*, 507–528.

Beach, S. R. H., Sandeen, E. E., & O'Leary, K. D. (1990). *Depression in marriage: A model for etiology and treatment.* New York: Guilford Press.

Beach, S. R. H., Smith, D. A., & Fincham, F. D. (1994). Marital interventions for depression: Empirical foundation and future prospects. *Applied and Preventive Psychology, 3*, 233–250.

Beardslee, W., Bemporad, J., Keller, M. B., & Klerman, G. L. (1983). Children of parents with a major affective disorder: A review. *American Journal of Psychiatry, 140*, 825–832.

Beardslee, W. R., Versage, E. M., Wright, E. J., Salt, P., Rothberg, P., Drezner, K., & Gladstone, T. (1997). Examination of preventive interventions for families with depression: Evidence of change. *Development and Psychopathology, 9*, 109–130.

Beck, A. (1976). *Cognitive therapy and the emotional disorders.* New York: International Universities Press.

Beck, A. T., Rush, A. J., Shaw, B. F., & Emery, G. (1979). *Cognitive therapy of depression.* New York: Guilford Press.

Beeghly, M., & Cicchetti, D. (1994). Child maltreatment, attachment, and the self system: Emergence of an internal state lexicon in toddlers at high social risk. *Development and Psychopathology, 6*, 5–30.

Bell, R. Q. (1968). A reinterpretation of the direction of effects in studies of socialization. *Psychological Review, 75*, 81–95.

Belsky, J. (1984). The determinants of parenting: A process model. *Child Development, 55*, 83–96.

Belsky, J. (1993). Etiology of child maltreatment: A developmental–ecological analysis. *Psychological Bulletin, 114*, 413–434.

Belsky, J., Campbell, S. B., Cohn, J. F., & Moore, G. (1996). Instability of infant–parent attachment security. *Developmental Psychology, 32*, 921–924.

Belsky, J., & Cassidy, J. (1994). Attachment: Theory and evidence. In M. Rutter, D. Hay, & S. Baron-Cohen (Eds.), *Developmental principles and clinical issues in psychology and psychiatry* (pp. 373–402). Oxford, UK: Blackwell.

Belsky, J., Gilstrap, B., & Rovine, M. (1984). The Pennsylvania Infant and Family Development Project: I. Stability and change in mother–infant and father–infant interaction in a family setting at one, three, and nine months. *Child Development, 55*, 692–705.

Belsky, J., Hsieh, K.-H., & Crnic, K. (1998). Mothering, fathering, and infant negativity as antecedents of boys' externalizing problems and inhibition at age 3 years: Differential susceptibility to rearing experience? *Development and Psychopathology, 10*, 301–319.

Belsky, J., & Rovine, M. (1990). Patterns of marital change across the transition to parenthood. *Journal of Marriage and the Family, 52*, 5–19.

Belsky, J., Rovine, M., & Fish, M. (1989). The developing family system. In M. Gunnar & E. Thelen (Eds.), *Minnesota Symposia on Child Psychology: Vol. 22. Systems and development* (pp. 119–166). Hillsdale, NJ: Erlbaum.

Belsky, J., Rovine, M., & Taylor, D. G. (1984). The Pennsylvania Infant and Family Development Project: III. The origins of individual differences in infant–mother attachment: Maternal and infant contributions. *Child Development, 55*, 718–728.

Belsky, J., Steinberg, L., & Draper, P. (1991). Childhood experience, interpersonal development, and reproductive strategy: An evolutionary theory of socialization. *Child Development, 62*, 647–670.

Belsky, J., Woodworth, S., & Crnic, K. (1996a). Trouble in the second year: Three questions about family interaction. *Child Development, 67*, 556–578.

Belsky, J., Woodworth, S., & Crnic, K. (1996b). Troubled family interaction during toddlerhood. *Development and Psychopathology, 8*, 477–495.

Benes, F. M. (1994). Developmental changes in stress adaptation in relation to psychopathology. *Development and Psychopathology, 6*, 723–739.

Bergeman, C. S., & Wallace, K. A. (1999). Resiliency in later life. In T. L. Whitman & T. V. Merluzzi (Eds.), *Life-span perspectives on health and illness* (pp. 207–225. Mahwah, NJ: Erlbaum.

Bergman, L. R., & Magnusson, D. (1997). A person-oriented approach in research on developmental psychopathology. *Development and Psychopathology, 9*, 291–319.

Biddle, B. J., & Marlin, M. M. (1987). Causality, confirmation, credulity, and structural equation modeling. *Child Development, 58*, 4–17.

Biederman, J., Newcorn, J., & Sprich, S. (1991). Comorbidity of attention deficit disorder with conduct, depressive anxiety, and other disorders. *American Journal of Psychiatry, 144*, 330–333.

Biglan, A. (1995). Choosing a paradigm to guide prevention research and practice. *Drugs and Society, 8*, 149–160.

Biglan, A., & Hayes, S. C. (1996). Should the behavioral sciences become more pragmatic? The case for functional contextualism in research on human behavior. *Applied and Preventive Psychology, 5*, 47–57.

Biglan, A., Hops, H., Sherman, L., Freidman, L., Arthur, J., & Osteen, V. (1985). Problem solving interactions of depressed mothers and their spouses. *Behavior Therapy, 16*, 431–451.

Bird, H. (1996). Epidemiology of childhood disorders in a cross-cultural context. *Journal of Child Psychology and Psychiatry, 37*, 35–50.

Biringen, Z., & Robinson, J. (1991). Emotional availability in mother–child interactions: A reconceptualization for research. *American Journal of Orthopsychiatry, 61*, 258–271.

Birmaher, B., Kaufman, J., Brent, D., Dahl, R., Perel, J., Al-Shabbout, M., Nelson, B., Stahl, S., Rao, U., Waterman, G., Williamson, D., & Ryan, N. (1997). Neuroendocrine response to 5-hydroxy-L-tryptophan in prepubertal children of high risk of major depressive disorder. *Archives of General Psychiatry, 54*, 1113–1119.

Black, M. M., & Krishnakumar, A. (1998). Children in low-income, urban settings: Interventions to promote mental health and well-being. *American Psychologist, 53*, 635–646.

Block, J. (1971). *Lives through time*. Berkeley, CA: Bancroft.

Block, J. H., Block, J., & Gjerde, P. J. (1986). The personality of children prior to divorce. *Child Development, 57*, 827–840.

Block, J. H., Block, J., & Morrison, A. (1981). Parental agreement–disagreement on child-rearing orientations and gender-related personality correlates in children. *Child Development, 52*, 965–974.

Booth, A., & Amato, P. R. (1994). Parental marital quality, parental divorce, and relations with parents. *Journal of Marriage and the Family, 56*, 21–34.

Bousha, D. M., & Twentyman, C. T. (1984). Mother–child interactional style in abuse, neglect, and control groups: Naturalistic observations in the home. *Journal of Abnormal Psychology, 93*, 106–114.

Bowlby, J. (1949). The study and reduction of group tensions in the family. *Human Relations, 2*, 123–128.

Bowlby, J. (1951). Maternal care and mental health. *Bulletin of the World Health Organization, 3*, 355–533.

Bowlby, J. (1958). The nature of the child's tie to his mother. *International Journal of Psychoanalysis, 39*, 350–373.

Bowlby, J. (1969). *Attachment and loss. Vol. 1. Attachment*. New York: Basic Books.

Bowlby, J. (1973). *Attachment and loss. Vol. 2. Separation: Anxiety and anger*. New York: Basic Books.

Bowlby, J. (1980). *Attachment and loss. Vol. 3. Loss: Sadness and depression*. New York: Basic Books.

Boyce, W. T., Alkon, A., Tschann, J. M., Chesney, M. A., & Alpert, B. S. (1995). Dimensions of psychobiologic reactivity: Cardiovascular responses to laboratory stressors in preschool children. *Annals of Behavioral Medicine, 17*, 315–323.

Boyce, W. T., Frank, E., Jensen, P., Kessler, R., Nelson, N., Steinberg, L., & the MacArthur Foundation Research Network on Psychopathology and Development. (1998). Social context in developmental psychopathology: Recommendations for future research from the MacArthur Network on Psychopathology and Development. *Developmental Psychopathology, 10*(2), 143–164.

Bradbury, T. N. (Ed.). (1998). *The developmental course of marital dysfunction*. Cambridge, UK, and New York: Cambridge University Press.

Bradbury, T. N., Cohan, C. L, & Karney, B. R. (1998). Optimizing longitudinal research for understanding and preventing marital dysfunction. In T. N. Bradbury (Ed.), *The developmental course of marital dysfunction* (pp. 279–311). Cambridge, UK, and New York: Cambridge University Press.

Brestan, E. V., & Eyberg, S. M. (1998). Effective psychosocial treatments of conduct-disordered children and adolescents: 29 years, 82 studies, and 5,272 kids. *Journal of Clinical Child Psychology, 27*, 180–189.

Bretherton, I. (1985). Attachment theory: Retrospect and prospect. In I. Bretherton & E. Waters (Eds.), Growing points in attachment theory and research. *Monographs of the Society for Research in Child Development, 50*(1–2, Serial No. 209), 3–35.

Bretherton, I., Walsh, R., Lependorf, M., & Goergeson, H. (1997). Attachment networks in postdivorce families: The maternal perspective. In L. Atkinson & K. J. Zucker (Eds.), *Attachment and psychopathology* (pp. 97–134). New York: Guilford Press.

Brody, G. H. (1998). Sibling relationship quality: Its causes and consequences. *Annual Review of Psychology, 49*, 1–24.

Brody, G. H., Flor, D. L., & Gibson, N. M. (1999). Linking maternal efficacy beliefs, developmental goals, parenting practices, and child competence in rural single-parent African American families. *Child Development, 70*, 1197–1208.

Brody, G. H., Stoneman, Z., & Burke, M. (1987). Family system and individual child correlates of sibling behavior. *American Journal of Orthopsychiatry, 57*, 561–569.

Brody, G. H., Stoneman, Z., & Gauger, K. (1996). Parent–child relationships, family problem-solving behavior, and sibling relationship quality: The moderating role of sibling temperaments. *Child Development, 67*, 1289–1300.

Brody, G. H., Stoneman, Z., & McCoy, J. K. (1992). Associations of maternal and paternal direct and differential behavior with sibling relationships: Contemporaneous and longitudinal analyses. *Child Development, 63*, 82–92.

Bronfenbrenner, U. (1979). *The ecology of human development: Experiments by nature and design.* Cambridge, MA: Harvard University Press.

Bronfenbrenner, U. (1986). Ecology of the family as a context for human development: Research perspectives. *Developmental Psychology, 22*, 723–742.

Brown, G. W., & Harris, T. O. (1978). *Social origins of depression: A study of psychiatric disorders in women.* London: Tavistock.

Brown, G. W., Lemyre, L., & Bifulco, A. (1992). Social factors and recovery from anxiety and depressive disorders: A test of specificity. *British Journal of Psychiatry, 161*, 44–54.

Browne, A., & Finkelhor, D. (1986). Impact of sexual abuse: A review of the research. *Psychological Bulletin, 99*, 66–77.

Bryk, A. S., & Raudenbush, S. W. (1987). Application of hierarchical linear models to assessing change. *Psychological Bulletin, 101*, 147–158.

Buchanan, C. M., Eccles, J. S., & Becker, J. B. (1992). Are adolescents the victims of raging hormones? Evidence for activational effects of hormones on moods and behavior at adolescence. *Psychological Bulletin, 111*, 62–107.

Buchanan, C. M., Maccoby, E. E., & Dornbusch, S. M. (1991). Caught between parents: Adolescents' experience in divorced homes. *Child Development, 62*, 1008–1029.

Bugental, D. B., Caporael, L., & Shennum, W. A. (1980). Experimentally produced child uncontrollability: Effects on the potency of adult communication patterns. *Child Development, 51*, 520–528.

Bugental, D. B., & Cortez, V. L. (1988). Physiological reactivity to responsive and unresponsive children as moderated by perceived control. *Child Development, 59*, 686–693.

Bugental, D. B., Lewis, J. C., Lin, E., Lyon, J., & Kopeikin, H. (1999). In charge but not in control: The management of teaching relationships by adults with low perceived power. *Developmental Psychology, 35*, 1367–1378.

Burack, J. A. (1997). The study of atypical and typical populations in developmental psychopathology: The quest for a common science. In S. S. Luthar, J. A. Burack, D.

Cicchetti, & J. R. Weisz (Eds.), *Developmental psychopathology: Perspectives on adjustment, risk, and disorder* (pp. 139–165). New York: Cambridge University Press.

Burbach, D. J., & Borduin, C. M. (1986). Parent–child relations and the etiology of depression: A review of methods and findings. *Clinical Psychology Review, 6,* 133–153.

Byng-Hall, J. (1999). Family and couple therapy: Toward greater security. In J. Cassidy & P. R. Shaver (Eds.), *Handbook of attachment: Theory, research, and clinical applications* (pp. 625–645). New York: Guilford Press.

Cairns, R. B. (1990). Developmental epistemology and self-knowledge: Towards a reinterpretation of self-esteem. In G. Greenberg & E. Tobach (Eds.), *The T. C. Schneirla Conference Series: Vol. 4. Theories of the evolution of knowing* (pp. 69–86). Hillsdale, NJ: Erlbaum.

Cairns, R. B. (1991). Multiple metaphors for a singular idea. *Developmental Psychology, 27,* 23–26.

Cairns, R. B., Cairns, B. D., & Neckerman, H. J. (1989). Early school dropout: Configurations and determinants. *Child Development, 60,* 1437–1452.

Cairns, R. B., Costello, E. J., & Elder, G. H., Jr. (1996). The making of developmental science. In R. B. Cairns, G. H. Elder, Jr., & E. J. Costello (Eds.), *Developmental science* (pp. 223–234). New York: Cambridge University Press.

Cairns, R. B., Elder, G. H., Jr., & Costello, E. J. (Eds.). (1996). *Developmental science.* New York: Cambridge University Press.

Cairns, R. B., Gariepy, J.-L., & Hood, K. E. (1990). Development, microevolution, and social behavior. *Psychological Review, 97,* 49–65.

Calkins, S. D., & Fox, N. A. (1992). The relations among infant temperament, security of attachment, and behavioral inhibition at twenty-four months. *Child Development, 63,* 1456–1472.

Calkins, S. D., Fox, N. A., & Marshall, T. R. (1996). Behavioral and physiological antecedents of inhibited and uninhibited behavior. *Child Development, 67,* 523–540.

Campbell, S. B. (1990). *Behavior problems in preschool children: Clinical and developmental issues.* New York: Guilford Press.

Campbell, S. B. (1995). Behavior problems in preschool children: A review of recent research. *Journal of Child Psychology and Psychiatry and Allied Disciplines, 36,* 113–149.

Campbell, S. B. (1997). Behavior problems in preschool children: Developmental and family issues. In T. H. Ollendick & R. Prinz (Eds.), *Advances in clinical child psychology* (Vol. 19, pp. 1–26). New York: Plenum Press.

Campbell, S. B. (1998). Developmental considerations in child psychopathology. In T. Ollendick & M. Hersen (Eds.), *Handbook of child psychopathology* (3rd ed., pp. 1–35). New York: Plenum Press.

Campbell, S. B. (2000). Developmental perspectives on attention deficit disorder. In M. Lewis, A. Sameroff, & S. Miller (Eds.), *Handbook of developmental psychopathology* (2nd ed., pp. 383–401). New York: Kluwer/Plenum.

Campbell, S. B., & Cohn, J. F. (1997). The timing and chronicity of postpartum depression: Implications for infant development. In L. Murray & P. J. Cooper (Eds.), *Postpartum depression and child development* (pp. 165–197). New York: Guilford Press.

Campbell, S. B., Cohn, J. F., & Meyers, T. (1995). Depression in first-time mothers: Mother–infant interaction and depression chronicity. *Developmental Psychology, 31,* 349–357.

Campbell, S. B., March, C. L., Pierce, E. W., Ewing, L. J., & Szumowski, E. K. (1991). Hard-to-manage preschool boys: Family context and the stability of externalizing behavior. *Journal of Abnormal Child Psychology, 19,* 301–318.

Campbell, S. B., Pierce, E. W., March, C. L., & Ewing, L. J. (1991). Noncompliant behavior, overactivity, and family stress as predictors of negative maternal control in preschool children. *Development and Psychopathology, 3,* 175–190.

Campbell, S. B., Pierce, E. W., March, C. L., Ewing, L. J., & Szumowski, E. K. (1994). Hard-to-manage preschool boys: Symptomatic behavior across contexts and time. *Child Development, 65,* 836–851.

Campbell, S. B., Pierce, E. W., Moore, G., Marakovitz, S., & Newby, K. (1996). Boys' externalizing problems at elementary school age: Pathways from early behavior problems, maternal control, and family stress. *Development and Psychopathology, 8,* 701–720.

Campbell, S. B., Shaw, D. S., & Gilliom, M. (in press). Early externalizing behavior problems: Toddlers and preschoolers at risk for later maladjustment. *Development and Psychopathology*

Campos, J. J., Campos, R. G., & Barrett, K. C. (1989). Emergent themes in the study of emotional development and emotion regulation. *Developmental Psychology, 25,* 394–402.

Campos, J. J., Mumme, D. L., Kermoian, R., & Campos, R. G. (1994). Commentary: A functionalist perspective on the nature of emotion. In N. Fox (Ed.), The development of emotion regulation: Biological and behavioral considerations. *Monographs of the Society for Research in Child Development, 59*(2–3, Serial No. 240), 284–303.

Cantwell, D. P. (1996a). ADHD: A review of the past 10 years. *Journal of the American Academy of Child and Adolescent Psychiatry, 35,* 978–987.

Cantwell, D. P. (1996b). Classification of child and adolescent psychopathology. *Journal of Child Psychology and Psychiatry, 37,* 3–12.

Capaldi, D. M., & Clark, S. (1998). Prospective family predictors of aggression: Towards female partners for at-risk men. *Developmental Psychology, 34*(6), 1175–1188.

Caplan, H. L., Cogill, S. R., Alexandra, H., Robson, K. M., Katz, R., & Kumer, J. (1989). Maternal depression and the emotional development of the child. *British Journal of Psychiatry, 154,* 818–822.

Carlson, E. A. (1998). A prospective longitudinal study of attachment disorganization/disorientation. *Child Development, 69,* 1107–1128.

Carlson, E. A., & Sroufe, L. A. (1995). Contribution of attachment theory to developmental psychopathology. In D. Cicchetti & D. Cohen (Eds.), *Developmental psychopathology: Theory and methods* (Vol. 1, pp. 581–617). New York: Wiley.

Carlson, V., Cicchetti, D., Barnett, D., & Braunwald, K. (1989). Disorganized/disoriented attachment relationships in maltreated infants. *Developmental Psychology, 25,* 525–531.

Caron, C., & Rutter, M. (1991). Co-morbidity in child psychopathology: Concepts, issues, and research strategies. *Journal of Child Psychology and Psychiatry, 32,* 1063–1079.

Caspi, A., & Moffitt, T. E. (1991). Individual differences are accentuated during periods of social change: The sample case of girls at puberty. *Journal of Personality and Social Psychology, 61,* 157–168.

Caspi, A., & Moffitt, T. E. (1995). The continuity of maladaptive behavior: From de scription to understanding in the study of antisocial behavior. In D. Cicchetti & D. J. Cohen (Eds.), *Developmental psychopathology: Vol. 2. Risk, disorder, and adaptation* (pp. 472–511). New York: Wiley.

Cassidy, J., Parke, R. D., Butkovsky, L., & Braungart, J. M. (1992). Family–peer connections: The roles of emotional expressiveness within the family and children's understanding of emotions. *Child Development, 63,* 603–618.

Chamberlain, P. (1996). Community based residential treatment for adolescents with conduct disorder. In T. Ollendick & R. Prinz (Eds.), *Advances in clinical child psychology* (Vol. 18, pp. 63–90). New York: Plenum Press.

Chamberlain, P., & Reid, J. B. (1998). Comparison of two community alternatives to incarceration for chronic juvenile offenders. *Journal of Consulting and Clinical Psychology, 66,* 624–633.

Chao, R. K. (1994). Beyond parental control and authoritarian parenting style: Understanding Chinese parenting through the cultural notion of training. *Child Development, 65,* 1111–1119.

Chase-Lansdale, P. L., Wakschlag, L. S., & Brooks-Gunn, J. (1995). A psychological perspective on the development of caring in children and youth: The role of family. *Journal of Adolescence, 18,* 515–556

Christensen, A. (1988). Dysfunctional interaction patterns in couples. In P. Noller & M. A. Fitzpatrick (Eds.), *Perspectives on marital interaction* (pp. 31–52). Clevedon, UK: Multlingual Matters.

Christensen, A., Phillips, S., Glasgow, R. E., & Johnson, S. M. (1983). Parental characteristics and interactional dysfunction in families with child behavior problems: A preliminary investigation. *Journal of Abnormal Child Psychology, 11,* 153–166.

Cicchetti, D. (1984). The emergence of developmental psychopathology. *Child Development, 55,* 1–7.

Cicchetti, D. (1989). How research on child maltreatment has informed the study of child development: Perspectives from developmental psychopathology. In D. Cicchetti & V. Carlson (Eds.), *Child maltreatment: Theory and research on the causes and consequences of child abuse and neglect* (pp. 377–431). New York: Cambridge University Press.

Cicchetti, D. (1990a). A historical perspective on the discipline of developmental psychopathology. In J. Rolf, A. Masten, D. Cicchetti, K. Nuchterlein, & S. Weintraub (Eds.), *Risk and protective factors in the development of psychopathology* (pp. 2–28). New York: Cambridge University Press.

Cicchetti, D. (1990b). Perspectives on the interface between normal and atypical development. *Development and Psychopathology, 2,* 329–333.

Cicchetti, D. (1991). Defining psychological maltreatment: Reflections and future directions. *Development and Psychopathology, 3,* 1–2.

Cicchetti, D. (1993). Fractures in the crystal: Developmental psychopathology and the emergence of self. *Developmental Review, 11,* 271–287.

Cicchetti, D. (1996). Child maltreatment: Implications for development theory and research. *Human Development, 39,* 18–39.

Cicchetti, D., & Aber, L. (1998). Editorial: Contextualism and psychopathology. *Developmental Psychopathology, 10*(2), 137–142.

Cicchetti, D., Ackerman, B. P., & Izard, C. E. (1995). Emotions and emotion regulation in developmental psychopathology. *Development and Psychopathology, 7,* 1–10.

Cicchetti, D., & Cohen, D. J. (1995a). Perspectives on developmental psychopathology.

In D. Cicchetti & D. J. Cohen (Eds.), *Developmental psychopathology: Vol. 1. Theory and methods* (pp. 3–20). New York: Wiley.

Cicchetti, D., & Cohen, D. J. (Eds.). (1995b). *Developmental psychopathology: Vol. 1. Theory and methods. Vol. 2. Risk, disorder, and adaptation.* New York: Wiley.

Cicchetti, D., Cummings, E. M., Marvin, R. S., & Greenberg, M. T. (1990). An organizational perspective on attachment beyond infancy. In M. T. Greenberg, D. Cicchetti, & E. M. Cummings (Eds.), *Attachment in the preschool years* (pp. 51–95). Chicago: University of Chicago Press.

Cicchetti, D., Ganniban, J., & Barnett, D. (1991). Contributions from the study of high risk populations to understanding the development of emotion regulation. In J. Garber & K. Dodge (Eds.), *The development of emotion regulation and dysregulation* (pp. 15–48). New York: Cambridge University Press.

Cicchetti, D., & Garmezy, N. (1993). Prospects and promises in the study of resilience. *Development and Psychopathology, 5*, 497–502.

Cicchetti, D., & Lynch, M. (1993). Toward an ecological/transactional model of community violence and child maltreatment: Consequences for children's development. *Psychiatry, 56*, 96–118.

Cicchetti, D., & Richters, J. E. (1997). Examining the conceptual and scientific underpinnings of research in developmental psychopathology. *Development and Psychopathology, 9*, 189–191.

Cicchetti, D., & Rogosch, F. A. (1996). Equifinality and multifinality in developmental psychopathology. *Development and Psychopathology, 8*, 597–600.

Cicchetti, D., & Rogosch, F. A. (1997). The role of self-organization in the promotion of resilience in maltreated children. *Development and Psychopathology, 9*, 797–815.

Cicchetti, D., Rogosch, F., & Toth, S. (1998). Maternal depressive disorder and contextual risk: Contributions to the development of attachment insecurity and behavior problems in toddlerhood. *Development and Psychopathology, 10*(2), 283–300.

Cicchetti, D., & Toth, S. L. (1991). A developmental perspective on internalizing and externalizing disorders. In D. Cicchetti & S. L. Toth (Eds.), *Rochester Symposium on Developmental Psychopathology: Vol. 2. Internalizing and externalizing expressions of dysfunction* (pp. 1–19). Hillsdale, NJ: Erlbaum.

Cicchetti, D., & Toth, S. L. (1995). A developmental psychopathology perspective on child abuse and neglect. *Journal of the American Academy of Child and Adolescent Psychiatry, 34*, 541–565.

Cicchetti, D., & Toth, S. L. (1998). The development of depression in children and adolescents. *American Psychologist, 53*, 221–241.

Cicchetti, D., Toth, S. L., & Hennessy, K. (1989). Research on the consequences of child maltreatment and its application to educational settings. *Topics in Early Childhood Special Education, 9*, 33–55.

Cicchetti, D., & Tucker, D. (1994). Development and self-regulatory structures of the mind. *Development and Psychopathology, 6*, 533–549.

Clarke-Stewart, K. A. (1973). Interactions between mothers and their young children: Characteristics and consequences. *Monographs of the Society for Research in Child Development, 38*(5–6, Serial No. 153).

Clarke-Stewart, K. A. (1988). Parents' effects on children's development: A decade of progress? *Journal of Applied Developmental Psychology, 9*, 41–84.

Cohn, J. F., & Campbell, S. (1992). Influence of maternal depression on infant affect regulation. In D. Cicchetti & S. Toth (Eds.), *Rochester Symposium in Developmental*

Psychopathology: Vol. 4. Developmental perspectives on depression (pp. 103–130). Rochester, NY: University of Rochester Press.

Cohn, J. F., Campbell, S. B., Matias, R., & Hopkins, J. (1990). Face-to-face interactions of postpartum depressed and nondepressed mother–infant pairs at 2 months. *Developmental Psychology, 26,* 15–23.

Cohn, J., & Tronick, E. (1983). Three-month-old infants' reaction to simulated maternal depression. *Child Development, 54,* 185–190.

Cohn, J. F., & Tronick, E. Z. (1989). Specificity of infants' response to mothers' affective behavior. *Journal of the American Academy of Child and Adolescent Psychiatry, 28,* 242–248.

Coie, J. D., & Dodge, K. A. (1998). Aggression and antisocial behavior. In N. Eisenberg (Ed.), *Handbook of child psychology. Vol. 3: Social, emotional, and personality development* (5th ed., pp. 779–862). New York: Wiley.

Coie, J. D., Dodge, K. A., & Kupersmidt, J. B. (1990). Peer group behavior and social status. In S. R. Asher & J. D. Coie (Eds.), *Peer rejection in childhood: Cambridge studies in social and emotional development* (pp. 17–59). New York: Cambridge University Press.

Coie, J. D., Terry, R., Lenox, K., Lochman, J. E., & Hyman, C. (1995). Childhood peer rejection and aggression as predictors of stable patterns of adolescent disorder. *Development and Psychopathology, 7,* 697–713.

Coie, J. D., Watt, N., West, S., Haskins, D., Asarnow, J., Markman, H., Ramey, S., Shure, M., & Long, B. (1993). The science of prevention: A conceptual framework and some directions for a national research program. *American Psychologist, 48,* 1013–1022.

Cole, D. A. (1991). Preliminary support for a competency-based model of depression in children. *Journal of Abnormal Psychology, 100,* 181–190.

Cole, D. A., Martin, J. M., Powers, B., & Truglio, R. (1997). Modeling causal relations between academic and social competence and depression: A multitrait–multimethod longitudinal study of children. *Journal of Abnormal Psychology, 105,* 258–270.

Cole, P. M., Michel, M., & Teti, L. (1994). The development of emotion regulation and dysregulation: A clinical perspective. In N. Fox (Ed.), The development of emotion regulation: Biological and behavioral considerations. *Monographs of the Society for Research in Child Development*(2–3, Serial No. 240), 73–102.

Cole, P. M., & Putnam, F. W. (1992). Effect of incest on self and social functioning: A developmental psychopathology perspective. *Journal of Consulting and Clinical Psychology, 60,* 174–184.

Cole, P. M., & Zahn-Waxler, C. (1992). Emotional dysregulation in disruptive behavior disorders. In D. Cicchetti & S. L. Toth (Eds.), *Rochester Symposium on Developmental Psychopathology: Vol. 4. Developmental perspectives on depression* (pp. 173–209). Rochester, NY: University of Rochester Press.

Cole, P. M., Zahn-Waxler, C., & Smith, K. D. (1994). Expressive control during a disappointment: Variations related to preschoolers' behavior problems. *Developmental Psychology, 30,* 835–846.

Coley, R. L., & Chase-Lansdale, P. L. (1998). Adolescent pregnancy and parenthood. *American Psychologist, 53,* 152–166.

Colin, V. L. (1996). *Human attachment.* New York: McGraw-Hill.

Collins, W. A., Gleason, T., & Sesma, A. (1997). Internalization, autonomy, and relationships: Development during adolescence. In J. E. Grusec & L. Kuczynski (Eds.),

Parenting and children's internalization of values: A handbook of contemporary theory (pp. 78–99). New York: Wiley.

Collins, W. A., Harris, M. L., & Susman, A. (1995). Parenting during middle childhood. In M. H. Bornstein (Ed.), *Handbook of parenting: Vol. 1. Children and parenting* (pp. 65–89). Mahwah, NJ: Erlbaum.

Collins, W. A., Hennighausen, K. C., Schmit, D. T., & Sroufe, L. A. (1997). Developmental precursors of romantic relationships: A longitudinal analysis. In S. Shulman & W. A. Collins (Eds.), Romantic relationships in adolescence: Developmental perspectives. *New Directions for Child Development, 78,* 69–84.

Compas, B. E., Hinden, B. R., & Gerhardt, C. A. (1995). Adolescent development: Pathways and processes of risk and resilience. *Annual Review of Psychology, 46,* 265–293.

Conduct Problems Prevention Research Group. (1992). A developmental and clinical model for the prevention of conduct disorder: The FAST Track Program. *Development and Psychopathology, 4,* 509–527.

Conduct Problems Prevention Research Group. (1999). Initial impact of the Fast Track Prevention Trial for conduct problems: I. The high risk sample. *Journal of Consulting and Clinical Psychology, 67,* 631–647.

Conger, K. J., & Conger, R. D. (1994). Differential parenting and change in sibling differences in delinquency. *Journal of Family Psychology, 8,* 287–302.

Conger, R. D., Conger, K. J., Elder, G. H., Lorenz, F. O., Simons, R. L., & Whitbeck, L. B. (1992). A family process model of economic hardship and adjustment of early adolescent boys. *Child Development, 63,* 526–541.

Conger, R. D., Conger, K. J., Elder, G. H., Lorenz, F. O., Simons, R. L., & Whitbeck, L. B. (1993). Family economic stress and adjustment of early adolescent girls. *Developmental Psychology, 29,* 206–219.

Conger, R. D., Elder, G. H., Lorenz, F. O., Conger, K. J., Simons, R. L., Whitbeck, L. B., Huck, S., & Melby, J. N. (1990). Linking economic hardship to marital quality and instability. *Journal of Marriage and the Family, 52,* 643–656.

Conger, R. D., Elder, G. H., Melby, J. N., Simons, R. L., & Conger, K. J. (1991). A process model of family economic pressure and early adolescent alcohol use. *Journal of Early Adolescence, 11,* 430–449.

Conger, R. D., Ge, X., Elder, G. H., Lorenz, F. O., & Simons, R. L. (1994). Economic stress, coercive family process, and developmental problems of adolescents. *Child Development, 65,* 541–561.

Conger, R. D., Patterson, G. R., & Ge, X. (1995). It takes two to replicate: A mediational model for the impact of parents' stress on adolescent adjustment. *Child Development, 66,* 80–97.

Connolly, J. A., & Johnson, A. M. (1996). Adolescents' romantic relationships and the structure and quality of their close interpersonal ties. *Personal Relationships, 3,* 185–195.

Cook, E. H., Stein, M. A., Krasnowski, M. D., Cox, N. J., Olkon, D. M., Kieffer, J. E., & Leventhal, B. L. (1995). Association of attention deficit hyperactivity disorder and the dopamine transporter gene. *American Journal of Human Genetics, 56,* 993–998.

Cooper, M. L., Peirce, R. S., & Tidwell, M. C. O. (1995). Parental drinking problems and adolescent offspring substance use: Moderating effects of demographic and familial factors. *Psychology of Addictive Behaviors, 9,* 36–52.

Courchesne, E., Chisum, H., & Townsend, J. (1994). Neural activity–dependent brain changes in development: Implications for psychopathology. *Development and Psychopathology*, 6, 697–722.

Cowan, C. P., Cowan, P. A., & Heming, G. (1999). *Two variations of a preventive intervention for couples: Effects on parents and children.* Unpublished manuscript.

Cowan, P. A., Cohn, D. A., Cowan, C. P., & Pearson, J. L. (1996). Parents' attachment histories and children's externalizing and internalizing behaviors: Exploring family systems models of linkage. *Journal of Consulting and Clinical Psychology*, 64, 53–63.

Cowan, P. A., & Cowan, C. P. (1999, August). *What an intervention design reveals about how parents affect their children's academic achievement and social competence.* Paper presented at the Conference Parenting and the Child's World: Multiple Influences on Intellectual and Social-Emotional Development, Bethesda, MD.

Cowan, P. A., Cowan, C. P., & Schulz, M. S. (1996). Thinking about risk and resilience in families. In E. M. Hetherington & E. Blechman (Eds.), *Risk and resilience: Advances in family research* (Vol. 5, pp. 1–38). Hillsdale, NJ. Erlbaum.

Cowan, P. A., Powell, D., & Cowan, C. P. (1998). Parenting interventions: A family systems perspective. In I. E. Sigel & K. A. Renninger (Eds.), *Handbook of child psychology: Vol. 4. Child psychology in practice* (5th ed., pp. 3–72). New York: Wiley.

Cowen, E. L. (1977). Baby steps toward primary prevention. *American Journal of Community Psychology*, 5, 1–22.

Cox, A. D., Puckering, C., Pound, A., & Mills, M. (1987). The impact of maternal depression in young people. *Journal of Child Psychology and Psychiatry*, 28, 917–928.

Cox, M. J., & Owen, M. T. (1993, March). Marital conflict and conflict negotiation: Effects on infant–mother and infant–father relationships. In M. Cox & J. Brooks-Gunn (Chairs), *Conflict in families: Causes and consequences.* Symposium conducted at the meeting of the Society for Research in Child Development, New Orleans, LA.

Cox, M. J., & Paley, B. (1997). Families as systems. *Annual Review of Psychology*, 48, 243–267.

Cox, M. J., Paley, B., & Payne, C. C. (1997, April). *Marital and parent–child relationships.* Paper presented at the biennial meeting of the Society for Research in Child Development, Washington, DC.

Coyne, J. C. (1976). Depression and the response of others. *Journal of Abnormal Psychology*, 85, 186–193.

Coyne, J. C., & Downey, G. (1991). Social factors and psychopathology: Stress, social support, and coping processes. *Annual Review of Psychology*, 55, 347–352.

Coyne, J. C., Schwoeri, L., & Downey, G. (1994). Depression, the marital relationship, and parenting: An interpersonal view. In G. P. Sholevar (Ed.), *The transmission of depression in families and children: Assessment and intervention* (pp. 31–57). Northvale, NJ: Aronson.

Crick, N. R. (1995). Relational aggression: The role of intent attributions, feelings of distress, and provocation type. *Development and Psychopathology*, 7, 313–322.

Crick, N. R., & Dodge, K. A. (1994). A review and reformulation of social information-processing mechanisms in children's social adjustment. *Psychological Bulletin*, 115, 74–101.

Crick, N. R., & Dodge, K. A. (1996). Social information-processing mechanisms in reactive and proactive aggression. *Child Development*, 67, 993–1002.

Crittenden, P. (1988). Relationships at risk. In J. Belsky & T. Nezworski (Eds.), *Clinical implications of attachment theory* (pp. 136–174). Hillsdale, NJ: Erlbaum.

Crittenden, P. M. (1992). Children's strategies for coping with adverse home environments: An interpretation using attachment theory. *Child Abuse and Neglect, 16,* 329–343.

Crittenden, P. M., & Ainsworth, M. D. S. (1989). Child maltreatment and attachment theory. In D. Cicchetti & V. Carlson (Eds.), *Child maltreatment: Theory and research on the causes and consequences of child abuse and neglect* (pp. 432–463). New York: Cambridge University Press.

Crittenden, P. M., Claussen, A. H., & Sugarman, D. B. (1994). Physical and psychological maltreatment in middle childhood and adolescence. *Development and Psychopathology, 6,* 145–164.

Crittenden, P. M., & DiLalla, D. L. (1988). Compulsive compliance: The development of an inhibitory coping strategy in infancy. *Journal of Abnormal Child Psychology, 5,* 585–599.

Crockenberg, S., & Litman, C. (1990). Autonomy as competence in 2-year-olds: Maternal correlates of child defiance, compliance and self-assertion. *Developmental Psychology, 6,* 961–971.

Crockenberg, S. B. (1986). Are temperamental differences in babies associated with predictable differences in caregiving? In J. V. Lerner & R. M. Lerner (Eds.), *Temperament and social interaction in infants and children* (pp. 53–73). San Francisco: Jossey-Bass.

Crockenberg, S. B., & Forgays, D. (1996). The role of emotion in children's understanding and emotional reactions to marital conflict. *Merrill–Palmer Quarterly, 42,* 22–47.

Cummings, E. M. (1987). Coping with background anger in early childhood. *Child Development, 58,* 976–984.

Cummings, E. M. (1990). Classification of attachment on a continuum of felt-security: Illustrations from the study of children of depressed parents. In M. T. Greenberg, D. Cicchetti, & E. M. Cummings (Eds.), *Attachment in the preschool years: Theory, research, and intervention* (pp. 311–338). Chicago: University of Chicago Press.

Cummings, E. M. (1994). Marital conflict and children's functioning. *Social Development, 3,* 16–36.

Cummings, E. M. (1995a). Security, emotionality, and parental depression. *Developmental Psychology, 31,* 425–427.

Cummings, E. M. (1995b). The usefulness of experiments for the study of the family. *Journal of Family Psychology, 9,* 175–185.

Cummings, E. M. (1998a). Children exposed to marital conflict and violence: Conceptual and theoretical directions. In G. Holden, B. Geffner, & E. Jouriles (Eds.), *Children exposed to marital violence: Theory, research, and applied issues* (pp. 55–94). Washington, DC: American Psychological Association.

Cummings, E. M. (1998b). Stress and coping approaches and research: The impact of marital conflict and violence. In B. B. R. Rossman & M. S. Rosenberg (Eds.), *Multiple victimization of children: Conceptual, developmental, research, and treatment issues* (pp. 31–50). New York: Haworth Press

Cummings, E. M. (1999). Some considerations on integrating psychology and health from a life-span perspective. In T. L. Whitman, T. V. Merluzzi, & R. D. White (Eds.), *Life-span perspectives on health and illness* (pp. 277–294). Mahwah, NJ: Erlbaum.

Cummings, E. M., Ballard, M., & El-Sheikh, M. (1991). Responses of children and adolescents to interadult anger as a function of gender, age, and mode of expression. *Merrill–Palmer Quarterly, 37,* 543–560.

Cummings, E. M., Ballard, M., El-Sheikh, M., & Lake, M. (1991). Resolution and children's responses to interadult anger. *Developmental Psychology, 27,* 462–470.

Cummings, E. M., & Cicchetti, D. (1990). Towards a transactional model of relations between attachment and depression. In M. Greenberg, D. Cicchetti, & E. M. Cummings (Eds.), *Attachment in the preschool years: Theory, research, and intervention* (pp. 339–372). Chicago: University of Chicago Press.

Cummings, E. M., & Cummings, J. S. (1988). A process-oriented approach to children's coping with adults' angry behavior. *Developmental Review, 3,* 296–321.

Cummings, E. M., & Davies, P. T. (1994a). *Children and marital conflict: The impact of family dispute and resolution.* New York: Guilford Press.

Cummings, E. M., & Davies, P. T. (1994b). Maternal depression and child development. *Journal of Child Psychology and Psychiatry, 35,* 73–112.

Cummings, E. M., & Davies, P. T. (1995). The impact of parents on their children: An emotional security hypothesis. *Annals of Child Development, 10,* 167–208.

Cummings, E. M., & Davies, P. T. (1996). Emotional security as a regulatory process in normal development and the development of psychopathology. *Development and Psychopathology, 8,* 123–139.

Cummings, E. M., & Davies, P. T. (1999). Depressed parents and family functioning: Interpersonal effects and children's functioning and development. In T. Joiner & J. C. Coyne (Eds.), *The interactional nature of depression: Advances in interpersonal approaches* (pp. 299–327). Washington, DC: American Psychological Association.

Cummings, E. M., Davies, P., & Simpson, K. (1994). Marital conflict, gender, and children's appraisal and coping efficacy as mediators of child adjustment. *Journal of Family Psychology, 8,* 141–149.

Cummings, E. M., & El-Sheikh, M. (1991). Children's coping with angry environments: A process-oriented approach. In E. M. Cummings, A. Greene, & K. Karraker (Eds.), *Life-span developmental psychology: Perspectives on stress and coping* (pp. 131–150). Hillsdale, NJ: Erlbaum.

Cummings, E. M., Goeke-Morey, M. C., & Graham, M. A. (1999, August). *Marital conflict as parenting.* Paper presented at the National Institute of Child Health and Human Development Parenting Conference, Bethesda, MD.

Cummings, E. M., Hennessy, K., Rabideau, G., & Cicchetti, D. (1994). Responses of physically abused boys to interadult anger involving their mothers. *Development and Psychopathology, 6,* 31–41.

Cummings, E. M., Iannotti, R., & Zahn-Waxler, C. (1985). The influence of conflict between adults on the emotions and aggression of young children. *Developmental Psychology, 21,* 495–507.

Cummings, E. M., Iannotti, R. J., & Zahn-Waxler, C. (1989). Aggression between peers in early childhood: Individual continuity and developmental change. *Child Development, 60,* 887–895.

Cummings, E. M., & O'Reilly, A. (1997). Fathers in family context: Effects of marital quality on child adjustment. In M. E. Lamb (Ed.), *The role of the father in child development* (3rd ed., pp. 49–65). New York: Wiley.

Cummings, E. M., Simpson, K., & Wilson, A. (1993). Children's responses to interadult anger as a function of information about resolution. *Developmental Psychology, 29,* 978–985.

Cummings, E. M., Vogel, D., Cummings, J. S., & El-Sheikh, M. (1989). Children's responses to different forms of expression of anger between adults. *Child Development, 60*, 1392–1404.

Cummings, E. M., & Wilson, A. G. (1999). Contexts of marital conflict and children's emotional security: Exploring the distinction between constructive and destructive conflict from the children's perspective. In M. Cox & J. Brooks-Gunn (Eds.), *Formation, functioning, and stability of families* (pp. 105–129). Mahwah, NJ: Erlbaum.

Cummings, E. M., & Zahn-Waxler, C. (1992). Emotions and the socialization of aggression: Adults' angry behavior and children's arousal and aggression. In A. Fraczek & H. Zumkley (Eds.), *Socialization and aggression* (pp. 61–84). New York and Berlin: Springer-Verlag.

Cummings, E. M., Zahn-Waxler, C., & Radke-Yarrow, M. (1981). Young children's responses to expressions of anger and affection by others in the family. *Child Development, 52*, 1274–1282.

Cummings, E. M., Zahn-Waxler, C., & Radke-Yarrow, M. (1984). Developmental changes in children's reactions to anger in the home. *Journal of Child Psychology and Psychiatry, 25*, 63–75.

Cummings, J. S., Pelligrini, D., Notarius, C., & Cummings, E. M. (1989). Children's responses to angry adult behavior as a function of marital distress and history of interparent hostility. *Child Development, 60*, 1035–1043.

Curran, P. J., & Chassin, L. (1996). A longitudinal study of parenting as a protective factor for children of alcoholics. *Journal of Studies on Alcohol, 57*, 305–313.

Dadds, M. R., Schwartz, S., & Sanders, M. R. (1987). Marital discord and treatment outcome in behavioral treatment of child problems. *Journal of Consulting and Clinical Psychology, 55*, 396–403.

Dahl, R. E. (1996). The regulation of sleep and arousal: Development and psychopathology. *Development and Psychopathology, 8*, 3–27.

Darling, N., & Steinberg, L. (1993). Parenting style as context: An integrative model. *Psychological Bulletin, 113*, 487–496.

Davidson, R. J., Ekman, P., Saron, C. D., & Senulis, J. A. (1990). Approach–withdrawal and cerebral asymmetry: I. Emotional expression and brain physiology. *Journal of Personality and Social Psychology, 58*, 330–341.

Davies, P. T. (1995). *Children's emotional security as a mediator in the link between marital conflict and child adjustment.* Unpublished doctoral dissertation, West Virginia University, Morgantown.

Davies, P. T., & Cummings, E. M. (1994). Marital conflict and child adjustment: An emotional security hypothesis. *Psychological Bulletin, 116*, 387–411.

Davies, P. T., & Cummings, E. M. (1995). Children's emotions as organizers of their reaction to interadult anger: A functionalist perspective. *Developmental Psychology, 31*, 677–684.

Davies, P. T., & Cummings, E. M. (1998). Exploring children's emotional security as a mediator of the link between marital relations and child adjustment. *Child Development, 69*, 124–139.

Davies, P. T., Dumenci, L., & Windle, M. (1999). The interplay between maternal depressive symptoms and marital distress in the prediction of adolescent adjustment. *Journal of Marriage and the Family, 61*, 238–254.

Davies, P. T., Myers, R. L., & Cummings, E. M. (1996). Responses of children and adolescents to marital conflict scenarios as a function of the emotionality of conflict endings. *Merrill–Palmer Quarterly, 42*, 1–21.

Davies, P. T., Myers, R. L., Cummings, E. M., & Heindel, S. (1999). Adult conflict history and children's subsequent responses to conflict. *Journal of Family Psychology*, 13, 610–628.

Davies, P. T., & Windle, M. (1997). Gender-specific pathways between maternal depressive symptoms, family discord, and adolescent adjustment. *Developmental Psychology*, 33, 657–668.

Davis, B. T., Hops, H., Alpert, A., & Sheeber, L. (1998). Child responses to parental conflict and their effect on adjustment: A study of triadic relations. *Journal of Family Psychology*, 12, 163–177.

Dawson, G., Frey, K., Panagiotides, H., Yamada, E., Hessl, D., & Osterling, J. (1999). Infants of depressed mothers exhibit atypical frontal electrical brain activity during interactions with mother and with a familiar, nondepressed adult. *Child Development*, 70, 1058–1066.

Dawson, G., Frey, K., Self, J., Panagiotides, H., Hessl, D., Yamada, E., & Rinaldi, J. (1999). Frontal brain electrical activity in infants of depressed and nondepressed mothers: Relation to variations in infant behavior. *Development and Psychopathology*, 11, 589–605.

Deater-Deckard, K., & Dodge, K. A. (1997a). Externalizing behavior problems and discipline revisited: Nonlinear effects and variation by culture, context, and gender. *Psychological Inquiry*, 8, 161–175.

Deater-Deckard, K., & Dodge, K. A. (1997b). Spare the rod, spoil the authors: Emerging themes in research on parenting and child development. *Psychological Inquiry*, 8, 230–235.

Deater-Deckard, K., Dodge, K. A., Bates, J. E., & Pettit, G. S. (1996). Physical discipline among African American and European American mothers: Links to children's externalizing behaviors. *Developmental Psychology*, 32, 1065–1072.

Denham, S. A. (1989). Maternal affect and toddlers' social-emotional competence. *American Journal of Orthopsychiatry*, 59, 368–376.

Denham, S. A., Renwick, S. M., & Holt, R. W. (1991). Working and playing together: Prediction of preschool social–emotional competence from mother–child interactions. *Child Development*, 62, 242–249.

Derryberry, D., & Reed, M. A. (1994). Temperament and the self-organization of personality. *Development and Psychopathology*, 6, 653–676.

De Wolff, M., & van Ijzendoorn, M. H. (1997). Sensitivity and attachment: A meta-analysis on parental antecedents of infant attachment. *Child Development*, 68, 571–591.

Dickstein, S., Seifer, R., Hayden, L. C., Schiller, M., Sameroff, A. J., Keitner, G., Miller, I., Rasmussen, S., Matzko, M., & Magee, K. D. (1998). Levels of family assessment: II. Impact of maternal psychopathology on family functioning. *Journal of Family Psychology*, 12, 23–40.

Dishion, T. J. (1990). The family ecology of boys' peer relations in middle childhood. *Child Development*, 61, 874–892.

Dishion, T. J., Andrews, D. W., & Crosby, L. (1995). Antisocial boys and their friends in early adolescence: Relationship characteristics, quality, and interactional process. *Child Development*, 66, 139–151.

Dishion, T. J., Patterson, G. R., Stoolmiller, M., & Skinner, M. L. (1991). Family, school, and behavioral antecedents to early adolescent involvement with antisocial peers. *Developmental Psychology*, 27, 172–180.

Dodge, K. A. (1990a). Nature versus nurture in childhood conduct disorder: It is time to ask a different question. *Developmental Psychology*, 26, 698–701.

Dodge, K. A. (1990b). Developmental psychopathology in children of depressed mothers. *Developmental Psychology, 26,* 3–6.

Dodge, K. A., & Coie, J. D. (1987). Social-information-processing factors in reactive and proactive aggression in children's peer groups. *Journal of Personality and Social Psychology, 53,* 1146–1158.

Dodge, K. A., Pettit, G. S., & Bates, J. E. (1994a). Socialization mediators of the relation between socioeconomic status and child conduct problems. *Child Development, 65,* 649–665.

Dodge, K. A., Pettit, G. S., & Bates, J. E. (1994). Effects of physical maltreatment on the development of peer relations. *Development and Psychopathology, 6,* 43–55.

Dodge, K. A., Pettit, G. S., Bates, J. E., & Valente, E. (1995). Social information-processing patterns partially mediate the effect of early physical abuse on later conduct problems. *Journal of Abnormal Psychology, 104,* 632–643.

Dornbusch, S. M., Ritter, P. L., Leiderman, P. H., Roberts, D. F., & Fraleigh, M. J. (1987). The relation of parenting style to adolescent school performance. *Child Development, 58,* 1244–1257.

Downey, G., & Coyne, J. C. (1990). Children of depressed parents: An integrative review. *Psychological Bulletin, 108,* 50–76.

Downey, G., Feldman, S., Khuri, J., & Friedman, S. (1994). Maltreatment and childhood depression. In W. M. Reynolds & H. F. Johnston (Eds.), *Handbook of depression in children and adolescents* (pp. 481–508). New York: Plenum Press.

Downey, G., & Walker, E. (1989). Social cognition and adjustment in children at risk for psychopathology. *Developmental Psychology, 25,* 835–845.

Dozier, M., & Kobak, R. R. (1992). Psychophysiology in attachment interviews: Converging evidence for deactivating strategies. *Child Development, 63,* 1473–1480.

Dumas, J. E., Prinz, R. J., Smith, E. P., & Laughlin, J. (1999). The EARLY ALLIANCE prevention trial: An integrated set of interventions to promote competence and reduce risk for conduct disorder, substance abuse, and school failure. *Clinical Child and Family Psychology Review, 2,* 37–53.

Dunn, J., & Plomin, R. (1990). *Separate lives: Why siblings are so different.* New York: Basic Books.

Dunn, J., & Stocker, C. (1989). The significance of differences in siblings' experiences within the family. In K. Kreppner & R. Lerner (Eds.), *Family systems and life-span development* (pp. 289–301). Hillsdale, NJ: Erlbaum.

Easterbrooks, M. A., Cummings, E. M., & Emde, R. N. (1994). Young children's responses to constructive marital disputes. *Journal of Family Psychology, 8,* 160–169.

Eccles, J. S., Lord, S., & Buchanan, C. M. (1996). School transitions in early adolescence: What are we doing to our young people? In J. A. Graber & J. Brooks-Gunn (Eds.), *Transitions through adolescence: Interpersonal domains and context* (pp. 251–284). Mahwah, NJ: Erlbaum.

Eccles, J. S., Lord, S., & Roeser, R. W. (1996). Round holes, square pegs, rocky roads, and sore feet: A discussion of stage–environment fit theory applied to families and school. In D. Cicchetti & S. L. Toth (Eds.), *Rochester Symposium on Developmental Psychopathology: Vol. 7. Adolescence: Opportunities and challenges* (pp. 47–92). Rochester, NY: University of Rochester Press.

Eccles, J. S., Midgley, C., Wigfield, A., Buchanan, C. M., Reuman, D., Flanagan, C., & MacIver, D. (1993). Development during adolescence: The impact of stage–environment fit on young adolescents' experiences in schools and in families. *American Psychologist, 48,* 90–101.

Eckenrode, J., Laird, M., & Doris, J. (1993). School performance and disciplinary problems among abused and neglected children. *Developmental Psychology, 29,* 53–62.

Edelbrock, C. S., Costello, A. J., Dulcan, M. J., Kalas, R., & Conover, N. C. (1985). Age differences in the reliability of the psychiatric interview of the child. *Child Development, 56,* 265–275.

Eder, R. A. (1990). Uncovering children's psychological selves: Individual and developmental differences. *Child Development, 61,* 849–863.

Edwards, C. P. (1996). Parenting toddlers. In M. H. Bornstein (Ed.), *Handbook of parenting: Vol. 1. Children and parenting* (pp. 41–63). Mahwah, NJ: Erlbaum.

Egeland, B., Carlson, E., & Sroufe, L. A. (1993). Resilience as process. *Development and Psychopathology, 5,* 517–528.

Egeland, B., & Farber, E. (1984). Infant–mother attachment: Factors related to its development and changes over time. *Child Development, 55,* 753–771.

Egeland, B., Pianta, R., & O'Brien, M. A. (1993). Maternal intrusiveness in infancy and child maladaptation in early school years. *Development and Psychopathology, 5,* 359–370.

Egeland, B., Pianta, R., & Ogawa, J. (1996). Early behavior problems: Pathways to mental disorders in adolescence. *Development and Psychopathology, 8,* 735–749.

Egeland, B., Sroufe, L. A., & Erickson, M. (1983). The developmental consequences of different patterns of maltreatment. *Child Abuse and Neglect, 54,* 1168–1175.

Eisenberg, N. (1996). Meta-emotion and socialization of emotion in the family: A topic whose time has come: Comment on Gottman et al. (1996). *Journal of Family Psychology, 10,* 269–276.

Eisenberg, N., & Fabes, R. A. (1994). Mothers' reactions to children's negative outcomes: Relations to children's temperament and anger behavior. *Merrill–Palmer Quarterly, 40,* 138–156.

Eisenberg, N., Fabes, R. A., Guthrie, I. K., Murphy, B. C., Maszk, P., Holmgren, R., & Suh, K. (1996). The relations of regulation and emotionality to problem behavior in elementary school children. *Development and Psychopathology, 8,* 141–162.

Eisenberg, N., Fabes, R. A., Shepard, S. A., Guthrie, I. K., Murphy, B. C., & Reiser, M. (1999). Parental reactions to children's negative emotions: Longitudinal relations to quality of children's social functioning. *Child Development, 70,* 513–534.

Eisenberg, N., Spinrad, T. L., & Cumberland, A. (1998). Parental socialization of emotion. *Psychological Inquiry, 9,* 241–273.

Elder, G. H. (1974). *Children of the Great Depression: Social change in life experience.* Chicago: University of Chicago Press.

Elicker, J., Englund, M., & Sroufe, L. A. (1992). Predicting peer competence and peer relationships in childhood from early parent–child relationships. In R. Parke & G. Ladd (Eds.), *Family–peer relationships: Modes of linkage* (pp. 77–106). Hillsdale, NJ: Erlbaum.

Elliott, D. S., Huizinga, D., & Ageton, S. S. (1985). *Explaining delinquency and drug use.* Beverly Hills, CA: Sage.

Elmer, E. (1977). *Fragile families, troubled children.* Pittsburgh, PA: University of Pittsburgh Press.

El-Sheikh, M. (1994). Children's emotional and physiological responses to interadult angry behavior: The role of history of interparental hostility. *Journal of Abnormal Child Psychology, 22,* 661–678.

El-Sheikh, M. (1997). Children's responses to adult–adult and mother–child arguments:

The role of parental marital conflict and distress. *Journal of Family Psychology, 11*, 165–175.

El-Sheikh, M., Ballard, M., & Cummings, E. M. (1994). Individual differences in preschoolers' physiological and verbal responses to videotaped angry interactions. *Journal of Abnormal Child Psychology, 22*, 303–320.

El-Sheikh, M., & Cheskes, J. (1995). Background verbal and physical anger: A comparison of children's responses to adult–adult and adult–child arguments. *Child Development, 66*, 446–458.

El-Sheikh, M., & Cummings, E. M. (1992). Availability of control and preschoolers' responses to interadult anger. *International Journal of Behavioral Development, 15*, 207–226.

El-Sheikh, M., & Cummings, E. M. (1995). Children's responses to angry adult behavior as a function of experimentally manipulated exposure to resolved and unresolved conflict. *Social Development, 4*, 75–91.

El-Sheikh, M., & Cummings, E. M. (1997). Marital conflict, emotional regulation, and the adjustment of children of alcoholics. In K. C. Barrett (Ed.), The communication of emotion: Current research from diverse perspectives. *New Directions for Child Development, 77*, 25–44. San Francisco: Jossey-Bass.

El-Sheikh, M., Cummings, E. M., & Goetsch, V. (1989). Coping with adults' angry behavior: Behavioral, physiological, and self-reported responding in preschoolers. *Developmental Psychology, 25*, 490–498.

El-Sheikh, M., Cummings, E. M., & Reiter, S. (1996). Preschoolers' responses to ongoing interadult conflict: The role of prior exposure to resolved versus unresolved arguments. *Journal of Abnormal Child Psychology, 24*, 665–679.

Emde, R. N. (1994). Individuality, context, and the search for meaning. *Child Development, 65*, 719–737.

Eme, R. F. (1979). Sex differences in childhood psychopathology: A review. *Psychological Bulletin, 86*, 574–595.

Emery, R. E. (1982). Interparental conflict and the children of discord and divorce. *Psychological Bulletin, 92*, 310–330.

Emery, R. E. (1988). *Marriage, divorce, and children's adjustment*. Newbury Park, CA: Sage.

Emery, R. E. (1989). Family violence. *American Psychologist, 44*, 321–328.

Emery, R. E. (1992). Family conflict and its developmental implications: A conceptual analysis of deep meanings and systemic processes. In C. U. Shantz & W. W. Hartup (Eds.), *Conflict in child and adolescent development* (pp. 270–298). London: Cambridge University Press.

Emery, R. E. (1994). *Renegotiating family relationships: Divorce, child custody, and mediation*. New York: Guilford Press.

Emery, R. E. (1999). *Marriage, divorce, and children's adjustment* (2nd ed.). Thousand Oaks, CA: Sage.

Emery, R. E., Fincham, F. D., & Cummings, E. M. (1992). Parenting in context: Systemic thinking about parental conflict and its influence on children. *Journal of Consulting and Clinical Psychology, 60*, 909–912.

Emery, R. E., & Forehand, R. (1994). Parental divorce and children's well-being: A focus on resilience. In R. J. Haggerty, L. R. Sherrod, N. Garmezy, & M. Rutter (Eds.), *Stress, risk, and resilience in children and adolescents: Processes, mechanisms, and interventions* (pp. 64–99). New York: Cambridge University Press.

Emery, R. E., & Kitzmann, K. M. (1995). The child in the family: Disruptions in family functions. In D. Cicchetti & D. J. Cohen (Eds.), *Developmental psychopathology. Vol. 2: Risk, disorder, and adaptation* (pp. 3–31). New York: Wiley.

Emery, R. E., & O'Leary, K. D. (1982). Children's perceptions of marital discord and behavior problems of boys and girls. *Journal of Abnormal Child Psychology, 10*, 11–24.

Emery, R. E., Waldron, M., Kitzmann, K. M., & Aaron, J. (1999). Delinquent behavior, future divorce or nonmarital childbearing, and externalizing behavior among offspring: A 14-year prospective study. *Journal of Family Psychology, 13*, 568–579.

Endicott, J., & Spitzer, R. L. (1978). A diagnostic interview: The Schedule for Affective Disorders and Schizophrenia. *Archives of General Psychiatry, 35*, 837–844.

Erel, O., & Burman, B. (1995). Interrelations of marital relations and parent–child relations: A meta-analytic review. *Psychological Bulletin, 188*, 108–132.

Erickson, M. F., Egeland, B., & Pianta, R. (1989). The effects of maltreatment on the development of young children. In D. Cicchetti & S. Toth (Eds.), *Child maltreatment: Theory and research on the causes and consequences of child abuse and neglect* (pp. 647–684). Cambridge, UK: Cambridge University Press.

Eyberg, S. M., Boggs, S., & Algina, J. (1995). Parent–child interaction therapy: A psychosocial model for the treatment of young children with conduct problem behavior and their families. *Psychopharmacology Bulletin, 31*, 83–91.

Fabes, R. A., Eisenberg, N., & Eisenbud, L. (1993). Behavioral and physiological correlates of children's reactions to others in distress. *Developmental Psychology, 29*, 655–663.

Fabes, R. A., Eisenberg, N., Smith, M. C., & Murphy, B. C. (1996). Getting angry at peers: Associations with liking of the provocateur. *Child Development, 67*, 942–956.

Farber, E. A., & Egeland, B. (1987). Invulnerability among abused and neglected children. In E. J. Anthony & B. J. Cohler (Eds.), *The invulnerable child* (pp. 253–288). New York: Guilford Press.

Fauber, R. E., Forehand, R., Thomas, A. M., & Wierson, M. (1990). A mediational model of the impact of marital conflict on adolescent adjustment in intact and divorced families: The role of disrupted parenting. *Child Development, 61*, 1112–1123.

Feldman, S., & Downey, G. (1994). Rejection sensitivity as a mediator of the impact of childhood exposure to family violence on adult attachment behavior. *Development and Psychopathology, 6*, 231–247.

Fendrich, M., Warner, V., & Weissman, M. M. (1990). Family risk factors, parental depression, and psychopathology in offspring. *Developmental Psychology, 26*, 40–50.

Fergusson, D. M., & Horwood, L. J. (1996). The role of adolescent peer affiliations in the continuity between childhood behavioral adjustment and juvenile offending. *Journal of Abnormal Child Psychology, 24*, 205–221.

Fergusson, D. M., Horwood, L. J., & Lynskey, M. T. (1995). Maternal depressive symptoms and depressive symptoms in adolescents. *Journal of Child Psychology and Psychiatry, 36*, 1161–1178.

Fergusson, D. M., & Lynskey, M. T. (1993). The effect of maternal depression on child conduct disorder and attention deficit behaviours. *Social Psychiatry and Psychiatric Epidemiology, 28*, 116–123.

Fergusson, D. M., & Lynskey, M. T. (1997). Physical punishment/maltreatment during childhood and adjustment in young adulthood. *Child Abuse and Neglect, 21*, 617–630.

Field, T. (1992). Infants of depressed mothers. *Development and Psychopathology, 4,* 49–66.

Field, T., Fox, N., Pickens, J., & Nawrocki, T. (1995). Relative right frontal EEG activation in 3- to 6-month-old infants of "depressed" mothers. *Developmental Psychology, 31,* 358–363.

Field, T., Pickens, J., Fox, N. A., Nawrocki, T., & Gonzalez, J. (1995). Vagal tone in infants of depressed mothers. *Development and Psychopathology, 7,* 227–231.

Field, T. M. (1984). Early interactions between infants and their postpartum depressed mothers. *Infant Behavior and Development, 7,* 517–522.

Fillmore, K. M. (1985). The social victims of drinking. *British Journal of Addiction, 80,* 307–314.

Fillmore, K. M., & Midanik, L. (1984). Chronicity of drinking problems among men: A longitudinal study. *Journal of Studies of Alcohol, 45,* 228–236.

Fincham, F. D. (1994). Understanding the association between marital conflict and child adjustment: Overview. *Journal of Family Psychology, 8,* 123–127.

Fincham, F. D. (1998). Child development and marital relations. *Child Development, 69,* 543–574.

Fincham, F. D., Beach, S. R. H., Harold, G. T., & Osborne, L. N. (1997). Marital satisfaction and depression: Different causal relationships for men and women? *Psychological Science, 8,* 351–357.

Fincham, F. D., Grych, J. H., & Osborne, L. N. (1994). Does marital conflict cause child maladjustment? Directions and challenges for longitudinal research. *Journal of Family Psychology, 8,* 128–140.

Fincham, F. D., & Osborne, L. N. (1993). Marital conflict and children: Retrospect and prospect. *Clinical Child Psychology, 13,* 75–88.

Finnegan, R. A., Hodges, E. V. E., & Perry, D. G. (1996). Preoccupied and avoidant coping during middle childhood. *Child Development, 67,* 1318–1328.

Fogas, B. S., Wolchik, S. A., Braver, S. L., Freedom, D. S., & Bay, X. (1992). Locus of control as a mediator of negative divorce-related events and adjustment problems in children. *American Journal of Orthopsychiatry, 62,* 589–598.

Folkman, S. (1991). Coping across the lifespan: Theoretical issues. In E. M. Cummings, A. Greene, & K. Karraker (Eds.), *Lifespan developmental psychology: Perspectives on stress and coping* (pp. 3–20). Hillsdale, NJ: Erlbaum.

Forehand, R., Lautenschlager, G. J., Faust, J., & Graziano, W. G. (1986). Parent perceptions and parent–child interactions in clinic-referred children: A preliminary investigation of the effects of maternal depressive moods. *Behaviour Research and Therapy, 24,* 73–75.

Forehand, R. L., & McMahon, R. J. (1981). *Helping the noncompliant child: A clinician's guide to parent training.* New York: Guilford Press.

Forehand, R., Wierson, M., Thomas, A. M., Armistead, L., Kempton, T., & Neighbors, B. (1991). The role of family stressors and parent reltionships on adolescent functioning. *Journal of the American Academy of Child and Adolescent Psychiatry, 30,* 316–322.

Fox, N. A. (1989). Psychophysiological correlates of emotional reactivity during the first year of life. *Developmental Psychology, 25,* 364–372.

Fox, N. A. (1994). Dynamic cerebral processes underlying emotion regulation. In N. A. Fox (Ed.), The development of emotion regulation: Biological and behavioral considerations. *Monographs of the Society for Research in Child Development, 59*(2–3, Serial No. 240), 152–166.

Fox, N. A., Calkins, S. D., & Bell, M. A. (1994). Neural plasticity and development in the first two years of life: Evidence from cognitive and socioemotional domains of research. *Development and Psychopathology, 6*, 677–696.

Fox, N. A., & Card, J. A. (1999). Psychophysiological measures in the study of attachment. In J. Cassidy & P. R. Shaver (Eds.), *Handbook of attachment: Theory, research, and clinical applications* (pp. 226–245). New York: Guilford Press.

Fuhrman, T., & Holmbeck, G. N. (1995). A contextual–moderator analysis of emotional autonomy and adjustment in adolescence. *Child Development, 66*, 793–811.

Fuligni, A. J., & Eccles, J. S. (1993). Perceived parent–child relationships and early adolescents' orientation toward peers. *Developmental Psychology, 29*, 622–632.

Fullinwider-Bush, N., & Jacobitz, D. B. (1993). The transition to young adulthood: Generational boundary dissolution and female identity development. *Family Process, 32*, 87–103.

Furman, W., & Wehner, E. A. (1994). Romantic views: Toward a theory of adolescent romantic relationships. In R. Montemayor & G. R. Adams (Eds.), *Personal relationships during adolescence: Vol. 6. Advances in adolescent development: An annual book series* (pp. 168–195). Newbury Park, CA: Sage.

Gable, S., Belsky, J., & Crnic, K. (1995). Coparenting during the child's 2nd year: A descriptive account. *Journal of Marriage and the Family, 57*, 609–616.

Garber, J. (1984). Classification of child psychopathology: A developmental perspective. *Child Development, 55*, 30–48.

Garber, J., Braafladt, N., & Zeman, B. (1991a). Affect regulation in depressed and nondepressed children and young adolescents. *Development and Psychopathology, 7*, 93–115.

Garber, J., Braafladt, N., & Zeman, J. (1991b). The regulation of sad affect: An information processing perspective. In J. Garber & K. A. Dodge (Eds.), *The development of emotion regulation and dysregulation* (pp. 208–240). New York: Cambridge University Press.

Garbutt, J. C., Mayo, J. P., Little, K. Y., Gillette, G. M., Mason, G. A., Dew, B., & Prange, A. J. (1994). Dose–response studies with protirelin. *Archives of General Psychiatry, 51*, 875–883.

Garcia-O'Hearn, C., Margolin, G., & John, R. (1997). Mothers' and fathers' reports of children's reactions to naturalistic marital conflict. *Journal of the American Academy of Child and Adolescent Psychiatry, 36*, 1366–1373.

Gardner, F. E. (1987). Positive interaction between mothers and conduct-problem children: Is there training for harmony as well as fighting? *Journal of Abnormal Child Psychology, 15*, 283–293.

Gardner, F. E. (1989). Inconsistent parenting: Is there evidence for a link with children's conduct problems? *Journal of Abnormal Child Psychology, 17*, 223–233.

Garmezy, N. (1985). Stress-resistant children: The search for protective factors. In J. E. Stevenson (Ed.), Recent research in developmental psychopathology. *Journal of Child Psychology and Psychiatry Book* (Suppl. 4, pp. 213–233). Oxford, UK: Pergamon Press.

Garmezy, N., & Masten, A. (1991). The protective role of competence indicators in children at risk. In E. M. Cummings, A. L. Greene, & K. K. Karraker (Eds.), *Life-span developmental psychology: Perspectives on stress and coping* (pp. 151–176). Hillsdale, NJ: Erlbaum.

Garmezy, N., Masten, A. S., & Tellegen, A. (1984). The study of stress and competence in children: A building block for developmental psychopathology. *Child Development, 55*, 97–111.

Garmezy, N., & Rutter, M. (1983). *Stress, coping, and development in children.* New York: McGraw-Hill.

Gassner, S., & Murray E. J. (1969). Dominance and conflict in the interaction between parents of normal and neurotic children. *Journal of Abnormal Psychology, 74,* 33–41.

Ge, X., Conger, R. D., Lorenz, F. O., Shanahan, M., & Elder, G. H. (1995). Mutual influences in parent and adolescent psychological distress. *Developmental Psychology, 31,* 406–419.

Gelfand, D. M., & Teti, D. M. (1990). The effects of maternal depression on children. *Clinical Psychology Review, 10,* 329–353.

Geller, J., & Johnson, C. (1995). Depressed mood and child conduct problems: Relationships to mothers' attributions for their own and their children's experiences. *Child and Family Behavior Therapy, 17,* 19–34.

Giovannoni, J., & Becerra, R. M. (1979). *Defining child abuse.* New York: Free Press.

Gittelman-Klein, R. (1986). Questioning the clinical usefulness of projective psychological tests for children. *Developmental and Behavioral Pediatrics, 7,* 378–382.

Glenn, N. D. (1998). Problems and prospects in longitudinal research on marriage: A sociologists perspective. In T. N. Bradbury (Ed.), *The developmental course of marital dysfunction* (pp. 427–440). Cambridge, UK: Cambridge University Press.

Glick, J. A. (1992). Werner's relevance for contemporary developmental psychology. *Developmental Psychology, 28,* 558–565.

Glick, M. (1997). The developmental approach to adult psychopathology. In S. S. Luthar, J. A. Burack, D. Cicchetti, & J. R. Weisz (Eds.), *Developmental psychopathology: Perspectives on adjustment, risk, and disorder* (pp. 227–247). New York: Cambridge University Press.

Gold, P., Goodwin, F., & Chrousos, G. (1988). Clinical and biochemical manifestations of depression: Relation to the neurobiology of stress (Part 1). *New England Journal of Medicine, 319,* 348–353.

Goldberg, W. A., & Easterbrooks, M. A. (1984). The role of marital quality in toddler development. *Developmental Psychology, 20,* 504–514.

Gonzales, N. A., Cauce, A. M., Friedman, R. J., & Mason, C. A. (1996). Family, peer, and neighborhood influences on academic achievement among African-American adolescents: One-year prospective effects. *American Journal of Community Psychology, 24,* 365–387.

Goodman, S. H., Adamson, L. B., Riniti, J., & Cole, S. (1994). Mothers' expressed attitudes: Associations with maternal depression and children's self-esteem and psychopathology. *Journal of the American Academy of Child and Adolescent Psychiatry, 33,* 1265–1274.

Goodwin, F., & Jamison, K. (1990). *Manic depressive illness.* New York: Oxford University Press.

Goodyer, I. M. (1990). *Life experiences, development, and childhood psychopathology.* Chichester, UK: Wiley.

Gordis, E. B., Margolin, G., & John, R. (1997). Marital aggression, observed parental hostility, and child behavior during triadic family interaction. *Journal of Family Psychology, 11,* 76–89.

Gotlib, I. H. (1982). Self-reinforcement and depression in interpersonal interaction: The role of performance level. *Journal of Abnormal Psychology, 93,* 19–30.

Gotlib, I. H., & Asarnow, R. F. (1979). Interpersonal and impersonal problem-solving skills in mildly and clinically depressed students. *Journal of Consulting and Clinical Psychology, 47,* 86–95.

Gotlib, I. H., & Robinson, L. A. (1982). Responses to depressed individuals: Discrepancies between self-report and observer-rated behavior. *Journal of Abnormal Psychology, 91*, 231–240.

Gottlieb, G. (1991a). Epigenetic systems view of human development. *Developmental Psychology, 27*, 33–34.

Gottlieb, G. (1991b). Experiential canalization of behavioral development: Theory. *Development Psychology, 27*, 4–13.

Gottman, J. M. (1994). *Why marriages succeed or fail.* New York: Simon & Schuster.

Gottman, J. M., Katz, L. F., & Hooven, C. (1996). Parental meta-emotion philosophy and the emotional life of families: Theoretical models and preliminary data. *Journal of Family Psychology, 10*, 243–268.

Gottman, J. M., Katz, L. F., & Hooven, C. (1997). *Meta-emotion: How families communicate emotionally.* Mahwah, NJ: Erlbaum.

Graber, J. A., & Brooks-Gunn, J. (1996). Transitions and turning points: Navigating the passage from childhood through adolescence. *Developmental Psychology, 32*, 768–776.

Granger, D. A., Weisz, J. R., McCracken, J. M., Ikeda, S. C., & Douglas, P. (1996). Reciprocal influences among adrenocortical activation, psychosocial processes, and the behavioral adjustment of clinic-referred children. *Child Development, 67*, 3250–3262.

Greenberg, M. T., Cicchetti, D., & Cummings, E. M. (1990a). History of a collaboration in the study of attachment. In M. Greenberg, D. Cicchetti, & M. Cummings (Eds.), *Attachment in the preschool years: Theory, research, and intervention* (pp. xiii–xix). Chicago: University of Chicago Press.

Greenberg, M. T., Cicchetti, D., & Cummings, E. M. (Eds.). (1990b). *Attachment during the preschool years: Theory, research, and intervention.* Chicago: University of Chicago Press.

Greenberg, M. T., Leguna, L. J., Coie, J. D., & Pinderhughes, E. E. (1999). Predicting developmental outcomes at school entry using a multiple-risk model: Four American communities. *Developmental Psychology, 35*, 403–417.

Greenberg, M. T., Speltz, M. L., & DeKlyen, M. (1993). The role of attachment in the early development of disruptive behavior problems. *Development and Psychopathology, 5*, 191–214.

Greenough, W. T. (1991). Experience as a component of normal development: Evolutionary considerations. *Developmental Psychology, 27*, 14–17.

Grolnick, W. S., & Slowiaczek, M. L. (1994). Parents' involvement in children's schooling: A multidimensional conceptualization and motivational model. *Child Development, 65*, 237–252.

Grossmann, K., Grossmann, K. E., Spangler, G., Suess, G., & Unzner, L. (1985). Maternal sensitivity and newborns' orientation responses as related to quality of attachment in northern Germany. In I. Bretherton & E. Waters (Eds.), Growing points in attachment theory and research. *Monographs of the Society for Research in Child Development, 50* (Serial No. 209), 233–257.

Grossmann, K. E., & Grossmann, K. (1990). The wider concept of attachment in cross-cultural research. *Human Development, 33*, 31–47.

Grusec, J. E., Dix, T., & Mills, R. (1982). The effects of type, severity, and victim of children's transgressions on maternal discipline. *Canadian Journal of Behavioural Science, 14*, 276–289.

Grusec, J. E., & Goodnow, J. J. (1994a). Impact of parental discipline methods on the child's internalization of values: A reconceptualization of current points of view. *Developmental Psychology, 30,* 4–19.

Grusec, J. E., & Goodnow, J. J. (1994b). Summing up and looking to the future. *Developmental Psychology, 30,* 29–31.

Grych, J. H. (1998). Children's appraisals of interparental conflict: situational and contextual influences. *Journal of Family Psychology, 12,* 437–453.

Grych, J. H., & Fincham, F. (1990). Marital conflict and children's adjustment: A cognitive–contextual framework. *Psychological Bulletin, 108,* 267–290.

Grych, J. H., & Fincham, F. (1993). Children's appraisals of marital conflict: Initial investigations of the cognitive–contextual framework. *Child Development, 64,* 215–230.

Grych, J., Seid, M., & Fincham, F. (1992). Assessing marital conflict from the child's perspective: The children's perceptions of intrerparental conflict scale. *Child Development, 63,* 558–572.

Gunnar, M. R., Porter, F., Wolf, C., Rigatuso, J., & Larson, M. (1995). Neonatal stress reactivity: Predictions to later emotional temperament. *Child Development, 66,* 1–13.

Haley, J. (1976). *Problem-solving therapy.* New York: Harper & Row.

Hall, E., & Cummings, E. M. (1997). The effects of marital and parent-child conflicts on other family members: Grandmothers and grown children. *Family Relations, 46,* 135–144.

Hall, E. J. (1997). *The relation of adult attachment and family conflict.* Unpublished doctoral dissertation, West Virginia University, Morgantown.

Hamilton, C. E. (in press). Continuity and discontinuity of attachment from infancy. *Child Development.*

Hamilton, E. B., Jones, M., & Hammen, C. (1993). Maternal interaction style in affective disordered, physically ill, and normal women. *Family Process, 32,* 329–340.

Hammen, C. L., Burge, D., Daley, S. E., Davila, J., Paley, B., & Rudolph, K. (1995). Interpersonal attachment cognitions and prediction of symptomatic responses to interpersonal stress. *Journal of Abnormal Psychology, 104,* 436–443.

Hardy, J. B., Astone, N. M., Brooks-Gunn, J., Shapiro, S., & Miller, T. L. (1998). Like mother, like child: Intergenerational patterns of age at first birth and associations with childhood and adolescent characteristics and adult outcomes in the second generation. *Developmental Psychology, 34,* 1220–1232.

Harlow, H. F. (1958). The nature of love. *American Psychologist, 13,* 673–685.

Harnish, J. D., Dodge, K. A., Valente, E., and the Conduct Problems Prevention Research Group. (1995). Mother–child interaction quality as a partial mediator of the roles of maternal depressive symptomatology and socioeconomic status in the development of child behavior problems. *Child Development, 66,* 739–753.

Harold, G. T., & Conger, R. D. (1997). Marital conflict and adolescent distress: The role of adolescent awareness. *Child Development, 68,* 333–350.

Harold, G. T., Fincham, F. D., Osborne, L. N., & Conger, R. D. (1997). Mom and dad are at it again: Adolescent perceptions of marital conflict and adolescent psychological distress. *Developmental Psychology, 33,* 333–350.

Harrington, R. C., Bredenkamp, D., Groothues, C., Rutter, M., Fudge, H., & Pickles, A. (1994). Adult outcomes of childhood and adolescent depression. III. Links with suicidal behaviours. *Journal of Child Psychology and Psychiatry, 35,* 1309–1319.

Harrington, R. C., Fudge, H., Rutter, M., Bredenkamp, D., Groothues, C., & Pridham, J.

(1993). Child and adult depression: a test of continuities with data from a family study. *British Journal of Psychiatry, 162,* 627–633.

Harrington, R. C., Fudge, H., Rutter, M., Pickles, A., & Hill, J. (1991). Adult outcomes of childhood and adolescent depression: II. Links with antisocial disorders. *Journal of the American Academy of Child and Adolescent Psychiatry, 30,* 434–439.

Harrington, R., Rutter, M., & Fombonne, E. (1996). Developmental pathways in depression: Multiple meanings, antecedents, and endpoints. *Development and Psychopathology, 8,* 601–616.

Harrington, R., Rutter, M., Weissman, M., Fudge, H., Groothues, C., Bredenkamp, D., Pickles, A., Rende, R., & Wickramaratne, P. (1997). Psychiatric disorders in the relatives of depressed probands: I. Comparison of prepubertal adolescent and early adult onset cases. *Journal of Affective Disorders, 42,* 9–22.

Harris, J. R. (1995). Where is the child's environment? A group socialization theory of development. *Psychological Review, 102,* 458–489.

Hart, C. H., DeWolf, M., & Burts, D. C. (1993). Parental disciplinary strategies and preschoolers' play behavior in playground settings. In C. H. Hart (Ed.), *Children on playgrounds: Research perspectives and applications* (pp. 271–313). Albany: State University of New York Press.

Hart, J., Gunnar, M., & Cicchetti, D. (1995). Salivary cortisol in maltreated children: Evidence of relations between neuroendocrine activity and social competence. *Development and Psychopathology, 7,* 11–26.

Hart, J., Gunnar, M., & Cicchetti, D. (1996). Altered neuroendocrine activity in maltreated children related to symptoms of depression. *Development and Psychopathology, 8,* 201–214.

Hauser, S. T., Powers, S. I., & Noam, G. G. (1991). *Adolescents and their families: Paths of ego development.* New York: Free Press.

Hauser, S. T., Vieyra, M. A., Jacobson, A. M., & Wertlieb, D. (1985). Vulnerability and resilience in adolescence: Views from the family. *Journal of Early Adolescence, 5,* 81–100.

Hawkins, J. D., Catalano, R. F., & Miller, J. Y. (1992). Risk and protective factors for alcohol and other drug problems in adolescence and early adulthood: Implications for substance abuse prevention. *Psychological Bulletin, 112,* 64–105.

Hayden, L. C., Schiller, M. Dickstein, S., Seifer, R., Sameroff, A. J., Miller, I., Keitner, G., & Rasmussen, S. (1998). Levels of family assessment: I. Family, marital, and parent–child interaction. *Journal of Family Psychology, 12,* 7–22.

Hazan, C., & Shaver, P. R. (1990). Love and work: An attachment–theoretical perspective. *Journal of Personality and Social Psychology, 59,* 270–280.

Hazelrigg, M. D., Cooper, H. M., & Borduin, C. M. (1987). Evaluating the effectiveness of family therapies: An integrative review and analysis. *Psychological Bulletin, 101,* 428–442.

Hebb, D. O. (1949). *The organization of behavior: A neuropsychological theory.* New York: Wiley.

Heinicke, C. M. (1995). Expanding the study of the formation of the child's relationship. In E. Waters, B. E. Vaughn, G. Posada, & K. Kondo-Ikemura (Eds.), Caregiving, cultural, and cognitive perspectives on secure-base behavior and working models: New growing points of attachment theory and research. *Monographs of the Society for Research in Child Development, 60*(2–3, Serial No. 244), 300–309.

Henggeler, S., Melton, G. B., & Smith, L. A. (1992). Family preservation using multisystemic therapy: An effective alternative to incarcerating serious juvenile offenders. *Journal of Consulting and Clinical Psychology, 60,* 953–961.

Henggeler, S. W., Schoenwald, S. K., & Pickrel, S. G. (1995). Multisystemic therapy: Bridging the gap between university- and community-based treatment. *Journal of Consulting and Clinical Psychology, 63,* 709–717.

Hennessy, K., Rabideau, G., Cicchetti, D., & Cummings, E. M. (1994). Responses of physically abused children to different forms of interadult anger. *Child Development, 65,* 815–828.

Herman, M. R., Dornbusch, S. M., Herron, M. C., & Herting, J. R. (1997). The influence of family regulation, connection, and psychological autonomy on six measures of adolescent functioning. *Journal of Adolescent Research, 12,* 34–67.

Hetherington, E. M. (1989). Coping with family transitions: Winners, losers, and survivors. *Child Development, 60,* 1–14.

Hetherington, E. M., Bridges, M., & Insabella, G. M. (1998). What matters? What does not? Five perspectives on the association between marital transitions and children's adjustment. *American Psychologist, 53,* 167–184.

Hetherington, E. M., & Clingempeel, W. G. (1992). Coping with marital transitions: A family systems perspective. *Monographs of the Society for Research in Child Development,57*(2–3, Serial number 227).

Hetherington, E. M., Henderson, S. H., & Reiss, D. (1999). Adolescent siblings in stepfamilies: Family functioning and adolescent adjustment. *Monographs of the Society for Research in Child Development, 57*(2–3, Serial No. 227).

Hetherington, E., & Martin, B. (1986). Family factors and psychopathology in children. In H. C. Quay & J. S. Werry (Eds.), *Psychopathological disorders of childhood* (3rd ed., pp. 332–391). New York: Wiley.

Hetherington, E. M., Stanley-Hagan, M., & Anderson, E. R. (1989). Marital transitions: A child's perspective. *American Psychologist, 44,* 303–312.

Hill, J. P., & Lynch, M. E. (1983). The intensification of gender-related role expectations during early adolescence. In J. Brooks-Gunn & A. C. Petersen (Eds.), *Girls at puberty: Biological and psychosocial perspectives* (pp. 201–228). New York: Plenum Press.

Hinde, R. A. (1992). Developmental psychology in the context of other behavioral sciences. *Developmental Psychology, 28,* 1018–1029.

Hinshaw, S. P. (1987). On the distinction between attentional deficits/hyperactivity and conduct problems/aggression in child psychopathology. *Psychological Bulletin, 101,* 443–463.

Hinshaw, S. P. (1994). *Attention deficits and hyperactivity in children.* Thousand Oaks, CA: Sage.

Hinshaw, S. P., Lahey, B. B., & Hart, E. (1993). Issues of taxonomy and comorbidity in the development of conduct disorder. *Development and Psychopathology, 5,* 31–49.

Hirschi, T. (1969). *Causes of delinquency.* Berkeley: University of California Press.

Hodges, K., Cools, J., & McKnew, D. (1989). Test-retest reliability of a clinical research interview for children: The Child Assessment Schedule. *Psychological Assessment, 1,* 317–322.

Hodges, K., Saunders, W. B., Kashani, J., Hamlett, K., & Thompson, R. J. (1990). Internal consistency of DSM-III diagnoses using the symptom scales of the Child Assessment Schedule. *Journal of the American Academy of Child and Adolescent Psychiatry, 29,* 635–641.

Hoffman, M. L. (1960). Power assertion by the parent and its impact on the child. *Child Development*, *31*, 129–143.

Hoffman, M. L. (1970). Conscience, personality, and socialization techniques. *Human Development*, *13*, 90–126.

Hoffman, M. L. (1983). Affective and cognitive processes in moral internalization: An information processing approach. In E. T. Higgins, D. Ruble, & W. Hartup (Eds.), *Social cognition and social development: A sociocultural perspective* (pp. 236–274). Cambridge, UK: Cambridge University Press.

Hoffman, M. L. (1994). Discipline and internalization. *Developmental Psychology*, *30*, 26–28.

Hoffman, M. L., & Saltzstein, H. D. (1967). Parent discipline and the child's moral development. *Journal of Personality and Social Psychology*, *5*, 45–57.

Hoffman-Plotkin, D., & Twentyman, C. T. (1984). A multimodal assessment of behavioral and cognitive deficits in abused and neglected preschoolers. *Child Development*, *55*, 794–802.

Hogue, A., & Steinberg, L. (1995). Homophily of internalized distress in adolescent peer groups. *Developmental Psychology*, *31*, 897–906.

Holden, G. W., & Miller, P. C. (1999). Enduring and different: A meta-analysis of the similarity in parents' child rearing. *Psychological Bulletin*, *125*, 223–254.

Holden, G. W., & Ritchie, K. L. (1991). Linking extreme marital discord, child rearing, and child behavior problems: Evidence from battered women. *Child Development*, *62*, 311–327.

Holden, G. W., Stein, J. D., Ritchie, K. L., Harris, S. D., & Jouriles, E. N. (1998). Parenting behaviors and beliefs of battered women. In G. W. Holden, R. A. Geffner, & E. N. Jouriles (Eds.), *Children exposed to marital violence: Theory, research, and applied issues* (pp. 289–334). Washington, DC: American Psychological Association.

Holmbeck, G. N. (1996). A model of family relational transformations during the transition to adolescence: Parent–adolescent conflict and adaptation. In J. A. Graber, J. Brooks-Gunn, & A. C. Petersen (Eds.), *Transitions through adolescence: Interpersonal domains and context* (pp. 167–199). Mahwah, NJ: Erlbaum.

Holmbeck, G. N. (1997). Toward terminology, conceptual, and statistical clarity in the study of mediators and moderators: Examples from the child clinical and pediatric psychology literatures. *Journal of Consulting and Clinical Psychology*, *65*, 599–610.

Holmbeck, G. N., Paikoff, G. N., & Brooks-Gunn, J. (1995). Parenting adolescents. In M. H. Bornstein (Ed.), *Handbook of parenting: Vol. 1. Children and parenting* (pp. 91–118). Mahwah, NJ: Erlbaum.

Hooley, J. M. (1986). Expressed emotion and depression: Interactions between patients and high versus low-expressed emotion spouses. *Journal of Abnormal Psychology*, *95*, 237–246.

Hooley, J. M., & Teasdale, J. D. (1989). Predictors of relapse in unipolar depressives: Expressed emotion, marital distress, and perceived criticism. *Journal of Abnormal Psychology*, *98*, 229–237.

Hops, H. (1995). Age- and gender-specific effects of parental depression: A commentary. *Developmental Psychology*, *31*, 428–431.

Hops, H. (in press). Intergenerational transmission of depressive symptoms: Gender and developmental considerations. In C. Mundt, M. Goldstein, K. Hahlweg, & P. Fiedler (Eds.), *Proceedings of the Symposium of Interpersonal Factors in the Origin and Course of Affective Disorders*. London: Royal College of Psychiatrists.

Hops, H., Biglan, A., Sherman, L., Arthur, J., Friedman, L., & Osteen, R. (1987). Home observations of family interactions of depressed women. *Journal of Consulting and Clinical Psychology, 55,* 341–346.

Hops, H., Sherman, L., & Biglan, A. (1990). Maternal depression, marital discord, and children's behavior: A developmental perspective. In G. R. Patterson (Ed.), *Depression and aggression in family interaction* (pp. 185–208). Hillsdale, NJ: Erlbaum.

Howes, P., & Markman, H. J. (1989). Marital quality and child functioning: A longitudinal investigation. *Child Development, 60,* 1044–1051.

Huesmann, L. R., Eron, L. D., Lefkowitz, M. M., & Walder, L. O. (1984). Stability of aggression over time and generations. *Developmental Psychology, 20,* 1120–1134.

Huffman, L. C., Bryan, Y. E., del Carmen, R., Pedersen, F. A., Doussard-Roosevelt, J. A., & Porges, S. A. (1998). Infant temperament and cardiac vagal tone: Assessments at twelve weeks of age. *Child Development, 69,* 624–635.

Hunt, J. M. (1961). *Intelligence and experience.* New York: Ronald Press.

Hussong, A. M., & Chassin, L. (1997). Substance use initiation among adolescent children of alcoholics: Testing protective factors. *Journal of Studies on Alcohol, 58,* 272–279.

Huston, A. C., McLoyd, V. C., & Garcia Coll, C. (1994). Children and poverty: Issues in contemporary research. *Child Development, 65,* 275–282.

Isabella, R. A., Belsky, J., & von Eye, A. (1989). Origins of infant–mother attachment: An examination of interactional synchrony during the infant's first year. *Developmental Psychology, 25,* 12–21.

Jackson, J. F. (1993). Multiple caregivers among African Americans and infant attachment: The need for an emic approach. *Human Development, 36,* 87–102.

Jacobson, N. S., Fruzzetti, A. E., Dobson, K., Whisman, M., & Hops, H. (1993). Couple therapy as a treatment for depression: 2. The effects of relationship quality and therapy on depressive relapse. *Journal of Consulting and Clinical Psychology, 57,* 5–10.

Jacobvitz, D., Morgan, E., Kretchmar, M., & Morgan, Y. (1992). The transmission of mother–child boundary disturbances across three generations. *Development and Psychopathology, 3,* 513–527.

Jacobvitz, D., & Sroufe, L. A. (1987). The early caregiver–child relationship and attention-deficit disorder with hyperactivity in kindergarten: A prospective study. *Child Development, 58,* 1488–1495.

Jaffe, P. G., Wolfe, D. A., & Wilson, S. K. (1990). *Children of battered women.* Newbury Park, CA: Sage.

Jaffe, P., Wolfe, D., Wilson, S. K., & Zak, L. (1986). Family violence and child adjustment: A comparative analysis of girls' and boys' behavioral symptoms. *American Journal of Psychiatry, 143,* 74–77.

Jenkins, J. M., & Smith, M. A. (1991). Marital disharmony and children's behaviour problems: Aspects of a poor marriage that affect children adversely. *Journal of Child Psychology and Psychiatry, 32,* 793–810.

Jensen, P. S., & Hoagwood, K. (1997). The book of names: DSM-IV in context. *Development and Psychopathology, 9,* 231–250.

Johnson, J. E., & McGillicudy-Dilisi, A. (1983). Family environment factors and children's knowledge of rules and conventions. *Child Development, 54,* 218–226.

Joiner, T. E. (1995). The price of soliciting and receiving negative feedback: Self-verification theory as a vulnerability to depression theory. *Journal of Abnormal Psychology, 104,* 364–372.

Joiner, T. E., & Metalsky, G. I. (1995). A prospective test of an integrative interpersonal theory of depression: A naturalistic study of college roommates. *Journal of Personality and Social Psychology, 69,* 778–788.

Josephs, R. A., Markus, H. R., & Tafarodi, R. W. (1992). Gender and self-esteem. *Journal of Personality and Social Psychology, 63,* 391–402.

Jouriles, E. N., Barling, J., & O'Leary, K. D. (1987). Predicting child behavior problems in maritally violent families. *Journal of Abnormal Child Psychology, 15,* 165–173.

Jouriles, E. N., Bourg, W., & Farris, A. (1991). Marital adjustment and child conduct problems: A comparison of the correlation across samples. *Journal of Consulting and Clinical Psychology, 59,* 354–357.

Jouriles, E. N., & Farris, A. M. (1992). Effects of marital conflict on subsequent parent–son interactions. *Behavior Therapy, 23,* 355–374.

Jouriles, E. N., McDonald, R., & Norwood, W. D. (1998). Knives, guns, and interparent violence: Relations with child behavior problems. *Journal of Family Psychology, 12,* 178–194.

Jouriles, E. N., McDonald, R., Stephens, N., Norwood, W., Spiller, L. C., & Ware, H. S. (1998). Breaking the cycle of violence: Helping families departing from battered women's shelters. In G. W. Holden, R. A. Geffner, & E. N. Jouriles (Eds.), *Children exposed to marital violence: Theory, research, and applied issues* (pp. 337–369). Washington, DC: American Psychological Association.

Kagan, J., Reznick, S., & Snidman, N. (1987). The physiology and psychology of behavioral inhibition in children. *Child Development, 58,* 1459–1473.

Kagan, J., Reznick, S., & Snidman, N. (1988). Biological bases of childhood shyness. *Science, 240,* 167–171.

Karney, B. R., & Bradbury, T. N. (1995). The longitudinal course of marital quality and stability: A review of theory, methods, and research. *Psychological Bulletin, 118,* 3–34.

Kaslow, N. J., & Thompson, M. P. (1998). Applying the criteria for empirically supported treatments to studies of psychosocial interventions for child and adolescent depression. *Journal of Clinical Child Psychology, 27,* 146–155.

Katz, J., & Beach, S. R. H. (1997). Self-verification and depressive symptoms in marriage and courtship: A multiple pathway model. *Journal of Marriage and the Family, 59,* 903–914.

Katz, L. F., & Gottman, J. M. (1995a). Vagal tone protects children from marital conflict. *Development and Psychopathology, 7,* 83–92.

Katz, L. F., & Gottman, J. M. (1995b, April). *Marital conflict and child adjustment: Father's parenting as a mediator of children's negative peer play.* Paper presented at the Meetings of the Society for Research in Child Development, Indianapolis, IN.

Katz, L. F., & Gottman, J. M. (1997a). Buffering children from marital conflict and dissolution. *Journal of Clinical Child Psychology, 26,* 157–171.

Katz, L. F., & Gottman, J. (1997b, April). *Positive parenting and regulatory physiology as buffers from marital conflict and dissolution.* Paper presented at the biennial metting of the Society for Research in Child Development, Washington, DC.

Kaufman, J., Cook, A., Arny, L., Jones, B., & Pittinsky, T. (1994). Problems defining resiliency: Illustrations from the study of maltreated children. *Development and Psychopathology, 6,* 215–229.

Kaufman, J., & Zigler, E. F. (1989). The intergenerational transmission of child abuse. In D. Cicchetti & V. Carlson (Eds.), *Child maltreatment: Theory and research on the causes and consequences of child abuse and neglect* (pp. 129–150). New York: Cambridge University Press.

Kazdin, A. E. (1993). Treatment of conduct disorder: Progress and directions in psychotherapy research. *Development and Psychopathology, 5,* 277–310.

Kazdin, A. E. (1994). Interventions for aggressive and antisocial children. In L. D. Eron, J. H. Gentry, & P. Schlegel (Eds.), *Reason to hope: A psychosocial perspective on violence and youth* (pp. 341–3820. Washington, DC: American Psychological Association.

Kazdin, A. E. (1995). *Conduct disorder in children and adolescents* (2nd ed.). Newbury Park, CA: Sage.

Kazdin, A. E. (1997a). A model for developing effective treatments: Progression and interplay of theory, research, and practice. *Journal of Clinical Child Psychology, 26,* 114–129.

Kazdin, A. E. (1997b). Conduct disorder across the life-span. In S. S. Luthar, J. A. Burack, D. Cicchetti, & J. R. Weisz (Eds.), *Developmental psychopathology: Perspectives on adjustment, risk, and disorder* (pp. 248–272). New York: Cambridge University Press.

Kazdin, A. E., Siegel, T. C., & Bass, D. (1990). Drawing upon clinical practice to inform research on child and adolescent psychotherapy. *Professional Psychology: Research and Practice, 21,* 189–190.

Kazdin, A. E. Mazurick, J. L., & Siegel, T. C. (1994). Treatment outcome among children with externalizing disorder who terminate prematurely versus those who complete psychotherapy. *Journal of the American Academy of Child and Adolescent Psychiatry, 33,* 549–557.

Kazdin, A. E. (1994). Interventions for aggressive and antisocial children. In L. D. Eron, J. H. Gentry, & P. Schlegel (Eds.), *Reason to hope: A psychosocial perspective on violence and youth* (pp. 341–382). Washington, DC: American Psychological Association.

Keenan, K., & Shaw, D. S. (1996). Developmental and social influences on young girls' behavioral and emoitonal problems. *Psychological Bulletin, 121,* 97–113.

Kellam, S. G., Ling, X., Mersica, R., Brown, C. H., & Ialongo, N. (1998). The effect of the level of aggression in the first grade classroom on the course and malleability of aggressive behavior into middle school. *Development and Psychopathology, 10,* 165–186.

Kellam, S. G., Rebok, G. W., Ialongo, N., & Mayer, L. (1994). The course and malleability of aggressive behavior from early first grade into middle school: Results of a developmental epidemiologically-based preventive trial. *Journal of Child Psychology and Psychiatry, 35,* 359–382.

Kellam, S. G., & van Horn, Y. V. (1997). Life course development, community epidemiology, and preventive trials: A scientific structure and prevention research. *American Journal of Community Psychology, 25,* 177–188.

Kerig, P. (1996). Assessing the links between interparental conflict and child adjustment: The conflicts and problem-solving scales. *Journal of Family Psychology, 10,* 454–473.

Kerig, P. (1997, April). *Gender and children's coping efforts as moderators of the effects of interparental conflict on children.* Paper presented at the biennial meeting of the Society for Research in Child Development, Washington, DC.

Kershner, J. G., & Cohen, N. J. (1992). Maternal depressive symptoms and child functioning. *Journal of Applied Developmental Psychology, 13,* 51–63.

Kim, L. S., Sandler, I. N., & Tein, J.-Y. (1997). Locus of control as a stress moderator and mediator in children of divorce. *Journal of Abnormal Child Psychology, 25,* 145–155.

Klaczynski, P. A., & Cummings, E. M. (1989). Responding to anger in aggressive and nonaggressive boys. *Journal of Child Psychology and Psychiatry, 30,* 309–314.

Klebanov, P. K., Brooks-Gunn, J., McCarton, C., & McCormick, M. C. (1998). The contribution of neighborhood and family income to developmental test scores over the first three years of life. *Child Development, 69,* 1420–1436.

Kobak, R., & Ferenz-Gillies, R. (1995). Emotion regulation and depressive symptoms during adolescence: A functionalist perspective. *Development and Psychopathology, 7,* 183–192.

Kobak, R., & Sceery, A. (1988). Attachment in later adolescence: Working models, affect regulation, and perceptions of self and others. *Child Development, 59,* 135–146.

Kochanska, G. (1995). A longitudinal study of the roots of preschoolers' conscience: Committed compliance and emerging internalization. *Child Development, 66,* 1752–1769.

Kochanska, G. (1997). Multiple pathways to conscience for children with different temperaments: From toddlerhood to age 5. *Developmental Psychology, 33,* 228–240.

Kochanska, G., Kuczynski, L., Radke-Yarrow, M., & Welsh, J. D. (1987). Resolution of control episodes between well and affectively ill mothers and their young child. *Journal of Abnormal Child Psychology, 15,* 441–456.

Kochanska, G., Murray, K., & Coy, K. C. (1997). Inhibitory control as a contributor to conscience in childhood: From toddler to early school age. *Child Development, 68,* 263–277.

Kochanska, G., & Thompson, R. A. (1997). The emergence and development of conscience in toddlerhood and early childhood. In J. E. Grusec & L. Kuczynski (Eds.), *Parenting and children's internalization of values: A handbook of contemporary theory* (pp. 53–77). New York: Wiley.

Kolberg, K. J. S. (1999a). Biological development and health risk. In T. L. Whitman, T. V. Merluzzi, & R. D. White (Eds.), *Life-span perspectives on health and illness* (pp. 23–45). Mahwah, NJ: Erlbaum.

Kolberg, K. J. S. (1999b). Environmental influences on prenatal development and health. In T. L. Whitman, T. V. Merluzzi, & R. D. White (Eds.), *Life-span perspectives on health and illness* (pp. 87–103). Mahwah, NJ: Erlbaum.

Kopp, C. B. (1982). Antecedents of self-regulation: A developmental perspective. *Developmental Psychology, 18,* 199–214.

Kopp, C. B. (1989). Regulation of distress and negative emotions: A developmental view. *Developmental Psychology, 25,* 343–354.

Kotchick, B. A., Forehand, R., Brody, G., Armistead, L., Simon, P., Morse, E., & Clark, L. (1997). The impact of maternal HIV infection on parenting in inner-city African American families. *Journal of Family Psychology, 11,* 447–461.

Kotchick, B. A., Summers, P., Forehand, R., & Steele, R. G. (1997). The role of parental and extrafamilial social support in the psychosocial adjustment of children with a chronically ill father. *Behavior Modification, 21,* 409–432.

Kovacs, M. (1991). *The Children's Depression Inventory (CDI).* North Tonawanda, NY: Multi-Health Systems.

Kovacs, M. (1998). Presentation and course of major depressive disorder during childhood and later years of the life span. In M. E. Hertzig & E. A. Farber (Eds.), *Annual progress in child psychiatry and child development: 1997* (pp. 285–298). Bristol, PA: Brunner/Mazel.

Krause, N. (1995). Stress, alcohol use, and depressive symptoms in later life. *Gerontologist, 35,* 296–307.

Krevans, J., & Gibbs, J. C. (1996). Parents' use of inductive discipline: Relations to children's empathy and prosocial behavior. *Child Development, 67,* 3263–3277.

Kuczynski, L., Radke-Yarrow, M., Kochanska, G., & Girnius-Brown, O. (1987). A developmental interpretation of young children's noncompliance. *Developmental Psychology, 23,* 799–806.

Kurdek, L. A., & Fine, M. A. (1994). Family acceptance and family control as predictors of adjustment in young adolescents: Linear, curvilinear, or interactive effects? *Child Development, 65,* 1137–1146.

Kurdek, L. A., Fine, M. A., & Sinclair, R. J. (1995). School adjustment in sixth graders: Parenting transitions, family climate, and peer norm effects. *Child Development, 66,* 430–455.

Ladd, G. W. (1992). Themes and theories: Perspectives on processes in family–peer relationships. In R. D. Parke & G. W. Ladd (Eds.), *Family–peer relationships: Modes of linkage* (pp. 3–34). Hillsdale, NJ: Erlbaum.

LaGreca, A. M., & Stone, W. L. (1993). The Social Anxiety Scale for Children-Revised: Factor structure and concurrent validity. *Journal of Clinical Child Psychology, 22,* 17–27.

Lahey, B. B., Applegate, B., McBurnett, K., Biederman, J., Greenhill, L., Hynd, G. W., Barkley, R. A. Newcorn, J., Jensen, P. S., & Richters, J. (1994). DSM-IV field trials for attention deficit hyperactivity disorder in children and adolescents. *American Journal of Psychiatry, 151,* 1673–1685.

Lahey, B. B., Loeber, R., Quay, H. C., Frick, P. J., & Grimm, J. (1992). Oppositional defiant and conduct disorders: Issues to be resolved for DSM-IV. *Journal of the American Academy of Child and Adolescent Psychiatry,* MI31, 539–546.

Lahey, B. B., Pelham, W. E., Stein, M. A., Loney, J., Trapani, C., Nugent, K., Kipp, H., Schmidt, E., Lee, S., Cale, M., Gold, E., Hartung, C. M., Willcutt, E., & Baumann, B. (1998). Validity of DSM-IV attention-deficit/hyperactivity disorder for younger children. *Journal of the American Academy of Child and Adolescent Psychiatry, 37,* 695–702.

Lamb, M. E. (Ed.). (1976). *The role of the father in child development.* New York: Wiley.

Lamb, M. E. (1987). Predictive implications of individual differences in attachment. *Journal of Consulting and Clinical Psychology, 55,* 817–824.

Lamb, M. E. (Ed.). (1997). *The role of the father in child development* (3rd ed.). New York: Wiley.

Lamb, M. E., & Elster, A. B. (1985). Adolescent mother–infant–father relationships. *Developmental Psychology, 21,* 768–773.

Lambert, M. C., & Weisz, J. R. (1992). Jamaican and American adult perspectives on child psychopathology: Further exploration of the threshold model. *Journal of Consulting and Clinical Psychology, 60,* 146–149.

Lamborn, S. D., Mounts, N. S., Steinberg, L., & Dornbusch, S. M. (1991). Patterns of competence and adjustment among adolescents from authoritative, authoritarian, indulgent, and neglectful families. *Child Development, 62,* 1049–1065.

Lamborn, S. D., & Steinberg, L. (1993). Emotional autonomy redux: Revisiting Ryan and Lynch. *Child Development, 64,* 483–499.

LaRoche, C. (1989). Children of parents with major affective disorders. *Psychiatric Clinics of North America, 12*, 919–932.

Laumakis, M., Margolin, G., & John, R. (1998). The emotional, cognitive, and coping responses of preadolescent children to different dimensions of marital conflict. In G. Holden, B. Geffner, & E. Jouriles (Eds.), *Children and family violence* (pp. 257–288). Washington, DC: American Psychological Association.

Lay, K., Waters, E., & Parke, K. A.(1989). Maternal responsiveness and child compliance: The role of mood as a mediator. *Child Development, 60*, 1405–1411.

Lazar, I., & Darlington, R. (1982). Lasting effects of early education: A report from the Consortium for Longitudinal Studies. *Monographs of the Society for Research in Child Development, 47* (Serial No. 195).

Lazarus, R. S., & Folkman, S. (1984). *Stress, coping, and appraisal.* New York: Springer.

Lee, C. M., & Gotlib, I. H. (1991). Family disruption, parental availability, and child adjustment. *Advances in Behavioral Assessment of Children and Families, 5*, 171–199.

Lefkowitz, M. M., & Burton, N. (1978). Childhood depression: A critique of the concept. *Psychological Bulletin, 85*, 716–726.

Lerner, J. V. (1983). The role of temperament in psychosocial adaptation in early adolescence: A test of a "goodness of fit" model. *Journal of Genetic Psychology, 143*, 149–157.

Lerner, R. M. (1979). A dynamic interactional concept of individual and social relationship development. In R. L. Burgess & T. L. Huston (Eds.), *Social exchange in developing relationships* (pp. 271–305). New York: Academic Press.

Lerner, R. M. (1996). Relative plasticity, integration, temporality, and diversity in human development: A developmental contextual perspective about theory, process, and method. *Developmental Psychology, 32*, 781–786.

Lerner, R. M., & Kauffman, M. B. (1985). The concept of development in contextualism. *Developmental Review, 5*, 309–333.

Lerner, R. M., & Lerner, J. V. (1989). Organismic and social contextual bases of development: The sample case of early adolescence. In W. Damon (Ed.), *Child development today and tomorrow* (pp. 69–85). San Francisco: Jossey-Bass.

Lewinsohn, P. M., Clarke, G. N., Hops, H., & Andrews, J. (1990). Cognitive-behavioral group treatment of depression in adolescents. *Behavior Therapy, 21*, 385–401.

Lewinsohn, P. M., Hops, H., Roberts, R. E., Seely, J. R., & Andrews, J. A. (1993). Adolescent psychopathology: I. Prevalence and incidence of depression and other DSM-III-R disorders in high school students. *Journal of Abnormal Psychology, 102*, 133–144.

Lewis, C. C. (1981). The effects of parental firm control: A reinterpretation of the findings. *Psychological Bulletin, 90*, 547–563.

Lewis, M., Feiring, C., & Rosenthal, S. (in press). Attachment over time. *Child Development.*

Lieberman, A. F. (1992). Infant–parent psychotherapy with toddlers. *Development and Psychopathology, 4*, 559–574.

Lindahl, K. M. (1998). Family process variables and children's disruptive behavior problems. *Journal of Family Psychology, 12*, 420–436.

Lindahl, K. M., & Malik, N. M. (1999). Marital conflict, family processes, and boys' externalizing behavior in Hispanic American and European American families. *Journal of Clinical Child Psychology, 28*(1), 12–24.

Lochman, J. (1992). Cognitive behavioral intervention with aggressive boys: Three year follow up and preventive effects. *Journal of Consulting and Clinical Psychology, 60*, 426–432.

Lochman, J. E., & Curry, J. F. (1986). Effects of social problem-solving training and self-instruction training with aggressive boys. *Journal of Clinical Child Psychology, 15*, 159–164.

Loeb, R. C., Horst, L., & Horton, P. (1980). Family interaction patterns associated with self-esteem in preadolescent girls and boys. *Merrill–Palmer Quarterly, 26*, 205–217.

Loeber, R. (1982). The stability of antisocial and delinquent child behavior: A review. *Child Development, 53*, 1431–1446.

Loeber, R. (1984). Patterns and development of antisocial child behavior. *Annals of Child Development, 2*, 77–116.

Loeber, R. (1991a). Antisocial behavior: More enduring than changeable? *Journal of the American Academy of Child and Adolescent Psychiatry, 30*, 393–397.

Loeber, R. (1991b). Questions and advances in the study of developmental pathways. In D. Cicchetti & S. L. Toth (Eds.), *Rochester Symposium on Developmental Psychopathology: Vol. 3. Models and integrations* (pp. 97–116). Rochester, NY: University of Rochester Press.

Loeber, R., & Dishion, T. J. (1984). Boys who fight at home and school: Family conditions influencing cross-setting consistency. *Journal of Consulting and Clinical Psychology, 52*, 759–768.

Loeber, R., Wung, P., Keenan, K., Giroux, B., Stouthamer-Loeber, M., Van Kammen, W. B., & Maughan, B. (1993). Developmental pathways in disruptive child behavior. *Development and Psychopathology, 5*, 103–133.

Loeber, R., & Stouthamer-Loeber, M. (1998a). Development of juvenile aggression and violence: Some common misconceptions and controversies. *American Psychologist, 53*, 242–259.

Loeber, R., & Stouthamer-Loeber, M. (1998b). Juvenile aggression at home and at school. In D. S. Elliott, B. A. Hamburg, & K. R. Williams (Eds.), *Violence in American schools: A new perspective* (pp. 94–126). New York: Cambridge University Press.

Lollis, S., & Kuczynski, L. (1997). Beyond one hand clapping: Seeing bidirectionality in parent–child relations. *Journal of Social and Personal Relationships, 14*, 441–461.

Londerville, S., & Main, M. (1981). Security of attachment, compliance, and maternal training methods in the second year of life. *Developmental Psychology, 17*, 289–299.

Lonigan, C. J., & Elbert, J. C. (Eds.). (1998). Empirically supported psychosocial interventions for children [Special issue]. *Journal of Clinical Child Psychology, 27* (2).

Lonigan, C. J., Elbert, J. C., & Johnson, S. B. (1998). Empirically supported psychosocial interventions for children: An overview. *Journal of Clinical Child Psychology, 27*, 138–145.

Luthar, S. S. (1991). Vulnerability and resilience: A study of high-risk adolescents. *Child Development, 62*, 600–616.

Luthar, S. S. (1993). Annotation: Methodological and conceptual issues in research on childhood resilience. *Journal of Child Psychology and Psychiatry, 34*, 441–453.

Luthar, S. S. (1995). Social competence in the school setting: Prospective cross-domain associations among inner-city teens. *Child Development, 66*, 416–429.

Luthar, S. S., & Cushing, G. (1999). Measurement issues in the empirical study of resilience: An overview. In M. D. Glantz & J. L. Johnson (Eds.), *Resilience and development: Positive life adaptations* (pp. 129–160). New York: Kluwer.

Luthar, S. S., Doernberger, C. H., & Ziegler, E. (1993). Resilience is not a unidimensional construct: Insights from a prospective study of inner-city adolescents. *Development and Psychopathology, 5*, 703–717.

Luthar, S. S., & Ziegler, E. (1993). Vulnerability and competence: A review of research on resilience in childhood. In M. E. Hertzig & E. A. Farber (Eds.), *Annual progress in child psychiatry and child development (1992)* (pp. 232–255). New York: Brunner/Mazel.

Lynch, M., & Cicchetti, D. (1998a). An ecological–transactional analysis of children and contexts: The longitudinal interplay among child maltreatment, community violence, and children's symptomatology. *Developmental Psychopathology, 10*(2), 235–258.

Lynch, M., & Cicchetti, D. (1998b). Trauma, mental representation, and the organization of memory for mother–referent material. *Development and Psychopathology, 10*, 739–759.

Lyons-Ruth, K. (1995). Broadening our conceptual frameworks: Can we reintroduce relational strategies and implicit representational systems to the study of psychopathology? *Developmental Psychology, 31*, 432–436.

Lyons-Ruth, K., Connell, D. B., Zoll, D., & Stahl, J. (1987). Infants at social risk: Relations among infant maltreatment, materal behavior, and infant attachment behavior. *Developmental Psychology, 23*, 223–232.

Lytton, H. (1990). Child and parent effects in boys' conduct disorder: A reinterpretation. *Developmental Psychology, 26*, 683–697.

Lytton, J. (1991). Parents' differential socialization of boys and girls: A meta-analysis. *Psychological Bulletin, 109*, 267–296.

MTA Cooperative Group. (1999a). A 14-month randomized clinical trial of treatment strategies for attention deficit hyperactivity disorder (ADHD). *Archives of General Psychiatry, 56*, 1073–1086.

MTA Cooperative Group. (1999b). Moderators and mediators of treatment response for children with ADHD: The MTA Study. *Archives of General Psychiatry, 56*, 1088–1096.

Maccoby, E. E. (1992). The role of parents in the socialization of children: An historical overview. *American Psychologist, 28*, 1006–1017.

Maccoby, E. E., Buchanan, C. M., Mnookin, R. H., & Dornbusch, S. M. (1993). Post-divorce roles of mothers and fathers in the lives of children. *Journal of Family Psychology, 7*, 24–28.

Maccoby, E., & Martin, J. (1983). Socialization in contexts of the family: Parent–child interaction. In E. M. Hetherington (Ed.), *Handbook of child psychology: Vol. 4. Socialization, personality, and social development* (4th ed., pp. 1–101). New York: Wiley.

MacDonald, K. (1987). Parent–child physical play with rejected, neglected, and popular boys. *Developmental Psychology, 23*, 705–711.

Macfie, J., Toth, S. L., Rogosch, F. A., Robinson, J., Emde, R. N., & Cicchetti, D. (1999). Effect of maltreatment on preschoolers' narrative representations of responses to relieve distress and of role reversal. *Developmental Psychology, 35*, 460–465.

Magnusson, D., & Cairns, R. B. (1996). Developmental science: Toward a unified framework. In R. B. Cairns, G. H. Elder, & G. J. Costello (Eds.), *Developmental science* (pp. 7–30). New York: Cambridge University Press.

Mahoney, A., Boggio, R., & Jouriles, E. (1996). Effects of verbal marital conflict on subsequent mother–son interactions in a child clinical sample. *Journal of Clinical Child Psychology, 25*, 262–271.

Main, M., & Goldwyn, R. (1984). Predicting rejection of her infant from mother's representation of her own experiences: Implications for the abused–abusing intergenerational cycle. *Child Abuse and Neglect, 8*, 203–217.

Main, M., Kaplan, N., & Cassidy, J. C. (1985). Security in infancy, childhood and adulthood: A move to the level of representation. In I. Bretherton & E. Waters (Eds.), Growing points of attachment theory and research. *Monographs of the Society for Research in Child Development, 50*(1–2, Serial No. 209), 66–104.

Main, M., & Solomon, J. (1990). Procedures for identifying infants as disorganized/disoriented during the Ainsworth Strange Situation. In M. T. Greenberg, D. Cicchetti, & E. M. Cummings (Eds.), *Attachment in the preschool years: Theory, research, and intervention* (pp. 121–160). Chicago: University of Chicago Press.

Mangelsdorf, S., Gunnar, M., Kestenbaum, R., Lang, S., & Andreas, D. (1990). Infant proneness-to-distress temperament, maternal personality, and mother–infant attachment: Associations and goodness of fit. *Child Development, 61*, 820–831.

Manly, J. T., Cicchetti, D., & Barnett, D. (1994). The impact of subtype, frequency, chronicity, and severity of child maltreatment on social competence and behavior problems. *Development and Psychopathology, 6*, 121–143.

Mannuzza, S., Klein, R. G., Bessler, A., Malloy, P., & LaPadula, M. (1993). Adult outcome of hyperactive boys: Educational achievement, occupational rank, and psychiatric status. *Archives of General Psychiatry, 50*, 565–576.

March, J. S., Parker, J. D. A., Sullivan, K., Stallings, P., & Conners, C. K. (1997). The Multidimensional Anxiety Scale for Children (MASC): Factor structure, reliability, and validity. *Journal of the American Academy of Child and Adolescent Psychiatry, 36*, 554–565.

Margolin, G., Christensen, A., & John, R. (1996). The continuance and spillover of everyday tensions in distressed and nondistressed families. *Journal of Family Psychology, 10*, 304–321.

Martin, J. A. (1981). A longitudinal study of the consequences of early mother–infant interaction: A microanalytic approach. *Monographs of the Society for Research in Child Development, 46*(3, Serial No. 46).

Mash, E. J., & Barkley, R. A. (Eds.). (1998). *Treatment of childhood disorders* (2nd ed.). New York: Guilford Press.

Mash, E. J., & Terdal, L. G. (1997). *Assessment of childhood disorders* (3rd ed.). New York: Guilford Press.

Mash, E. J., & Wolfe, D. A. (1999). *Abnormal child psychology*. Belmont, CA: Wadsworth.

Mason, C. A., Cauce, A. M., Gonzales, N., & Hiriaga, Y. (1996). Neither too sweet nor too sour: Problem peers, maternal control, and problem behavior in African American adolescents. *Child Development, 67*, 2115–2130.

Masten, A. S., Best, K., & Garmezy, N. (1990). Resilience and development: Contributions from the study of children who overcome adversity. *Development and Psychopathology, 2*, 425–444.

Masten, A. S., & Coatsworth, J. D. (1995). Competence, resilience, and psychopathology. In D. Cicchetti & D. Cohen (Eds.), *Developmental psychopathology, Vol. 2: Risk, disorder, and adaptation* (pp. 715–752). New York: Wiley.

Masten, A. S., & Coatsworth, J. D. (1998). The development of competence in favorable and unfavorable environments. *American Psychologist, 53,* 205–220.

Masten, A. S., Garmezy, N., Tellegen, A., Pellegrini, D. S., Larkin, K., & Larsen, A. (1988). Competence and stress in school chidlren: The moderating effects of individual and family qualities. *Journal of Child Psychology and Psychiatry, 29,* 745–764.

Masters, J. C., & Wellman, H. M. (1974). The study of human infant attachment: A procedural critique. *Psychological Bulletin, 81,* 218–237.

Maxwell, S. E., & Delaney, H. D. (1990). *Designing experiments and analyzing data: A model comparison perspective.* Belmont, CA: Wadsworth.

McCord, J. (1979). Some child-rearing antecedents of criminal behavior in adult men. *Journal of Personality and Social Psychology, 37,* 1477–1486.

McCord, J. (1993). Conduct disorder and antisocial behavior: Some thoughts about processes. *Development and Psychopathology, 5,* 321–329.

McFadyen-Ketchum, S. A., Bates, J. E., Dodge, K. A., & Pettit, G. S. (1996). Patterns of change in early childhood aggressive–disruptive behavior: Gender differences in predictions from early coercive and affectionate mother–child interactions. *Child Development, 67,* 2417–2433.

McGee, R. A., & Wolfe, D. A. (1991a). Psychological maltreatment: Toward an operational definition. *Development and Psychopathology, 3,* 3–18.

McGee, R. A., & Wolfe, D. A. (1991b). Between a rock and a hard place: Where do we go from here in defining psychological maltreatment? *Development and Psychopathology, 3,* 119–124.

McGue, M., Sharma, A., & Benson, P. (1996). The effect of common rearing on adolescent adjustment: Evidence from a U.S. adoption cohort. *Developmental Psychology, 32,* 604–613.

McGuffin, P., Katz, R., Watkins, S., & Rutherford, J. (1996). A hospital-based twin register of the heritability of DSM-IV unipolar depression. *Archives of General Psychiatry, 53,* 129–136.

McGuire, S., Dunn, J., & Plomin, R. (1995). Maternal differential treatment of siblings and children's behavioral problems: A longitudinal study. *Development and Psychopathology, 7,* 515–528.

McHale, J. P. (1994). *Co-parenting and family-level dynamics.* Colloquium presented at the University of Illinois, Champaign.

McHale, J. P. (1995). Co-parenting and triadic interactions during infancy: The roles of marital distress and child gender. *Developmental Psychology, 31,* 985–996.

McHale, J. P., & Rasmussen, J. L. (1998). Co-parental and family group-level dynamics during infancy: Early family precursors of child and family functioning during preschool. *Development and Psychopathology, 10,* 39–59.

McHale, S. M., & Crouter, A. C. (1996). The family contexts of children's sibling relationships. In G. H. Brody (Ed.), *Sibling relationships: Their causes and consequences* (pp. 173–195). Norwood, NJ: Ablex.

McHale, S. M., & Pawletko, T. M. (1992). Differential treatment of siblings in two family contexts. *Child Development, 63,* 68–81.

McLanahan, S., & Sandefur, G. (1994). *Growing up with a single parent: What hurts, what helps.* Cambridge, MA: Harvard University Press.

McLeod, J. D., Kessler, R. C., & Landis, K. R. (1992). Speed of recovery from major depressive episodes in a community sample of married men and women. *Journal of Abnormal Psychology, 101,* 277–287.

McLoyd, V. C. (1990). The impact of economic hardship on black families and children: Psychological distress, parenting, and socioemotional development. *Child Development, 61,* 311–346.

McLoyd, V. C. (1998). Socioeconomic disadvantage and child development. *American Psychologist, 53,* 185–204.

McNeal, E. T., & Cimbolic, P. (1986). Antidepressants and biochemical theories of depression. *Psychological Bulletin, 99,* 361–374.

Mendelson, W. B., Johnson, N. E., & Stewart, M. A. (1971). Hyperactive children as teenagers: A follow-up study. *Journal of Nervous and Mental Disease, 153,* 273–279.

Miller, N. B., Cowan, P. A., Cowan, C. P., Hetherington, E. M., & Clingempeel, W. G. (1993). Externalizing in preschoolers and early adolescents: A cross-study replication of a family model. *Developmental Psychology, 29,* 3–18.

Miller-Tutzauer, C., Leonard, K. E., & Windle, M. (1991). Marriage and alcohol use: A longitudinal study of "maturing out." *Journal of Studies on Alcohol, 52,* 434–440.

Minuchin, S. (1974). *Families and family therapy.* Cambridge, MA: Harvard University Press.

Minuchin, P. (1985). Families and individual development: Provocations from the field of family therapy. *Child Development, 56,* 289–302.

Moffitt, T. E. (1990). Juvenile delinquency and attention deficit disorders: Boys' developmental trajectories from age 3 to age 15. *Child Development, 61,* 893–910.

Moffitt, T. E. (1993a). Adolescence-limited and life-course-persistent antisocial behavior: A developmental taxonomy. *Psychological Review, 100,* 674–701.

Moffitt, T. E. (1993b). The neuropsychology of conduct disorder. *Development and Psychopathology, 5,* 135–151.

Moffitt, T. E., Caspi, A., Belsky, J., & Silva, P. A. (1992). Childhood experience and the onset of menarche: A test of a sociobiological model. *Child Development, 63,* 47–58.

Moffitt, T. E., Caspi, A., Dickson, N., Silva, P., & Stanton, W. (1996). Childhood-onset versus adolescent-onset antisocial conduct problems in males: Natural history from ages 3 to 18 years. *Development and Psychopathology, 8,* 399–424.

Moos, R. H., Cronkite, R. C., & Moos, B. S. (1998). The long-term interplay between family and extrafamily resources and depression. *Journal of Family Psychology, 12,* 326–343.

Moschell, M. (1991, August). Wanted: Parent. *Family Times,* p. 3.

Murray, L. (1992). The impact of postnatal depression on infant development. *Journal of Child Psychology and Psychiatry, 33,* 543–561.

Myers, B. J. (1984). Mother–infant bonding: The status of this critical period hypothesis. *Developmental Review, 4,* 240–274.

Myers, R. L. (1997). *Relations between marital conflict, children's internal working models of parental relations, and the quality of their long-term episodic memory of interadult conflict.* Unpublished master's thesis, West Virginia University, Morgantown.

Neeman, J., Hubbard, J., & Masten, A. S. (1995). The changing importance of romantic relationship involvement to competence from late childhood to late adolescence. *Development and Psychopathology, 7,* 727–750.

NICHD Early Child Care Research Network. (1998). Early child care and self control, compliance, and behavior problems at 24 and 36 months. *Child Development, 69,* 1145–1170.

NICHD Early Child Care Research Network. (1999). Chronicity of maternal depressive symptoms, maternal sensitivity, and child functioning at 36 months. *Developmental Psychology, 35,* 1297–1310.

Nixon, C. L., & Cummings, E. M. (1999). Sibling disability and children's reactivity to conflicts involving family members. *Journal of Family Psychology, 13,* 274–285.

Notarius, C., & Markman, H. (1993). *We can work it out: Making sense of marital conflict.* New York: Putnam's Sons.

Nottelman, E. D., & Jensen, P. S. (1995). Comorbidity of disorders in children and adolescents: Developmental perspectives. In T. H. Ollendick & R. J. Prinz (Eds.), *Advances in clinical child psychology, Vol. 17* (pp. 109–156). New York: Plenum Press.

O'Brien, M., Bahadur, M., Gee, C., Balto, K., & Erber, S. (1997). Child exposure to marital conflict and child coping responses as predictors of child adjustment. *Cognitive Therapy and Research, 21,* 39–59.

O'Brien, M., Margolin, G., & John, R. S. (1995). Relation among marital conflict, child coping, and child adjustment. *Journal of Clinical Child Psychology, 24,* 346–361.

O'Brien, M., Margolin, G., John, R. S., & Krueger, L. (1991). Mothers' and sons' cognitive and emotional reactions to simulated marital and family conflict. *Journal of Consulting and Clinical Psychology, 59,* 692–703.

O'Connor, T. G., Hetherington, E. M., & Reiss, D. (1998). Family systems and adolescent development: Shared and nonshared risk and protective factors in nondivorced and remarried families. *Development and Psychopathology, 10,* 353–375.

Offord, D. R., Boyle, M. H., Fleming, J., Blum, H. M., & Rae Grant, N. (1989). Ontario Child Health Study: Summary of selected results. *Canadian Journal of Psychiatry, 34,* 483–491.

Okun, A., Parker, J. G., & Levendosky, A. A. (1994). Distinct and interactive contributions of physical abuse, socioeconomic disadvantage, and negative life events to children's social, cognitive, and affective adjustment. *Development and Psychopathology, 6,* 77–98.

Olds, D. L., Henderson, C. R., Chamberlin, R., & Tatelbaum, R. (1986). Preventing child abuse and neglect: A randomized trial of nurse home visitation. *Pediatrics, 78,* 65–78.

Olds, D. L., Henderson, C. R., Kitzman, H., & Cole, R. (1995). Effects of prenatal and infancy nurse home visitation on surveillance of child maltreatment. *Pediatrics, 95,* 365–372.

O'Leary, K. D., Christian, J. L., & Mendell, N. R. (1994). A closer look at the link between marital discord and depressive symptomatology. *Journal of Social and Clinical Psychology, 13,* 33–41.

O'Leary, K. D., Riso, L. P., & Beach, S. R. H. (1990). Attributions about the marital discord/depression link and therapy outcome. *Behavior Therapy, 21,* 413–422.

Ollendick, T. H. (1983a). Reliability and validity of the Revised Fear Survey Schedule for Children (FSSC-R). *Behaviour Research and Therapy, 21,* 685–692.

Ollendick, T. H. (1983b). Development and validation of the Children's Assertiveness Inventory. *Child and Family Behavior Therapy, 5,* 1–15.

Ollendick, T. H., & King, N. J. (1998) Empirically supported treatments for children with phobic and anxiety disorders: Current status. *Journal of Clinical Child Psychology, 27,* 156–167.

Olweus, D. (1979). Stability of aggressive reaction patterns in males: A review. *Psychological Bulletin, 86,* 852–875.

Oppenheim, D., Emde, R. N., & Warren, S. (1997). Children's narrative representations of mothers: Their development and associations with child and mother adaptation. *Child Development, 68*, 127–138.

Oppenheim, D., Nir, A., Warren, S., & Emde, R.N. (1997). Emotion regulation in mother–child narrative co-construction: Associations with children's narratives and adaptation. *Developmental Psychology, 33*, 284–294.

Osborne, L. A., & Fincham, F. D. (1996). Marital conflict, parent–child relationships, and child adjustment: Does gender matter? *Merrill–Palmer Quarterly, 42*, 48–75.

Overton, W. F., & Horowitz, H. A. (1991). Developmental psychopathology: Integrations and differentiations. In D. Cicchetti & S. Toth (Eds.), *Rochester Symposium on Developmental Psychopathology: Vol. 3. Models and integrations* (pp. 1–42). Rochester, NY: University of Rochester Press.

Owen, M. T., & Cox, M. J. (1997). Marital conflict and the development of infant–parent attachment relationships. *Journal of Family Psychology, 11*, 152–164.

Pan, H. S., Neidig, P. H., & O'Leary, K. D. (1994). Predicting mild and severe husband-to-wife physical aggression. *Journal of Consulting and Clinical Psychology, 62*, 975–981.

Parke, R. D. (1979). Interactional designs. In R. B. Cairns (Ed.), *The analysis of social interactions: Methods, issues, and illustrations* (pp. 15–35.) New York: Erlbaum.

Parke, R. D. (1988). Families in life-span perspectives: A multi-level developmental approach. In E. M. Hetherington, R. M. Lerner, & M. Perlmutter (Eds.), *Child development in life-span perspective* (pp. 159–190). Hillsdale, NJ: Erlbaum.

Parke, R. D. (1996). *Fatherhood*. Cambridge, MA: Harvard University Press.

Parke, R. D., & Buriel, R. (1998). Socialization in the family: Ethnic and ecological perspectives. In N. Eisenberg (Ed.), *Handbook of child psychology: Vol. 3. Social, emotional and personality development* (pp. 463–552). New York: Wiley.

Parke, R. D., Cassidy, J., Burks, V. M., Carson, J. L., & Boyum, L. (1992). Familial contribution to peer competence among young children: The role of interactive and affective processes. In R. D. Parke & G. W. Ladd (Eds.), *Family–peer relationships: Modes of linkage* (pp. 107–134). Hillsdale, NJ: Erlbaum.

Parke, R. D., & Ladd, G. W. (Eds.). (1992). *Family–peer relationships: Modes of linkage*. Hillsdale, NJ: Erlbaum.

Parke, R. D., & Slaby, R. C. (1983). The development of aggression. In P. H. Mussen (Series Ed.) & E. M. Hetherington (Vol. Ed.), *Handbook of child psychology: Vol. 4. Socialization, personality, and social development* (pp. 547–641). New York: Wiley.

Pasch, L. A., & Bradbury, T. N. (1998). Social support, conflict, and the development of marital dysfunction. *Journal of Consulting and Clinical Psychology, 66*, 219–230.

Patterson, G. R. (1982). *Coercive family process*. Eugene, OR: Castalia.

Patterson, G. R. (1997). Performance models for parenting: A social interactional perspective. In J. E. Grusec & L. Kuczynski (Eds.), *Parenting and children's internalization of values: A handbook of contemporary theory* (pp. 193–226). New York: Wiley.

Patterson, G. R. (1998). Continuities—a search for causal mechanisms: Comments on the Special Section. *Developmental Psychology, 34*(6), 1263–1269.

Patterson, G. R., DeBaryshe, B., & Ramsey, E. (1989). A developmental perspective on antisocial behavior. *American Psychologist, 44*, 329–335.

Patterson, G. R., & Stouthamer-Loeber, M. (1984). The correlation of family management practices and delinquency. *Child Development, 55*, 1299–1307.

Patterson, G. R., & Yoerger, K. (1997). A developmental model for late-onset delinquency. *Nebraska Symposium on Motivation, 44,* 119–177.

Pelham, W. E., & Hoza, B. (1996). Intensive treatment: Summer treatment program for children with ADHD. In E. D. Hibbs & P. S. Jensen (Eds.), *Psychosocial treatment research of child and adolescent disorders: Empirically based strategies for clinical practice* (pp. 311–340). Washington, DC: American Psychological Association.

Pelham, W. E., & Lang, A. R. (1993). Parental alcohol consumption and deviant child behavior: Laboratory studies of reciprocal effects. *Clinical Psychology Review, 13,* 763–784.

Pelham, W. E., Milich, R., Cummings, E. M., Murphy, D. A., Schaughency, E. A., & Greiner, A. R. (1992). Effects of background anger, provocation, and methylphenidate on emotional arousal and aggressive responding in attention deficit/hyperactivity disordered boys with and without concurrent aggressiveness. *Journal of Abnormal Child Psychology, 19,* 407–426.

Pelham, W. E., Wheeler, T., & Chronis, A. (1998). Empirically supported psychosocial treatments for attention deficit hyperactivity disorder. *Journal of Clinical Child Psychology, 27,* 190–205.

Pellegrini, D. S. (1990). Psychosocial risk and protective factors in childhood. *Developmental and Behavioral Pediatrics, 11,* 201–209.

Pepper, S. C. (1942). *World hypotheses, a study in evidence.* Berkeley: University of California Press.

Petersen, A. C., Sarigiani, P. A., & Kennedy, R. E. (1991). Adolescent depression: Why more girls? *Journal of Youth and Adolescence, 20,* 247–271.

Pettit, G. S. (1997). The developmental course of violence and aggression: Mechanisms of family and peer influence. *Psychiatric Clinics of North America, 20,* 283–299.

Pettit, G. S., & Bates, J. E. (1989). Family interaction patterns and children's behavior problems from infancy to 4 years. *Developmental Psychology, 25,* 413–420.

Pettit, G. S., Bates, J. E., & Dodge, K. A. (1993). Family interaction patterns and children's conduct problems at home and school: A longitudinal perspective. *School Psychology Review, 22,* 403–420.

Pettit, G. S., Bates, J. E., & Dodge, K. A. (1997). Supportive parenting, ecological context, and children's adjustment: A seven-year longitudinal study. *Child Development, 68,* 908–923.

Pettit, G. S., Clawson, M. A., Dodge, K. A., & Bates, J. E. (1996). Stability and change in peer-rejected status: The role of child behavior, parenting, and family ecology. *Merrill–Palmer Quarterly, 42,* 267–294.

Phares, V. (1997). Psychological adjustment, maladjustment, and father–child relationships. In M. E. Lamb (Ed.), *The role of the father in child development* (pp. 261–283). New York: Wiley.

Phares, V., & Compas, B. E. (1992). The role of fathers in child and adolescent psychopathology: Make room for Daddy. *Psychological Bulletin, 111,* 387–412.

Phillips, D. A., Voran, M., Kisker, E., Howes, C., & Whitebrook, M. (1994). Child care for children in poverty: Opportunity or inequity. *Child Development, 65,* 472–492.

Pierce, E. W., Ewing, L. J., & Campbell, S. B. (1999). Diagnostic status and symptomatic behavior of hard-to-manage preschool children in middle childhood and early adolescence. *Journal of Clinical Child Psychology, 28,* 44–57.

Pike, A., McGuire, S., Hetherington, E. M., Reiss, D., & Plomin, R. (1996). Family environment and adolescent depressive symptoms and antisocial behavior: A multivariate genetic analysis. *Developmental Psychology, 32,* 590–603.

Pinsof, W. M., & Wynne, L. C. (1995). The efficacy of marital and family therapy: An empirical overview, conclusions, and recommendations. *Journal of Marital and Family Therapy, 21,* 585–613.

Plomin, R. (1994a). *Genetics and experience: The interplay between nature and nurture.* Thousand Oaks, CA: Sage.

Plomin, R. (1994b). Nature, nurture, and social development. *Social Development, 3,* 37–53.

Plomin, R. (1995a). Genetics and children's experiences in the family. *Journal of Child Psychology and Psychiatry and Allied Disciplines, 36,* 33–68.

Plomin, R. (1995b). Genetics, environmental risks, and protective factors. In J. R. Turner, L. R. Cardon, & J. K. Hewitt (Eds.), *Behavior genetic approaches in behavioral medicine* (pp. 217–235). New York: Plenum Press.

Plomin, R. (1995c). Molecular genetics and psychology. *Current Directions in Psychological Science, 4,* 114–117.

Pollak, S. D., Cicchetti, D., Klorman, R., & Brumaghim, J. T. (1997). Cognitive brain event-related potentials and emotion processing in maltreated children. *Child Development, 68,* 773–787.

Pollak, S., Cicchetti, D., & Klorman, R. (1998). Stress, memory, and emotion: Developmental considerations from the study of child maltreatment. *Development and Psychopathology, 10,* 811–828.

Porges, S. W. (1996). Physiological regulation in high-risk infants: A model for assessment and potential intervention. *Development and Psychopathology, 8,* 43–58.

Porges, S. W. (1997). Emotion: An evolutionary by-product of the neural regulation of the autonomic nervous system. In C. S. Carter & I. I. Lederhendler (Eds.), *The integrative neurobiology of affiliation* (pp. 62–77). New York: New York Academy of Sciences.

Porter, B., & O'Leary, K. D. (1980). Marital discord and childhood behavior problems. *Journal of Abnormal Child Psychology, 8,* 287–295.

Posada, G., Gao, Y., Wu, F., Posada, R., Tascon, M., Schoelmerich, A., Sagi, A., Kondo-Ikemura, K., Haaland, W., & Synnevaag, B. (1995). The secure-base phenomenon across cultures: Children's behavior, mothers' preferences, and experts' concepts. In E. Waters, B. E. Vaughn, G. Posada, & K. Kondo-Ikemura (Eds.), Caregiving, cultural, and cognitive perspectives on secure-base behavior and working models: New growing points of attachment theory and research. *Monographs of the Society for Research in Child Development, 60*(2–3, Serial No. 244), 27–48.

Post, R. M., Rubinow, D. R., & Ballenger, J. C. (1986). Conditioning and sensitization in the longitudinal course of affective illness. *British Journal of Psychiatry, 149,* 191–201.

Post, R. M., & Weiss, S. R. B. (1997). Emergent properties of neural systems: How focal molecular neurobiological alterations can affect behavior. *Development and Psychopathology, 9,* 907–929.

Post, R. M. Weiss, S. R. B., & Leverich, G. S. (1994). Recurrent affective disorder: Roots in developmental neurobiology and illness progression based on changes in gene expression. *Development and Psychopathology, 6,* 781–813.

Powers, J. L., & Eckenrode, J. (1988). The maltreatment of adolescents. *Child Abuse and Neglect, 12,* 189–199.

Puig-Antich, J., Goetz, D., Davies, M., Kaplan, T., Davies, S., Ostrow, L., Asnis, L., Twonmey, J., Iyengar, S., & Ryan, N. D. (1989). Imipramine in prepubertal major depressive disorders. *Archives of General Psychiatry, 46,* 406–418.

Quiggle, N. L., Garber, J., Panak, W. F., & Dodge, K. A. (1992). Social information processing in aggressive and depressed children. *Child Development, 63,* 1344–1350.

Quinton, D., & Rutter, M. (1988). *Parenting breakdown: The making and breaking of intergenerational links.* Aldershot, England, and Brookfield, VT: Avebury.

Quittner, A. L., & Opipari, L. C. (1994). Differential treatment of siblings: Interview and diary analyses comparing two family contexts. *Child Development, 65,* 800–814.

Radke-Yarrow, M., Cummings, E. M., Kuczynski, L., & Chapman, M. (1985). Patterns of attachment in two- and thee-year-olds in normal families and families with parental depression. *Child Development, 56,* 884–893.

Radke-Yarrow, M., Nottleman, E., Belmont, B., & Welsh, J. D. (1993). Affective interactions of depressed and nondepressed mothers and their children. *Journal of Abnormal Child Psychology, 21,* 683–695.

Radke-Yarrow, M., Zahn-Waxler, C., & Chapman, M. (1983). Children's prosocial dispositions and behavior. In P. H. Mussen (Series Ed.) & E. H. Hetherington (Vol. Ed.), *Handbook of child psychology: Vol. IV. Socialization, personality, and social development* (pp. 469–546). New York: Wiley.

Rae-Grant, N., Thomas, B. J., Offord, D. R., & Boyle, M. H. (1989). Risk, protective factors, and prevalence of behavioral and emotional disorders in children and adolescents. *Journal of the Academy of Child and Adolescent Psychiatry, 28,* 262–268.

Ramey, C. T., Bryant, D. M., Wasik, B. H., Sparling, J. J., Fendt, K. H., & LaVange, L. M. (1992). The Infant Health and Development Program for low birth weight, premature infants: Program elements, family participation, and child intelligence. *Pediatrics, 89,* 454–465.

Ramey, C. T., & Ramey S. L. (1998). Early intervention and early experience. *American Psychologist, 53,* 109–120.

Ramey, S. L., & Ramey, C. T. (1992). Early educational intervention with disadvantaged children—to what effect? *Applied and Preventive Psychology, 1,* 131–140.

Reese, H. W., & Overton, W. F. (1970). Models of development and theories of development. In L. R. Goulet & P. B. Baltes (Eds.), *Life-span developmental psychology: Research and theory* (pp. 115–145). New York: Academic Press.

Reid, J. (1993). Prevention of conduct disorder before and after school entry: Relating interventions to developmental findings. *Development and Psychopathology, 5,* 243–262.

Reiss, D., Hetherington, E. M., Plomin, R., Howe, G. W., Simmens, S. J., Henderson, S. H., O'Connor, T. J., Bussell, D. A., Anderson, E. R., & Law, T. (1995). Genetic questions for environmental studies: Differential parenting of siblings and its associations with depression and antisocial behavior in adolescents. *Archives of General Psychiatry, 52,* 925–936.

Rende, R. D., & Plomin, R. (1990). Quantitative genetics and developmental psychopathology: Contributions to understanding normal development. *Development and Psychopathology, 2,* 393–407.

Rende, R., & Plomin, R. (1993). Families at risk for psychopathology: Who becomes affected and why? *Development and Psychopathology, 5,* 529–540.

Rende, R. D., Plomin, R., Reiss, D., & Hetherington, E. M. (1993). Genetic and environmental influences on depressive symptomatology in adolescence: Individual differences and extreme scores. *Journal of Child Psychology and Psychiatry and Allied Disciplines, 34,* 1387–1398.

Rende, R., Weissman, M., Rutter, M., Wickramaratne, P., Harrington, R., & Pickles, A. (1997). Psychiatric disorders in the relatives of depressed probands: II. Familial loading for comorbid non-depressive disorders based upon proband age of onset. *Journal of Affective Disorders, 42*, 23–28.

Repetti, R. L., McGrath, E., & Ishikawa, S. (1995). Daily stress and coping in childhood and adolescence. In A. J. Goreczny & M. Hersen (Eds.), *Handbook of pediatric and adolescent health psychology* (pp. 3–32). New York: Allyn & Bacon.

Repetti, R. L., & Wood, J. (1997). Families accommodating to chronic stress: Unintended and unnoticed processes. In B. Gottlieb (Ed.), *Coping with chronic stress* (pp. 191–220). New York: Plenum.

Reynolds, C. R., & Kamphaus, R. W. (1992). *Behavior Assessment System for Children (BASC)*. Circle Pines, MN: American Guidance Services.

Reynolds, W. M., & Mazza, J. J. (1994). Suicide and suicidal behaviors in children and adolescents. In W. M. Reynolds, & H. F. Johnston (Eds.), *Handbook of depression in children and adolescents* (pp. 525–580). New York: Plenum Press.

Richters, J. E. (1997). The Hubble hypothesis and the developmentalist's dilemma. *Develoment and Psychopathology, 9*, 193–229.

Richters, J. E., & Cicchetti, D. (1993). Toward a developmental perspective on conduct disorder. *Development and Psychopathology, 5*, 1–4.

Roberts, M. C. (1996). *Model programs in child and family mental health*. Mahwah, NJ: Erlbaum.

Rogers, M. J., & Holmbeck, G. N. (1997). Effects of interparental aggression on children's adjustment: The moderating role of cognitive appraisal and coping. *Journal of Family Psychology, 11*, 125–130.

Rogosch, F. A., Cicchetti, D., & Aber, J. L. (1995). The role of child maltreatment in early deviations in cognitive and affective processing abilities and later peer relationship problems. *Development and Psychopathology, 7*, 591–609.

Rothbart, M. K., Ahadi, S., & Hershey, K. L. (1994). Temperament and social behavior in children. *Merrill–Palmer Quarterly, 40*, 21–39.

Rothbart, M. K., Posner, M. I., & Rosnicky, J. (1994). Orienting in normal and pathological development. *Development and Psychopathology, 6*, 635–652.

Rothbaum, F. (1988). Maternal acceptance and child functioning. *Merrill–Palmer Quarterly, 34*, 163–184.

Rubin, K. H., Coplan, R. J., Fox, N. A., & Calkins, S. D. (1995). Emotionality, emotion regulation, and preschoolers' social adaptation. *Development and Psychopathology, 7*, 49–62.

Rutter, M. (1970). Sex differences in response to family stress. In E. J. Anthony & C. Koupernik (Eds.) *The child in his family* (pp. 165–196). New York: Wiley.

Rutter, M. (1980). *Changing youth in a changing society*. Cambridge, MA: Harvard University Press.

Rutter, M. (1981). Stress, coping, and development: Some issues and some questions. *Journal of Child Psychology and Psychiatry, 22*, 323–356.

Rutter, M. (1983). Statistical and personal interactions: Facets and perspectives. In D. Magnusson & V. Allen (Eds.), *Human development: An interactional perspective* (pp. 295–319). New York: Academic Press.

Rutter, M. (1985). Resilience in the face of adversity. *Psychiatry, 147*, 598–611.

Rutter, M. (1986). The developmental psychopathology of depression: Issues and perspectives. In M. Rutter, C. E. Izard, & P. B. Read (Eds.), *Depression in young people: Developmental and clinical perspectives* (pp. 3–30). New York: Guilford Press.

Rutter, M. (1987). Psychosocial resilience and protective mechanisms. *American Journal of Orthopsychiatry, 57*, 316–331.

Rutter, M. (1988). Epidemiological approaches to developmental psychopathology. *Archives of General Psychiatry, 45,* 486–495.

Rutter, M. (1989a). Age as an ambiguous variable in developmental research: Some epidemiological considerations from developmental psychopathology. *International Journal of Behavioral Development, 12,* 1–34.

Rutter, M. (1989b). Pathways from childhood to adult life. *Journal of Child Psychology and Psychiatry, 30,* 23–51.

Rutter, M. (1990). Commentary: Some focus and process considerations regarding the effects of parental depression on children. *Developmental Psychology, 26,* 60–67.

Rutter, M. (1992). Adolescence as a transition period: Continuities and discontinuities in conduct disorder. *Journal of Adolescent Health, 13,* 451–460.

Rutter, M. (1993). Resilience: Some conceptual considerations. *Journal of Adolescent Health, 14,* 626–631.

Rutter, M. (1994). Stress research: Accomplishments and tasks ahead. In R. J. Haggerty, L. R. Sherrod, N. Garmezy, & M. Rutter (Eds.), *Stress, risk, and resilience in children and adolescents; Processes, mechanisms, and interventions* (pp. 354–385). New York: Cambridge University Press.

Rutter, M. (1996). Developmental psychopathology: Concepts and prospects. In M. F. Lenzenweger & J. J. Haugaard (Eds.), *Frontiers of developmental psychopathology* (pp. 209–237). New York: Oxford University Press.

Rutter, M. (1997). Antisocial behavior: Developmental psychopathology perspectives. In D. M. Stoff, J. Breiling, & J. D. Maser (Eds.), *Handbook of antisocial behavior* (pp. 115–124). New York: Wiley.

Rutter, M. (1998). Some research considerations on intergenerational continuation and discontinutation: Comments on the Special Section. *Developmental Psychology, 34*(6), 1269–1273.

Rutter, M., Dunn, J., Plomin, R., Simonoff, E., Pickles, A., Maughan, B., Ormel, J., Meyer, J., & Eaves, L. (1997). Integrating nature and nurture: Implications of person–environment correlations and interactions for developmental psychopathology. *Development and Psychopathology, 9,* 335–364.

Rutter, M., & Pickles, A. (1991). Person–environment interactions: Concepts, mechanisms, and implications for data analysis. In T. D. Wachs & R. Plomin (Eds.), *Conceptualization and measurement of organism–environment interaction* (pp. 105–136). Washington, DC: American Psychological Association.

Rutter, M., & Quinton, D. (1984). Parental psychiatric disorder: Effects on children. *Psychological Medicine, 14,* 853–880.

Rutter, M., Tizard, J., Yule, W., Graham, P., & Whitmore, K. (1977). Research report: Isle of Wight Studies 1964–1974. *Psychological Medicine, 6,* 313–332.

Ryan, R. M., Deci, E. L., & Grolnick, W. S. (1995). Autonomy, relatedness, and the self: Their relation to development and psychopathology. In D. Cicchetti & D. J. Cohen (Eds.), *Developmental psychopathology: Vol. 1. Theory and methods* (pp. 618–655). New York: Wiley.

Safer, D. J., Zito, J. M., & Fine, E. M. (1996). Increased methylphenidate usage for attention deficit disorder in the 1990s. *Pediatrics, 98,* 1084–1088.

St. Pierre, R. G., & Layzer, J. I. (1998). *Improving the life chances of children in poverty: Assumptions and what we have learned* (SRCD Social Policy Report, XII). Ann Arbor, MI: Society for Research in Child Development.

Sameroff, A. J. (1995). General systems theories and developmental psychopathology. In

D. Cicchetti & D. J. Cohen (Eds.), *Developmental psychopathology: Vol. 1. Theory and methods* (pp. 659–695). New York: Wiley.

Sameroff, A. J., Seifer, R., Baldwin, A., & Baldwin, C. P. (1993). Stability of intelligence from preschool to adolescence: The influence of social and family risk factors. *Child Development, 64*, 80–97.

Sandler, I. N., Tein, J.-Y., & West, S. G. (1994). Coping, stress, and the psychological symptoms of children of divorce: A cross-sectional and longitudinal study. *Child Development, 65*, 1744–1763.

Sandler, I. N., Wolchik, S. A., Braver, S. L., & Fogas, B. (1991). Stability and quality of life events and psychological symptomatology of children of divorce. *American Journal of Community Psychology, 19*, 501–520.

Sattler, J. M. (1992). Assessment of children's intelligence. In C. E. Walker & M. C. Roberts (Eds.), *Handbook of clinical child psychology* (2nd ed., pp. 85–100). New York: Wiley.

Schaffer, H. R., & Emerson, P. E. (1964). The development of social attachments in infancy. *Monographs of the Society for Research in Child Development, 29*(3, Serial No. 94).

Schneider, M. L., Clarke, A. S., Kraemer, G. W., Roughton, E. C., Lubach, G. R., Rimm-Kaufman, S., Schmidt, D., & Ebert, M. (1998). Prenatal stress alters brain biogenic amine levels in primates. *Development and Psychopathology, 10*, 427–440.

Schulenberg, J., Maggs, J. L., & Hurrelmann, K. (1997). Negotiating developmental transitions during adolescence and young adulthood: Health risks and opportunities. In J. Schulenberg & J. L. Maggs (Eds.), *Health risks and developmental transitions during adolescence* (pp. 1–19). New York: Cambridge University Press.

Schwartz, D., Dodge, K. A., Pettit, G. S., & Bates, J. E. (1997). The early socialization of aggressive victims of bullying. *Child Development, 68*, 665–675.

Schwoeri, L., & Shoolevar, G. P. (1994). The family transmission of depression. In G. P. Sholevar (Ed.), *The transmission of depression in families and children: Assessment and intervention* (pp. 123–144). Northvale, NJ: Aronson.

Seifer, R. (1995). Perils and pitfalls of high-risk research. *Developmental Psychology, 31*, 420–424.

Serbin, L. A., Cooperman, J. M., Peters, P. L., Lehoux, P. M., Stack, D. M., & Schwartzman, A. E. (1998). Intergenerational transfer of psychosocial risk in women with childhood histories of aggression, withdrawal, or aggression and withdrawal. *Developmental Psychology, 34*, 1246–1262.

Serbin, L. A., & Stack, D. M. (1998). Introduction to the Special Section: Stuying intergenerational continuity and the transfer of risk. *Developmental Psychology, 34*(6), 1159–1161.

Shadish, W. R., Montgomery, L. M., Wilson, P., Wilson, M. R., Bright, I., & Okwumabua, T. (1993). Effects of family and marital psychotherapies: A meta-analysis. *Journal of Consulting and Clinical Psychology, 61*, 992–1002.

Shaffer, D., Fisher, P., Dulcan, M. K., & Davies, M. (1996). The NIMH Diagnostic Interview Schedule for Children Version 2.3 (DISC-2.3): Description, acceptability, prevalence rates, and performance in the MECA study. *Journal of the American Academy of Child and Adolescent Psychiatry, 35*, 865–877.

Shaffer, D., Fisher, P., Piacentini, J., Schwab-Stone, M., & Wicks, J. (1993). *Diagnostic interview schedule for children*. New York: Columbia University Press.

Shaffer, D. R. (1994). *Social and personality development* (3rd ed.). Pacific Grove, CA: Brooks/Cole.

Shantz, C. (1987). Conflicts between children. *Child Development, 58,* 283–305.

Shaw, D. S., & Bell, R. Q. (1993). Developmental theories of parental contributors to antisocial behavior. *Journal of Abnormal Child Psychology, 21,* 493–518.

Shaw, D. S., Owens, E. B., Vondra, J. I., Keenan, K., & Winslow, E. B. (1996). Early risk factors and pathways in the development of early disruptive behavior problems. *Development and Psychopathology, 8,* 679–700.

Shaw, D. S., & Vondra, J. I. (1993). Chronic family adversity and infant attachment security. *Journal of Child Psychology and Psychiatry, 34,* 1205–1215.

Sheeber, L. B., & Johnson, J. H. (1992). Child temperament, maternal adjustment, and changes in family life style. *American Journal of Orthopsychiatry, 62,* 178–185.

Sheets, V., Sandler, I., & West, S. G. (1996). Appraisals of negative events by preadolescent children of divorce. *Child Development, 67,* 2166–2182.

Sher, K. J. (1991). *Children of alcoholics: A critical appraisal of theory and research.* Chicago: University of Chicago Press.

Shields, A. M., Cicchetti, D., & Ryan, R. M. (1994). The development of emotional and behavioral self-regulation and social competence among maltreated school-age children. *Development and Psychopathology, 6,* 57–75.

Shifflett-Simpson, K., & Cummings, E. M. (1996). Mixed message resolution and children's responses to interadult conflict. *Child Development, 67,* 437–448.

Sim, H., & Vuchinich, S. (1996). The declining effects of family stressors on antisocial behavior from childhood to adolescence and early adulthood. *Journal of Family Issues, 17,* 408–427.

Simmons, R. G., & Blyth, D. A. (1987). *Moving into adolescence: The impact of pubertal change and school context.* Hawthorne, NY: Aldine De Gruyter.

Smetana, J. G. (1995). Context, conflict, and constraint in adolescent–parent authority relationships. In M. Killen & D. Hart (Eds.), *Morality in everyday life: Developmental perspectives* (pp. 225–255). New York: Cambridge University Press.

Smetana, J. G., Toth, S. L., Cicchetti, D., Bruce, J., Kane, P., & Daddis, C. (1999). Maltreated and nonmaltreated preschoolers' conceptions of hypothetical and actual moral transgressions. *Developmental Psychology, 35,* 269–281.

Smolak, L., Levine, M. P., & Gralen, S. (1993). The impact of puberty and dating on eating problems among middle school girls. *Journal of Youth and Adolescence, 22,* 355–368.

Snyder, J. (1991). Discipline as a mediator of the impact of maternal stress and mood on child conduct problems. *Development and Psychopathology, 3,* 263–276.

Snyder, J., Schrepferman, L., & St. Peter, C. (1997). Origins of antisocial behavior: Negative reinforcement and affect dysregulation of behavior as socialization mechanisms in family interaction. *Behavior Modification, 21,* 187–215.

Sonuga-Barke, E. J. S. (1998). Categorical models of childhood disorder: A conceptual and empirical analysis. *Journal of Child Psychology and Psychiatry, 39,* 115–133.

Spangler, G., & Grossmann, K. E. (1993). Biobehavioral organization in securely and insecurely attached infants. *Child Development, 64,* 1439–1450.

Speiker, S. J., & Bensley, L. (1994). Roles of living arrangements and grandmother social support in adolescent mothering and infant attachment. *Developmental Psychology, 30,* 102–111.

Speiker, S. J., Larson, N. C., Lewis, S. M., Keller, T. E., & Gilchrist, L. (1999). Developmental trajectories of disruptive behavior problems in preschool children of adolescent mothers. *Child Development, 70,* 443–458.

Speltz, M. L. (1990). The treatment of preschool conduct problems. In M. T. Greenberg, D. Cicchetti, & E. M. Cummings (Eds.), *Attachment in the preschool years: Theory, research, and intervention* (pp. 399–426). Chicago: University of Chicago Press.

Speltz, M. L., Greenberg, M. T., & DeKlyen, M. (1990). Attachment in preschoolers with disruptive behavior: A comparison of clinic-referred and nonproblem children. *Development and Psychopathology, 2,* 31–46.

Sroufe, L. A. (1979). The coherence of individual development: Early care, attachment, and subsequent developmental issues. *American Psychologist, 34,* 834–841.

Sroufe, L. A. (1985). Attachment classification from the perspective of infant–caregiver relationships and infant temperament. *Child Development, 56,* 1–14.

Sroufe, L. A. (1988). The role of infant–caregiver attachment in development. In J. Belsky & T. Nezworski (Eds.), *Clinical implications of attachment* (pp. 18–38). Hillsdale, NJ: Erlbaum.

Sroufe, L. A. (1989). Relationships, self, and individual adapation. In A. J. Sameroff & R. N. Emde (Eds.), *Relationship disturbances in early childhood: A developmental approach* (pp. 70–94). New York: Basic Books.

Sroufe, L. A. (1990). Considering normal and abnormal together: The essence of developmental psychopathology. *Development and Psychopathology, 2,* 335–347.

Sroufe, L. A. (1997). Psychopathology as an outcome of development. *Development and Psychopathology, 9,* 251–268.

Sroufe, L. A., Carlson, E. A., Levy, A. K., & Egeland, B. (1999). Implications of attachment theory for developmental psychopathology. *Development and Psychopathology, 11,* 1–13.

Sroufe, L. A., & Egeland, B. (1991). Illustrations of person–environment interaction from a longitudinal study. In T. D. Wachs & R. Plomin (Eds.), *Conceptualization and measurement of organism–environment interaction* (pp. 68–84). Washington, DC: American Psychological Association.

Sroufe, L. A., Egeland, B., & Carlson, E. A. (1999). One social world: The integrated development of parent–child and peer relationships. In W. A. Collins & B. Laursen (Eds.), *The Minnesota Symposia on Child Psychology: Vol. 30. Relationships as developmental contexts* (pp. 241–261). Mahwah, NJ: Erlbaum.

Sroufe, L. A., Egeland, B., & Kreutzer, T. (1990). The fate of early experience following developmental change: Longitudinal approaches to individual adaptation in childhood. *Child Development, 61,* 1363–1373.

Sroufe, L. A., & Jacobitz, D. (1989). Diverging pathways, developmental transformations, multiple etiologies, and the problem of continuity in development. *Human Development, 32,* 196–203.

Sroufe, L. A., Jacobvitz, D., Mangelsdorf, S., DeAngelo, E., & Ward, M. J. (1985). Generational boundary dissolution between mothers and their preschool children: A relationship systems approach. *Child Development, 56,* 316–325.

Sroufe, L. A., & Rutter, M. (1984). The domain of developmental psychopathology. *Child Development, 55,* 17–29.

Sroufe, L. A., & Waters, E. (1977a). Attachment as an organizational construct. *Child Development, 48,* 1184–1199.

Sroufe, L. A., & Waters, E. (1977b). Heart rate as a convergent measure in clinical and developmental research. *Merrill–Palmer Quarterly, 23,* 3–27.

Stansbury, K., & Gunnar, M. R. (1994). Adrenocrotical activity and emotion regulation.

In N. A. Fox (Ed.), The development of emotion regulation: Biological and behavioral considerations. *Monographs of the Society for Research in Child Development, 59*(2–3, Serial No. 240), 108–134.

Stayton, D. J., Hogan, R., & Ainsworth, M. D. (1971). Infant obedience and maternal behavior: The origins of socialization reconsidered. *Child Development, 42,* 1057–1069.

Steele, B. (1976). Violence within the family. In R. E. Helfer & C. H. Kempe (Eds.), *Child abuse and neglect: The family and the community* (pp. 3–24). Cambridge, MA: Ballinger.

Steinberg, L. (1988). Reciprocal relation between parent–child distance and pubertal maturation. *Developmental Psychology, 24,* 122–128.

Steinberg, L. (1990). Autonomy, conflict, and harmony in the family relationship. In S. S. Feldman & G. R. Elliot (Eds.), *At the threshold: The developing adolescent* (pp. 255–276). Cambridge, MA: Harvard University Press.

Steinberg, L., Dornbusch, S. M., & Brown, B. B. (1992). Ethnic differences in adolescent achievement: An ecological perspective. *American Psychologist, 47,* 723–729.

Steinberg, L., Elmen, J. D., & Mounts, N. S. (1989). Authoritative parenting, psychosocial maturity, and academic success among adolescents. *Child Development, 60,* 1424–1436.

Steinberg, L., Lamborn, S. D., Darling, N., Mounts, N. S., & Dornbusch, S. M. (1994). Over-time changes in adjustment and competence among adolescents from authoritative, authoritarian, indulgent, and neglectful families. *Child Development, 65,* 754–770.

Steinberg, L., Lamborn, S., Dornbusch, S., & Darling, N. (1992). Impact of parenting practices on adolescent achievement: Authoritative parenting, school involvement, and encouragement to succeed. *Child Development, 63,* 1266–1281.

Steinberg, L., Mounts, N. S., Lamborn, S. D., & Dornbusch, S. M. (1991). Authoritative parenting and adolescent adjustment across varied ecological niches. *Journal of Research on Adolescence, 1,* 19–36.

Stice, E., & Barrera, M. (1995). A longitudinal examination of reciprocal relations between perceived parenting and adolescents' substance use and externalizing behaviors. *Developmental Psychology, 31,* 322–334.

Stifter, C. A., Fox, N. A., & Porges, S. W. (1989). Facial expressivity and vagal tone in 5- and 10-month-old infants. *Infant Behavior and Development, 12,* 127–137.

Stocker, C. M. (1995). Differences in mothers' and fathers' relationships with siblings: Links with children's behavior problems. *Development and Psychopathology, 7,* 499–513.

Stocker, C. M., & Youngblade, L. (1999). Marital conflict and parental hostility: Links with children's sibling and peer relationships. *Journal of Family Psychology, 13,* 598–609.

Stoneman, Z., Brody, G. H., & Burke, M. (1989). Marital quality, depression, and inconsistent parenting: Relationship with observed mother–child conflict. *American Journal of Orthopsychiatry, 59,* 105–117.

Stormshak, E. A., Bierman, K. L., & the Conduct Problems Prevention Research Group. (1998). The implications of different developmental patterns of disruptive behavior problems for school adjustment. *Development and Psychopathology, 10,* 451–468.

Strack, S., & Coyne, J.C. (1983). Social confirmation of dysphoria: Shared and private reactions to depression. *Journal of Personality and Social Psychology, 44,* 798–806.

Sullivan, M. L. (1998). Integrating qualitative and quantitative methods in the study of developmental psychopathology in context. *Development and Psychopathology*, *10*(2), 377–394.

Swann, W. B. (1983). Self-verification: Brining social reality into harmony with the self. In J. Suls & A. G. Greenwald (Eds.), *Social psychological perspectives on the self* (Vol. 2, pp. 33–66). Hillsdale, NJ : Erlbaum.

Takahashi, K. (1990). Are the key assumptions of the "Strange Situation" procedure universal: A view from Japanese research. *Human Development, 33*, 23–30.

Tannenbaum, L., & Forehand, R. (1994). Maternal depressive mood: The role of the father in preventing adolescent problem behaviors. *Behavioral Research and Therapy, 32*, 321–325.

Tarullo, L. B., DeMulder, E. K., Martinez, P. E., & Radke-Yarrow, M. (1994). Dialogues with preadolescents and adolescents: Mother/child interaction patterns in affectively ill and well dyads. *Journal of Abnormal Child Psychology, 22*, 33–51.

Teti, D., Gelfand, D. M., Messinger, D. S., & Isabella, R. (1995). Maternal depression and the quality of early attachment: An examination of infants, preschoolers, and their mothers. *Developmental Psychology, 31*, 364–376.

Teti, D. M., Gelfand, D. M., & Pompa, J. (1990). Depressed mothers' behavioral competence with their infants: Demographic and psychosocial correlates. *Development and Psychopathology, 2*, 259–270.

Teti, D. M., Sakin, J. W., Kucera, E., & Corns, K. M. (1996). And baby makes four: Predictors of attachment security among preschool-age firstborns during the transition to siblinghood. *Child Development, 67*, 579–596.

Thomas, A. M., & Forehand, R. (1991). The relationship between paternal depressive mood and early adolescent functioning. *Journal of Family Psychology, 4*, 260–271.

Thompson, R. A. (1986). Temperament, emotionality, and infant social cognition. In J. V. Lerner & R. M. Lerner (Eds.), *Temperament and social interaction in infants and children* (pp. 35–52). San Francisco: Jossey-Bass.

Thompson, R. A. (1994). Emotion regulation: A theme in search of definition. In N. A. Fox (Ed.), The development of emotion regulation: Biological and behavioral considerations. *Monographs of the Society for Research in Child Development, 59*(2–3, Serial No. 240), 25–52.

Thompson, R. A. (2000). Legacy of early attachment. *Child Development, 71*, 145–152.

Thompson, R. A., & Calkins, S. D. (1996). The double-edged sword: Emotional regulation for children at risk. *Development and Psychopathology, 8*, 163–182.

Thompson, R. A., Flood, M. F., & Lundquist, L. (1995). Emotional regulation: Its relations to attachment and developmental psychopathology. In D. Cicchetti & S. L. Toth (Eds), *Rochester Symposium on Developmental Psychopathology: Vol. 6. Emotion, cognition, and representation* (pp. 261–299). Rochester, NY: University of Rochester Press.

Thompson, R. A., & Jacobs, J. E. (1991). Defining psychological maltreatment: Research and policy perspectives. *Development and Psychopathology, 3*, 93–102.

Tickamyer, A. R., & Duncan, C. M. (1990). Poverty and opportunity structure in rural America. *Annual Review of Sociology, 16*, 67–86.

Toth, S. L., & Cicchetti, D. (1996). The impact of relatedness with mother on school functioning in maltreated children. *Journal of School Psychology, 34*, 247–266.

Toth, S. L., Cicchetti, D., Macfie, J., & Emde, R. N. (1997). Representations of self and other in the narratives of neglected, physically abused, and sexually abused preschoolers. *Development and Psychopathology, 9*, 781–796.

Tout, K., de Haan, M., Campbell, E. K., & Gunnar, M. R. (1998). Social behavior correlates of cortisol activity in child care: Gender differences and time-of-day effects. *Child Development, 69,* 1247–1262.

Towle, C. (1931). The evaluation and management of marital status in foster homes. *American Journal of Orthopsychiatry, 1,* 271–284.

Trevarthen, C., & Aiken, K. J. (1994). Brain development, infant communication, and empathy disorders: Intrinsic factors in child mental health. *Development and Psychopathology, 6,* 597–633.

Trickett, P. K., Aber, J. L., Carlson, V., & Cicchetti, D. (1991). Relationship of socioeconomic status to the etiology and developmental sequelae of physical child abuse. *Developmental Psychology, 27,* 148–158.

Trickett, P. K., & Kuczynski, L. (1986). Children's misbehaviors and parental discipline strategies in abusive and nonabusive families. *Developmental Psychology, 22,* 115–123.

Trickett, P. K., & McBride-Chang, C. (1995). The developmental impact of different forms of child abuse and neglect. *Developmental Review, 15,* 311–337.

Tronick, E. Z. (1989). Emotions and emotional communication in infants. *American Psychologist, 44,* 112–119.

Tubman, J. G., Windle, M., & Windle, R. C. (1996). Cumulative sexual intercourse patterns among middle adolescents: Problem behavior precursors and concurrent health risk behaviors. *Journal of Adolescent Health, 18,* 182–191.

Turkheimer, E., & Gottesman, I. I. (1991). Individual differences and the canalization of human behavior. *Developmental Psychology, 27,* 18–22.

Valenzuela, M. (1990). Attachment in chronically underweight young children. *Child Development, 62,* 1984–1996.

Valenzuela, M. (1997). Maternal sensitivity in a developing society: The context of urban poverty and infant chronic undernutrition. *Developmental Psychology, 33,* 845–855.

van den Boom, D. C. (1994). The influence of temperament and mothering on attachment and exploration: An experimental manipulation of sensitive responsiveness among lower-class mothers with irritable infants. *Child Development, 65,* 1457–1477.

van der Kamp, L. J., & Bijleveld, C. C. J. (1998). Methodological issues in longitudinal research. In C. C. J. Bijleveld & L. J. van der Kamp (Eds.), *Longitudinal data analysis* (pp. 1–45). Thousand Oaks, CA: Sage.

van IJzendoorn, M. H., & Kroonenberg, P. M. (1988). Cross-cultural patterns of attachment: A meta-analysis of the Strange Situation. *Child Development, 59,* 147–156.

Vaughn, B. E., Egeland, B. R., Sroufe, L. A., & Waters, E. (1979). Individual differences in infant/mother attachment at twelve and eighteen months: Stability and change in families under stress. *Child Development, 50,* 971–975.

Vaughn, B. E., Stevenson-Hinde, J., Waters, E., Kotsaftis, A., Lefeuer, G. B., Shouldice, A., Trudel, M., & Belsky, J. (1992). Attachment security and temperament in infancy and early childhood: Some conceptual clarifications. *Developmental Psychology, 28,* 463–473.

Verhulst, F. C., & Koot, H. M. (1994). *Child psychiatric epidemiology.* Thousand Oaks, CA: Sage.

Vitaro, F., Brendgen, M., Pagani, L., Tremblay, R. E., & McDuff, P. (1999). Disruptive behavior, peer association, and conduct disorder: Testing the developmental links through early intervention. *Development and Psychopathology, 11,* 287–304.

Vitaro, F., & Tremblay, R. E. (1994). Impact of a prevention program on aggressive children's friendships and social adjustment. *Journal of Abnormal Child Psychology, 2,* 457–476.

Vitaro, F., Tremblay, R. E., Gagnon, C., & Pelletier, D. (1994). Predictive accuracy of behavioral and sociometric assessments of high-risk kindergarten children. *Journal of Clinical Child Psychology, 23,* 272–282.

Vitaro, F., Tremblay, R. E., Kerr, M., Pagani, L., & Bukowski, W. M. (1997). Disruptiveness, friends' characteristics, and delinquency in early adolescence: A test of two competing models of development. *Child Development, 68,* 676–689.

Volling, B. L., & Elins, J. L. (1998). Family relationships and children's emotional adjustment as correlates of maternal and paternal differential treatment: A replication with toddler and preschool siblings. *Child Development, 69,* 1640–1656.

Vondra, J., Barnett, D., & Cicchetti, D. (1989). Perceived and actual competence among maltreated and comparison school children. *Development and Psychopathology, 1,* 237–255.

Wachs, T. D. (1991a). Environmental considerations in studies with nonextreme groups. In T.D. Wachs & R. Plomin (Eds.), *Conceptualization and measurement of organism–environment interaction* (pp. 44–67). Washington, DC: American Psychological Association.

Wachs, T. D. (1991b). Synthesis: Promising research designs, measures, and strategies. In T. D. Wachs & R. Plomin (Eds.), *Conceptualization and measurement of organism–environment interaction* (pp. 162–182). Washington, DC: American Psychological Association.

Wachs, T. D. (1996). Known and potential processes underlying developmental trajectories in childhood and adolescence. *Developmental Psychology, 32,* 796–801.

Wachs, T. D., & Gandour, M. J. (1983). Temperament, environment, and six-month cognitive-intellectual development: A test of the organismic specificity hypothesis. *International Journal of Behavioural Development, 6,* 135–152.

Waddington, C. H. (1957). *The strategy of genes.* London: Allen & Unwin.

Wahler, R. G., & Dumas, J. E. (1986). Maintenance factors in coercive mother–child interactions: The compliance and predictability hypotheses. *Journal of Applied Behavior Analysis, 19,* 13–22.

Wakefield, J. (1997). When is development disordered? Developmental psychopathology and the harmful dysfunction analysis of mental disorder. *Development and Psychopathology, 9,* 269–290.

Wallerstein, J. S., & Blakeslee, S. (1989). *Second chances: Men, women, and children a decade after divorce.* New York: Ticknor & Fields.

Wandersman, A., & Nation, M. (1998). Urban neighborhoods and mental health: Psychological contributions to understanding toxicity, resilience, and interventions. *American Psychologist, 53,* 647–656.

Wangby, M., Bergman, L. R., & Magnusson, D. (1999). Development of adjustment problems in girls: What syndromes emerge? *Child Development, 70,* 678–699.

Waters, E. (1978). The reliability and stability of individual differences in infant–mother attachment. *Child Development, 49,* 483–494.

Waters, E., & Cummings, E. M. (2000). A secure base from which to explore close relationships. *Child Development, 71,* 164–172.

Waters, E., Merrick, S., Treboux, D., Crowell, J., & Albersheim, L. (in press). Attachment security in infancy and early adulthood: A 20-year longitudinal study. *Child Development.*

Waters, E., & Sroufe, L. A. (1983). Social competence as a developmental construct. *Developmental Review, 3,* 79–97.

Waters, E., Weinfield, N. S., & Hamilton C. (in press). The stability of attachment security from infancy to adolescence and early adulthood. *Child Development.*

Watson, J. B. (1925). *Behaviorism.* New York: Norton.

Webster-Stratton, C. (1984). Randomized trial of two parent training programs for families with conduct disordered children. *Journal of Consulting and Clinical Psychology, 52,* 666–678.

Webster-Stratton, C. (1985). The effects of father involvement in parent training for conduct problem children. *Journal of Child Psychology and Psychiatry, 26,* 801–810.

Weinfield, N., Sroufe, L. A., & Egeland, B. (in press). Attachment from infancy to early adulthood in a high-risk sample. *Child Development.*

Weiss, B., Dodge, K. A., Bates, J. E., & Pettit, G. S. (1992). Some consequences of early harsh discipline: Child aggression and a maladaptive social information processing style. *Child Development, 63,* 1321–1335.

Weiss, G., & Hechtman, L.T. (1993). *Hyperactive children grown up: ADHD in children, adolescents, and adults* (2nd ed.). New York: Guilford Press.

Weissman, M. M. (1987). Advances in psychiatric epidemiology: Rates and risks for major depression. *American Journal of Public Health, 77,* 445–451.

Weissman, M., Warner, V., Wickramaratne, P., Moreau, D., & Olfson, M. (1997). Offspring of depressed parents 10 years later. *Archives of General Psychiatry, 54,* 932–940.

Weisz, J. R., Chayaisit, W., Weiss, B., Eastman, K. L., & Jackson, E. W. (1995). A multimethod study of problem behavior among Thai and American children in school: Teacher reports versus direct observations. *Child Development, 66,* 402–415.

Weisz, J. R., Donenberg, G. R., Han, S. S., & Weiss, B. (1995). Bridging the gap between laboratory and clinic in child and adolescent psychotherapy. *Journal of Consulting and Clinical Psychology, 63,* 688–701.

Weisz, J. R., & Hawley, K. M. (1998). Finding, evaluating, refining, and applying empirically supported treatments for children and adolescents. *Journal of Clinical Child Psychology, 27,* 206–216.

Weisz, J. R., & Weiss, B. (1993). *Effects of psychotherapy with children and adolescents.* Newbury Park, CA: Sage.

Weisz, J. R., Weiss, B., & Donenberg, G. R. (1992). The lab versus the clinic: Effects of child and adolescent psychotherapy. *American Psychologist, 47,* 1578–1585.

Wekerle, C., & Wolfe, D. A. (1998). The role of child maltreatment and attachment style in adolescent relationship violence. *Development and Psychopathology, 10,* 571–586.

Wells, K. C., Pelham, W. E., Kotkin, R. A., Hoza, B., Abikoff, H. B., Abramowitz, A., Arnold, L. E., Cantwell, D. P., Conners, C. K., Del Carmen, R., Elliott, G., Greenhill, L. L., Hechtman, L., Hibbs, E., Hinshaw, S. P., Jensen, P. S., March, J. S., Schiller, E., Severe, J., & Swanson, J. B. (in press). Psychosocial treatment strategies in the MTA Study: Rationale, methods, and critical issues in design and implementation. *Journal of Abnormal Child Psychology.*

Werner, E. E. (1986). Resilient offspring of alcoholics: A longitudinal study from birth to age 18. *Journal of Studies on Alcohol, 47,* 34–40.

Werner, E. E. (1993). Risk, resilience, and recovery: Perspectives from the Kauai Longitudinal Study. *Development and Psychopathology, 5,* 503–515.

Werner, H. (1948). *Comparative psychology of mental development.* New York: International Universities Press.

Werner, H. (1957). The concept of development from a comparative and organismic point of view. In D. B. Harris (Ed.), *The concept of development* (pp. 125–148). Minneapolis: University of Minnesota Press.

West, M. O., & Prinz, R. J. (1987). Parental alcoholism and childhood psychopathology. *Psychological Bulletin, 102*, 204–218.

Whiffen, V., & Gotlib, I. (1989). Infants of postpartum depressed mothers: Temperament and cognitive status. *Journal of Abnormal Psychology, 98*, 274–279.

Whisman, M. (2000). Marital distress and depression: Findings from community and clinical studies. In S. R. H. Beach (Ed.), *Marital and family processes in depression: A scientific foundation for clinical practice.* Washington, DC: American Psychological Association.

Willett, J. B., Singer, J. D., & Martin, N. C. (1998). The design and analysis of longitudinal studies of development and psychopathology in context: Statistical models and methodological recommendations. *Development and Psychopathology, 10*, 395–426.

Wilson, B. J., & Gottman, J. M. (1995). Marital interaction and parenting: The role of repair of negativity in families. In M. H. Bornstein (Ed.), *Handbook of parenting: Vol. 4. Applied and practical considerations of parenting* (pp. 33–56). Hillsdale, NJ: Erlbaum.

Windle, M. (1992). A longitudinal study of stress buffering for adolescent problem behaviors. *Developmental Psychology, 28*, 522–530.

Windle, M. (1999). Critical conceptual and measurement issues in the study of resilience. In M. D. Glantz & J. L. Johnson (Eds.), *Resilience and development: Positive life adaptations* (pp. 161–176). New York: Kluwer.

Windle, M., & Davies, P. T. (1999). Developmental theory and research. In K. E. Leonard & H. T. Blane (Eds.), *Psychological theories of drinking and alcoholism* (2nd ed., pp. 164–202). New York: Guilford Press.

Windle, M., Hooker, K., Lenerz, K., East, P. L., Lerner, J. V., & Lerner, R. M. (1986). Temperament, perceived competence, and depression in early and late adolescents. *Developmental Psychology, 22*, 384–392.

Windle, M., & Tubman, J. G. (1999). Children of alcoholics. In W. K. Silverman & T. H. Ollendick (Eds.), *Developmental issues in the clinical treatment of children* (pp. 393–414). Boston: Allyn and Bacon.

Windle, M., & Windle, R. C. (1993). The continuity of behavioral expression among disinhibited and inhibited childhood subtypes. *Clinical Psychology Review, 13*, 741–761.

Wolfe, D. A., Jaffe, P., Wilson, S., & Zak, L. (1985). Children of battered women: The relation of child behavior to family violence and maternal stress. *Journal of Consulting and Clinical Psychology, 53*, 657–665.

Wolfe, D. A., & McGee, R. (1994). Dimensions of child maltreatment and their relationship to adolescent adjustment. *Development and Psychopathology, 6*, 165–181.

Wolfe, D. A., Wekerle, C., Reitzel-Jaffe, D., & Lefebvre, L. (1998). Factors associated with abusive relationships among maltreated and nonmaltreated youth. *Development and Psychopathology, 10*, 61–85.

Zahn-Waxler, C. (1993). Warriors and worriers: Gender and psychopathology. *Development and Psychopathology, 5*, 79–90.

Zahn-Waxler, C., Cole, P. M., Welsh, J. D., & Fox, N. A. (1995). Psychophysiological correlates of empathy and prosocial behaviors in preschool children with behavior problems. *Development and Psychopathology, 7*, 27–48.

Zahn-Waxler, C., Cummings, E. M., McKnew, D. H., & Radke-Yarrow, M. (1984). Altruism, aggression, and social interactions with a manic–depressive parent. *Child Development, 55*, 112–122.

Zahn-Waxler, C., Iannotti, R. J., Cummings, E. M., & Denham, S. (1990). Antecedents of problem behaviors in children of depressed mothers. *Development and Psychopathology, 2*, 271–291.

Zahn-Waxler, C., & Radke-Yarrow, C. (1982). The development of altruism: Alternative research strategies. In N. Eisenberg (Ed.), *The development of prosocial behavior* (pp. 109–137). New York: Academic Press.

Zahn-Waxler, C., Radke-Yarrow, M., & King, R. A. (1979). Child rearing and children's prosocial initiations toward victims of distress. *Child Development, 50*, 319–330.

Zaslow, M. J., & Hayes, C. D. (1986). Sex differences in children's response to psychosocial stress: Toward a cross-context analysis. In M. E. Lamb, A. L. Bron, & B. Rogoff (Eds.), *Advances in developmental psychology* (Vol. 4, pp. 285–337). Hillsdale, NJ: Erlbaum.

Zero to Three/National Center for Clinical Infant Programs. (1994). *Diagnostic classification, 0–3: Diagnostic classification of mental health and developmental disorders of infancy and early childhood*. Arlington, VA: Author.

Zigler, E., & Gilman, E. (1996). Not just any care: Shaping a coherent child care policy. In E. F. Zigler, S. L. Kagan, & N. W. Hall (Eds.), *Children, families, and government* (pp. 94–116). New York: Cambridge University Press.

Zigler, E., & Glick, M. (1986). *A developmental approach to adult psychopathology*. New York: Wiley.

Zigler, E., Taussig, C., & Black, K. (1992). Early childhood intervention: A promising preventative for juvenile delinquency. *American Psychologist, 47*, 997–1006.

Zigler, E., & Valentine, J. (1979). *Project Head Start: A legacy of the war on poverty*. New York: Free Press.

Zucker, R. A. (1986). The four alcoholisms: A developmental account of the etiologic process. *Nebraska Symposium on Motivation, 34*, 27–83.

Zucker, R. A. (1994). Pathways to alcohol problems and alcoholism: A developmental account of the evidence for multiple alcoholisms and for contextual contributions to risk. In R. A. Zucker, G. M. Boyd, & J. Howard (Eds.), *The development of alcohol problems: Exploring the biopsychosocial matrix of risk* (NIAAA Research Monograph 26, pp. 255–289). Rockville, MD: Department of Health and Human Services.

Zucker, R. A., Ellis, D. A., Fitzgerald, H. E., Bingham, C. R., & Sanford, K. (1996). Other evidence for at least two alcoholisms: II. Life course variation in antisociality and heterogeneity of alcoholic outcome. *Development and Psychopathology, 8*, 831–848.

Zucker, R. A., Fitzgerald, H. E., & Moses, H. D. (1995). Emergence of alcohol problems and the several alcoholisms: A developmental perspective on etiologic theory and life course trajectory. In D. Cicchetti & D. J. Cohen (Eds.), *Developmental psychopathology: Vol. 2. Risk, disorder, and adaptation* (pp. 677–711). New York: Wiley.

Index